# Paediatrics and Child Health

To our children: Aaron and Rebecca Krom;
Sophie, Jake, and Naomi Lee;
Alysa, Katie, Ilana, Hannah and David Levene.

To our spouses: Michael, Sue, and Alison.

To those individuals who over the course of years have influenced our approach to children in health and disease:
Ben Berliner, Victor Dubowitz, David Hall, Ze'ev Hochberg, Hugh Jolly, Jim Littlewood, Esther Rudolf, Hedva Steiner, Myron Winick.

# Paediatrics and Child Health

## Third edition

**Mary Rudolf**
Consultant Paediatrician and Professor of Child Health
Head of Studies, MSc in Child Health, University of Leeds
NHS Leeds and University of Leeds

**Tim Lee**
Consultant in Paediatric Respiratory Medicine
Organiser, MSc in Child Health, University of Leeds
Leeds Teaching Hospital Trust and University of Leeds

**Malcolm Levene**
Emeritus Professor of Paediatrics and Child Health
University of Leeds

**WILEY-BLACKWELL**
A John Wiley & Sons, Ltd., Publication

Blackwell Publishing was acquired by John Wiley & Sons in February 2007. Blackwell's publishing program has been merged with Wiley's global Scientific, Technical and Medical business to form Wiley-Blackwell.

*Registered office:* John Wiley & Sons Ltd, The Atrium, Southern Gate, Chichester, West Sussex, PO19 8SQ, UK

*Editorial offices:*   9600 Garsington Road, Oxford, OX4 2DQ, UK
The Atrium, Southern Gate, Chichester, West Sussex, PO19 8SQ, UK
111 River Street, Hoboken, NJ 07030-5774, USA

For details of our global editorial offices, for customer services and for information about how to apply for permission to reuse the copyright material in this book please see our website at www.wiley.com/wiley-blackwell.

*Library of Congress Cataloging-in-Publication Data*

Rudolf, Mary, author.
    Paediatrics and child health / Mary Rudolf, Consultant paediatrician and Professor of Child Health NHS Leeds and University of Leeds, Tim Lee, Consultant in Paediatric Respiratory Medicine, Co-organiser MSc in Child Health West Yorkshire, Lead, Medicines for Children Research Network, Malcolm Levene, Leeds General Infirmary. – Third Edition.
        p. ; cm.
    Includes bibliographical references and index.
    ISBN 978-1-4051-9474-7 (pbk. : alk. paper)   1. Pediatrics.   2. Children–Health and hygiene.   I. Lee, Tim, (Pediatrician), author.   II. Levene, Malcolm   I. (Malcolm Irvin), author.   III. Title.
    [DNLM:   1. Pediatrics.   2. Child Welfare. WS 200]
    RJ45.R86 2011
    618.92–dc22
                                                                                                    2010047404

A catalogue record for this book is available from the British Library.

Set in 10/12 pt Adobe Garamond Pro by Toppan Best-set Premedia Limited

Printed and bound in Malaysia by Vivar Printing Sdn Bhd

1  2011

# Contents

**Companion website**
This book is accompanied by a companion website:

# www.wiley.com/go/rudolf/paediatrics

with:
• Fully downloadable figures and illustrations

# Preface to the third edition

*Experience is the child of Thought, and Thought is the child of Action. We cannot learn men from books.*
                                    Benjamin Disraeli.

Was Disraeli right? Are books a very limited resource? Certainly the only way to become competent as a doctor is to encounter children and their medical problems on the wards, in clinics and their homes. It is only through these Experiences that Thought and understanding can lead you to the Action required to meet children's needs.

But of course reading must accompany experience. This book has always been seen of value in complementing your paediatric rotation and ensuring that you are well equipped for paediatric examinations as well as clinical practice.

As before, it aims first and foremost, to provide you with the necessary tools to arrive at a diagnosis and to care for children in the context of their family and school. Unlike most medical textbooks which use diseases as their building blocks, this textbook uses symptoms and signs at its core. Competences you must acquire are highlighted in each chapter, a logical approach to important presenting symptoms follows and the correct technique you need to develop for examining children is shown in the accompanying video. The book ends with self assessment so you can test your knowledge and understanding.

This third edition has been fully revised so that it allows you to work through the curriculum organ system by organ system. As before there are features that allow you to readily recognize the important, common or serious conditions that you must not miss. An exciting development has been the provision of free access to a Desktop Edition so that you can view and interact with the book electronically, including videos on clinical examination. A companion website allows you to download figures and illustrations.

The words of Benjamin Disraeli are a reminder that no book can substitute for clinical experience but we hope that this book can indeed 'learn' students, and help you get the most out of your paediatric experience, guiding you to appropriate Thought and Action.

# Acknowledgements

We are grateful to the following who have contributed illustrations: Dr Rosemary Arthur, Mr P.D. Bull, Dr Tony Burns, Professor Martin Curzon, Dr Mark Goodfield, Dr Phillip Holland, Mr Tim Milward, Dr P.R. Patel, Dr John Puntis, Mr Mark Stringer, Dr David Swirsky, Ms Clare Widdows, Dr Susan Wyatt and Dr Jane Wynne. We would like to thank the Royal College of Paeditrics and Child Health and Harlow Printing for permission to reproduce their growth charts. We would like to thank the following: Extract of 'Henry King who chewed string and was cut off in dreadful Agonies' from *Cautionary Verses* by Hilaire Belloc (Copyright © The Estate of Hilaire Belloc 1930) is reproduced by permission of PFD (www.pfd.co.uk) on behalf of the Estate of Hilaire Belloc. Extract of 'Rebecca who slammed doors for fun, and perished miserably' from *Cautionary Verses* by Hilaire Belloc (Copyright © The Estate of Hilaire Belloc) is reproduced by permission of PFD (www.pfd.co.uk) on behalf of the Estate of Hilaire Belloc. Extract from 'Now We Are Six' © A.A. Milne. Published by Egmont UK Limited, London and used with permission. Published by Dutton's Children's Books, a division of Penguin Young Readers Group, a member of Penguin Group (USA) Inc, 345 Hudson Street, New York, NY 10014, and used with permission. All rights reserved. Extract from *When We Were Very Young* © A.A. Milne. Published by Egmont UK Limited, London and used with permission. Published by Dutton's Children's Books, a division of Penguin Young Readers Group, a member of Penguin Group (USA) Inc, 345 Hudson Street, New York, NY 10014, and used with permission. All rights reserved.

# How to get the best out of your textbook

Welcome to the new edition of *Paediatrics and Child Health*. Over the next two pages you will be shown how to make the most of the learning features included in the textbook

## An interactive textbook ▶

For the first time, your textbook gives you free access to a Wiley Desktop Edition – a digital, interactive version of this textbook. You can view your book on a PC, Mac, laptop and Apple mobile device, and it allows you to:

**Search:** Save time by finding terms and topics instantly in your book, your notes, even your whole library (once you've downloaded more textbooks)

**Note and Highlight:** Colour code highlights and make digital notes right in the text so you can find them quickly and easily

**Organize:** Keep books, notes and class materials organized in folders inside the application

**Share:** Exchange notes and highlights with friends, classmates and study groups

**Upgrade:** Your textbook can be transferred when you need to change or upgrade your computer or device

**Link:** Link directly from the page of your interactive textbook to all of the material contained on the companion website

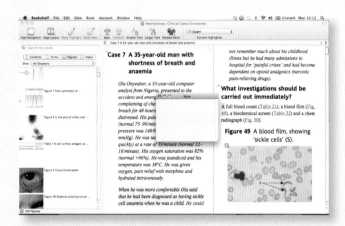

Simply log on to
**www.wiley.com/go/rudolf/paediatrics**
for full instructions on how to get started

## Video showing you how to ▶ examine children

A unique feature of the textbook is a detailed video taking you step by step through the examination of the child. Salient features are captured and the correct technique demonstrated for each organ system – essential for eliciting signs, coming to a diagnosis and showing your competence in OSCE examinations.

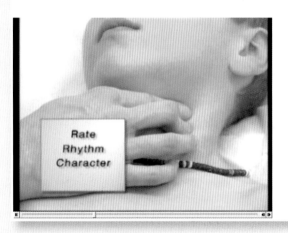

## FREE companion website

Your textbook is also accompanied by a FREE companion website that contains:

- Fully downloadable figures and illustrations

Log on to **www.wiley.com/go/rudolf/paediatrics** to find out more

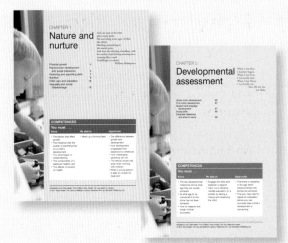

## Features contained within your textbook

Chapters are organized by organ system. Each opens with the competences you need to acquire as well as the key topics covered. The first part of each chapter goes through the most important symptoms and guides you through the differential diagnosis and the features of the history, examination and investigations that will help you come to a competent diagnosis. Full details of common and important conditions and disorders follow.

Throughout your textbook you will find a series of icons highlighting the learning features in the book:

Red flags: Worrying symptoms and signs indicative of serious conditions that you must not miss are highlighted with red flags.

Clues to the diagnosis boxes: The conditions you need to consider when encountering a sick child are shown with clues for key symptoms and signs that will help you come to the correct diagnosis.

At a Glance boxes: These boxes concisely summarize the aetiology, clinical features, investigations and management of common and important conditions for quick re-cap.

Key points boxes: Key points boxes highlight the `take-home' messages you need to remember.

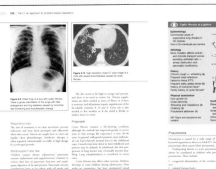

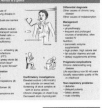

Your textbook is full of useful photographs, illustrations and tables. The Desktop Edition version of your textbook will allow you to copy and paste any photograph or illustration into assignments, presentations and your own notes.

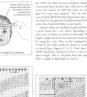

We hope you enjoy using your new textbook. Good luck with your studies!

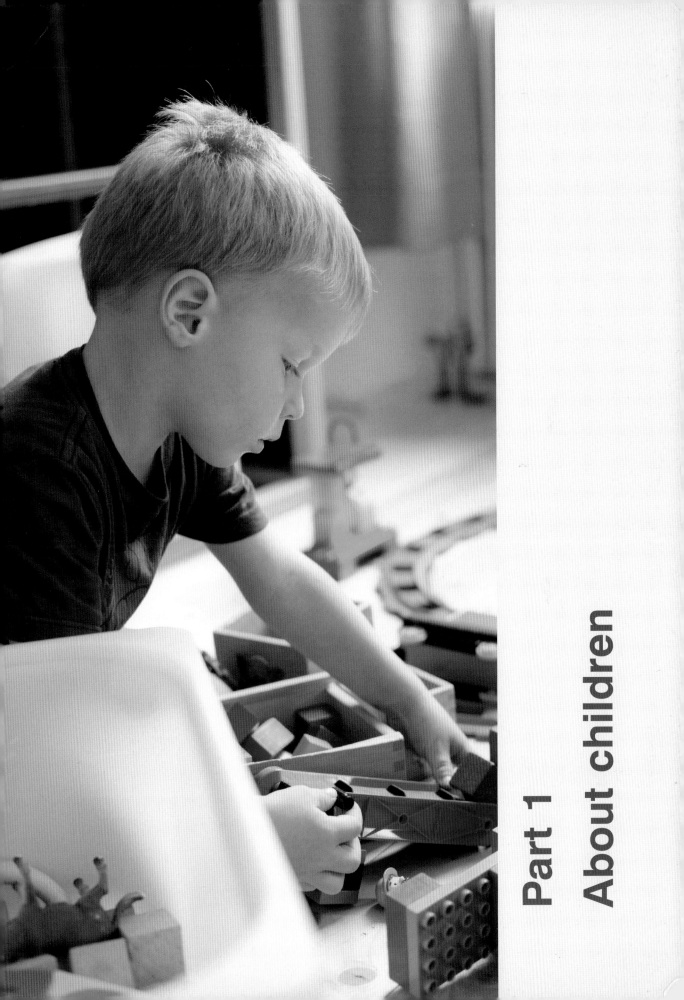

Part 1
About children

# CHAPTER 1
# Nature and nurture

And one man in his time
plays many parts,
His acts being seven ages. At first
the infant,
Mewling and puking in
the nurse's arms.
And then the whining schoolboy, with
his satchel,
And shining morning face,
creeping like a snail
Unwillingly to school.

*William Shakespeare*

## COMPETENCES

### You must . . .

| Know | Be able to | Appreciate |
|---|---|---|
| • The factors that affect growth<br>• The influence that the quality of parenting has on a child's development<br>• The advantages of breast-feeding<br>• The components of a balanced healthy diet<br>• The effects of poverty on health | • Make up a formula feed | • The difference between growth and development<br>• How development progresses from babyhood to childhood<br>• How challenging parenting can be<br>• The ethical issues that arise when working with children<br>• When a young person is able to consent to treatment |

*Paediatrics and Child Health*, Third Edition. Mary Rudolf, Tim Lee, Malcolm Levene.
© 2011 Mary Rudolf, Tim Lee and Malcolm Levene. Published 2011 by Blackwell Publishing Ltd.

Paediatrics is the branch of medicine that covers the childhood years. In general, the younger the child the more the physiology and metabolism differ from those of adults, but in older children these differences become less pronounced. There are, however, two areas that are unique to paediatrics: physical growth and development. A good understanding of how children change in terms of growth and development in the early years is very important, and without this understanding it is not possible to practice paediatrics well. This chapter discusses how the child develops physically, neurologically, psychologically and emotionally from birth through to full maturity. The chapter also discusses the importance of parenting and how this influences a child's well-being, how nutritional needs change through childhood and how poverty impacts on children's health.

## Physical growth

### Growth vs. development
Growth and development are intimately related, but are not necessarily dependent on one another. *Growth* is a combination of increase both in the number of cells (hyperplasia) and in the size of cells (hypertrophy). *Development* is an increase in complexity of the organism due to the maturation of the nervous system. A child may develop normally but be retarded in growth, and vice versa. Brain injury does not necessarily cause impaired somatic growth, although many children who are severely intellectually retarded are small. Growth can be measured accurately, but the measurement of development is much more difficult to quantify.

### Factors that affect growth (see Box 1.1)
Growth is influenced by a number of semi-independent factors, but growth itself is a continuum from early fetal life through to the end of adolescence. The following are the major factors affecting growth:

---

**Box 1.1 Factors necessary for normal growth**

- Genetic potential (mid-parental height)
- Optimal intrauterine nutrition
- Appropriate postnatal nutrition
- Good health
- Normal psychosocial factors (nurture)
- Normal hormonal milieu

---

- *Genetics.* Growth patterns and final height are largely determined by genetic factors. A normal child's final height can be predicted as falling close to the centile midway between the parents' centiles.
- *Hormones.* The principal hormones influencing early growth are growth hormone and thyroid hormone. Growth hormone in childhood and the sex hormones play an important part in the pubertal growth spurt. Disturbance of any of these affects a child's growth.
- *Nutrition.* World-wide, malnutrition is an important factor that influences children's growth, and is the major factor accounting for the differences in height observed between populations in developing and more developed countries. In many developed countries (including Britain and the USA), malnutrition is still a cause of poor growth, and is sometimes associated with neglect. Overnutrition, a leading cause of obesity, is on the increase.
- *Illness.* Illness causes a child's growth to slow down. If the illness is short-lived, rapid catch-up occurs. Chronic illness can affect growth profoundly and irreversibly.
- *Psychosocial factors.* Sociodemographically, children and adults from higher socioeconomic classes are taller than their peers from the lower classes. An adverse psychosocial environment, particularly if there is emotional neglect, can have a profound negative effect on a child's growth.

### Growth in infancy
The rate of growth in the first year of life is more rapid than at any other age. Between birth and 1 year of age, children on average increase their length by 50%, and triple their birthweight. Head circumference increases by one third. During the second year of life the rate of growth slows down and the baby changes shape to take on the appearance of the leaner and more muscular child.

### Growth in the preschool and school years
In the preschool years a child continues to gain weight and height steadily. Beyond the age of 2 or 3 years until puberty, the growth rate is steady at about 3–3.5 kg and 6 cm per year.

### Growth in adolescence
Adolescence is characterized by a growth spurt which occurs under the influence of rising sex hormone levels. During the 3 or 4 years of puberty boys grow about 25 cm and girls 20 cm. Growth in the pubertal years is discussed in Chapter 23.

## Catch-up growth

During a period of illness or starvation the rate of growth is slowed. After the incident the child usually grows more rapidly, catching up towards, or actually to, the original growth ('catch-up growth'). The degree to which catch-up is successful depends on the timing of the onset of slow growth and its duration. This is particularly important in infants who have suffered intrauterine growth retardation (see pp. 407–9), and who may have reduced growth potential.

In nutritionally compromised children, weight falls before height is impaired, and head growth is the last to be affected. If growth has been slowed for too long or into puberty, complete catch-up is not achieved. Early detection of children with abnormal growth velocity patterns has important therapeutic implications. Early treatment is more likely to ensure that acceptable adult height is achieved.

## Organ growth

Not all body systems grow at the same rate, and in some respects the growth rates of some organs are independent of others. Full maturation is not complete until the end of the second decade.

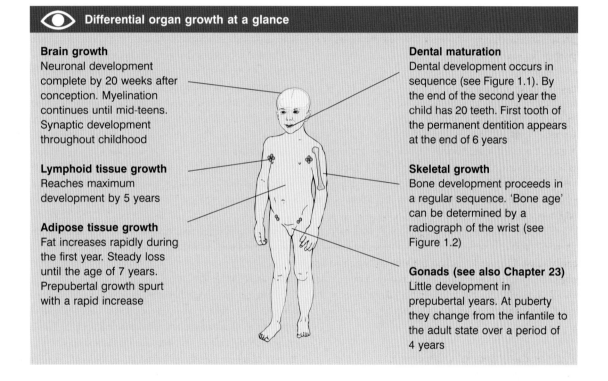

### 👁 Differential organ growth at a glance

**Brain growth**
Neuronal development complete by 20 weeks after conception. Myelination continues until mid-teens. Synaptic development throughout childhood

**Lymphoid tissue growth**
Reaches maximum development by 5 years

**Adipose tissue growth**
Fat increases rapidly during the first year. Steady loss until the age of 7 years. Prepubertal growth spurt with a rapid increase

**Dental maturation**
Dental development occurs in sequence (see Figure 1.1). By the end of the second year the child has 20 teeth. First tooth of the permanent dentition appears at the end of 6 years

**Skeletal growth**
Bone development proceeds in a regular sequence. 'Bone age' can be determined by a radiograph of the wrist (see Figure 1.2)

**Gonads (see also Chapter 23)**
Little development in prepubertal years. At puberty they change from the infantile to the adult state over a period of 4 years

# Psychomotor development and social interaction

Babies are born into a social world and learn to interact initially with their parents, then other close relatives and eventually with other children and adults. In order to achieve full social development children must achieve neurodevelopmental milestones that help them make contact with the outer world.

Early social development is divided into discrete periods corresponding to developmental landmarks; each period is an important milestone leading towards developing into a social being. More detail about developmental milestones and how to assess them are covered in Part 2. Here you are provided with an outline of a child's development through the stages of childhood. It is important to remember that each stage is dependent on the growing maturity of the nervous system. Development cannot be accelerated from outside, but external factors, particularly environment and to a lesser extent illness, can retard it.

## Babyhood and the preschool years

### 0–2 months

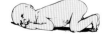

Mothers of new babies learn to 'bond' with their baby during the first hours and days after birth. This is not an automatic process

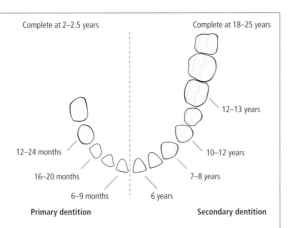

Complete at 2–2.5 years

Complete at 18–25 years

12–13 years

12–24 months

10–12 years

16–20 months

7–8 years

6–9 months

6 years

**Primary dentition**

**Secondary dentition**

**Figure 1.1** Dental development, showing the age at which teeth generally erupt.

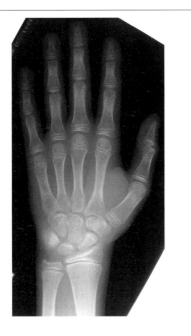

**Figure 1.2** X-ray of the left wrist taken for bone age. The development of the various bones is assessed, to give an estimate of the child's skeletal maturity.

babies often suffer feelings of guilt because they have never been told that this is a common experience.

The infant is born with a variety of needs that must be met by the parents. In the first 2 months the baby starts to adapt his or her behaviour into states of arousal. Sleep and wake cycles begin to emerge at this time and are influenced by the routine in the house. The longest period of sleep usually occurs in the night.

Infants show a great degree of alertness and are particularly attracted to human faces and the spoken word. Contact is achieved with the mother particularly during feeding. Mothers and babies coordinate their behaviour and take turns to initiate contact by means of alternating sucking with pauses for eye contact. It appears that infants are programmed to respond to their carers in particular ways, and in turn the carer is profoundly influenced by her own programming to stimulate the infant and to respond to the baby's contact. A major milestone in the development of a baby as a social being in these early weeks is the beginning of the first smile (at around 6 weeks).

### 2–5 months

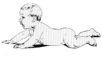

A major developmental change that occurs at the beginning of this period is the infant's visual development. At 2 months a baby can sustain eye contact and this is a vital stimulus for parent–child interaction. Over time infants show progressively more gaze interaction, and parents respond with facial expression, speech and intonation.

Another important milestone is the beginning of vocalization. When babies start to babble, carers respond as if engaging in 'conversation'. They respond to their baby's sounds by questioning or talking to the infant, with pauses for a response. Although infants do not understand the meaning of their carer's speech, the pattern and interaction are essential for the child's own language and social development. Studies have shown that if mothers do not respond appropriately to their infants by smiling and talking *en face*, babies become distressed and may withdraw from further interaction. Sensitive parental response at this age is essential for normal social development.

and is facilitated by close physical contact. Mothers who are separated from their babies after birth (e.g. because they are premature and require admission to a neonatal unit) find bonding more difficult. For this reason, parents should be encouraged to handle their babies even when their baby is receiving intensive care. Parents who find they do not immediately love their

### 5–8 months

At this age children begin to pay more detailed attention to objects. They begin to reach for toys and so start to explore the inanimate world. Through interaction with their carers, simple play starts to

emerge. At 6 weeks of age babies spend about 70% of contact time regarding their carers, but by 6 months two thirds of the time is taken up with regarding the rest of the world. First contact with objects is by gaze and later by pointing.

At this stage infants transform from being egocentric to realizing that they live in a world which is shared with people and objects.

### 8–18 months

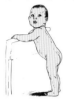

During this period mobility rapidly develops and children start to leave the safety of their carer to interact further with the environment. They begin to initiate contact rather than simply reacting to it, and the concept of reciprocating begins to emerge. They can initiate an enjoyable game such as 'peek-a-boo' and can control the game by adapting their response to the adult's. They begin to 'learn the rules' of the game and of social interaction in general. They begin to use carers to obtain desired objects, and can also manipulate objects to attract adults' attention.

At this stage children also learn to associate their cry with response and, for example, know that if they are uncomfortable due to a dirty nappy, relief will be provided. Babies who are institutionalized become apathetic if their cries are unanswered, because communication has been extinguished.

In the first half of the second year babies begin to take more interest in other children. Initially children play side by side, occasionally sharing a toy. By 18 months they may play together, but there is less vocal contact than when they are engaged with an adult. Carers, particularly parents, are the main influence in social training at this stage.

### 18 months and beyond

By 18 months children begin to communicate verbally using speech to describe an event or effect a wish. Make-believe play develops by 2 years, when children use familiar objects to reconstruct events. They also develop the ability to recognize shapes, including letters (which is the first stage of reading), and then to copy shapes with a pencil.

### School age children

Motor, language and social skills continue to develop rapidly during the school years. Horizons are broadened by starting school, and often for the first time children need to learn to function outside the security and safety of their own home. Expectations for appropriate behaviour in a variety of situations increase. During school years the child also begins to develop a conscience and an understanding of right and wrong.

Socialization is particularly important at this age, and children need to learn to relate to a variety of other children and adults. Play is an extremely important part of this process and brings benefits far beyond its impact on physical development and motor skills. It is necessary for children's happiness and well-being, impacts on the quality of friendships, cultural understanding and social, emotional and cognitive functioning, and allows the development of imagination, creativity and exploration. Through play children practice adult roles, learn a variety of competences, enhance their academic performance, and work out how to handle challenges, work in groups, make decisions and develop leadership skills.

### Adolescence

Adolescence, the period which bridges childhood and maturity, is a period of biological, psychological and sociological maturation. This is discussed in detail in Chapter 23.

## Parenting and parenting skills

Parenting is arguably the most important factor contributing to the health and well-being of children. Yet it is assumed that it comes naturally and does not need to be taught. The breakdown of the extended family compounds the situation as parents are often isolated in bringing up children, and responsibilities go unshared. Where parenting is good, children in quite adverse circumstances develop resilience to the adversity. Where parenting is poor, particularly where it is neglectful or abusive, difficulties are passed from generation to generation.

Psychologists have defined four styles of parenting as shown in Figure 1.3 depending on how responsive a parent is to their child's physical and emotional needs and the extent to which they are 'in charge'. The *authoritative style* is optimal and involves being sensitive and responsive while remaining in charge and able to maintain appropriate limits for behaviour. By contrast, the *authoritarian style* takes control to extremes, and is coupled with low responsiveness. Restrictions and demands are made without the

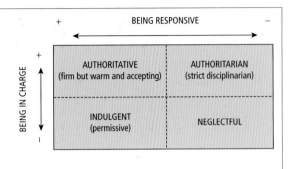

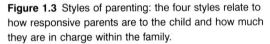

**Figure 1.3** Styles of parenting: the four styles relate to how responsive parents are to the child and how much they are in charge within the family.

child's needs, feelings and preferences being taken into account. An *indulgent style* is a kind but weak approach to parenting, where the parent is responsive to the child's wishes and demands even when they are not in the child's best interests. It is linked to an inability to set limits and maintain boundaries. A *neglectful style* is one where the parent is neither in charge nor responsive to the child.

The authoritative style is the ideal as it promotes healthy development and a feeling of security where children know that their needs will be respected and their views considered within a consistent framework. Research shows that authoritative parenting is linked to a large number of positive outcomes such as social development, self-esteem and mental health, higher academic achievement, lower levels of problem behaviour, increased ability to self-regulate, less depression and less risk taking, The other styles have been associated with lower academic grades, lower levels of self-control, poorer psychosocial and emotional development, behavioural problems and substance abuse.

It is now being recognized that parenting should be taught to young people while at school. The curriculum should address emotional well-being and discipline as much as the practicalities of caring for babies and young children. Schools are beginning to acknowledge this, although it has to be said that teenagers may find it hard to relate to the issues. A further opportunity to impart good principles and practice comes at antenatal classes. An important part of well child care is to support parents in developing their parenting skills. Parenting groups are often available for parents and the evidence is clear that they can be helpful, particularly in improving the quality of home life and the management of difficult behaviour.

Common parenting difficulties and how they can be addressed are discussed in Chapter 19.

## Nutrition

Milk is the food of babies and it is capable of meeting the infant's nutritional needs for the first 6 months of life. Breast milk is the ideal food for human babies, but may be unavailable for some infants, in which case alternative formulae are available.

### *Nutritional requirements in infancy*

#### Water
Over 70% of a newborn infant's weight is water, compared with 60% for an adult. Infants are less able to conserve water and consequently their fluid requirements are considerably higher than those of older children.

#### Energy
Newborn infants require approximately 110 kcal/kg per day (462 kJ/kg per day) for normal growth, and these energy requirements are provided by a balance of carbohydrate, fat and protein.

- *Carbohydrate.* Almost all the carbohydrate in both human and formula milk is lactose, and about 40% of the total energy requirement comes from carbohydrate sources.
- *Fat.* Fat is the most important source of energy in milk and provides approximately one half of an infant's energy requirement.
- *Protein.* Milk protein can be divided into curd and whey. Curd consists predominantly of casein and precipitates in the stomach. Whey contains mainly lactalbumin and lactoferrin. Colostrum is the very thin watery milk produced by the breast in the first few days after giving birth. It has a very high proportion of immunoglobulins.

#### Minerals
The mineral requirements change as babies mature. At birth the renal conservation of sodium is poor and newborn babies lose more in their urine than older infants. Premature babies, in turn, require a higher sodium intake than full-term babies because of the functional immaturity of the kidneys.

Calcium and phosphate absorption in infancy is high as a result of the rapid growth rate. The relative ratio of these two minerals is important in determining adequate absorption.

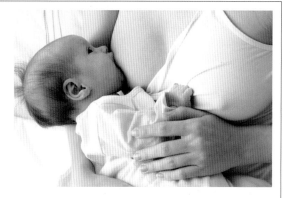

**Figure 1.4** Mother breast-feeding her 6-week-old baby.

| Table 1.1 Factors associated with successful breast-feeding |
| --- |
| High socioeconomic class |
| Intention to breast-feed whilst pregnant |
| Paternal support |
| Whether the mother herself has been breast-fed |

### Vitamins

All babies require essential vitamins. Surprisingly, breast milk is deficient in vitamin K. All newborn infants should be given vitamin K at birth to prevent haemorrhagic disease of the newborn.

### Trace elements

There are a large number of essential trace elements present in milk which are essential for normal growth and development. Iron is one of the most important, and breast milk contains sufficient iron for dietary needs over the first 6 months of life.

### *Breast-feeding (see Figure 1.4)*

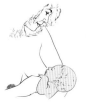 The proportion of women breast-feeding varies widely throughout the world. The World Health Organization reports that in some countries it is usual for all mothers to breast-feed for up to 1 year. In Britain only two thirds of women offer their babies any breast milk at all, and less than half continue to breast-feed by the time the baby is 4 months old. These figures are influenced by socioeconomic class: 97% of women in the highest socioeconomic class feed their first baby compared with less than 50% in a group of less advantaged women.

In order to support breast-feeding more widely, the World Health Organization and UNICEF established The Baby Friendly Initiative as a worldwide programme to encourage maternity hospitals and community services to promote successful breast-feeding and to practise in accordance with the International Code of Marketing of Breastmilk Substitutes. This has helped to ensure a higher stand-

ard of care for pregnant women and breast-feeding mothers and babies.

The factors that predict successful breast-feeding are shown in Table 1.1.

In developed countries the benefits of breast-feeding are psychological as much as physical. In developing countries the argument for breast-feeding is very strong: formula feeds may easily be contaminated by polluted water used in making up the feed, with the risk of fatal gastroenteritis. Everywhere, breast-feeding has the advantages of being free of cost and convenient.

### Physiology of lactation

During pregnancy there is a marked increase in the number of ducts and alveoli within the breast, in response to changes in maternal and placental hormones. The size of the nipple also increases. In the third trimester prolactin sensitizes the glandular tissue, causing small amounts of colostrum to be secreted.

At birth, oestrogen levels fall rapidly while prolactin rises. This is stimulated further by the infant's sucking at the breast. The prolactin secretion from the anterior pituitary maintains milk production from the breast alveoli. The volume of milk produced relates to the frequency, duration and intensity of sucking.

The flow of milk from the breast is under the control of the let-down reflex. The baby's rooting at the nipple causes afferent impulses to pass to the posterior pituitary, which secretes oxytocin. This acts on the smooth muscle fibres surrounding the alveoli so that milk is forced into the large ducts. As the baby takes less milk, the stimulus for prolactin production reduces and lactation is inhibited. The hormonal maintenance of lactation is summarized in Figure 1.5.

The let-down reflex is stimulated by contact with the baby, including hearing the baby cry and handling the child. Dripping of milk from the breast not being suckled is caused by reflex action; this diminishes after the first few weeks. Anxiety and embarrassment

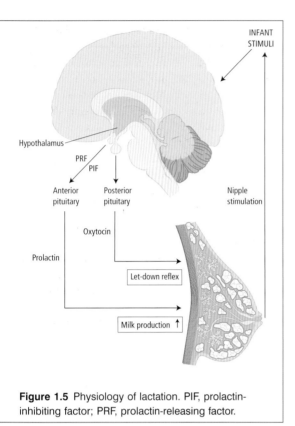

**Figure 1.5** Physiology of lactation. PIF, prolactin-inhibiting factor; PRF, prolactin-releasing factor.

suppress the reflex by action of the sympathetic nervous system. Every step possible should therefore be taken to put the mother at her ease and avoid unnecessary anxiety.

**Colostrum.** The milk produced in the first few days after birth is called colostrum and is a thin, yellowish fluid. It is particularly valuable for the establishment of lactobacilli in the bowel and contains less fat and energy but more immunoglobulins than later milk.

The constituents of milk do not reach their mature proportions until 10–14 days after birth. The secretion from the breast between colostrum and mature milk is referred to as transitional milk.

## Technique of breast-feeding
The majority of the milk taken by a baby from the breast is consumed in the first 5 minutes of the feed. Much of the rest of the time at the breast is spent in non-nutritive sucking. Mothers should be aware of the feeling of her breast being 'emptied' by her baby shortly after commencement of suckling, but the time spent at the breast following this is also very important.

Mothers should be encouraged to put the baby to the breast directly after birth. A normal baby immediately attempts to suck. Little milk is produced, but the stimulation is important in the establishment of lactation. Mothers should then be encouraged to put the baby to the breast on demand and should also feed the baby during the first night. The time the baby spends on the breast should be gradually increased so that the nipples become accustomed to the baby sucking.

Trauma to the nipple in the first few days after birth has to be minimized. The baby exerts strong suction on the nipple and a baby should never be pulled off the breast. The mother should be shown how to release the baby by using her finger to depress the breast away from the corner of the baby's mouth. Feeds should commence on alternate breasts.

Babies are often given complement formula feeds in the early days of life by well-meaning staff in order to let the mother rest, but this is counterproductive and should be avoided. If a baby appears to be hungry and it is considered not appropriate to put him or her to the breast, a solution of dextrose and water may be given.

It is common for mothers to encounter difficulties in establishing breast-feeding in the first weeks, and to feel that their milk is inadequate. The difficulties often relate to positioning of the baby, and expert support from breast-feeding counsellors can often help resolve the problems.

## Advantages of breast-feeding
The advantages of breast-feeding are summarized in Table 1.2, and ways to encourage successful breast-feeding are shown in Box 1.2.

| **Table 1.2** Advantages of breast-feeding |
| --- |
| Perfect balance of milk constituents |
| Little risk of bacterial contamination |
| Anti-infective properties |
| Ideal food for brain growth and optimal development |
| Convenience |
| No expense to purchase milk |
| Psychological satisfaction |
| Possibly reduces risk of atopic disorders |
| Exposes baby to a variety of flavours |

## Box 1.2 Ways to encourage successful breast-feeding

• Introduce the concept to both parents antenatally
• Place the baby on the breast immediately after delivery
• Allow the baby to feed on demand, in the early days especially
• Avoid offering any formula feeds
• Ensure the mother receives good nutrition and plenty of rest

**Table 1.3** Role of anti-infective agents in breast milk

| | |
|---|---|
| Cells | Milk is teeming with white cells, mainly macrophages, polymorphs and both T- and B-lymphocytes |
| Immunoglobulins | Secretory IgA is the predominant immunoglobulin. Particularly high concentration in colostrum |
| Lysozyme | Lyses bacterial cell walls |
| Lactoferrin | Binds iron necessary for the replication of some bacteria and reduces bacterial growth |
| Interferon | Present in low concentrations in breast milk and has antiviral properties |
| Bifidus factor | The carbohydrate bifidus factor encourages lactobacilli to flourish in the bowel, inhibiting overgrowth of *Escherichia coli* |

Breast-fed infants have a significantly lower risk of respiratory and gastrointestinal infections in the early months of life compared with formula-fed infants. Breast milk has a number of important anti-infective properties which are summarized in Table 1.3.

### Contraindications to breast-feeding

For the average healthy infant there are no disadvantages to breast-feeding. Infants born with anomalies such as severe cleft lip and palate and obstructive bowel problems may not be able to feed, although every effort should be made to provide them with expressed breast milk rather than formula feeds.

Similarly, there are very few contraindications to breast-feeding for the mother. The most important reason to prevent a mother from breast-feeding is if she is HIV-positive: the risk of transmitting the HIV virus to her baby is doubled by breast-feeding. A mother who is excreting *Mycobacterium tuberculosis* should also not breast-feed.

Mastitis (inflammation of the breast) is a common problem but, far from contraindicating, it is alleviated by continued and frequent breast-feeding.

### Drugs in breast milk

Most drugs given to the mother are excreted to some degree in her milk, but the exposure to the infant is usually so little that the risk is minimal. Examples of drugs that are definitely contraindicated in a breast-feeding mother are tetracyclines (which stain developing teeth), antimetabolites (impair cell growth) and opiates (drug addiction).

### *Formula feeds*

Formula milks are based on cow's milk, but are highly adjusted to meet the basic nutritional requirements of growing immature infants. A variety of components of cow's milk are utilized. Skimmed milk is produced by removing the fat content, and the curd can be separated, leaving whey and lactose together with minerals. These are the building blocks of infant milk formula.

Virtually all formula feeds have added carbohydrate, usually lactose or maltodextrins. Most milk manufacturers replace the fat with polyunsaturated vegetable oil or butterfat blend. This alters the fatty acid profile to resemble breast milk more closely. The protein base of formula milk is usually demineralized whey to which the appropriate mixture of minerals, vitamins and trace elements are added. Casein-predominant milks are usually given as a supplement to babies of 4–6 months who are perceived to be still hungry. This process produces a formula milk product that is similar in its basic proportions to that of mature breast milk.

It is clear that although there are similarities between breast and formula milks, the constituents are chemically quite different. The protein in formula milk is based on cow's milk protein and the fat content is quite different to breast milk fat content. The major differences between breast and formula milk are shown in Table 1.4.

**Table 1.4** Comparisons between breast and formula milk

| Breast milk | Formula milk |
|---|---|
| Sterile | May be contaminated by 'bad' water |
| Contains anti-infective properties (see p. 11) | |
| Reduces risk of infection | |
| No cost | Expensive |
| Perfectly adapted to human babies | Foreign protein |
| | Non-human fat content |
| Allergic disorders reduced | May increase risk of allergy |
| Possible IQ enhancement | |
| Some protection from obesity | |

## Additives

Formula or bottle-fed babies require no vitamin supplementation.

Fluoride drops are advised for babies from 6 months if the drinking water is not fluoridated.

## Preparation of feeds

The preparation of formula feeds is summarized in Figure 1.6. Some parents find it more convenient to make up the day's supply of feeds at one time, and to store the milk in a refrigerator. Parents need to understand and be instructed to use a level measure of powder and not a heaped one, as this would produce too concentrated a feed, especially in its electrolyte content, and could lead to hypernatraemic dehydration (see p. 95). To obtain a level measure the excess powder is removed with the blade of a knife.

Scrupulous attention should be paid to sterility: bottles and teats should be sterilized either by boiling or by an antiseptic solution such as mild sodium hypochlorite (Milton). It is essential that the bottles are filled with the solution and the teats are totally immersed. The Milton solution should be made up each day.

Most parents like to give the milk warm, although babies will take a cold feed just as well. To ensure that the feed is not too hot it should be tested by shaking out a little onto the back of the hand. The teat should not be touched or it will become contaminated. The hole in the teat should be large enough so that when the bottle is inverted, milk comes out rapidly in drops, but not in a stream. Too large a hole causes the baby to choke on the feed, and too small a hole leads to excessive air swallowing as a result of the baby's vigorously sucking to obtain the milk.

### Weaning (see Boxes 1.3 and 1.4)

Healthy infants do not require weaning until 6 months of age. Breast or formula milk provide all their nutritional requirements in the early months. Too early an introduction of mixed feeding may be associated with obesity.

In developed countries there is a wide choice of weaning foods. In Britain cereals and rusks are the favoured first solid food, but package foods to which water is added may also be used. All modern cereals for babies are gluten free, and this may be associated with a fall in the incidence of coeliac disease (pp. 180–1). The semi-solid food is given by spoon before offering the bottle or breast. Its timing should be whatever suits the mother. Alternative weaning foods are purées of cooked vegetables, fish or meat. These can be purchased in pre-prepared containers or be liquidized at home in a food blender.

Babies are conservative individuals and dislike change. The earlier a new-tasting food is introduced, the more likely it is to be accepted. It is often recommended that one new food should be introduced at a time. Babies may well be reluctant to accept new tastes at first, which can be interpreted as dislike. Repeated offerings generally result in acceptance. When weaning, cup and spoon feeding should be introduced early in order to make the change easier and reduce the possibility of the baby refusing to give up the bottle (see Figure 1.7).

As children get older their diet will become more like that of the rest of the family. The child will now begin to try to hold the spoon him- or herself, although he or she is likely to go through a stage of wanting to use fingers only. A baby who has started to chew his or her fingers, even before any teeth have erupted, can be given toast or a hard rusk to chew on. It is good to encourage self-feeding as this helps ensure that the baby is not over- or underfed. At no time should the child be left alone while feeding, however, for fear of choking.

By the age of 9 months, most babies are ready to eat at least one meal a day with the family. The food

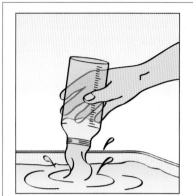

1. Sterilize the feeding bottle

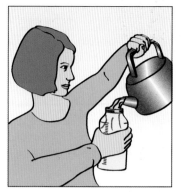

2. Add the appropriate volume of cooled boiled water to the bottle

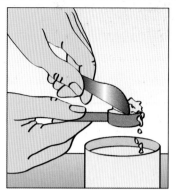

3. Add 1 level scoop of milk powder to each 30 ml of water

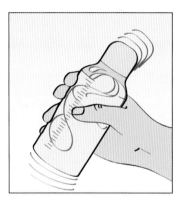

4. Shake bottle well

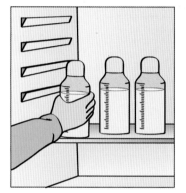

5. Keep in fridge until ready to feed

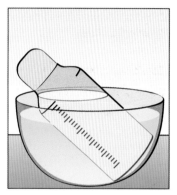

6. Rewarm the feed to room temperature or body temperature prior to feeding

**Figure 1.6** Preparation of formula feed.

## Box 1.3 Principles of infant nutrition

- Breast milk is the ideal sole feed for the first 4–6 months
- Continue breast or formula milk for the first year
- Introduce solid foods from 6 months
- Once a baby is able to chew, mashed and then cut up food can be given
- Babies can usually feed themselves biscuits or rusks at 7 months
- Cup feeds should replace breast-feeds, and bottles be discouraged beyond the age of 1 year
- Vitamin supplements should be given once weaning is well established

## Box 1.4 The weaning process

| | |
|---|---|
| 0–6 months | Breast or formula milk only |
| 6 months | Introduce solid foods – pureed and finger feeds |
| 7–9 months | Give more soft feeds before milk feeds. Encourage finger feeding. Give fruit juices in a cup |
| 9–12 months | Mash food with a fork. Three meals a day, at least one with the family |
| 1 year and beyond | Undiluted cow's milk in a cup |

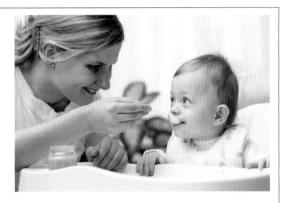

**Figure 1.7** Mother feeding her 6-month-old baby. She is seated so she can interact with him and pick up on his hunger and fullness cues, ensuring that she does not under- or over-feed him.

should be similar to what the rest of the family is eating, but without added sugar or salt. It should be presented in an attractive and appropriate way: cut up into small pieces or mashed. Children can be given undiluted and unboiled bottled cow's milk from 12 months of age. This can be served cold, but as many children are used to warm milk they may initially reject it.

At 6 months a multivitamin preparation should be started once weaning is well established to ensure adequate intake as young children often do not achieve adequate intake through their diet.

### Nutrition in the preschool years (see Box 1.5)

As toddlers children become increasingly dextrous and coordinated and should be eating independently using a spoon and drinking from a cup. Alongside this independence comes a change in eating habits and it is normal for a toddler to eat unpredictably, consuming large meals on some occasions and almost negligible amounts at others. It is also usual for them to develop a wariness of new foods and become 'picky' about what they eat.

Milk is now no longer the main source of nutrition, although the child should still drink 1 pint of milk per day. In these early years, it is important to ensure that the child becomes used to eating a well-balanced diet. This should include foods from the four basic food groups:

• meat, fish, poultry and eggs;
• dairy products (milk and cheese products);
• fruits and vegetables;
• cereals, grains, potatoes and rice.

In encouraging a good diet, it must be stressed that children of this age have different requirements from adults. A diet low in fat and high in fibre is unlikely to provide the calorie content that is essential for active, rapidly growing children. For this reason whole-fat milk rather than semi-skimmed milk should be given until the age of 2 years. It is also important to discourage children from developing a taste for sweet and salty foods.

The development of independence and inconsistent eating habits often causes problems within the family (see pp. 356–7). Parents may become very anxious about the child's diet and resort to a variety of tactics to make their child eat. This can be extremely stressful for all concerned and may be associated with weight faltering (see pp. 257–9).

The other common problem of this period is iron-deficiency anaemia (see p. 345) resulting from low iron stores. These may be inadequately maintained by a low intake of iron-rich foods and so fail to keep up with the growth of the child. Excessive milk intake may contribute by leading to a reduction in appetite for other nutrients, and may also be responsible for poor weight gain.

### Nutrition in the school years

In the school years children have to learn to eat food other than that provided at home, and usually have a midday meal at school. The principles of healthy eating should be maintained. The Food Standards Agency has produced the 'Eatwell Plate' (see Figure 1.8) to guide families on how to balance their diet. It

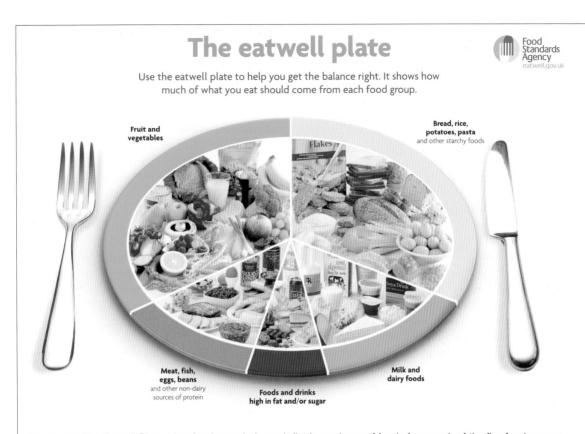

**Figure 1.8** The Eatwell Plate, showing how a balanced diet is made up of foods from each of the five food groups. © Crown copyright.

clearly shows how prominent fruit and vegetables should be, and how little fat and sugar is required relative to the other foods. The challenges of maintaining healthy eating are compounded when children are introduced to snacking on sugary and salty foods by their peers. Schools are well placed to educate about nutrition and provide well-balanced meals, and regulations are in place to make sure that food eaten on the premises is nutritious.

As important as *what* children eat is *how* they eat. Too often children help themselves to meals or 'graze' through out the day. Family mealtimes (Figure 1.9) are associated with many benefits including enhanced language development, psychosocial well-being, fewer high-risk behaviours, reduced obesity levels and lower academic dropout rates.

The adolescent years bring increased requirements for energy, calcium, nitrogen and iron. Unfortunately, in this critical period, when good nutrition is so important, modern teenagers often develop lifestyles which lead to a very poor nutritional intake. Particular problems include an increase in snacking

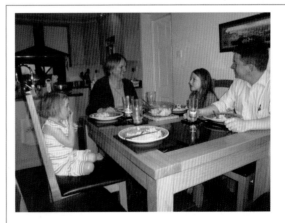

**Figure 1.9** A family mealtime. Eating regularly together as a family is associated with a broad range of benefits in such areas as social behaviour, language development and academic achievement.

and skipping meals, an inappropriate consumption of fast foods, dieting and restrictive cult diets. The problems of obesity (see pp. 259–62) and eating disorders (see pp. 441–2) often have their onset at this time, while teenage pregnancy has nutritional consequences for both the baby and the mother.

## Child care and education

Increasingly, mothers are working outside the home and have to find alternative care for their young children. Options include a nanny or minder in the home, or child care outside the home. Child-minders who take other children into their own home have to be legally approved and registered with the Department of Social Services.

Alternative care is available in **day nurseries** staffed by nursery nurses. These may be run by Social Care, privately or by voluntary organizations. Unfortunately they are in limited supply and are often expensive. In disadvantaged areas family centres may be provided, which not only provide child care but are also attended by parents with the aim of improving parenting skills.

The majority of children grow up away from an extended family network, and many parents appreciate the opportunities for their children to mix with other children from a young age. **Mother and toddler groups** and **playgroups** are available in most areas. The former are attended by children accompanied by a carer. Playgroups are run by trained and registered leaders, where children attend for a few sessions per week and have the opportunity to meet, play and socialize with others. **Sure Start** programmes are a UK government initiative that provide a variety of facilities and programmes for young families in disadvantaged areas, including daycare.

In Britain compulsory education begins at the age of 5 years, although there is limited availability of **nursery school** places from the age of 3 years. From 5 to 11 years children attend **primary school**, then move to **secondary school** until the school-leaving age of 16 years. At 16 years teenagers have the option to continue their education in a **secondary school sixth form, sixth form college** or **college of further education**.

Educational provision for children with special needs is discussed on pages 46–7.

## Inequality and social disadvantage

A large and increasing number of children, in both developed and developing countries, grow up socially disadvantaged. Disadvantage may arise as a consequence of poverty, poor housing, homelessness, inadequate parenting and problems resulting from immigration. It is important to appreciate that these all have a significant impact on children's health. Alleviation of these problems is mainly a political issue for society, but doctors need to understand the impact of the problems and, where necessary and possible, to act as the child's advocate in improving their circumstances.

### Poverty

It is hard to bring up a family on a low income. Not only is it hard to feed and clothe children, and provide them with the care and conditions required for them to develop and thrive, but poverty also often diminishes the capacity of parents to be supportive, consistent and involved with their children.

Poverty has a strong effect on the physical health of children, and children from poor families have higher than average rates of death and illness from almost all causes (Table 1.5). Many factors are responsible for the increased morbidity, including overcrowding, poor hygiene and health care, poor diet, environmental pollution, poor education and stress.

### Housing

Housing conditions have a profound effect on children's health and development. Dampness and mould are associated with an increase in a wide variety of symptoms and illnesses. Overcrowding and poor sanitary conditions are related to the spread of

| **Table 1.5** Morbidity associated with poverty |
| --- |
| Low birthweight |
| Poor growth |
| Respiratory infections |
| Iron-deficiency anaemia |
| Lead poisoning |
| Poor vision |
| Hearing disorders |
| Psychological problems |
| More and longer hospitalizations |
| Lower survival in some malignancies (e.g. leukaemia) |
| Lower educational attainment |
| More likely to attend special school |

gastroenteritis and respiratory infections. Inadequate housing may lead to parental depression, affecting a child's psychosocial development and behaviour. Poor housing is also linked to a higher rate of accidents, including road traffic accidents as a result of a lack of safe supervised areas for play outside.

## Homelessness

Homelessness exacerbates the problems of poverty. Homeless families have very restricted facilities, often living in bed and breakfast or hostel accommodation, with little space or privacy and little possibility of cooking. Moves are frequent, with disruption in the provision of health and social services and schooling for the children. Homeless children suffer from increased frequency of illness (infections, anaemia), neurological conditions and learning disorders, fits, mental illness, dental problems, trauma and substance abuse, and are more likely to be victims of abuse and neglect.

## Family structure

There have been major changes in the structure of society in recent years. Fewer children in developed countries now live with both natural parents, and there are increasing numbers of parents bringing up children single-handedly. Although this does not necessarily imply that the children are disadvantaged, single parenting is difficult, particularly if it is associated, as it often is, with a reduced income, lack of support with resultant stress and depression, and family tensions and arguments. These all may have an effect on the child.

## Ethnic minorities and immigrants

The other major change that has occurred in developed countries is absorption of a variety of different ethnic and cultural groups. While immigrant families are often well supported within their cultural framework, children may be disadvantaged in a variety of ways of which health professionals need to be aware.

Language and cultural barriers often lead to high degrees of social stress and isolation, and families may find it difficult to access services including health care. Specific health problems affecting some groups include nutritional deficiencies, higher perinatal and infant mortality rates, and inherited diseases if consanguinity is common practice.

# CHAPTER 2

# Health care and child health promotion

The fundamental objective of pediatrics is to guide children safely and happily through childhood so that they will become healthy, well adjusted, normal young adults—to enable them to achieve their maximum potential physically, intellectually, psychologically and socially.

*James G. Hughes, MD*

## COMPETENCES

### You must . . .

| Know | Be able to | Appreciate |
|---|---|---|
| • The roles that different health professionals take in providing health care to children<br>• The screening tests that are routinely carried out on children<br>• The immunizations that are routinely given and the diseases they protect against<br>• Contraindications to immunizations<br>• When to be concerned about a child's growth pattern<br>• The role of health professionals in protecting children from neglect and abuse | • Undertake a systematic examination of the newborn<br>• Examine for congenital dislocation of the hips<br>• Palpate for testicular descent<br>• Advise parents about common problems relating to child care | • That liaison with other professionals is key in providing good health care<br>• That growth is an indicator of a child's health<br>• That health professionals have an obligation to report suspected child abuse<br>• The special ethical issues that arise when working with children<br>• When a young person is able to consent to treatment |

*Paediatrics and Child Health*, Third Edition. Mary Rudolf, Tim Lee, Malcolm Levene.
© 2011 Mary Rudolf, Tim Lee and Malcolm Levene. Published 2011 by Blackwell Publishing Ltd.

# The Healthy Child programme

The Healthy Child Programme is the national child health promotion programme in the UK. It aims to promote children's health and development, prevent illness and work in partnership with parents to achieve physical, social and emotional well-being for all children. The Programme is underpinned by the principle of progressive universalism whereby all children receive a basic package of care which is increased progressively according to the needs of the child and family.

The Programme (see Table 2.1) has many facets which include:

- guidance on important child health topics such as parenting, development, behavioural problems, nutrition and the use of services for children;
- a focus on vulnerable children, with identification of children in need, whether socially disadvantaged or with disabilities;
- monitoring of developmental progress;
- prevention of disease by immunization;

**Table 2.1** The Healthy Child Programme

| Age | Health guidance | Observation and examination | Screening procedure |
|---|---|---|---|
| Newborn | Feeding and nutrition<br>Parenting<br>Injury prevention<br>Baby care<br>Crying and sleep problems<br>Passive smoking<br>Car seats<br>Reducing risk of SIDS | Full physical examination<br>Weight<br>Head circumference | Hip examination<br>Testicular descent<br>Red reflex<br>Phenylketonuria<br>Thyroid<br>Haemoglobinopathies<br>Cystic fibrosis<br>MCADD<br>Hearing test |
| 6 weeks–6 months | Parenting<br>Maternal mental health<br>Nutrition and weaning<br>Development<br>Play<br>Immunization<br>Recognition of illness in babies<br>Accidents: fires, falls and scalds, baths | Weight, length at 6–8 weeks (and 3–4 months if concern)<br>Head circumference<br>Eyes<br>Development<br>Cardiac examination | Hip examination at 6–8 weeks<br>Testicular descent at 6–8 weeks |
| 6 months–1 year | Children's physical, emotional and social needs<br>Parenting<br>Accident prevention<br>Nutrition<br>Passive smoking<br>Developmental needs, language and play<br>Behaviour problems<br>Dental health | Monitor growth<br>Evaluate development | |
| 1–3 years | Children's physical, emotional and social needs<br>Parenting<br>Behaviour<br>Language development<br>Nutrition, play and sleep<br>Dental care<br>Accident prevention<br>Toilet training | At 2-year review:<br>• monitor growth<br>• evaluate development | |

| Age | Health guidance | Observation and examination | Screening procedure |
|-----|-----------------|-----------------------------|---------------------|
| **Table 2.1** The Healthy Child Programme (cont'd) | | | |
| 3–5 years | Parental and teacher concerns<br>Nutrition, play and sleep<br>Accident prevention<br>Dental health<br>Medical or developmental problems<br>   that may interfere with education<br>Review immunization status | | |
| Primary school | Health education in school | Height and weight for the National Child Measurement Programme at school entry and at age 11 years | At school entry:<br>• Vision (Snellen chart)<br>• Hearing (sweep test) |
| Secondary school | Health education in school<br>Self-referrals to school doctor or nurse<br>Careers advice | | Visual acuity in disadvantaged areas<br>*Chlamydia* |

- detection of abnormalities through physical examination and screening tests, and facilitating early recognition by parents;
- measurement and recording of physical growth;
- health promotion and education.

## Professionals involved in child health promotion in the UK

### Health visitors

Health visitors are nurses who are specially trained in child care and development. They generally work within the framework of a health centre, often with GPs or children's centres, and carry out the bulk of the child health promotion programme for preschool children. This includes running child health clinics, visiting at home and providing support, particularly for those children and families identified as being in need or at risk.

### School nurses

School nurses are specially trained nurses who work in the framework of schools. They are responsible for identifying children with medical needs, facilitating their care at school, providing liaison between professionals and supplying medical information to school staff. As school doctors are no longer required to see every child at school entry, the school nurse is now responsible for reviewing all children and selecting those who need to be seen by the community paediatrician.

### Community paediatricians

Community paediatricians are doctors who specialize in working in the community. They are responsible for evaluating children identified through the child health promotion programme or school as having problems. Some have specialized roles such as audiology, child protection or developmental paediatrics.

### General practitioners

In recent years GPs have taken over responsibility for the routine aspects of most of the preschool child health promotion programme.

### Parents

Parents have a central role in enhancing the health of their children and they should be seen as partners in child health promotion.

## Child health records

### Parent-held child health records

Every child is issued a child health record at birth which is kept by the parents. The advantages of this are that the child's record is available wherever and whenever the child is seen, confidentiality rests with the parents and, most importantly, it involves parents centrally in child health promotion. The parent-held record consists of a record of child health checks, the child's growth chart, parental observations, a record of primary care and dental and hospital visits, and health education and advice. Parents have welcomed this development and have been shown to be effective in ensuring that the record is kept up to date.

### Other records

In addition to the parent-held record, each professional keeps their own record of contact with the child. Computer-based systems are increasingly being used and are particularly effective in child health promotion.

### Special registers

Many districts keep registers of children with special needs or chronic illness. They are useful in providing parents with information about services, keeping track of referral and review, anticipating needs and auditing the service. The parents' permission is required before placing a child on such a register.

### Detection of medical and developmental problems

An important part of child health promotion involves identification of subtle or latent defects and disorders that may seriously affect the child later in life. These defects and disorders are usually identified in one of the following ways:

- Child health checks.
- Follow-up of infants and children who have suffered various forms of trauma or illness.
- Detection by parents or relatives, who are often the first to recognize that their child has a problem. When such suspicions are reported to a health professional they should be taken seriously, as parents are often right.
- Detection by other professionals such as nursery nurses, playgroup leaders and teachers. Playgroup leaders and nursery nurses play an important part in child care, particularly in deprived areas, and become expert at recognizing the child whose health or development requires further evaluation.

## Health education and promotion

Increasingly, young families are growing up isolated and without the support of an extended family. Parenting skills and confidence are often lacking, and the Healthy Child Programme is therefore particularly valuable in providing information and advice to inexperienced parents. In disadvantaged areas this often takes place through Sure Start centres (p. 16). The following issues are addressed by the programme.

### Baby care

Young parents are likely to need advice about simple issues such as clothing, bathing, handling and positioning their baby. They need to know about common medical problems, and to learn the appropriate responses when the baby is unwell. As time goes by, they need to know about normal development, what to expect from their child, how to promote learning and how to recognize developmental difficulties.

### Nutrition (see Chapter 1)

If a good nutritional environment is provided in the early years, the ground is laid for healthy eating later in childhood and beyond. Addressing nutritional issues is a major focus of a health visitor's work. It includes promoting breast-feeding, advising about weaning, dealing with toddlers' eating difficulties and education about healthy diets for the entire family.

### Behavioural problems

Behavioural concerns are universal. Advice and support in the early stages can avoid their developing into major problems. Crying, sleep problems and temper tantrums are particularly common issues of concern.

### Dental care

Information should be provided about dental hygiene and regular dental check-ups.

### Passive smoking

Children exposed to passive smoking are at greatly increased risk of respiratory disorders. Avoidance of passive smoking is an important health promotion issue.

### Unintentional injury

Accidents are the commonest cause of mortality in the childhood years and an important cause of morbidity. The term 'accident' is actually inappropriate as it implies the injury occurred by chance. In fact most accidents are predictable and could be avoided with appropriate strategies. As most accidents occur in the home, education of parents has an important impact on the prevention of accidents. Areas which should be addressed in the course of health education are shown in Table 2.2.

## Health promotion in school

School provides an invaluable opportunity to educate the young about healthy living. The school years are a time when adjustments in lifestyle can be made more easily than later on in life. Issues of particular importance which are addressed are:

- nutrition;
- physical activity;
- drugs and alcohol abuse;

- contraception and safe sex;
- sexually transmitted diseases;
- smoking;
- healthy relationships;
- parenting skills.

## Screening (see Table 2.1)

Screening is the identification of unrecognized disease or defects by the application of tests, examinations and other procedures. Screening tests sort out apparently well children who may have a problem from those who do not. A screening test is not intended to be diagnostic.

Various criteria have been established to determine whether there is a value in screening for a particular condition. These criteria include a recognizable latent or early symptomatic stage of the condition, and the availability of some form of treatment or intervention that can influence the course and prognosis. Cost inevitably must be considered and needs to be balanced against the cost of medical care as a whole and the cost of treatment if the patient does not present until later.

The following screening tests have been incorporated into the child health promotion programme in the UK.

### Congenital hypothyroidism

- *Age at which the test is performed.* Neonates (5–8 days of age).
- *The test.* A few drops of blood are obtained by heel prick, dripped onto a filter paper and sent to a central laboratory for analysis of thyroid hormone ($T_4$) or thyroid-stimulating hormone (TSH) (Figure 2.1).
- *Significance of the test.* Approximately one in 4000 infants is born with congenital hypothyroidism. If untreated, cretinism with severe learning disability (mental retardation) results (see p. 269). If treated early with thyroid hormone, the child grows and develops normally.
- *Action if the test is abnormal.* The baby must be referred urgently to a paediatric endocrinologist.

### Guthrie test for phenylketonuria

- *Age at which the test is performed.* Neonates (5–8 days of age).
- *The test.* The test is carried out on the same sample as that taken for thyroid testing. The baby must be on full milk feeds for 3 days prior to testing.

**Table 2.2** Strategies for the reduction of injuries in childhood

| Injury | Prevention strategy |
|---|---|
| Road traffic injuries | Use of car seats and belts |
| | Road safety instruction from age 2 years |
| | Cycle helmets |
| Falls | Gate on stairs |
| | Guards on windows |
| | Safe playground surfaces |
| Burns | Exercise caution in the kitchen |
| | Reduce home hot water temperature |
| | Install smoke detectors |
| | Install fire guards |
| | Have flameproof clothing |
| | Cover electric sockets |
| | Avoid trailing flexes on kettles and irons |
| Drowning | Never leave young children alone in bath |
| | Fence pools |
| | Swim only with lifeguard present |
| Poisoning | Keep medicines/poisons out of reach |
| | Have locks on cupboards |
| | Have safety caps on bottles |
| Choking | Keep small toys away from toddlers |
| | Do not give nuts before age 5 years |
| | Teach Heimlich manoeuvre (p. 377) |

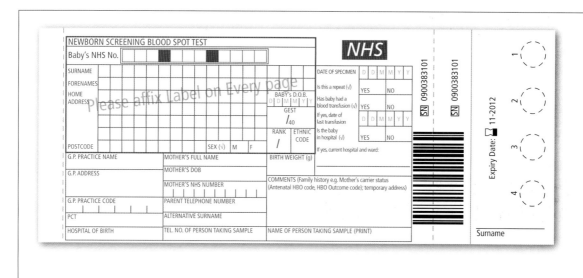

| NEWBORN SCREENING BLOOD SPOT TEST | | |
|---|---|---|
| Baby's NHS No. | | |

**NHS**

| SURNAME | | | DATE OF SPECIMEN | D D M M Y Y |
| FORENAMES | | | Is this a repeat (√) | YES | NO |
| HOME ADDRESS | | | Has baby had a blood transfusion (√) | YES | NO |
| | | BABY's D.O.B. | If yes, date of last transfusion | D D M M Y Y |
| | | GEST | Is the baby in hospital (√) | YES | NO |
| POSTCODE | SEX (√) M F | | If yes, current hospital and ward: |
| G.P. PRACTICE NAME | MOTHER'S FULL NAME | BIRTH WEIGHT (g) |
| G.P. ADDRESS | MOTHER'S DOB | |
| | MOTHER'S NHS NUMBER | COMMENTS (Family history e.g. Mother's carrier status (Antenatal HBO code, HBO Outcome code); temporary address) |
| G.P. PRACTICE CODE | PARENT TELEPHONE NUMBER | |
| PCT | ALTERNATIVE SURNAME | |
| HOSPITAL OF BIRTH | TEL. NO. OF PERSON TAKING SAMPLE | NAME OF PERSON TAKING SAMPLE (PRINT) |

Please affix Label on Every page

SN 090083101   SN 090083101

Expiry Date: 11-2012

Surname

**Figure 2.1** Neonatal screening blood test for phenylketonuria (Guthrie test) and hypothyroidism.

- *Significance of the test.* One in 10 000 babies is born with phenylketonuria (PKU). This causes severe learning disability (mental retardation). Introduction of a low-phenylalanine diet prevents the build-up of phenylalanine metabolites which cause brain damage.
- *Action if the test is abnormal.* Referral to a metabolic clinic for dietary advice and long-term follow-up.

### Other newborn screening tests

**Cystic fibrosis.** Immunoreactive trypsin levels in blood are used as a screening test for cystic fibrosis.

**Haemoglobinopathies (sickle cell disease and thalassaemia).** These are common in some ethnic communities. Screening is carried out in some parts of the country.

**Medium-chain acyl-coA dehydrogenase deficiency (MCADD).** A metabolic disorder where there is a deficiency of a mitochondrial enzyme, making it difficult for the body to break down fatty acids and produce energy. It can cause hypoglycaemia and sudden death in infants. Treatment involves ensuring that children do not go for long periods without food.

### Eliciting the red reflex using an ophthalmoscope (see also p. 81)

- *Age at which the test is performed.* Neonates, 6–8 weeks.

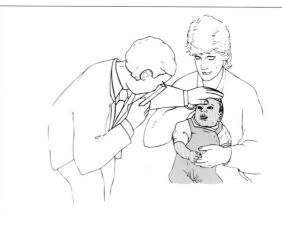

**Figure 2.2** Eliciting the red reflex using an ophthalmoscope.

- *The test.* The examiner looks through an ophthalmoscope, held approximately 50 cm from the baby, and directs the light into the baby's eyes. A red reflection is normally seen as the light is reflected back from the vascular retina (Figure 2.2).
- *Significance of the test.* If white light is reflected instead of red, it is a serious sign and suggests the presence of a cataract or other intraocular pathology, preventing the reflex from being elicited.
- *Action if the test is abnormal.* Immediate referral to an ophthalmologist is required, as in those conditions that are treatable, amblyopia (pp. 223–4) can only be avoided if treatment is given early.

## Examination for congenital dislocation of the hips (see also pp. 430–1)

- *Age at which the test is performed.* Neonates, 6–8 weeks.
- *The test.* The Ortolani and Barlow procedures (see Figures 22.10, 22.11) for babies up to the age of 3 months are described on pp. 430–1. Limited hip abduction, shortening of the leg and limp (once walking) are found beyond 3 months.
- *Significance of the test.* Approximately three babies per 1000 are born with dislocated, subluxed or dysplastic hips. Orthopaedic treatment given early is likely to be more effective in preventing limp in childhood and painful disability later in life.
- *Action if the test is abnormal.* Orthopaedic referral is required. Ultrasound is useful to confirm the diagnosis. Treatment involves the use of a harness or splint to maintain the hip in flexion and abduction. If this conservative treatment fails, surgery is required.

## Palpation for testicular descent

- *Age at which the test is performed.* Neonates, 6–8 weeks.
- *The test.* The testes are palpated when the baby is relaxed (Figure 2.3).
- *Significance of the test.* Non-palpable testes suggest maldescent (see pp. 315–6). If corrected early, the risks of the sequelae of infertility and malignancy are minimized.
- *Action if the test is abnormal.* If on repeat examination the testes are impalpable, referral to a paediatric surgeon is required. Surgery should be performed before the age of 2 years.

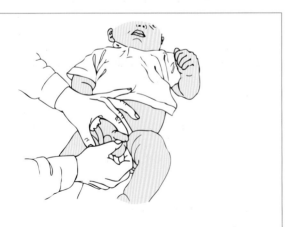

**Figure 2.3** Palpation for testicular descent.

## Hearing test (oto-acoustic emissions)

Oto-acoustic emission testing to identify hearing impairment is now carried out on all babies throughout the UK.

- *Age at which the test is performed.* Neonates.
- *The test.* An ear probe is attached to a portable computer. A 'cochlear echo' is detected if the cochlea is functioning normally.
- *Significance of the test.* Significant sensorineural hearing loss occurs in one to two babies per 1000. If it is not identified early before language is acquired, permanent impairment of language development can result.
- *Action if the test is abnormal.* A diagnostic brainstem evoked response test is carried out by the audiology service. If neurosensory deafness is confirmed, hearing aids and speech and language therapy are provided (see pp. 247–50).

## Later hearing screening

- *Age at which test is performed.* School entry.
- *The test.* Sweep audiometry tests the child's ability to hear sounds at a set level across the main speech frequencies.
- *Significance of the test.* As most cases of sensorineural deafness have already been detected through neonatal screening or distraction testing, this test principally identifies children with hearing impairment caused by secretory otitis media (see p. 120) that may have educational implications.
- *Action if the test is abnormal.* The ears should be examined for otitis media. Referral to an ear, nose and throat (ENT) surgeon and more sophisticated audiological evaluation is required.

## Visual acuity using a Snellen chart

- *Age at which the test is performed.* School entry, and repeated through the school years in some parts of the country.
- *The test.* The child's visual acuity is tested 6 m from the Snellen chart, with each eye occluded in turn (Figure 2.4). In young children a letter-matching card can be used instead of asking them to name the letters.
- *Significance of the test.* Myopia is very common in childhood. If the child can only read letter size 6/12 or less, he or she is likely to be myopic.
- *Action if the test is abnormal.* Referral to an optician for prescription of spectacles is required.

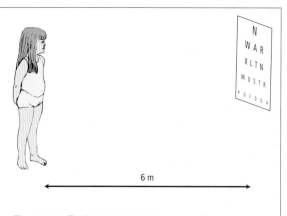

**Figure 2.4** Testing visual acuity using a Snellen chart.

## Growth and development

Growth during childhood is discussed in some detail in Chapter 13, and monitoring of children's growth is a part of child health promotion. Normal growth reflects a child's well-being, and any deviation may be indicative of adverse physical or psychosocial factors.

### Normal growth
A baby's weight and length at birth are influenced by intrauterine and to a lesser extent by genetic factors and so do not correlate well with parental heights. Over the next year or two the baby's growth adjusts, so that by the age of 2 years most children have attained their genetically destined centile. From the age of 2 years until the onset of puberty it is usual for a child to grow steadily along their centile with little deviation. During puberty it is normal for centiles to be crossed again until final height is achieved.

### Growth monitoring
In the past, growth monitoring through childhood has been an important part of routine child care. It is still maintained elsewhere, but in Britain it has been pruned down so that it is principally carried out only in the younger years, and as a means for identifying those at risk of obesity. Current recommendations for monitoring of growth are shown in Table 2.1. Growth monitoring has a number of benefits:

- *Identification of endocrine conditions.* Conditions leading to hormone excess or deficiencies profoundly affect growth, and may be missed if growth is not monitored (see p. 254).

- *Identification of other treatable conditions.* Although chronic illness usually presents with obvious signs and symptoms, some may only be detected by a fall-off in growth (see p. 256).
- *Identification of obesity and excessive weight gain.* A principal purpose of the National Child Measurement Programme is to monitor the prevalence of obesity and identify children at most risk (see pp. 259–60).
- *Identification of eating disorders.* Growth monitoring can identify the child with an eating disorder, whether anorexia (see p. 441) or excessive eating (see pp. 259–60).
- *Monitoring chronic diseases.* Chronic disease affects growth as a result of a number of factors. In some diseases, monitoring growth is an important part of management, e.g. in diabetes it reflects the adequacy of diabetic control.
- *Focus for discussion of health issues with parents.* Most parents are interested in their children's growth, particularly in the early years, and this can provide a good opportunity to discuss a variety of health issues with them.
- *Access to children at risk.* Children at risk may be identified through monitoring growth, which also serves to provide acceptable access to a family that might not otherwise welcome contact.
- *Public health issues.* The growth of a population reflects the population's health, and growth records can be an important source for epidemiological studies.

Guidance as to when one should become concerned about a child's growth are given in Chapter 13. In general, height or weight beyond the dotted lines on a growth chart (>99.6th or <0.4th centiles, see Figure 13.1) are outside the normal range and an evaluation needs to be considered, particularly if they are outside the range expected for parental height. Crossing of centile lines are of particular concern and a cause should be sought. In addition, a good clinical evaluation should be carried out in any child where the parents or other professionals are concerned about growth. Where a child is obese or overweight (BMI > 98th centile or between the 91st and 98th centile, respectively), guidance needs to be given about risk and the special importance of a healthy lifestyle.

### Common growth problems
Common problems identified through growth monitoring are shown in Table 2.3.

**Table 2.3** Problems seen in growth monitoring

*Common problems*

Short stature (see p. 266)

Failure to thrive (see p. 266)

Obesity (see p. 267)

*Less common problems*

Tall stature (see p. 262)

Fall-off in height (see p. 256)

Weight loss

## Developmental evaluation

Evaluation of a child's development involves a developmental history, observation of the child's behaviour and the assessment of developmental skills (pp. 84–9). The purpose is to ensure that the child's development is progressing at a normal rate, and to recognize deviations from the normal pattern; it is usually performed by the health visitor. Beyond early infancy developmental screening is no longer routine, but is targeted at needy or at-risk families, or where there is parental concern. If the child is delayed or is demonstrating abnormal development, referral is made to the appropriate therapist or, if difficulties seem to be complex, to a child development team (see p. 45–7).

# Immunization

Immunizations have changed the entire picture of paediatrics. In the past, family life and medical care were dominated by epidemics of infectious diseases that caused serious morbidity and mortality for the childhood population. These diseases are now rare, but if immunization rates fall, they re-emerge. A high level of uptake of immunizations is important to ensure both protection for the individual and also, for some diseases, herd immunity.

An important example where a disease has made a recurrence is measles. Recently epidemiological studies raised concerns (now recognized as unfounded) that the measles component of the MMR (measles, mumps, rubella) vaccine was responsible for increasing numbers of children suffering from autism and inflammatory bowel disease. There was broad coverage in the media, many parents declined immunization, and as a result, immunization rates fell to worryingly low levels. Major efforts were required to inform the public of the situation and restore immunization rates back to acceptable levels.

Table 2.4 shows the recommended schedule in the UK for immunizations at each age. There are few contraindications. Guidelines include those listed below.

## General immunization guidelines

• Immunizations should not be given at a younger age than indicated in the schedule.
• Vaccines which require repeat immunization should not be given at shorter intervals than indicated.
• If for any reason a child misses an immunization or immunizations, it should be given at a later stage. There is no need to restart the course.
• Immunizations should not be given if a child is acutely unwell with fever.
• Immunizations should not be given if there has been a serious reaction following a previous dose of the same vaccine.
• Live attenuated vaccines (e.g. measles, mumps, rubella, BCG) should not be given to immunodeficient children such as those on cytotoxic therapy or high-dose steroids because of the risk of severe generalized infection.

## Routine immunizations

### Diphtheria

Diphtheria is now very rare in developed countries. It is caused by the organism *Corynebacterium diphtheriae*. Infection occurs in the throat, forming a pharyngeal exudate, which leads to membrane formation and obstruction of the upper airways. An exotoxin released by the bacterium may cause myocarditis and neuritis with paralysis.

**The vaccine.** The vaccine is an inactivated toxin (toxoid), given as an intramuscular injection combined with tetanus, pertussis, polio and HiB vaccines at 2, 3 and 4 months, with boosters at school entry and in secondary school. A more dilute form is given to individuals over the age of 10 years.

### Tetanus

Tetanus is caused by an anaerobic organism, *Clostridium tetani*, found universally in the soil, which enters the body through open wounds. Progressive painful muscle spasms are caused by a neurotoxin produced by the organism. Involvement of the respiratory muscles results in asphyxia and death.

**Table 2.4** Routine childhood immunization programme in the UK

| When to immunize | Diseases protected against | Vaccine given |
|---|---|---|
| Birth | Tuberculosis<br>Hepatitis B | BCG for babies likely to come into close contact with tuberculosis<br>Given 3 times in infancy if mother is a carrier |
| 2 months | Diphtheria, tetanus, pertussis, polio, HiB<br>Pneumococcal infection | DTaP/IPV/HiB and PCV |
| 3 months | Diphtheria, tetanus, pertussis, polio, HiB<br>Meningitis C | DTaP/IPV/HiB and MenC |
| 4 months | Diphtheria, tetanus, pertussis, polio, HiB<br>Meningitis C<br>Pneumococcal infection | DTaP/IPV/HiB and MenC and PCV |
| Around 12 months | HiB<br>Meningitis C | HiB/MenC |
| Around 13 months | Measles, mumps, rubella<br>Pneumococcal infection | MMR and PCV |
| 3 years and 4 months or soon after | Diphtheria, tetanus, pertussis, polio<br>Measles, mumps, rubella | DtaP/IPV or dTaP/IPV and MMR |
| Girls aged 12–13 years | Cervical cancer caused by human papillomavirus types 16 and 18 | HPV |
| 13–18 years | Tetanus, diphtheria, polio | Td/IPV |

Each vaccination is given as a single injection into the muscle of the thigh or upper arm. From www.immunisation.nhs.uk.
BCG, bacille Calmette–Guérin; DTaP, diphtheria, tetanus and pertussis; HiB, *Haemophilus influenzae* type B; IPV, inactivated polio vaccine; MenC, meningococcal C; PCV, pneumococcal conjugate vaccine; Td, tetanus and diphtheria.

**The vaccine.** The vaccine is an inactivated toxin (toxoid) given combined with diphtheria, pertussis, polio and HiB vaccines at 2, 3 and 4 months by intramuscular injection. After a primary course of three injections in infancy and a booster at school entry, a further two boosters 10 years apart are required. If a dirty wound is incurred more than 10 years after the last injection, a further booster is required. If an unimmunized individual sustains a dirty wound, tetanus immunoglobulin is given and a full course of the inactivated toxoid initiated.

## Pertussis (whooping cough)

Whooping cough is caused by the bacterium *Bordetella pertussis*. It is an upper respiratory illness which lasts for 6–8 weeks, consisting of three stages: catarrhal, paroxysmal and convalescent. The child experiences paroxysms of coughing, followed by a whoop (a sudden massive inspiratory effort against a narrowed glottis), with vomiting, dyspnoea and sometimes seizures. Manifestations are most severe in children under the age of 2 years, where there is a high morbidity and mortality. Complications include bronchopneumonia, convulsions, apnoea and bronchiectasis. The diagnosis must be suspected clinically, and confirmed by special culture of nasopharyngeal swabs. Erythromycin given early in the catarrhal stage shortens the illness, but is ineffective if given when the whoop is heard.

**The vaccine.** The vaccine is made from the killed organism, given in three doses with diphtheria, tetanus, polio and HiB vaccines at 2, 3 and 4 months, and at school entry. Mild reactions consisting of local pain and swelling, irritability and pyrexia are common. The risks of naturally acquired pertussis far exceed any

## Whooping cough (pertussis) at a glance

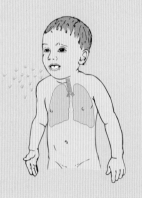

**Epidemiology**
Endemic, with epidemics every
   3–5 years

**Aetiology/pathophysiology**
*Bordetella pertussis* infection
Droplet spread

**Prevention**
Immunization with killed
   organism given at 2, 3 and 4
   months and at school entry

**History**
Paroxysms of coughing
Characteristic inspiratory whoop
   at end of paroxysm (absent in
   infants)
Fever*
Vomiting at end of paroxysm*
Seizures*

**Physical examination**
Very distressed during a
   paroxysm
Infant is very sick
Dyspnoea
Nasal discharge
Apathetic
Weight loss

**Confirmatory investigations**
Diagnosis is clinical
Confirmed by pernasal swab
   culture early in disease

**Differential diagnosis**
Pertussis is readily clinically
   recognized during the
   paroxysmal stage
Other causes of cough

**Management**
Erythromycin given early
   shortens the illness, but is
   ineffective later

**Complications**
Bronchopneumonia
Convulsions
Apnoea
Bronchiectasis

**Course/prognosis**
Lasts 6–8 weeks
High morbidity and mortality for
   children <2 years

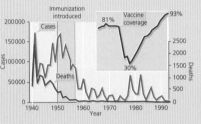

*NB Signs and symptoms are variable

risks of the vaccination and it is recommended for all babies, other than when a severe reaction has followed a previous immunization or if a progressive neurological disease is present.

## Polio
Polio is caused by the poliomyelitis virus, which produces a mild febrile illness, progressing to meningitis in some children. Paralysis in association with pain and tenderness develops as a result of anterior horn cell damage, and may lead to respiratory failure and bulbar paralysis. Residual paralysis is common in those who survive.

**The vaccine.** The IPV (inactivated polio vaccine) has now replaced the oral live vaccine and is given in three doses with diphtheria, tetanus, pertussis and HiB vaccines at 2, 3 and 4 months. The vaccine can cause irritability and fever within 12–24 hours.

## Haemophilus influenzae B
*Haemophilus influenzae* type B was the main cause of meningitis (p. 208) in young children, leading to severe neurological sequelae such as profound deafness, cerebral palsy and epilepsy in 10–15% of cases and death in 3%.

**The vaccine.** The HiB vaccine consists of the polysaccharide capsule of the killed organism conjugated with a protein, and is given with diphtheria, tetanus, pertussis and polio vaccines at 2, 3 and 4 months and again preschool and at age 13–18 years. It is only effective against type B infection. The vaccine is highly effective with a low incidence of side-effects.

## Meningococcus C
Meningococcus C (*Neisseria meningitidis*) causes a purulent meningitis in young children with a pur-

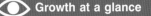
## Growth at a glance

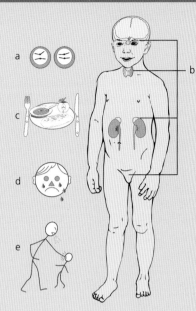

### General
Growth reflects a child's well-being and deviation suggests abnormal physical or psychosocial factors.
Between the age of 2 years and puberty, growth is usually steady along a centile

### Factors that affect growth
- Genetics (**a**)
- Hormones (**b**)
- Nutrition (**c**)
- Illness (**d**)
- Psychosocial factors (**e**)

### Growth standards
Charts for boys and girls give centile lines ranging from the 99.6th to the 0.4th centile

### National Child Measurement Programme (NCMP)
The NCMP was introduced in 2006 to monitor the rising problem of obesity.
Children are measured at school entry and at the age of 11 years.
Parents are provided with information if their child is overweight or obese

### Plotting a child's growth
Correction for gestational age must be made up to the age of 24 months

### Growth monitoring
Benefits include:
- identification of endocrine conditions
- identification of other treatable conditions
- identification of eating disorders
- monitoring chronic diseases
- focus for discussion of health issues with parents
- access to children at risk
- public health issues

### Guidelines for concern beyond the age of 2 years
Height or weight >99.6th or <0.4th centile
Crossing of centiles
Discrepancy between height and weight
Discrepancy with parental heights
Parental or professional concern
BMI > 98th centile (obesity)
BMI between 91st and 98th centile (overweight)

---

puric rash and septicaemic shock. Mortality is as high as 10% and morbidity includes hearing loss, seizures, brain damage, organ failure and tissue necrosis.

**The vaccine.** The vaccine is a conjugated polysaccharide antigen which is combined with tetanus toxoid as a carrier protein. It is given at 3, 4 and 12 months in a separate injection from the combined diphtheria, tetanus, pertussis, polio and HiB vaccine. The vaccine may cause some local swelling, fever, vomiting and irritability.

## Pneumococcal infection
Invasive pneumococcal infection is a cause of pneumonia, septicaemia and meningitis, which carry a high mortality and morbidity, particularly in babies.

**The vaccine.** The vaccine is a polyvalent vaccine containing purified capsular polysaccharide from each of the 23 types of pneumococcus. It is given at 2, 4 and 13 months. These 23 types are responsible for the vast majority of serious pneumococcal infections seen in this country. The vaccine may cause a sore arm and fever.

## Measles
Measles is characterized by a maculopapular rash, fever, coryza, cough and conjunctivitis (see p. 123). Complications include encephalitis leading to neurological damage and a high mortality rate.

**The vaccine.** The vaccine is a live attenuated virus given at around 13 months and again at 3 years 4 months with mumps and rubella (MMR), and before school entry. It is common for children to develop a rash and fever 5–10 days after the immunization. Children who are immunodeficient and those severely allergic to eggs (the vaccine is grown on chick embryo tissue) should not receive the vaccine.

### Mumps

Mumps causes a febrile illness with enlargement of the parotid glands (see p. 122). Complications include aseptic meningitis, sensorineural deafness and orchitis in adults.

**The vaccine.** The vaccine is a live attenuated virus grown on chick embryo tissue and is given with measles and rubella (MMR) at around 13 months and again at 3 years 4 months. It should not be given to immunodeficient children or those severely allergic to eggs.

### Rubella (German measles)

Rubella is a mild illness causing rash and fever (see p. 124). Its importance lies in the devastating effects it has on the fetus if infection occurs in the early stages of pregnancy. These include multiple congenital defects such as cataracts, deafness and congenital heart disease.

**The vaccine.** The vaccine is a live attenuated virus given with measles and mumps vaccines (MMR) at around 13 months and again at 3 years 4 months. A mild form of rubella sometimes occurs following vaccination. In the past it was given to girls only at the age of 11 years, but this policy has changed in order to try to achieve herd immunity and stop epidemics. The vaccine, like all live virus vaccines, is contraindicated in pregnancy.

### Tuberculosis

Tuberculosis (TB) remains a major problem in many developing countries and still occurs in developed countries, particularly in immigrant communities from endemic areas such as Asia and Africa. Most children with TB are identified because they are contacts of infected adults. Tuberculosis affects many organs including the lungs, meninges, bones and joints. The diagnosis is not always easy, and often relies on demonstration of tuberculin sensitivity, which develops within 4–8 weeks after infection. This is demonstrated by Heaf or Mantoux testing where purified protein derivative (PPD) is injected into the skin. The result is read 3–10 days later.

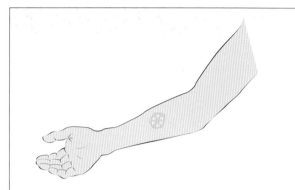

**Figure 2.5** The Heaf test. In tuberculin-positive individuals six raised papules surrounded by a wheal are seen at 3–10 days.

Tuberculin sensitivity causes severe induration at the site (Figure 2.5), and if this is found the child requires a chest X-ray and follow-up. Active TB requires treatment which must be continued over many months.

**BCG vaccination.** BCG (bacille Calmette–Guérin) is a live attenuated virus strain of *Mycobacterium tuberculosis*, which is given intradermally. It causes formation of a papule that enlarges over a few weeks and may ulcerate. It heals over 6–8 weeks, leaving a residual scar. It is given at birth to babies who are likely to come into close or prolonged contact with family members who have TB. In many parts of Britain, Asian babies are immunized in the first week of life.

### Cervical cancer

Infection with human papillomavirus (HPV) is common, with over 50% of sexually active women infected over the course of their lifetime. Two strains of HPV (16 and 18) are the cause of cervical cancer in over 70% of cases.

**The vaccine.** The HPV vaccine protects against the HPV 16 and 18. Given to 12–13-year-old girls, it does not protect against any other sexually transmitted infections or against pregnancy. Side effects include swelling, redness and pain at the injection site and other very mild side effects, such as fever and dizziness. Very rarely anaphylaxis can occur.

## Safeguarding children

In any aspect of paediatrics and child health care, concerns often arise regarding the possibility that a

## ◉ Tuberculosis at a glance

**Epidemiology**
TB still occurs in the UK, especially in the Asian community

**Aetiology/pathophysiology**
Infection with *Mycobacterium tuberculosis*
Primary infection may occur in the lung, skin or gut
Miliary TB (bloodstream spread) is the most serious complication in childhood

**Prevention**
Bacille Calmette–Guérin (live attenuated virus) given intradermally at birth to babies from high-risk families

**History**
Prolonged fever
Malaise
Anorexia
Cough
Weight loss
Contact with infected adult*

NB *Signs and symptoms are variable

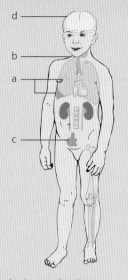

**Physical examination**
Signs depend on focus of infection:
• primary in lung – signs of bronchial obstruction, pleural effusion, etc. (a)
• primary in tonsils – cervical adenitis (b)
• primary in small bowel – malabsorption, peritonitis (c)
• miliary TB – meningitis, chest signs, hepatosplenomegaly (d)

**Confirmatory investigations**
Demonstration of tuberculin sensitivity by Heaf or Mantoux testing
Chest X-ray evidence of pulmonary TB
Culture of gastric washings

**Management**
Even if asymptomatic, tuberculinpositive children require treatment
Active TB requires treatment over many months

**Prognosis/complications**
Postprimary TB may present as local or disseminated (miliary) disease affecting:
• bones
• joints – arthritis
• kidneys – haematuria, renal failure
• pericardium – constrictive pericarditis
• CNS – mental retardation, hydrocephalus Morbidity and mortality is significant if TB is detected late

child is the victim of neglect, non-accidental injury, or emotional or sexual abuse. In this circumstance, it is the duty of the professional (and indeed any individual) to report these concerns to the authorities so that appropriate investigations can be made. Child health promotion goes beyond detecting abuse and also includes its management and prevention.

In a preventive role guidance and support are provided for families, reducing the likelihood of children becoming victims of abuse and neglect. The health visitor is ideally positioned to follow children who are at risk. She is usually seen as being a non-threatening and supportive professional, who is a visitor to all homes. Social Care also provides essential support for families in need, but by contrast may be seen to be an imposition.

When a child is found to be in need of child protection the health visitor, school nurse and community paediatrician have an important role in determining how the interests of the child are best met (p. 366). This involves close liaison with the family and other professionals. If the child is placed in care or has a Child Care Plan, the child health service provides continuous surveillance and support to ensure that the needs of the child are met.

The clinical presentation and care of children presenting actual or suspected child abuse or neglect is covered in detail in Chapter 20 ('Social paediatrics').

### The role of the child health service in safeguarding children

• Reporting suspected victims of abuse and neglect.
• Following children at risk of abuse and neglect. Health visitors are particularly well placed for this.
• Providing guidance to reduce the risk of abuse.

- Liaison with social services.
- Following children in care and on the child protection register.

# Ethical issues in paediatrics

Ethics is the science of morals, and morals are the personal framework that dictates right and wrong. The law defines what an individual in a society may and may not do, and a moral approach to a situation depends on an individual's conscience, religious views and previous experience.

Paediatrics is a speciality where there are many ethical issues to be considered, such as withdrawal of intensive care, consent and parental rights. You need to be aware of some of these issues, and it is the responsibility of every practising doctor to have established his or her own *modus vivendi* for working in these difficult areas (see Box 2.1).

Three important concepts underlie an understanding of ethical issues. These are the sanctity of life, the concept of omission vs. commission, and the quality of life. Each is briefly discussed here.

## Sanctity of life

Life is sacred, and any act intended to end a life is illegal. Those with some particular religious points of view think that every effort must be made to preserve life, under all circumstances, but this is not accepted

---

### Box 2.1 Principles of medical ethics

- The clinician can only act within the legal code
- Ethical decisions usually do not need to be made rapidly, only after full discussion and consideration
- It is usually inappropriate to make decisions which conflict with the views of the patient's relatives
- All members of staff must be involved in discussions before a decision is made
- Discuss all options with the parents so that they know that all the possible courses of treatment have been considered
- Where the child is mature enough, he or she should be involved in ethical decisions
- Adolescents may receive treatment without parental knowledge, provided they are deemed mature enough to appreciate its consequences
- Where dispute remains between clinical staff and parents, the courts should be asked to make a final decision

---

by others. Most people would agree that to offer an anencephalic baby intensive care would be wrong because the prognosis for life is so poor: intensive care simply delays the time when the heart will stop beating. Others believe that it is acceptable not to feed a patient in a persistent vegetative state, so that the patient dies of dehydration, albeit appropriately sedated. The concept of the sanctity of life alone is thus too broad to be the ultimate benchmark, and there is much scope within the law for making decisions that affect life and death.

## Omission vs. commission

This concept considers the method of a patient's death. It is illegal to undertake an act that kills a patient: this is an *act of commission*. An example would be giving a patient a lethal injection: this is both illegal and immoral. Many would argue that giving a powerful narcotic injection to a patient who is dying in extreme pain is acceptable, despite knowing that an outcome of this injection is death by respiratory depression. This is not illegal as the primary aim of the treatment is to alleviate pain, not to kill.

There is a moral difference between causing someone to die by a positive action and allowing death to occur by failing to act. An example of the latter is leaving septicaemia untreated in a patient on a ventilator who has a very poor prognosis, knowing that death will occur as a result of non-treatment with antibiotics. This is legal and, most would argue, ethical. An *act of omission* may be illegal if failure to treat causes a patient to die who might otherwise have fully recovered.

Both acts of commission and omission may therefore be acceptable in one framework and unacceptable (and illegal) in another.

## Quality of life

Most people would agree that ventilating a baby who has no chance of independent survival without a ventilator is wrong. The quality of life the child would have if he or she were to survive is a factor to be considered. This is usually what causes the most controversy within an ethical context.

'Quality of life' is a nebulous concept. It has been suggested that the quality of life is encapsulated within the idea of individual 'humanhood'. The qualities of humanhood are those that make us individual. These include:

- awareness of oneself;
- concept of time, both future and past;

- ability to communicate;
- care and concern for others;
- curiosity.

### Withdrawal of intensive care

Uncritical application of intensive care is one of the most frequent areas of ethical uncertainty in medicine and is particularly relevant to paediatrics. The physician must consider the following issues within the ethical context of offering or continuing intensive care:

- *What is the prognosis?* Intensive care that only acts to put off the time of death is unlikely to be in the best interest of the patient, but this may help relatives come to terms with the impending death. Long-term intensive care of a patient with a hopeless prognosis is often thought to be wrong. Withdrawal of intensive care should be considered, refocusing the emphasis of care from the child to the family, to help the parents with the process of mourning.
- *Quality of life.* If the patient survives, will the quality of life be acceptable? The answer to this question often depends on the family. Some parents may say that life of any quality is acceptable, even if their child is very severely damaged with blindness, severe spasticity and very low intelligence. Other parents may find a child with only moderate disability unacceptable.
- *Pain and suffering.* One may question whether treatment which is very painful or where the child has to suffer severely to overcome a life-threatening disorder is justified. The management of cancer is an example of a protracted course of unpleasant and distressing treatment. If the ultimate prognosis is good then this may be easy to justify, but if the prognosis is uncertain or poor then it may be unfair to put the child through the distress of treatment.
- *Use of scarce resources.* In most developed health care services there is an unequal balance between demand on facilities and their availability. There may only be one intensive care ventilator with two patients needing it. This often causes major dilemmas in neonatal intensive care, where a less acceptable form of therapy must be given because the resources are limited. A judgement may have to be made as to which patient is most likely to benefit from the treatment.

### Guidelines from the Royal College of Paediatrics and Child Health

Recommendations have been produced by the Royal College of Paediatrics and Child Health to help doctors decide when medical treatment should be withdrawn from children (although not intended for the newborn). The situations when withdrawal should be considered include:

- when the child is brain dead;
- when the child is in a permanent vegetative state;
- when care delays death without easing suffering;
- when the child survives so physically or mentally impaired that it is unreasonable to expect him or her to suffer further;
- when the illness is so progressive and irreversible that further treatment is intolerable.

### Consent and parental rights

Another area of ethical concern is the issue of consent. For adults, it is accepted that a competent patient has the right to accept or refuse health care. Many paediatric patients are not competent to make their own decisions and therefore parents traditionally have made such decisions on their behalf. This is acceptable in most situations and the majority of parents act in the best interests of their child, but the issue arises regarding the age at which an individual becomes competent to make his or her own decisions.

Whereas many people feel that a child's views should be taken into account, it is not possible to define a precise age at which a child will have the maturity to decide whether he or she wishes to be investigated or treated for an illness, particularly if this is at variance with the parents' views. An important concept regarding children's ability to give their own consent is that of 'Gillick competence' – where the law recognizes that if a doctor considers that a child under 16 years is mature enough to understand the implications of a procedure or treatment, he or she does not have to inform the parent.

The issue causing particular controversy in this regard relates to the prescription of contraceptives to adolescents. Strict requirements for parental consent may deter adolescents from seeking health care, with consequences in terms of teenage pregnancies and sexually transmitted disease. However, in Britain legal precedent allows a physician to prescribe contraceptives without parental consent, provided the adolescent is deemed mature enough to understand the risks and benefits.

Another difficult issue concerns situations where parents fail to act in the best interests of their child. Not many years ago it was accepted that parents had absolute rights over their child and that these rights should not and could not be interfered with by external agencies. In fact, the first court case prosecuting a parent for abusing a child had to be brought on the grounds of cruelty to an animal as there was no procedure for prosecuting a parent who was abusing a child. Society has changed its views and laws now exist whereby children can be protected and parental rights and authority curtailed (p. 366). However, debate continues as to the extent to which society and the law can intervene in parental practices, particularly where cultural issues are involved. An example of this is female circumcision.

## Ethical conflicts

The nature of ethical dilemmas means that there can be no right or wrong answers. Each case is different and its circumstances must be carefully reviewed. The parents' wishes must be very carefully considered and it is, in general, unwise to act against their wishes. Sometimes, however, it is necessary to do so if the parents' wishes are clearly unreasonable or unrealistic. In these circumstances it is usually appropriate to take the legal precaution of making the child a ward of court so that the decision is taken out of the clinician's direct control.

A second major source of ethical conflict arises when one clinical view conflicts with another. An example may be in withdrawing care, when the doctor thinks it a reasonable option but a senior nurse disagrees. These differences must be reconciled; it is a failure of clinical management if major disagreement continues to exist. It is important that the opinion of every member of the clinical team is heard and that no-one feels left out of the process. Ultimately a decision must be made by the senior clinician, but it is his or her role to ensure as far as possible that no-one feels that the decision is wrong.

The essence of decision making in medical ethics is effective communication. Communication should involve the child (when appropriate), parents, other relatives and staff, and, if necessary, lawyers and possibly clergy. Decisions cannot be made by committee but neither can they be made by diktat. Sometimes prolonging intensive care with no prospect of the patient surviving is the appropriate course of management in order to buy time for relatives to accept the appropriateness of the decision.

# CHAPTER 3

# Children with long-term medical conditions

Physicians of the utmost fame
Were called at once; but when they came
They answered, as they took their fees,
There is no cure for this disease.

*'Henry King', Cautionary Tales, Hilaire Belloc*

## COMPETENCES

### You must . . .

| Know | Be able to | Appreciate |
|---|---|---|
| • The principles involved in the paediatric care of children with chronic illness or disabilities<br>• The impact that cancer has on the child and the family, and the long-term issues for the child<br>• How the major disabilities in childhood present<br>• How 'bad news' should be broken<br>• The role of health professionals in the care of children with disabilities<br>• The pros and cons of mainstream vs. special education for children with disabilities | • Take a full and sensitive history from a child with a long-term medical condition, including psychosocial circumstances | • The impact that disability or a chronic illness has on the child and the family<br>• The principles involved in managing long-term medical conditions<br>• The stigma that some chronic conditions have<br>• The difficulties and stress of bringing up a disabled child<br>• The doctor's role in supporting the family<br>• The importance of multidisciplinary team work |

*Paediatrics and Child Health*, Third Edition. Mary Rudolf, Tim Lee, Malcolm Levene.
© 2011 Mary Rudolf, Tim Lee and Malcolm Levene. Published 2011 by Blackwell Publishing Ltd.

# Chronic illness

There is no universally accepted definition of childhood chronic conditions; however, the following definition is useful:

*a chronic illness is a physical condition that lasts longer than 3 months and is of sufficient severity to interfere with a child's ordinary activities to some degree.*

According to the UK General Household Survey, as many as 10–20% of children experience a long-standing medical condition at some point in childhood, with 5–10% having a moderately to severely handicapping long-term illness or disability (Table 3.1).

Children with chronic disease have many needs in common with each other, irrespective of what disease they may have. It is important to understand the impact that chronic illness has on a child and the family, and the physical, emotional and social stresses which may result. These psychosocial factors not only affect how the child functions in the family, with peers and at school, but can also affect the very course of the medical condition.

## The effect of chronic illness on the child

The impact that a chronic illness has on a child will vary depending on the age of the child and the age at which the condition developed. Interestingly, factors other than the severity and prognosis of the condition affect the child's adjustment. In fact there appears to be little relationship between the severity of the condi-

**Table 3.2** Factors affecting a child's adjustment to a chronic illness

| *The child* |
| The age of the child |
| The age at which the illness developed. School entry and adolescence are particularly vulnerable periods |
| Low intelligence or unattractiveness increase the probability of maladjustment |
| *The illness* |
| Conditions with unpredictable flare-ups or recurrences are more stressful than stable conditions |
| 'Invisible' conditions (e.g. diabetes) may be concealed by the family and lead to lack of acceptance |
| *The family* |
| The family's attitude and ability to function is the most critical factor in determining the child's adjustment |

tion and the degree of psychosocial difficulties encountered. Children with mild disabilities may suffer as much or more than those in whom the condition is severe. Factors which may influence a child's adjustment are shown in Table 3.2.

Given the impact that chronic illness has on a child, it is perhaps not surprising that the chronically ill child is two to three times more likely to experience emotional, behavioural and educational difficulties than healthy peers. Low self-esteem, impaired self-image, behavioural problems, depression, anxiety and school dysfunction are all common. These problems may occur as a result of the child's own reaction to his or her chronic illness or the reaction of parents, peers, professionals and society as a whole.

## The child and school

School is a central part of any child's life. Acquiring academic and vocational skills, and the development of work-related habits are only one component. An equally important part is the development of social interactions with peers and adults outside the family.

When ability to perform at school is affected by illness, children are placed at risk of becoming underachievers and failures in their own eyes and the eyes of their peers. This can be compounded by the amount of school missed through acute exacerbations,

**Table 3.1** Prevalence of chronic conditions in childhood

| Condition | Rates per 1000 |
| --- | --- |
| Asthma (moderate and severe) | 10.0 |
| Epilepsy | 8.0 |
| Congenital heart disease | 7.0–8.0 |
| Diabetes mellitus | 2.0 |
| Arthritis | 1.0 |
| Cystic fibrosis | 0.4 |
| Chronic renal failure | 0.1 |
| Malignancy | 0.1 |

outpatient appointments and hospitalizations. If the child has adapted poorly, further days may be missed in addition.

Chronic illness affects the social aspects of school life too. Frequent illness episodes and restrictions can exclude the child from activities. Physical appearance, acute medical problems, taking medications at school and special diets all make the child different. As a result children can be made fun of, and come to feel inferior to and isolated from their classmates.

In addition to contending with the special problems of the condition and the reaction of others, children are also likely to experience in aggravated form the concerns and difficulties that beset all children at school, such as peer acceptance, competition, anxiety about academic achievement and athletic prowess and concerns about physical appearance and sexual development.

### The effect of chronic illness on the family

The development of a long-term medical condition in a child can affect a family on a number of levels: practical, social and psychological. Altered daily routines, outpatient visits and hospitalizations, unexpected exacerbations and the administration of medications require organization, time and energy. Socially, the family may experience isolation from neighbours and friends, difficulty in finding babysitters, and may have to forgo activities and holidays and even change career plans.

#### The parents

Parents usually have a common response on learning that their child has a chronic illness, which is not dissimilar to that of bereavement. The initial reaction is one of shock or disbelief, which is followed by denial, anger and resentment. These feelings often induce a sense of guilt and then sadness. Acceptance eventually follows, although this may not occur if the parent gets stuck at an earlier stage.

It is not surprising that clinical anxiety, depression, guilt and grief are common problems particularly for mothers, who often take the major role in caring for the child. It is also not surprising that marriages are more subject to dissatisfaction, differences and arguments, and that marital problems are often exacerbated.

#### Siblings

Although siblings often develop kind and considerate relationships, they may also suffer. Parents are likely to be less available, and they may neglect, overindulge or develop unrealistic expectations for their healthy children. Anxiety, embarrassment, resentment and guilt are common, as are fears about their own well-being and the cause and nature of their sibling's health problems.

In discussing chronic illness in childhood the focus is often on psychopathology and psychosocial problems; however, it must be emphasized that the impact is not always negative. Some families seem to grow closer to each other, and in working with families the question often arises: 'How do some families of chronically ill children survive so well?'

## Paediatric care of children with chronic illness

When seeing children with chronic illnesses it is essential to develop rapport and have the skills necessary to assess the psychosocial consequences of the condition on the family. It is important to allow adequate time for this, particularly at the onset of the condition, and when important changes occur, such as at school entry and in adolescence. If there are problems, parents must be given the opportunity to express themselves without the child being present, and adolescents should be offered the possibility to be seen alone as well as with their parents. This is important, not only to allow the adolescent to talk about problems, but also as it transmits the message that they should begin to be responsible for their own health care.

In evaluating the child at an initial or follow-up visit a full picture of the child's physical, emotional and behavioural condition must be obtained. Key points in the assessment are shown in Box 3.1.

---

**Box 3.1 Key points to address when seeing a child with a chronic condition**

- What is the extent of the disease and its complications in the child?
- What understanding does the child have of the condition and of the difference treatment makes?
- What are the physical effects (e.g. poor growth, delayed puberty) of the illness on the child?
- How has the illness affected the child's performance at home, at school and with peers?
- How has the child adjusted to the illness?
- What impact does the child's illness have on the family and its members?
- How has the family adjusted to the special impact or burden of the illness?

## Principles of management (see Box 3.2)

Too often the management of chronic illness by medical professionals focuses on the relatively simple clinical management alone. It cannot be emphasized enough that the child must be seen as a whole. If this is ignored, the child's and family's needs are not met, thus increasing their difficulties, which in itself is likely to impact adversely the course of the illness.

### Counselling

In an age of technological medical advances there is still no substitute for the old-fashioned quality of caring for the child and the family. It is always remarkable how a thorough assessment is in itself a therapeutic intervention, and concern and empathy go a long way in assisting the family to make the best of the circumstances they face. It is important to note that it is rarely helpful to try to conceal chronic conditions (where this is possible), as it encourages the child to believe that the illness is a secret and something of which to be ashamed.

### Education

A vital aspect of management is education of the family about the condition. Gone are the days when doctors paternalistically 'protected' their patients from knowing about the condition and its prognosis. Including the parents increases their trust and also provides them with the skills to self-manage many aspects of the condition. This is particularly critical in conditions such as asthma, cystic fibrosis and diabetes.

### Coordination

Very often in chronic illness the child is looked after by a variety of health professionals: consultants, therapists and dietitians, not to mention teachers and social workers. Liaison and coordination is very important as differing opinions and advice can be very confusing for the family. The development of specialist clinics for the more common medical conditions has improved this problem, especially as clinics usually include specialist nurses whose role is one of support, education and liaison.

### Genetic issues

Most parents have questions regarding genetic implications for subsequent children and the affected child's own chances of fertility. It is important that these are addressed and, where necessary, referred to a geneticist.

### Support

An assessment of support available to the family must be made. Chronic illness can be an isolating experience and many families do not have the support of the extended family and friends. Referrals to a social worker may be needed in order to advise on benefits and services offered by social services (see p. 30). If the child has emotional and behavioural difficulties, referral for counselling may be required. Self-help and voluntary organizations such as the British Diabetes or Epilepsy Association can be helpful and often run support groups and activities allowing families with similar problems to meet.

### School

Involvement of the child's school is essential for a number of reasons.

- *Medical.* The school staff need to understand the child's condition well in order for them to cope competently with problems arising. The greatest concern is usually the handling of acute exacerbations, but other requirements such as dispensing medication and dietary restrictions must be discussed. Asking teachers to report untoward events such as symptoms or drug side effects can be helpful.
- *Educational.* These children are at risk of underachieving, for the reasons explained above. This risk can be minimized with appropriate support, such as help in making up with school work lost through illness or hospital visits, or providing preferential seating in class. Children may need extra encouragement, but care must be taken that this does not result in preferential treatment, which may have social repercussions. Some children may have special educational requirements that need to be met (see p. 46).
- *Social.* Teachers can be instrumental in helping the child cope and integrate socially into school life. Emotional and behavioural difficulties are likely to be expressed at school, and the teachers need to be sensitive to this. For the child whose family is failing to cope effectively, the school has a particularly important role.

## The child with a chronic medical condition at a glance

**Epidemiology**
10–20% of children have a chronic medical problem at some time in childhood, 5–10% have a severe or moderate condition

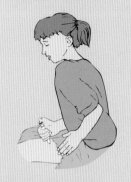

**Effect on the child**
Chronic illness:
• Impacts on the child psychologically
• Increases the risk of emotional, behavioural and educational difficulties
• Is associated with dysfunction at school

**Effect on the family**
The initial parental response is akin to bereavement. Parents must cope with:
• demands of appointments
• drug administration
• unexpected exacerbations
• social difficulties
  Siblings may suffer from altered attention and expectations, and experience more emotional and behavioural problems

**Effect on the child at school**
Academic performance, achievements and social life may be affected
Concerns and difficulties experienced by any child are likely to be aggravated

**Approach to the child**
Time, rapport and skill required
A holistic approach is essential

**Management**
Management must extend beyond the medical to:
• counselling and support
• education
• coordination and liaison between professionals
• genetic issues
• medical, educational and social issues at school

## The child with cancer

Cancer is a rare occurrence in childhood, and in the majority of cases the prognosis is good. Nonetheless, the diagnosis is inevitably one of the hardest for a family to come to terms with. Given its rarity, requirements for sophisticated investigation and treatment, and the need for longterm monitoring, paediatric cancer care should only take place in specialist centres. The management of cancer in children presents unique challenges as treatment with chemotherapy, surgery and radiation can adversely affect growth and development.

### Prevalence

In childhood the incidence of malignant disorders is about one in 10 000 children per year, and causes 19% of all deaths in children. Throughout childhood and adolescence the commonest malignancies are acute leukaemia, lymphomas and brain tumours.

Overall there has been a significant decrease in mortality in recent years, although this is very dependent on the type of malignancy. The various types of cancer are shown in Table 3.3.

### Aetiology and pathophysiology

In most cases of cancer, environmental and host factors are involved. In children, host factors may be more important than environmental factors, as cancers tend to occur in tissues (e.g. the haemopoietic and the nervous tissue) that are not exposed directly to the environment. The majority of solid tumours are embryonic in appearance, presumably because they are caused by malignant transformation of embryonic tissues.

### Initial presentation of the child with cancer

The presenting clinical features differ for each type of cancer (Table 3.3). However, certain less specific

**Table 3.3** Childhood cancers

| Type | Site | Peak age | Presentation |
|------|------|----------|--------------|
| Acute lymphoblastic leukaemia (p. 350) | White cell precursors | Throughout childhood Peak 5 years | Non-specific anorexia, lethargy, pallor, fever, bleeding |
| Hodgkin's disease | Lymph tissue | Late childhood, adolescence | Enlarged lymph nodes, systemic upset |
| Non-Hodgkin's lymphoma | Lymph tissue | Young children | Rapidly enlarging lymph node |
| Neuroblastoma | Any part of the sympathetic nervous system | First 2 years | Failure to thrive, abdominal mass, bleeding |
| Brain tumours | Infratentorial, supratentorial, hypothalamic–pituitary axis | School age | Cerebellar/brainstem dysfunction, endocrine/visual impairment, epilepsy/hemiplegia |
| Wilm's tumour | Kidney | Under 5 years | Abdominal mass |
| Rhabdomyosarcoma | Muscle | <5 years, late adolescence | Painful mass |
| Osteosarcoma | Femur, humerus | Adolescents | Bone pain, limp |
| Ewing's sarcoma | Bone | <10 years | Bone pain |
| Retinoblastoma | Retina | <2 years | White pupil, squint |
| Gonad/germ cell tumours | Ovaries/testis | <3 years, puberty | Scrotal mass, vomiting, nausea, pain in girls |

signs are suggestive of malignancy. These include atypical courses of apparently common childhood conditions, unexplained or prolonged fever (>3–4 weeks), and unexplained (and especially growing) masses, particularly when associated with weight loss.

A tentative diagnosis can often be inferred from the presenting symptoms, the location of the tumour and the age of the child, and then confirmed by biopsy. It is usually appropriate to search for metastatic disease first, so allowing the surgeon/oncologist to judge whether diagnostic biopsy or complete resection is the best procedure. The studies carried out depend on the tumour, and may be non-invasive or invasive.

## Staging

At the time of diagnosis it is critical that the extent of disease be accurately defined. This delineation is called staging. A system of staging has to be designed for each tumour on the basis of the extent of the disease at diagnosis and the subsequent clinical course. Staging helps to determine prognosis and treatment plans.

## Histology

At the core of diagnosis is the histological examination. The surgeon has to search carefully at biopsy, excision or exploration for evidence of regional dissemination to lymph node groups or adjacent organs. If an attempt is made to remove the whole tumour, the pathologist has to examine the margins of the specimen to ensure that no microscopic residue remains.

### Goals of management (see Box 3.3)

The goal of medical management is to eradicate the malignancy whenever possible. In so doing, the

## Box 3.3 Goals in managing cancer

- Eradicate the malignancy whenever possible, inflicting the least damage on normal tissues
- Sustain the child through the toxic effects of treatment
- Ensure that the nutritional status of the child is maintained
- Provide support for the family
- Follow the child for development of late sequelae related to the malignancy or the treatment

minimum of damage should be inflicted on normal tissues. As cancer therapy is invariably toxic, the child must be actively sustained through the effects of the treatment, and special attention paid to nutritional status. The diagnosis of malignancy is always devastating, and management must include good support for the child and family. Once treated, the child must be followed up long term for development of sequelae to the cancer or the treatment.

### Treatment

The most appropriate place for management of children with cancer is a specialized paediatric oncology centre. Centralizing care allows for the systematic assessment of new treatments, collaborative trials and the specialized support that families need. The treatment of childhood cancer rests on the initial diagnostic studies, and involves surgical removal, irradiation and/or chemotherapy. In many children all three therapies are necessary.

### Surgery

Surgery used to be the first-line treatment for most solid tumours. Chemotherapy is now usually initially used to shrink the tumour and so permit more limited and successful resection. Surgery is also required for insertion of indwelling central venous lines giving access for intensive chemotherapy, fluids and blood sampling.

### Radiotherapy

Radiotherapy is effective in the region to which it is applied, and so is principally used to treat areas of known disease. It is also used in total body irradiation in conjunction with bone marrow rescue techniques.

Unfortunately, it damages local tissue, and local effects can not only be disfiguring but also affect function (see Prognosis, p. 42).

### Chemotherapy

The drugs used in chemotherapy kill cancer cells by interfering with the replication and division of DNA during cell division. They are most commonly given intravenously, although some individual agents are given orally, topically or intrathecally. Their effectiveness depends on their being more cytotoxic to the malignant cells than they are to normal dividing cells. The use of several agents simultaneously reduces the likelihood of chemoresistance developing. Chemotherapeutic agents are toxic substances. The common side effects are hair loss, and bone marrow and immune suppression.

### Bone marrow transplantation

Haemopoietic suppression is the side effect that limits the use of many cytotoxic agents. The technique of bone marrow transplantation overcomes this problem, and so allows high doses of these agents to be used. Bone marrow is either harvested from a histocompatible donor or from the patient prior to treatment and then implanted after chemotherapy has finished. Profound immunosuppression, organ toxicity and graft-vs.-host disease are hazards. None the less, this treatment has been successful, particularly now it is being used earlier for patients in remission rather than with florid disease. Peripheral blood stem cell harvest and re-infusion is a similar procedure being used more frequently.

### Management of acute problems and supportive treatment

#### Management of the effects of cancer and therapy

**Metabolic consequences.** The breakdown of malignant tissue either before or as a result of therapy can precipitate uric acid crystals in the renal tubules, causing impaired renal function. Uric acid and creatinine levels must therefore be monitored and adequate hydration and allopurinol (a xanthine oxidase inhibitor) given to maintain uric acid in the normal range. Phosphates and potassium can also be released into the circulation and symptomatic hypocalcaemia and hyperkalaemia can be a problem.

**Bone marrow suppression.** Bone marrow suppression with consequent pancytopenia can occur as a result of bone marrow invasion in some cancers, or as a result of therapy. Anaemia is treated by transfusion of packed red cells, and thrombocytopenia by infusion of platelets. Granulocyte infusions, however, are toxic and rarely used. The febrile neutropenic (<500 cells/mm³) patient needs appropriate cultures and intravenous broad-spectrum antibiotic coverage.

**Immunosuppression.** Immunosuppression is a consequence of some tumours and treatment regimens, and may persist for months after treatment has stopped. Viruses normally of low pathogenicity can then produce serious disease. As a result, patients should not be given vaccines containing live virus, and if exposed to live varicella should receive immunoglobulin. If chicken pox develops they must be hospitalized and treated with aciclovir. Fungal infections are common, particularly candida, and opportunistic organisms such as *Pneumocystis jiroveci* can produce fatal disease.

### Nutrition

Patients undergoing cancer therapy commonly lose weight, particularly if undergoing intensive chemotherapy, total body irradiation or radiotherapy to the head and neck. Attention must be paid to their nutritional status. Parenteral nutrition is sometimes required.

### Symptom management

Cancer and its investigation and treatment produce distress, discomfort and sometimes pain. The effective use of analgesics, local anaesthetics and chemotherapy/radiotherapy should ensure control of almost all distressing symptoms.

### Emotional support

The child and family need support in coming to terms with the diagnosis. This process is helped by being told as soon as possible about the nature of the cancer, its prognosis and treatment. The child should be told all that he or she can understand and would find useful to know. Explanations may have to be repeated several times before distraught families feel that they really understand. Support is particularly essential for the dying child, who should wherever possible receive care at home with the back-up of the community paediatric nursing service and ready access to a familiar children's hospice or ward.

## Monitoring and the management of relapses

The child needs monitoring both for relapse of the malignancy and the adverse effects of treatment. Acute problems include febrile neutropenia, bone marrow suppression and immunosuppression.

Patients who have been successfully treated for childhood cancer should be examined annually and should be carefully assessed for the late effects of therapy (see 'Prognosis' below). The principles involved in the follow-up of any child with a chronic medical condition (p. 37) are particularly important for the child with cancer.

## Prognosis

The patient's prognosis varies with the type of tumour and the extent of disease at the time of diagnosis, as well as with the adequacy of treatment. More than 70% of the patients diagnosed today will be cured, and approximately 80% of children with acute lymphoblastic leukaemia survive more than 5 years.

However, the late consequences of therapy may result in serious morbidity (Figure 3.1), which may

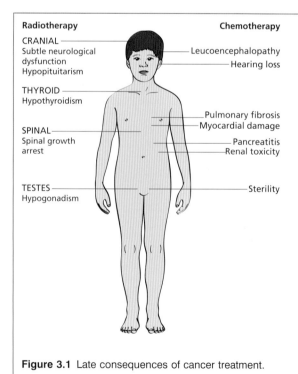

**Figure 3.1** Late consequences of cancer treatment.

only become evident when the child is fully grown. Radiotherapy may produce irreversible damage to organs, so that irradiation to one extremity can cause marked asymmetry. Spinal irradiation can cause spinal growth arrest and along with growth hormone deficiency contribute to short stature. Cranial radiation can cause subtle neurological dysfunction such as short-term memory defects, difficulties with mental arithmetic and poor attention span. Repeated radiation for relapses of leukaemia, or high-dose radiotherapy for intracranial malignancies, may damage the hypothalamic–pituitary axis, leading to a variety of endocrine disturbances such as growth hormone deficiency or pubertal delay. Irradiation of endocrine organs such as the thyroid gland or testes can destroy their endocrine function. Chemotherapeutic agents can also have long-term effects such as leucoencephalopathy, sterility, myocardial damage, renal toxicity, pulmonary fibrosis, pancreatitis and hearing loss.

Another late problem is the occurrence of second cancers in patients successfully cured of a first. The risk is in the order of 10% for patients who are 25 years beyond their treatment. This is probably caused by a combination of factors including an underlying genetic predisposition and the carcinogenic effects of radiotherapy and chemotherapeutic agents.

### Issues for the family

There are intense issues for the family of both a practical and emotional nature. The diagnosis and treatment of cancer demand the involvement of the parents at all stages. Although centralizing the care of paediatric oncology results in a superior service, the distances involved in reaching the centre can be problematic for many families. Residential facilities are often available, but these do not resolve the problems of child care for siblings, and separate families from normal family and friend support systems. Financial difficulties are common, and in many families a parent may have to give up or change jobs. Input from community nurses and social workers is important.

The emotional needs of the family are likely to be greater than the practical. The child and family need expert help to contend with facing life-threatening illness, ongoing fears of relapse and, for some, the process of dying and death. Relationships within a family are bound to be disturbed, and feelings of anxiety, depression, guilt and anger are common in all members.

The child has to cope not only with the effects of the cancer, but also with the debilitating effects of treatment and changes in appearance, such as alopecia, which can make reintegration into normal life all the more difficult.

### Issues at school

Whenever possible the child should remain in school and with classmates. Because most treatment regimens are intensive, considerable amounts of schooling are usually missed in the first year or two after diagnosis. Help should be provided so that the child does not fall too far behind.

School staff need preparation to help them understand the child's condition and prognosis, and to enable them to help the child reintegrate socially as well as academically.

## The child with cancer at a glance

### Epidemiology
One in 10 000 children.
Commonest cancers are acute lymphoblastic leukaemia, lymphoma and brain tumours

### Aetiology/pathophysiology
Host factors may be more important than environmental factors in childhood cancers

### How the diagnosis is made
The presentation depends on the individual malignancy. Nonspecific signs include unexplained or prolonged fever, unexplained (especially growing) masses and weight loss. Diagnosis is confirmed by histology. Staging is needed to determine treatment and prognosis

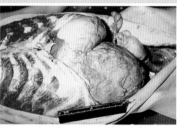

Postmortem photograph of an infant with Wilm's tumour

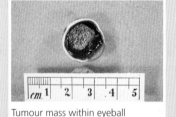

Tumour mass within eyeball

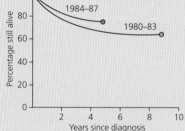

Survival curves for lymphoblastic leukaemia based on the United Kingdom Children's Cancer Study Group (UKCCSG)

### General management
Treatment must take place in a paediatric oncology centre
**Specific treatment** involves a combination of:
• Surgery
• Radiotherapy
• Chemotherapy
• Bone marrow transplantation
**Supportive treatment** required for:
• Effects of cancer and Rx:
• Metabolic disturbances
• Immunosuppression
• Bone marrow suppression
Nutrition
Symptom management including pain
Emotional support

### Liaison with school:
Missed schooling
Reintegration following treatment

### Management of acute problems
Fever — cultures and IV antibiotics
Immunosuppression — no live vaccines, treat chicken pox
Bone marrow suppression — packed red cells and platelet transfusion
Relapse

### Points for routine follow-up
Close monitoring is required for relapse of cancer and adverse effects of treatment. Once in full remission, annual routine follow-up is required indefinitely

### Prognosis
Varies with type and extent of cancer. Some 60% are cured. Overall, 80% survive >5 years. Late effects of treatment can be debilitating. Second cancers are not uncommon

# The child with a disability

The prevalence of physical and multiple disabilities in children is approximately 5–10 per 10 000. In this section the child with long-lasting and complex needs is considered. The commoner causes of disability are shown in Table 3.4.

## How disability presents

Children with disabilities are identified either as a result of parental suspicion, concern by health professionals or child health surveillance. This occurs at different times, depending on the problem. A syndrome or central nervous system abnormality may be identified in the antenatal period or at birth. Deafness, motor handicaps and severe learning disabilities often become apparent during the first year. Moderate or even severe learning disabilities, language disorder and autism may not be recognized until the child is two or three, when the family or health visitor question the child's developmental progress. Finally, children may present after life-threatening events such as head injury or encephalopathy.

## Assessment of disability

Identifying the underlying medical problem is only one aspect of the child's diagnosis. A detailed assessment of the child's development and how the difficulties are likely to impinge on his or her life is also needed. When the difficulties are complex, the paediatrician alone is unlikely to be able to make a sufficiently detailed assessment, or advise on appropriate management. In this circumstance the child should be referred to a child development team.

### The child development team

The child development team is a multidisciplinary team of professionals who are involved in assessing and managing children with complex difficulties (Figure 3.2). The members of the team (see Table 3.5) and the manner in which they work may vary from centre to centre, and their roles may overlap considerably in practice.

### Principles of management (see Box 3.4)

Management of a child with a disability goes beyond diagnosis, explanation of the problem and providing therapeutic input. It involves supporting the family while they come to terms with the child's difficulties and learn how to cope. It also involves a great deal of liaison work with other professionals both medical and non-medical.

The major benefit of the team approach lies in the coordination of care, so ensuring that the various professionals communicate with each other well and that the family does not receive a mixture of contradictory advice.

#### Breaking the news

The diagnosis of a disability is usually devastating, and the way that the news is initially broken is of long-lasting importance to the family. The session should be conducted in private by a senior doctor in the presence of both parents. There should be plenty of opportunity for questions, and a follow-up session should be arranged shortly after. If a baby is born with congenital anomalies, the first session should take place directly after birth, when possible with the baby present.

#### Medical management

Once the child's difficulties have been fully assessed, appropriate therapeutic input is required. This may be delivered in the child development centre, at home or at nursery. Once the child is in full-time school, the services are delivered there by community therapists, whose task is not only to work with the child but also to advise school staff.

#### Genetic counselling

When a child has been diagnosed as having a disability, the family will want to know the genetic implications for themselves and their relatives. Many disabilities

**Table 3.4** Commoner causes of disability among school children

| |
|---|
| *Physical and multiple disabilities* |
| Cerebral palsy |
| Spina bifida |
| Muscular dystrophy |
| *Severe learning difficulties* |
| Chromosomal abnormalities |
| Central nervous system abnormality |
| Idiopathic |
| *Special senses* |
| Severe visual handicap |
| Severe hearing loss |

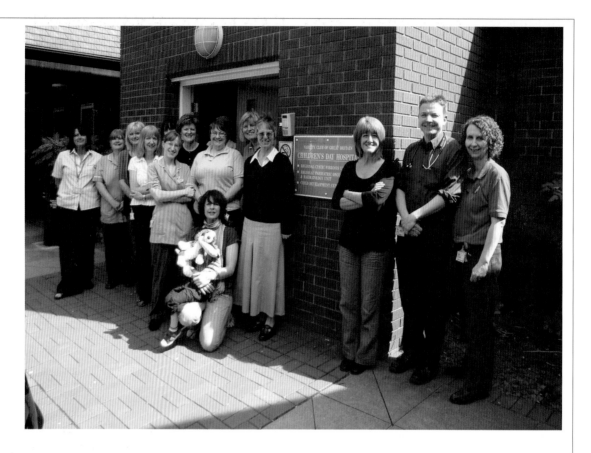

**Figure 3.2** Example of multidisciplinary team, consisting of specialist nurses, dietitian, physiotherapist, psychologist and clerical staff as well as medical staff.

have a genetic basis, in which case informed advice must be provided. However, even if there is no specific underlying genetic cause, the family will need to discuss the risk of further children being affected.

### Provision of services

Agencies other than health agencies are involved in providing services to the family:

- *Education services.* Education services are responsible for assessing learning difficulties, providing preschool home teaching, nursery schooling and education in both mainstream and special schools.
- *Social Care.* Social Care is responsible for providing preschool child care, relief care, advice about benefits and assessment for services needed on leaving school. Child protection concerns also fall into its remit.
- *Voluntary organizations.* Voluntary organizations provide support and information for families, run play facilities and provide educational opportunities and sitting services. Some are large national agencies with

numerous local branches, others are smaller groups concerned with a local issue or a single diagnosis.

### Education

Schools are required to provide extra provision for children with special needs and have the resources to provide additional help, whether individual or in small groups. When difficulties are severe or complex, the education authority is obliged to carry out a full formal assessment by an educational psychologist, including a medical report and reports from any other involved professionals such as therapists and the child's nursery or school. The child's educational needs and the provision which must be made to meet them are clearly outlined in a legally binding document known as the Statement of Special Educational Needs. The statement is reviewed on an annual basis.

**Mainstream and special schools**

Where possible, children with special needs are educated in mainstream schools, with extra help provided in the classroom as needed. This often involves the

**Table 3.5** The child development team

| Professional | Role |
|---|---|
| Developmental paediatrician | Diagnosis of medical problems |
| | Advice on medical issues |
| Physiotherapist | Assessment and management of gross motor difficulties, abnormal tone and prevention of deformities in cerebral palsy |
| | Provision of special equipment |
| Occupational therapist | Assessment and management of fine motor difficulties |
| | Advice on toys, play and appliances to aid daily living |
| Speech and language therapist | Advice on feeding |
| | Assessment and management of speech, language and all aspects of communication |
| Psychologist | Support and counselling of family and team |
| Special needs teacher | Advice on special educational needs |
| Social worker | Support for the family |
| | Advice on social service benefits, respite care, etc. |
| Health visitor | Support for the family |
| | Liaison with local health visitor |

**Box 3.4 Managing a child with a disability**

- Obtain a detailed assessment of the child's difficulties and abilities
- Explain the nature and possible causes of the child's disability
- Devise a programme to cover the child's and family's needs
- Help the family cope practically and emotionally
- Advise on educational needs and schooling

employment of a special needs assistant for the child, along with physiotherapy, occupational therapy and speech and language therapy support. Mainstream placement has the advantage of integrating children with special needs into a normal peer group in their own locality, and encouraging their adaptation to normal society at an early age. It is also advantageous for other children to learn to live alongside children with disabilities. However, there are some disadvantages as mainstream schools usually suffer from comparatively large classes, may have inadequate support, and the buildings may be poorly adapted for the child with physical difficulties.

Special schools, on the other hand, provide expert teaching in small classes, by staff who have an understanding of handicapping conditions. Transport and health service support are also provided. The disadvantage lies in the child's limited exposure to 'normal life'. Often, a good compromise between mainstream and special schooling is to establish special units for children with disabilities in the mainstream setting.

## Support

Having a child with a disability places extra pressure and stresses on any family. It is important, therefore, to determine how much support is available. Informal support in terms of family and friends can be variable, and additional support is often appreciated. This may take a number of forms. Voluntary organizations and parent support groups give families the opportunity to meet others in similar circumstances and so can reduce the sense of isolation. Sitting services and respite care give parents a break from the burden of constantly caring for the child, and help in the home can also be provided. As regards financial benefits, a child with disabilities is entitled to receive the Disability Living Allowance, with a mobility component from the age of 5 years, and the parents may receive the Invalid Care Allowance provided they are not in full-time work.

## Issues for the family

Families differ greatly in their reaction to having a child with a disability. However, on first receiving the news, they all tend to pass through similar emotional stages to those experienced in coping with bereavement. The first reaction is one of shock, when often only a small proportion of what is said is taken in. Negative feelings of fear and loss, anger and guilt then follow. Gradually adaptation follows and leads to the final stage of acceptance. Some parents have difficulty in reaching this last stage, in which case supportive counselling by a psychologist may be necessary.

The family needs to adapt again at each stage of the child's development. Independence becomes an issue at each step, but particularly so at adolescence. An important part of the child's education is to foster independence, and this is usually addressed well at special schools. Young adult disability teams provide a service to advise about options beyond secondary school.

## Issues for the school

When a child with a disability is accepted at a mainstream school, the school needs to be prepared and informed about any anticipated difficulties. If the child needs occupational therapy, physiotherapy or speech and language therapy, the staff will need to work with the therapists in order to implement their recommendations. In some circumstances the school may need to make alterations to accommodate physical disabilities. Special guidance or counselling may be required and help may be needed to integrate the child into the classroom.

---

### 👁 The child with a disability at a glance

**Epidemiology**
5–10 per 1000

**Presentation and how the diagnosis is made**
Antenatally or at birth if
  anomalies are present
In the first year for motor
  handicaps and severe
  learning disabilities
In the second or third year for
  moderate learning disabilities,
  language disorder and
  autism
After cranial insults

**Assessment of the disability**
• Detailed assessment of the
  child's abilities
• Recognition of the child's
  underlying medical problem
• Assessment of the likely
  long-term effects
• When difficulties are complex,
  a multi-disciplinary approach
  is needed.
  This involves the **child
  development team**: paediatrician, physiotherapist,
  occupational therapist,
  speech and language
  therapist, psychologist,
  teacher, social worker, health
  visitor

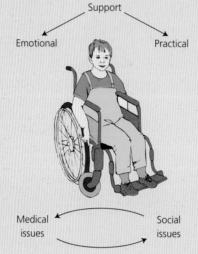

Support
Emotional        Practical

Medical          Social
issues           issues

**Issues for the family**
The initial impact is similar to
  bereavement
The impact of disability is
  similar to that of chronic
  illness (see pp. 36–7)

**Issues for the school**
School needs information and
  guidance, and may need to
  make adaptations

**Breaking the news**
Must be done by an
  experienced senior
  professional

**Medical management**
Usual paediatric care
If therapeutic input is needed, it
  should be provided initially at
  home, and then in nursery
  and school

**Genetic counselling**
Required for many families,
  even if no genetic cause is
  identified

**Provision of services**
Additional services are provided
  by education, social services
  and voluntary agencies

**Education**
The Statement of Special
  Educational Needs describes
  the provision that must be
  made for children with
  disabilities
Where possible, children with
  disabilities should be
  integrated into mainstream
  school

**Support**
Includes informal support,
  voluntary organizations,
  sitting services, respite care,
  home help, and social service
  allowances

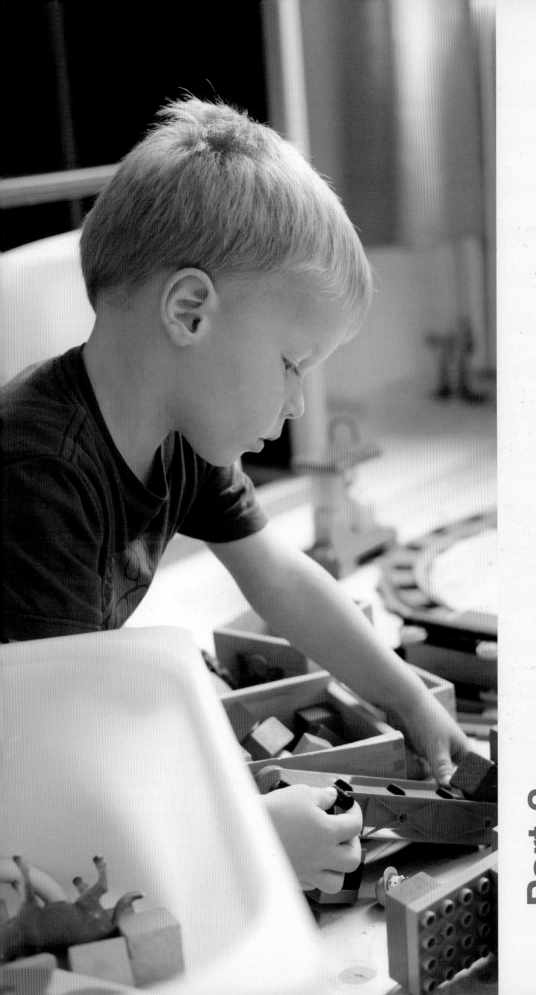

**Part 2**
**A paediatric tool kit**

# CHAPTER 4

# History taking and clinical examination

Studies of medical out-patient consultations show that 86% of diagnosis depends entirely on what the patient says; their own story. What doctors find on examination adds a further 6%; and technical investigations (X-rays, blood tests, etc.) add another 8%.

*British Medical Journal, 1975*

## COMPETENCES

### You must . . .

| Know | Be able to | Appreciate |
|---|---|---|
| • How to measure and weigh children accurately | • Engage the child and establish a rapport<br>• Carry out a competent physical examination demonstrating good technique<br>• Plot measurements accurately on a growth chart | • That children are likely to be wary of a physical examination<br>• That you may need to be flexible rather than strictly systematic in your approach<br>• It is best to leave unpleasant parts of the examination to the end |

In clinical medicine, history taking and physical examination are the keystones of diagnosis and subsequent therapy. The first contact between the child, the family and the doctor sets the scene for the future professional relationship. Very little may be remembered by the child and his or her family about the first visit except whether the doctor gave the impression of being an approachable and sympathetic person. When the patient is a child, the doctor's approach is of special importance and techniques must be altered in light of the patient's age.

Every child should have a personal child health record (see p. 20) held by a parent. This should be maintained as an individual record of a child's health, growth and development as well as contacts with doctors and health care workers. The record is particularly useful when the child is the subject of a new referral to a doctor, and should be brought to the appointment so that details of immunization, growth and development are readily available.

## The consultation

Before you start, you need to work at gaining the child's trust and co-operation. Start by introducing yourself to the child and parents, and try to put them at ease. You obviously need to talk to the child in a manner appropriate to their age. While you take the history observe the child as you can learn a great deal from how he or she looks and plays. It helps to make the room child-friendly and have toys available for children of different ages, so they can play while you talk to the parents.

Many parents and children cannot express their particular fears. For example, the presenting complaint of headache may represent fears about brain tumour, and enlarged glands may arouse anxiety about cancer. It is very important that you anticipate these problems and ask specifically about them. These fears can be elicited by asking questions such as: 'Is there anything in particular you are worried about?' or 'In my experience some parents worry about cancer in a child with tummy pain. Is this a fear of yours?'

When taking the history, you should decide whether it would be better for the child to leave the room to play rather than to hear him- or herself being discussed, but you should always make it clear that he or she can always return to the consulting room to prevent anxiety. A sensitive doctor should anticipate the parents' wish not to talk in front of the child, as some parents feel too embarrassed to ask, with the result that they may withhold important information.

Adolescents require particular sensitivity. It is ideal practice to offer both parent and child the opportunity to talk to you alone and then come back together to conclude the consultation. Time often does not permit this, but there will be circumstances where it is essential to talk to each alone, making it clear what aspects of the session are confidential.

### How to take a history

The history is usually given by the parents, although you should include the child if old enough. It is important to make the family feel they have your full attention and that you are listening to their concerns. It is very important that you develop a structured approach to make sure that you do not miss important points, but do not make this too rigid as it is sometimes necessary to pursue a different line to elicit important information. A suggested approach is shown in Box 4.1.

**Presenting complaint(s).** Record the chronology of the presenting complaint in a systematic manner with a heading for each date line starting from when the child was last '100%' or 'their normal self':

- 4 weeks ago: onset of cough;
- 3 days ago: sore throat;
- today: convulsion.

Don't write the days of the week in the history as they give no indication of the duration of the disease. It is important that you gain a clear idea in your mind of the chronology of the problem, so make sure you have done so by 'playing back' the history to the family.

**Previous medical history.** The GP's referral letter is often helpful in determining previous visits to the doctor's surgery and details of any medication the child has been given. Ask about all admissions to hospital. Enquire about allergies and determine how severe any previous allergic reactions have been. Ask specifically about asthma, eczema and hay fever.

**Perinatal history.** Ask about birthweight and the duration of pregnancy. Enquire about any problems during the pregnancy such as hypertension, smoking, drug ingestion, influenza-like illnesses, and details of the birth, type of delivery and condition at birth. If the mother cannot provide medical details, the following questions are helpful:

## Box 4.1 What to ask about when taking a history

| | |
|---|---|
| **Presenting complaint** | Record the main problems in the family's own words as they describe them |
| **History of presenting complaint** | Try to get an exact chronology from the time the child was last completely well. Allow the family to describe events themselves, using questions to direct them, and probe for specific information. Try to use open questions: 'Tell me about the cough' rather than 'Is the cough worse in the mornings?' |
| **Past medical history** | In young children and infants this should start from the pregnancy and include birthweight and details of the delivery and neonatal period, including any feeding or breathing problems<br>Ask about all illnesses, hospital attendances including accidents and admissions, and immunizations |
| **Drugs and allergies** | What drugs is the child taking and are there any allergies? |
| **Developmental history** | Ask about milestones and school performance. Are there any areas of concern? |
| **Family history** | Who is in the family and who lives at home? Ask about consanguinity, as cousin marriages increase the risk of genetic disorders. Ask if there are any illnesses that run in the family. Does anyone have a disability, and have there been any deaths in childhood? Draw up a family tree (see Figure 4.1) |
| **Social history** | Which school or nursery does the child attend? Ask about jobs and smoking, and try to get a feel for the financial situation at home. The social context of illness is very important in paediatrics |
| **Review of systems** | Ask screening questions for symptoms within systems other than the presenting system (see Box 4.2) |

- Did the baby need any special treatment at birth, for example, help with breathing?
- Was the baby taken away from you after birth? If so, for how long?
- How long was it before you could feed your baby?
- How old was the baby when he or she went home?
- Did the baby suffer from any fits in the newborn period?
- Did the baby have breathing problems requiring oxygen?

**Family history.** You should include a family tree (as shown in Figure 4.1) in your notes.

Ask specifically about:

- Whether there is a member of the family with a similar condition to that being complained of by the child.
- Whether there have been any disabled children or deaths in childhood.
- Consanguinity. This is particularly common in some ethnic groups.

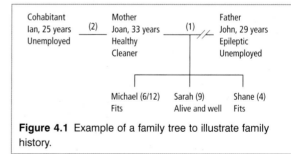

**Figure 4.1** Example of a family tree to illustrate family history.

- Establish how the family works. Who is the main carer? What are the parental occupations? If there is a man in the house, is he the father of the patient and/or the other children?

**Social history.** Social problems may strongly influence the health of children in a family. An absent father may be a source of unhappiness and you should find out about the relationship the child has with the natural father. School is another potential source of conflict and anxiety. Bullying may be a particular problem which is unknown to the parents. Find out if the symptoms are related to school days and how much time is missed from school.

**Review of systems.** Having explored the presenting complaint, past medical history and family circumstances, you should go on to cover all the other organ systems to make sure that you have not missed any details. A scheme is shown in Box 4.2.

| Box 4.2 Review of systems | |
|---|---|
| **General** | Activity, tiredness |
| | Sleep |
| | School absence |
| | Weight loss |
| **Cardiovascular** | Faints |
| | Murmurs |
| | Cyanosis |
| **Respiratory** | Cough |
| | Wheeze |
| **Gastrointestinal** | Diet |
| | Appetite |
| | Vomiting |
| | Diarrhoea |
| | Constipation |
| | Abdominal pain |
| **Genitourinary** | Enuresis |
| | Dysuria |
| | Frequency |
| | Age at menarche |
| | Dysmenorrhoea |
| **ENT** | Earache |
| | Hearing impairment |
| | Recurrent sore throat |
| | Enlarged glands |
| **Neurological** | Fits |
| | Faints/funny turns |
| | Headaches |
| | Hearing and vision |
| **Skin** | Any lesions or rashes |
| **Musculoskeletal** | Joint pain or swelling |
| **Development** | Gross motor |
| | Fine motor |
| | Speech and language |
| | Social |

## Examining the child

When you come to examine the child remember the following principles:

- **Rapport** — Develop a rapport with the child and gain their confidence. With younger children, complimenting them on their shoes or outfit is often a good start

- **Observation** — You should have already gained a good deal of information by your informal observation while taking the history

- **Undress the child** — The child should usually be undressed down to underwear so that you can maximize your chances of finding physical signs

- **Be systematic** — You need to follow a systematic structure to your examination. Leave unpleasant aspects such as the ears and throat to the end. Don't dive for your stethoscope but follow the order of

  - Observation
  - Palpation
  - Percussion
  - Auscultation

- **Right side of the bed** — Remember that if you are right-handed you should if possible examine the child on the right-hand side of the bed

Older children can be examined like adults, but younger children, particularly if fretful or anxious, must be approached quite differently. Any uncomfortable procedure such as examination of ears and throat should be left until last in order to avoid upsetting the child. Time spent initially gaining the child's confidence is never wasted. It may help if you keep up a 'running commentary' during the examination, asking questions as you go along. However, if the child fails to answer you should immediately move on. Children can become acutely embarrassed by a silence, but may be reassured by continuing chatter.

To avoid upset, ask the mother to undress the child. Vary your routine to suit the child – it may be necessary to examine the back before the front or the abdomen before the chest. This flexibility in routine means that parts of the examination may get forgotten, but you can avoid this by systematically recording your findings, so that it is immediately obvious if you have overlooked something.

Children are sometimes put off by a stethoscope. It is often helpful to put it first on the child's knee, or on a teddy bear, to show that they need not be frightened.

### Notes, problem lists and plans of action

When you have taken the history you should write your notes clearly following the systematic approach given above. Take a moment to draw up a provisional problem or issues list. This allows you to focus on parts of the physical examination that are particularly relevant to the child. Then examine the child and write up your examination in a systematic way, organ system by organ system. Draw up a brief summary paragraph delineating the key points from the history and physical examination.

Now you are in a position to revise your problem list. This should be itemized clearly and should be comprehensive. You should include all the factors including family and school difficulties. For example a problem list might read:

1  Abdominal pain
2  Constipation
3  Bullying at school
4  Sibling with cerebral palsy
5  Father unemployed

Having developed a problem list, a plan of action should follow logically. Itemize each action so that it is clear to others what you have undertaken to do. Actions should be considered under the following headings:

- Investigations to be carried out
- Treatment initiated
- Plans for follow-up and review

Finally, the parents need a full explanation, which should be recorded in the notes. Ensure that the parents understand what your view of the problem is, agree on what needs to be done and agree when the child should be seen again. It is often helpful to provide information leaflets, and contact with support organizations of families with similar problems where appropriate. If the plan is complicated you should provide the parents with notes, and write them a letter outlining what has been decided and what needs to be done.

### Hospital notes

Hospital notes serve a number of functions. They are a legal record of the consultation, and it is important that notes are clearly written and legible. They also serve as the principal mode of communication with colleagues. Providing a clear problem list means that all are aware of the issues.

The initial intake consultation should be laid out as described above. Follow-up notes during admission or in the outpatient clinic should also be structured. It is usually most helpful if these notes follow the format of the problem list. Some doctors use the 'SOAP' method of recording: for each problem they comment on:

- **S**ymptom
- **O**bservation
- **A**ssessment
- **P**lan

# An approach to examination

The remainder of this chapter provides you with a system by system approach to examining children, along with an explanation of how to elicit signs and interpret them..

## Growth

Accurate measurement of height, weight and head circumference is a vital part of the assessment of all children referred for a medical opinion. Growth can only accurately be assessed by taking at least two measurements of various growth parameters (e.g. length, weight and head circumference) and observing the relative points at which these measurements fall on a growth chart appropriate to the child's age and sex.

### Weight

Use a weighing scale that has been calibrated accurately. Infants should be laid in a pannier scale and older children weighed standing up. Babies should be weighed naked without a nappy, and older children in light clothing or (preferably) underwear only.

### Height and length

The measurement of height should be precise; it is only accurate if made with care using the appropriate equipment.

In the first 2 years of life, length is measured on a measuring frame or mat (Figure 4.2). From the age of two, providing the child can stand, height is measured against a specially calibrated standing frame.

Consistent technique is necessary to estimate standing height accurately (Figure 4.3). Check the heels are against the wall and the feet flat on the floor with the knees straight. Gently extend the neck and ensure the eyes are in line with the external auditory meatus.

### Head (occipitofrontal) circumference (OFC)

This should be measured accurately to the nearest millimetre. Use a flexible, non-stretchable tape measure and measure around the occipitofrontal circumference. Take three successive measurements at slightly different points. The widest is taken to be the OFC (Figure 4.4).

### Growth standards

In order to interpret a child's growth, comparison must be made with population standards. These standards are presented in the form of growth charts, which demonstrate the population's growth as centiles. The growth charts currently in use in the UK are

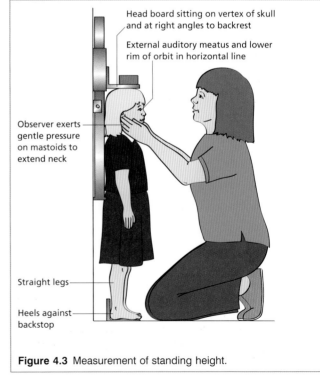

Head board sitting on vertex of skull and at right angles to backrest

External auditory meatus and lower rim of orbit in horizontal line

Observer exerts gentle pressure on mastoids to extend neck

Straight legs

Heels against backstop

**Figure 4.3** Measurement of standing height.

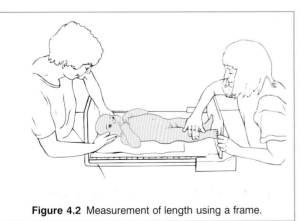

**Figure 4.2** Measurement of length using a frame.

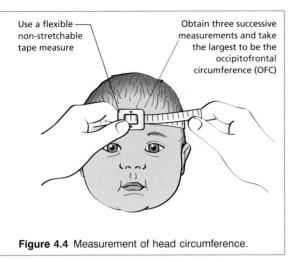

Figure 4.4 Measurement of head circumference.

the 1990 UK Child Growth Standards, which were constructed from detailed data collected on children across the country. In 2009 the charts for children aged 0–4 years were updated. They are now constructed from World Health Organization data, which was based on the growth of healthy breast-fed babies, rather than bottle-fed babies as previously.

Separate charts are available for girls and boys. Age is given along the *x* axis which, depending on the chart, may be shown in months or decimally. Height, length, weight and head circumference measurements lie along the *y* axis. Nine centiles ranging from the 99.6th to the 0.4th centile are shown as continuous or dotted lines (Figures 4.5–4.7). Body mass index (BMI) should be calculated if there is any concern about weight. This is calculated from the equation:

$$BMI = weight~in~kg/(height~in~metres)^2$$

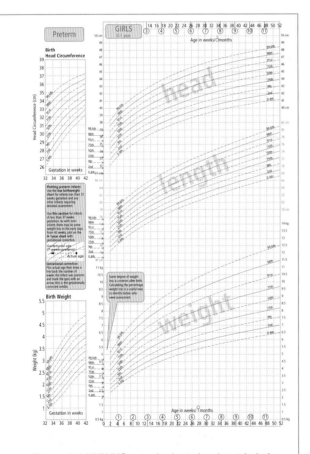
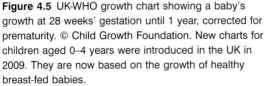

Figure 4.5 UK-WHO growth chart showing a baby's growth at 28 weeks' gestation until 1 year, corrected for prematurity. © Child Growth Foundation. New charts for children aged 0–4 years were introduced in the UK in 2009. They are now based on the growth of healthy breast-fed babies.

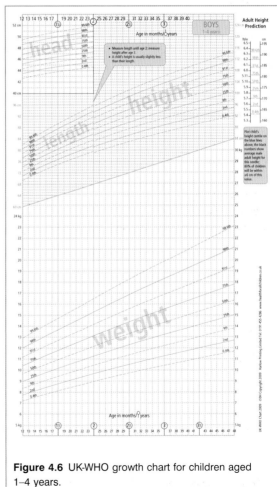

Figure 4.6 UK-WHO growth chart for children aged 1–4 years.

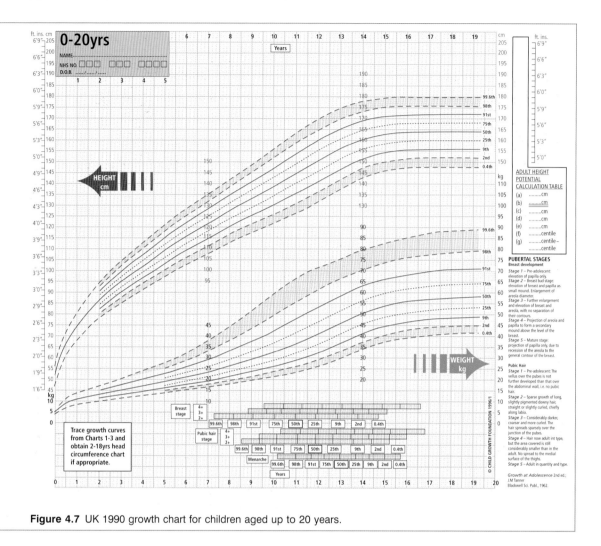

**Figure 4.7** UK 1990 growth chart for children aged up to 20 years.

## Plotting a child's growth (see Box 4.3)

In order to interpret a child's growth measurements, they must be plotted on the appropriate growth chart. If the child was born prematurely, two points are plotted up to the age of 2 years: the child's actual age and the corrected age (post-term age) are connected by an arrow. The centile along which the point falls relates the child's growth to the rest of the population. Thus, if a boy's weight falls on the 50th centile, he is average, and 50% of the population will be heavier and 50% lighter than him. If his height falls on the 9th centile, he is relatively short with 91% of the population taller and only 9% smaller.

The further a child's growth falls away from the normal population the more likely it is that he or she has a problem. Thus, measures falling between the 0.4th and 2nd centiles may be normal, whereas those

---

### Box 4.3 Principles of plotting a child's growth

- In the UK use the 1990 UK-WHO growth charts
- Mark the child's measurement with a dot (not a cross or circle)
- If a baby is born prematurely, indicate corrected (post-term) age up to the age of 2 years too
- Assess the *rate* of growth by measuring on two occasions at least 4–6 months apart
- Plateauing of growth and weight, or heights below the 0.4th centile, merit evaluation (see p. 256)
- A child's final height is expected to fall midway between the parent's centile lines.

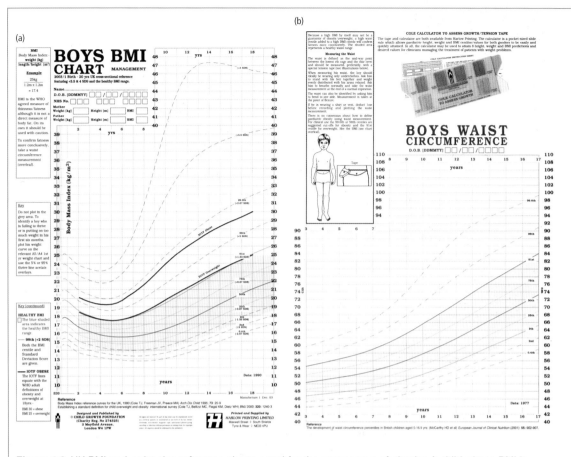

**Figure 4.8** UK BMI and waist circumference charts, used for the assessment of obesity. A child whose BMI is above the 98th centile is considered obese, and one with a BMI between the 91st and 98th centile is overweight.

below the 0.4th centile are more likely to be abnormal. Furthermore, crossing centiles over time is concerning (other than in the first 2 years or at puberty) and needs evaluation. Interpretation of growth in babyhood and at puberty is important and requires skill. Values for BMI should be plotted in the UK on the UK 1990 BMI charts, which have waist circumference charts on the reverse (see Figure 4.8).

### Interpretation of growth charts

After the first 2 years of life a child should continue to grow along the same centile, although infants in the first few months of life may follow a centile quite different to their subsequent growth centiles. It is important to relate the height to weight and head circumference and so gain an idea of the child's build. In general children are expected to reach a final height midway between their parents' centiles. This sometimes called target height. You can either simply

estimate this from the parents' position on the charts or calculate it using the formula given on the growth charts. Interpretation of children's patterns of growth is discussed in Chapter 13.

### General observation

Much can be learnt by watching the child while he or she is being undressed and by how the child plays. Observation starts from when the child and the child's family enter the room, and should not be confined to the course of the physical examination.

Formal observation should include:

- *Well or ill?* The first point to note is whether the child looks ill or well. Is she full of energy or does she prefer to cuddle up against the parent? Does she appear flushed or irritable?
- *Dysmorphism* Look at the child for evidence of dysmorphic features or asymmetry. This may be

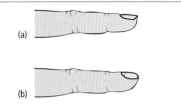

(a)

(b)

**Figure 4.9** Nail bed angle: (a) normal and (b) clubbing.

| Table 4.1 Commoner causes of finger clubbing | |
|---|---|
| Familial | Benign condition |
| Cardiovascular disease | Cyanotic heart disease, e.g. Fallot's tetralogy |
| Respiratory disease | Chronic suppurative lung disease, e.g. cystic fibrosis |
| Bowel disease | Chronic inflammatory bowel disease, e.g. ulcerative colitis |

obvious if there are major anomalies, or you may simply have a sense that the features are unusual.
• *Colour* Examine the lips and tongue for central cyanosis and pallor. Evert the lower eyelid to assess the colour of the mucosal membrane for anaemia or the conjunctiva for jaundice.
• *Hands* Examine the hands. Look at the palmar creases, and the nail beds for colour (cyanosis, anaemia). Look for clubbing. The most sensitive way to detect early clubbing is to look at the profile of the nail bed, as the normal nailbed angle is lost very early in the clubbing process (Figure 4.9). You can also appose the index finger nails, nail facing nail. In clubbing you do not see light between the nails. The commoner causes of clubbing are listed in Table 4.1.

## Cardiovascular examination

### Observation

When you examine the cardiovascular system (Box 4.4), make sure you take note of growth, as significant heart disease restricts growth and weight gain. Cyanosis is a major sign of cardiovascular disease. It also occurs as the result of respiratory disease, and you should examine both systems sequentially. Central cyanosis is always abnormal. This is determined by

**Box 4.4 How to examine the cardiovascular system**

**Growth** Measure the child and plot on to centile charts
**Observation** Look for
  Central cyanosis
  Anaemia
  Breathlessness
  Chest shape and scars
  Clubbing
**Palpation**
  Pulse
    • rate
    • rhythm
    • character
    • volume
  Absent or delayed femoral pulse
  Praecordium
    • parasternal heave (? right ventricular hypertrophy)
    • thrills
    • apex beat (? left ventricular hypertrophy)
  Hepatomegaly
  Oedema
  Capillary refill
**Auscultation**
  Heart sounds
  Murmurs
    • systolic or diastolic?
    • character
    • grade
    • site of maximum intensity
    • radiation
**Blood pressure**

examining the tongue. Lips and fingers may be blue because of non-cardiac causes such as cold, and are not uncommon in babies. Anaemia and clubbing can both be seen by examining the child's hands.

Check if the child is breathless, pale or sweating as these are signs of heart failure. Pectus carinatum (see Figure 4.15) is the only abnormal shape associated with heart disease.

### Palpation

#### Pulse

Examine the radial, femoral, brachial and carotid pulses for rate, rhythm and character. It is easier to assess the right brachial pulse in young children than the radial.

| Table 4.2 Range of heart rates in normal children | |
|---|---|
| **Age** | **Normal heart rate (beats per minute)** |
| <3 months | 100–180 |
| 3–24 months | 80–150 |
| 2–10 years | 70–110 |
| >10 years | 55–90 |

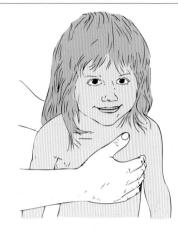

**Figure 4.10** Position to place hand to assess for a parasternal heave.

- *Rate.* The rate should be timed over 15 seconds and converted to a rate per minute. Normal heart rate depends on the child's age (Table 4.2).
- *Rhythm.* Children often show sinus arrhythmia, where the heart rate varies with the respiratory cycle, and this is normal. Occasional ectopic beats are also normal in children.
- *Pulse character.* This is detected by the pulse volume. A *collapsing pulse* (*waterhammer pulse*) occurs with a wide pulse pressure, most usually in children with patent ductus arteriosus. The increased pulse volume is best felt by elevating the limb. A *slow rising pulse* has a slow upstroke and rapid fall off. It is caused by left ventricular outflow obstruction.
- *Volume.* Is the pulse full, or weak and thready, as in shock?
- *Radiofemoral delay.* It is always important to compare the radial or brachial pulse in the right arm with the femoral pulse. In coarctation of the aorta, either the pulse in the right limb is felt before the femoral (or left radial pulse) or the femoral pulse is absent.

### Praecordium

- *Parasternal heave.* Right ventricular hypertrophy can be detected by placing the palm of your hand over the lower half of the sternum (Figure 4.10). An abnormal impulse is felt by a heaving sensation under the heel of your hand.
- *A thrill.* A thrill is a palpable murmur felt as a vibration and is always abnormal. Place your fingertips over the four valve areas and in the suprasternal notch (Figure 4.11).
- *Apex beat.* Place your hand over the chest with the fingertips in the anterior axillary line (Figure 4.12). The maximal lateral impulse is found with one fingertip. Define its position by counting down the ribs starting at the sternal angle, which corresponds to the

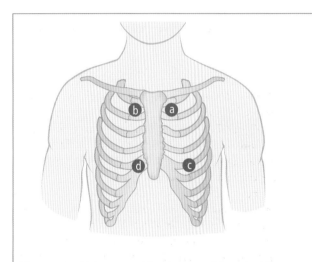

**Figure 4.11** Valve areas: (a) pulmonary, (b) aortic, (c) mitral, (d) tricuspid.

second rib. The apex beat is normally in the midclavicular line in the fifth intercostal space (fourth interspace in children less than 5 years old). A forceful apex or displacement of the apex to the left suggests left ventricular hypertrophy or lung disease distorting the mediastinal position.

### Liver

Palpate the lower edge of the liver and percuss the upper edge (see p. 67). Hepatomegaly suggests heart failure.

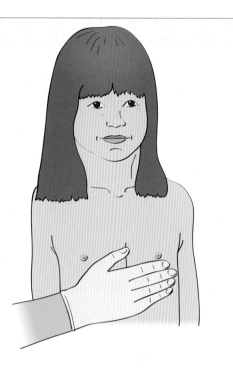

**Figure 4.12** Palpation of the apex beat by the index finger.

### Ankle oedema

Look for pitting oedema, although peripheral oedema and raised jugular venous pressure (JVP) are rarely seen in children.

### Capillary refill

Poor skin perfusion is a sign of shock. Apply moderate pressure with your finger on a warm periphery for 5 seconds and watch for the colour to return. The normal capillary refill time is up to 2 seconds; a time longer than this is suggestive of poor peripheral circulation or otherwise shock.

### *Auscultation*

Auscultate carefully with both the bell and the diaphragm of the stethoscope. The bell is particularly important in picking up low-pitched murmurs. Listen first for heart sounds and then for murmurs. Listen in the four valve areas (see Figure 4.11) and over the back.

### Heart sounds

The first heart sound is heard when the mitral and tricuspid valves close and the second when the aortic and pulmonary valves close. When the child breathes in, blood is sucked into the right side of the heart and right pulmonary ejection is prolonged, causing the pulmonary valve to close slightly after the aortic valve. During expiration the two valves close together. Normally, you can hear 'splitting' of the second heart sound in the pulmonary area on inspiration. In an atrial septal defect there is wide and fixed splitting of the second heart sound (i.e. it does not vary with respiration). A loud and single second heart sound is heard with a large left-to-right shunt (e.g. a ventricular septal defect). Listen for added sounds such as gallop rhythm in heart failure or ejection click in aortic stenosis.

### Murmurs (see also p. 192)

Murmurs are caused by turbulence of blood flow and may be innocent or pathological. If you hear a murmur:

- check for radiation in the axilla, over the carotid arteries and the back;
- listen again in inspiration and expiration;
- listen with the child lying down and sitting up;
- turn the child on the left side, as some murmurs change with position.

Murmurs can be graded according to their loudness and presence of a thrill (see Table 4.3), but the loudness may not correlate with severity. The murmur may occur during systole or diastole. Systolic murmurs may be either ejection (diamond-shaped in intensity) or pansystolic (Figure 4.13). Diastolic murmurs are always pathological, and are caused by increased blood flow through a normal atrioventricular valve, narrowing (stenosis) of an atrioventricular valve or incompetence (leak) of the pulmonary or aortic valves.

**Table 4.3** Grading of cardiac murmurs. Grades 1 and 2 are usually innocent, grades 5 and 6 are always significant and grades 3 and 4 are suspect

|  | Murmur | Thrill |
|---|---|---|
| Grade 1 | Barely audible | None |
| Grade 2 | Soft and variable in nature | None |
| Grade 3 | Easily heard | None |
| Grade 4 | Loud | Present |
| Grade 5 | Very loud | Present |
| Grade 6 | Heard without a stethoscope | Present |

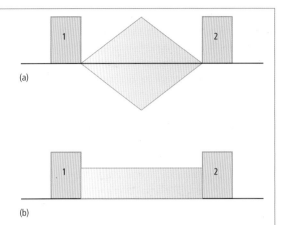

**Figure 4.13** Shape of cardiac murmurs: (a) ejection systolic murmur and (b) pansystolic murmur. 1, 2 denote the first and second heart sounds.

| Table 4.4 Upper limit of normal (above 2 standard deviations from the norm) for systolic blood pressure through childhood ||
| --- | --- |
| **Age of child** | **Abnormal systolic pressure (mmHg)** |
| Neonate | 90 |
| 1–12 months | 100 |
| 1–5 years | 110 |
| 6–9 years | 120 |
| 10–12 years | 130 |
| 13–14 years | 140 |

Describe the murmur according to the following characteristics:

- Is it systolic or diastolic?
- Character – is it blowing or harsh?
- The grade
- The site of maximum intensity
- The radiation

Most murmurs in children are innocent and you should be able to distinguish them from a pathological murmur (see p 192).

### Blood pressure

Measuring the child's blood pressure is an essential part of the physical examination, but is left to last to avoid upsetting the younger child. Use an appropri-

---

> **Key points: The cardiovascular system**
>
> - Sinus arrhythmia is normal in children
> - Radiofemoral delay or absent femoral pulses are always abnormal
> - A systolic ejection murmur denotes no cardiac pathology in at least 50% of cases
> - A thrill is always abnormal

ately sized cuff – it should be wide enough to cover two thirds of the upper arm and the bladder should completely encircle the arm. It is important to have a range of cuff sizes available in every paediatric clinic.

Oscillometric devices to measure blood pressure non-invasively are now readily available and are easily used even on the smallest child. It is still important to choose the appropriate cuff size.

The upper limit of normal for blood pressure in childhood is shown in Table 4.4.

## Respiratory system

> **Box 4.5 How to examine the respiratory system**
>
> **Observation** Look for
> Restlessness or drowsiness
> Abnormal shape of the chest
> Count the respiratory rate
> Audible respiratory sounds
> Signs of respiratory distress
> - subcostal/intercostal recession
> - use of accessory muscles
> - nasal flaring
> - tachypnoea
> Cyanosis and anaemia
> Clubbing
> **Palpation**
> Mediastinal deviation
> - tracheal position
> - apex beat
> Chest expansion
> **Percussion**
> For resonance
> To define the upper edge of liver dullness
> **Auscultation**
> Listen for
> breath sounds
> any adventitious noises (crepitations, wheezing)
> tactile vocal fremitus and vocal resonance
> Describe findings according to chest zones

In children, interpretation of physical signs relating to the respiratory system requires care (Box 4.5). The child with obvious sounds on auscultation may have no significant disease, whereas the child with more subtle signs, such as tachypnoea and intercostal recession, is likely to have a significant respiratory condition even if auscultation is unremarkable.

### Observation

#### Respiratory distress

Observe the child for signs of respiratory distress. Is there an audible wheeze or stridor? Is there tachypnoea, use of accessory muscles, nasal flaring or recession? Expiratory grunting is a particularly worrying sign associated with severe respiratory distress. The sites of chest recession are shown in Figure 4.14. Restlessness and drowsiness suggest hypoxia/hypercapnoea (increase in $pCO_2$). Count the respirations. The respiratory rate varies with age and is shown in Table 4.5.

### Signs of chronic disease

Examine the hands for clubbing, cyanosis or anaemia. The causes of clubbing are shown in Table 4.1.

Describe the chest shape. The commoner abnormalities are illustrated in Figure 4.15: barrel chest (because of air trapping) has an increased anteroposterior diameter and is best observed by looking at the chest from the side. Harrison's sulcus is caused by diaphragmatic overactivity and is shown by grooves parallel to and 2–3 cm above the costal margin. It is seen in chronic asthma. Pectus excavatum (also known as funnel chest) and pectus carinatum (also known as pigeon chest) are relatively common and may cause concern due to their cosmetic appearance, but are usually idiopathic and not associated with underlying respiratory disease.

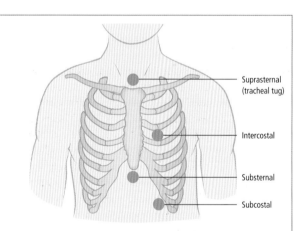

**Figure 4.14** Sites of chest recession in a young child with respiratory distress.

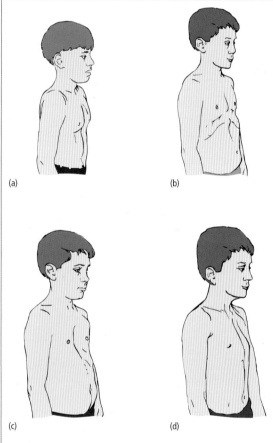

**Figure 4.15** Commoner types of chest wall deformity: (a) barrel chest, (b) Harrison's sulcus, (c) pectus excavatum, and (d) pectus carinatum.

| Table 4.5 Normal respiratory rate at different ages | |
|---|---|
| **Age** | **Awake respiratory rate (breaths per minute)** |
| 0–12 months | 25–40 |
| 1–5 years | 20–30 |
| 6 years and above | 15–25 |

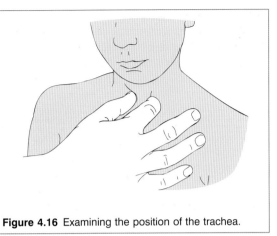

**Figure 4.16** Examining the position of the trachea.

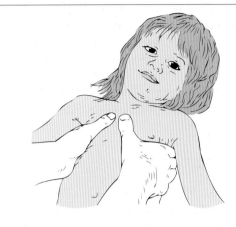

**Figure 4.17** Assessing chest expansion.

### Chest asymmetry

Look to see if one half of the chest is more prominent. This may be a result of scoliosis and is assessed by examining the spine (pp. 79).

### *Palpation*

#### Mediastinal deviation

Look for deviation of the trachea and the apex beat. The tracheal position is palpated by identifying the trachea in the suprasternal notch between two fingers (Figure 4.16). The apex impulse is detected by the method described on p. 61. Dextrocardia can be associated with chronic chest problems due to primary ciliary dyskinesia.

#### Chest expansion

Place your hands on the child's chest with your thumbs just touching at the sternum and your fingers lightly resting on the skin over the ribs (Figure 4.17). Ask the child to take a deep breath – the distance your thumbs move apart gives the degree of chest expansion. In a 5-year-old, 1 cm or more is normal.

### *Percussion*

The degree of resonance is assessed by percussion. Place the middle finger of your left hand (if you are right-handed) along the line of the rib and strike it with the first finger of the right hand as if it were a hammer hitting a small nail. Percuss the entire chest back and front in a systematic way, including the clavicles and in the axillae. The percussion note should be resonant across the chest, with normal liver dullness starting just below the nipple.

- *Hyper-resonance* occurs with hyperinflation due to air trapping, particularly seen in chronic asthma.

- *Dullness* to percussion is found in consolidation or lung collapse.
- *Stony dullness* occurs with pleural effusion.

Percussion is not very useful in children below 1 year of age.

### *Auscultation*

Ask the child to breathe in and out through the mouth. Upper airway sounds are often transmitted over the whole chest in children, but asking the child to cough may clear them. Listen for breath sounds using the diaphragm of the stethoscope. Start at the top of the chest, comparing one side with the other, and then listen over the back in a similar way. In young children, sounds transmitted from the upper airway may be confused with lower respiratory sounds, particularly wheezes. It may help to listen first to the noise of breathing without the stethoscope. Sometimes, when the upper airway sounds are soft, applying the stethoscope close to the child's mouth, nose or larynx may help to clarify whether the sounds are coming from the upper airway or the chest itself.

### Breath sounds

Normal breath sounds are called *vesicular* and there is a distinct interval between inspiration and expiration. *Bronchial breathing* has no break and has a harsher sound; it is heard normally over the trachea, but also occurs pathologically with pneumonia.

### Added sounds

*Crepitations* (crackles) sound like the soft rustling of leaves. These are heard with acute consolidation and chronic bronchiectasis, but are likely to be normal if cleared by coughing. *Rhonchi* (wheezes) indicate bronchial narrowing as heard in asthma and bronchiolitis. They are usually expiratory.

### Absent breath sounds

An absence of breath sounds in one area suggests pleural effusion, pneumothorax or dense consolidation.

### Tactile vocal fremitus and vocal resonance

If you find signs of consolidation, examine for vocal fremitus and resonance by palpating and listening when the child says 'ninety-nine'. The sounds and vibration are increased over an area of consolidation and decreased or absent over effusion or collapse.

### *Location in the chest*

If you detect any physical signs you should describe them according to their location in the chest (see Figure 4.18).

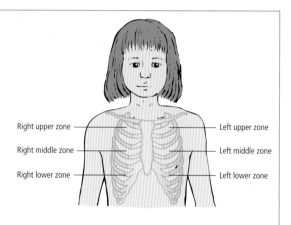

Right upper zone — Left upper zone

Right middle zone — Left middle zone

Right lower zone — Left lower zone

**Figure 4.18** How to describe the location of physical signs in the chest.

---

#### 🔑 Key points: The respiratory system

- In children, the observation of respiratory distress is more important than auscultatory findings
- The respiratory rate in infants is normally faster than in older children
- Percussion and auscultation may be unreliable in delineating consolidation in the young child
- In children, transmitted sounds from the upper airways may be easily confused with adventitious sounds

---

# The abdomen

---

#### Box 4.6 How to examine the abdomen

**Growth** Measure the child and plot on to centile charts
**Observation** Look for
  General appearance
  Clubbing
  Jaundice and anaemia
  Oedema
  Mouth
  Spider naevi
  Wasted buttocks
  Abdominal distension
**Palpation**
  Ask if the abdomen is tender
  Palpate lightly for obvious masses, deeply for other masses
  • liver
  • spleen
  • kidneys
  • groin (for hernia)
**Percussion**
  For resonance
  To define the upper edge of liver dullness
  ascites
  • shifting dullness
  • fluid thrill
**Auscultation**
  Note absent or tinkling bowel sounds
**Blood pressure**
**Rectal examination**
  Not routinely performed.
**Stool and urine specimens**
  Describe findings according to site in the abdomen

---

This section describes how to examine the abdomen if there is no acute problem (Box 4.6). The child with an 'acute abdomen' requires a different approach, which is described on p. 169.

A particularly important part of examining the gastrointestinal system is to plot the child's height and weight on a centile chart, as this is a critically important measure of gastrointestinal function.

In order to examine the abdomen, you must make sure the child is relaxed, otherwise the abdominal muscles contract and palpation becomes difficult. If necessary, small children can be examined on their parent's lap. Older children should lie on a couch. You should be at eye level with the abdomen, which may mean kneeling beside the couch. It may be necessary to examine some children standing up, if the alternative is to have them crying when lying down.

### Observation

Look for the following signs:

- *Jaundice and anaemia.* Look at the sclerae and conjunctiva. The colour of the urine should also be observed (p. 96).
- *Oedema.* This may be a feature of renal or liver disease. In children it is first noticed in the face, and the mother may remark on puffy features. Unlike oedema in adults, it is not usually seen in the feet or over the sacrum.
- *Mouth.* Check the state of the teeth and any abnormal smell
- *Skin lesions.* Pruritus is a common feature of cholestatic jaundice, and scratch marks may be very obvious. Look for palmar erythema and spider naevi, seen in children with chronic liver disease. These are small surface blood vessels that radiate out from a central point and sometimes resemble a small red spider. They blanch on pressure (unlike petechial haemorrhages) and then rapidly refill once the pressure is removed.
- *Wasted buttocks.* Look for loose skin folds over the buttocks, which suggest recent significant weight loss.
- *Abdominal distension.* Any distension (either generalized or localized) and visible peristalsis should be noted in particular. Remember that toddlers normally have a protuberant abdomen because of an exaggerated lordosis and relaxed abdominal musculature.
- *Hernias.* Umbilical herniae are common particularly in black infants. These usually require no treatment as they rarely obstruct or incarcerate. Examine the groin for the bulge of an inguinal hernia or maldescended testes (see p. 314 and p. 315).

### Palpation

The aim of palpation is to see if there is tenderness, any masses, or enlargement of the liver, spleen or kidneys. Before touching the child you should warm your hands and ask if there is any tenderness. Get down to the child's level and watch the child's face for any grimacing or wincing in response to pain. Palpate lightly first and then more deeply, using two or four fingers depending on the child's size. All four quadrants should be palpated in turn.

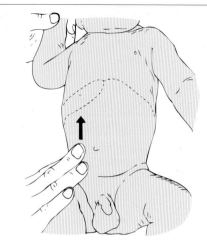

**Figure 4.19** Palpation for an enlarged liver.

### Liver

In children under 2 years old, you can normally palpate the liver 1–2 cm below the right costal margin. It enlarges down to the right iliac fossa, so start in the right lower quadrant. Use your right hand and palpate with the lateral side of your whole right index finger (see Figure 4.19). Gradually move your hand up towards the right costal margin until you feel the liver edge. If the child is fretful, it may help to place his or her hand under your own and palpate through it. You can confirm liver size by percussing the upper and lower borders. The liver may appear to be large if there is lung overinflation.

### Spleen

Usually the spleen is only modestly enlarged and palpable just under the left costal margin. As it enlarges it extends towards the right iliac fossa. There are two useful techniques to increase the chance of detecting a modestly enlarged spleen.

Start palpating in the right iliac fossa and move your hand up towards the left costal margin (see Figure 4.20), asking the child to take deep breaths. On inspiration you can feel a large spleen being pushed down towards your hand. You can also turn the child on to his or her right side towards you, causing the spleen to drop towards your right hand (see Figure 4.21).

### Kidneys

Examine the kidneys by bimanual palpation. Place one hand on the loin and press upwards. Place the other on the abdomen and palpate firmly. You should

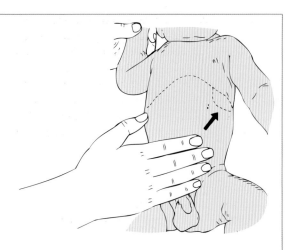

**Figure 4.20** Palpation for an enlarged spleen.

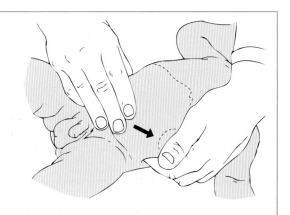

**Figure 4.21** Bimanual examination for a moderately enlarged spleen.

be able to feel an enlarged kidney. The lower pole of the right kidney may also be felt in thin, healthy individuals.

## Other masses

Carefully palpate for other masses and check for constipation, which you can feel as an indentable mass in the left iliac fossa.

## Hernias

Check if there is a hernia present (see p. 314).

## Percussion

Percuss the entire abdomen. The note is normally resonant, but hyper-resonant if the bowel is distended with gas. It is dull over the liver and spleen, and their size can be checked this way. It is also dull over a full bladder.

## Ascites

Ascites is suspected if you find dullness on percussion in the flanks and a resonant note in the midline. Confirm this by looking for:

- *Shifting dullness.* Roll the child over onto his or her side and percuss in the midline again. If the note is now dull, this indicates that ascitic fluid has shifted with the child's position to give a dull note.
- *A fluid thrill.* Place your hands on either side of the abdomen. Flick your finger on one side. You can feel the movement of the fluid against your other hand when ascites is present. The thrill can be blocked by asking the parent or child to place their hand firmly in the midline.

## Auscultation

Auscultation is useful in children with an acute abdomen (p. 169). The bowel sounds are absent if there is ileus, and increased or tinkling if there is bowel obstruction.

## Rectal examination

This is not routinely performed in children, and if needed must be left until last. Look at the anus for fissures or signs of trauma. Lubricate the tip of your index finger and press it flat against the edge of the anus before insertion – this causes less discomfort than inserting direct into the centre of the orifice. Use your little finger for infants.

You may need to examine the stool or urine specimens

## Location in the abdomen

Describe any symptoms or signs according to their location in the abdomen (see Figure 4.22).

---

**Key points: The abdomen**

- A protuberant abdomen is normal in toddlers
- Light palpation precedes deep palpation to assess areas that are acutely painful
- The liver edge is normally palpable in children below 2 years
- An underdeveloped scrotum suggests undescended testes

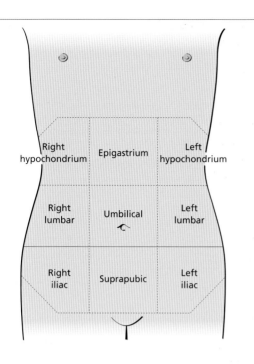

**Figure 4.22** How to describe the location of physical signs in the abdomen.

## Reticuloendothelial system

**Box 4.7 How to examine the reticuloendothelial system**

**General**
  Anaemia
  Jaundice
**Lymph nodes**
  Neck
  Axillae
  Groin
    • size
    • position
    • texture
    • mobility
**Focus of infection**
  Throat
  Limbs
**Liver**
**Spleen**

The reticuloendothelial system consists of the lymph glands, the liver and the spleen. Lymph node enlargement is very common and is usually due to local infection. In preschool children, small, 'shotty' (usually no larger than the size of a pea), firm, mobile and discrete glands are common. If one gland is enlarged you should check for lymphadenopathy elsewhere and hepatosplenomegaly. Describe a large node in terms of:

- **Size.**
- **Position.**
- **Texture** – is it hard or rubbery?
- **Mobility** – is it mobile or fixed to other tissues?

### General
Look for anaemia and jaundice (Box 4.7).

### Neck (see also swellings in the neck, p. 114)
The sternomastoid muscle divides the neck into the anterior and posterior triangles. Examine the lymph nodes in these two triangles (see Figure 4.23). Stand in front of the child to feel the pre- and post-auricular nodes, occipital nodes and those along the anterior cervical chain. Place your hands at the angle of the jaw and work them forward and down. Stand behind the child to feel the submental, submandibular and posterior cervical nodes.

Remember to examine the throat if you find cervical lymphadenopathy.

Enlarged cervical glands are most commonly caused by tonsil or, less commonly, middle ear infection, and both should be carefully examined. Occipital nodes enlarge as a result of scalp infection (eczema is a common cause), and rubella causes posterior auricular and occipital node enlargement.

### Axillae
Examine the axillae with the child sitting facing you. Support the child's flexed arm at the elbow, with your left hand holding the right arm. Place your right hand in the right axilla and feel for the presence of enlarged nodes against the chest wall. Reverse the process for the other side.

If there is lymphadenopathy check the hands or arms for a focus of infection.

### Groin
Lie the child down and gently palpate the groin for enlarged nodes. They are usually small, discreet and mobile.

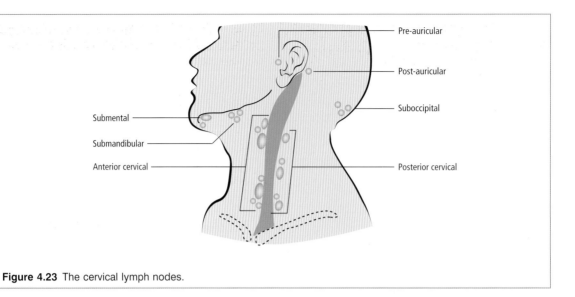

**Figure 4.23** The cervical lymph nodes.

If they are enlarged, look for infection in the feet or legs.

## Hepatosplenomegaly
Look for liver and spleen enlargement as described in the section on the abdomen.

---

> ### (⌀) Key points: Lymph node enlargement
>
> • *'Shotty' mobile nodes:* are common and of no concern
> • *If one gland is found to be enlarged:* carefully examine for lymphadenopathy elsewhere
> • *If lymphadenopathy is generalized:* examine for hepatosplenomegaly; blood tests are essential

---

## Genitalia

Baby boys need to be examined for undescended testicles (see also p. 315). Otherwise, genitalia are not usually examined unless there is a particular reason.

### Observation
Inspect the scrotum. If it is underdeveloped, this suggests undescended testicles. An enlarged scrotum may

indicate a hydrocoele. Look at the groin for swellings; look for hypospadias.

### Palpation
Palpate the testes with warm hands. If you cannot feel them, they may have retracted or they may be undescended. Retracted testes can usually be milked down from the inguinal area into the scrotum. If you are unsuccessful, it may help to examine the child squatting or sitting cross-legged (see Figure 2.3, p. 24).

Swelling in the groin is usually caused by enlarged lymph nodes, hernia or a gonad (see also p. 313). You should be able to distinguish them clinically. An *inguinal hernia* extends into the groin and the testis is palpable separate from the swelling. In a *hydrocoele* the testis cannot be palpated through the fluid. Lymph nodes have clear borders.

### Transillumination
This is useful to distinguish a hydrocoele from a hernia. When you hold a light to the scrotum, a hydrocoele transilluminates, whereas a hernia does not.

## Neurological examination of children

Neurological assessment in infants is discussed on p. 75. The interpretation of neurological signs is shown in Box 4.9.

| Box 4.8 How to examine the nervous system in an older child | |
|---|---|
| **Observation** | |
| Dysmorphic signs | |
| Abnormal movements | |
| Gait | |
| Gower's sign | |
| Posture | |
| **Motor examination** | |
| Muscle bulk | |
| Tone | |
| Power | |
| Coordination | |
| **Reflexes** | |
| Deep tendon jerks | |
| Plantar reflex | |
| Clonus | |
| **Sensation** | |
| Light touch | |
| Pain | |
| Temperature | |
| Proprioception | |
| **Cerebellar signs and coordination** | |
| Tremor | |
| Nystagmus | |
| Finger–nose test | |
| Heel–shin test | |
| Dysdiadochokinesis | |
| Ataxia – heel–toe walking | |
| Romberg's test | |
| Dysarthria | |
| **Cranial nerves** | |
| I | Smell |
| II | Fundi and vision |
| III, IV, VI | Eye movements |
| V | Clench teeth |
| | Facial sensation (Corneal reflex) |
| VII | Shut eyes |
| | Show teeth |
| VIII | Hearing |
| IX, X, XII | Stick out tongue. Uvular deviation (gag reflex) |
| XI | Turn head against resistance |
| | Shrug shoulders |

| Box 4.9 Interpretation of neurological signs |
|---|
| **Cerebellar signs** |
| Nystagmus |
| Intention tremor |
| Incoordination |
| Ataxia |
| Dysarthria |
| **Upper motor neurone lesion, e.g. cerebral palsy** |
| Hypertonia/spasticity |
| Increased deep tendon reflexes |
| Positive Babinski sign |
| Clonus |
| **Peripheral disease, e.g. muscular dystrophy** |
| Hypotonia |
| Weakness |
| Reduced/absent deep tendon jerks |
| Gower's sign |

## Abnormal movements

These may occur in children with neurological disorders. The commonest is choreoathetosis (writhing movements of the limbs), usually associated with facial grimacing. Sudden jerking movements may be due to myoclonic epilepsy or, in infants, infantile spasms (pp. 210, 211).

## Gait

In ambulant children, observing the way they walk (gait) is very important. An abnormal gait can be accentuated by asking the child to walk on tiptoes or run. Abnormal gait patterns include:

- *Stiffness.* This is the commonest major abnormality and suggests an upper motor neurone lesion, usually cerebral palsy (Figure 4.24). In mild cases you may only see it by asking the child to run. The patterns of movement in different types of cerebral palsy are discussed in Chapter 12.
- *Waddling.* The child with spastic diplegia has a more knock-kneed gait (Figure 4.25). The predominant feature is adduction of both thighs, so that the knees are flexed and knock together with the ankles apart. The child tends to take weight on the toes or anterior part of the foot. Waddling is also seen in Duchenne muscular dystrophy or congenital dislocation of the hips.
- *Ataxia.* The child walks unsteadily with a broad-based gait.

## Observation

### Dysmorphic signs

Look for unusual facial or other features that may suggest a genetic disorder or syndrome (Box 4.8).

## Gower's sign

Weakness is suspected if the child finds it difficult to get up from a sitting position on the floor. In Gower's

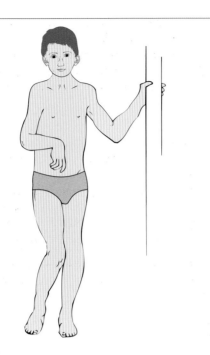

**Figure 4.24** A child with hemiplegia. The gait can be exaggerated by asking the child to run.

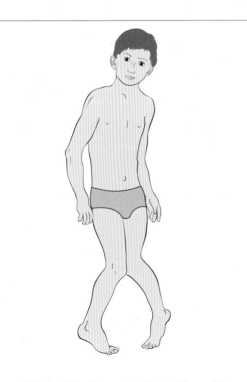

**Figure 4.25** A child with spastic diplegia. The gait is waddling.

sign, the child 'climbs up' his or her legs to a standing position (Figure 12.4).

## Muscle bulk

Look for muscle wasting and compare one side with the other. Wasting of muscle groups occurs in both upper motor neurone disorders (cerebral palsy) and in lower motor neurone lesions (spina bifida, nerve palsies).

## Posture

Observe the child's posture and look for evidence of contractures.

### Motor examination

## Tone

Muscle tone is defined as resistance to passive stretch. Lie the child down and move the major joints through their passive range of movement, feeling for resistance. *Hypertonia* (increased tone) suggests an upper motor neurone lesion and *hypotonia* (reduced tone, floppiness) a lower motor neurone lesion. *Spasticity* is the term used to describe spasm in a muscle group with increased tone. In cerebral palsy, the thigh adductors in the legs are most affected. To test for this, grasp the ankles (see Figure 4.26), abduct the legs and assess resistance. Then passively dorsiflex and plantarflex the foot. Resistance occurs particularly in dorsiflexion.

## Power

If the child can cooperate, test opposing muscle groups in both the arms and the legs. The muscle

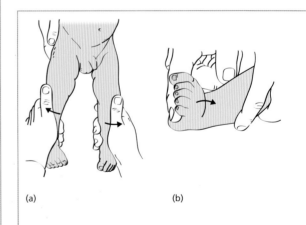

(a)  (b)

**Figure 4.26** Assessment of tone in the lower limbs: (a) assessment of adductor tone and (b) tone assessed at ankle by dorsiflexion/plantarflexion.

power around each joint should be assessed Ask the child to do the following manoeuvres against resistance:

*Upper limbs*
    Arms out to the side
    Bend your elbows
    Push out straight
    Squeeze fingers
    Hold the fingers out straight
    Spread fingers apart
*Lower limbs*
    Lift up your leg
    Bend your knee
    Straighten your leg
    Bend your foot down
    Cock up your foot

## Coordination

Coordination is part of the motor examination and is discussed below with other cerebellar signs.

### Reflexes

The reflexes may be normal, exaggerated (upper motor neurone lesion), reduced (lower motor neurone lesion) or absent. Before you conclude that a reflex is absent try *distraction* (reinforcement): ask the child to clench their teeth hard or to grasp their hands together and pull them apart, then try to elicit the reflex again.

    Check the following deep tendon reflexes:

- Biceps
- Triceps
- Supinator
- Knee
- Ankle

In young children, the ankle jerk is most easily elicited by gently holding the foot in a slightly dorsiflexed position with your thumb over the ball of the foot. You tap the hammer on your thumb and observe the elicited plantarflexion of the foot (Figure 4.27).

**Plantar reflex.** Use your thumb nail to stroke the lateral border of the sole of the foot firmly from the heel to the little toe. The response may be upgoing in infants until the age of 8 months, but thereafter downgoing is normal. A positive Babinski sign is an asymmetrical response or an upgoing response beyond the age of 8 months, and suggests an upper motor neurone lesion; clonus may also be present.

**Clonus.** Grasp the foot and sharply dorsiflex it. Clonus is present if repetitive jerking movements occur.

### Sensation

In older, cooperative children, sensation is tested in the same way as it is for adults, but sensory loss is not a common finding in children with upper motor neurone lesions. Compare one side with the other and make sure you ask the child to close his or her eyes so that there are no visual clues. Check for:

- *Light touch* using cotton wool
- *Pain* with a blunt needle
- *Temperature*
- *Proprioception* (position sense). Grasp the sides of the distal phalanx of the toe or thumb between your thumb and index finger. Move it up and down and ask the child which position it is in when you stop.

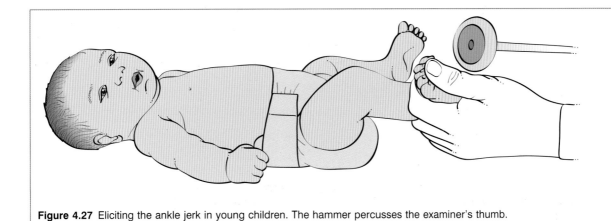

**Figure 4.27** Eliciting the ankle jerk in young children. The hammer percusses the examiner's thumb.

## Cerebellar signs and coordination

### Tremor
Ask the child to hold his or her arms outstretched and observe if there is a tremor.

### Nystagmus
Ask the child to look at your finger and move it from one side to the other, and up and down. Nystagmus is an involuntary rapid horizontal movement of the eye and is a sign of cerebellar, vestibular or brainstem dysfunction.

### Nose–finger test
Ask the child to touch the tip of their nose and then the tip of your finger. Once they have the idea, ask them to do this as quickly as possible while you move your finger. In ataxia the child will find it difficult to touch their nose or your finger accurately. Test both hands separately. *Intention tremor* is characteristic of damage to the posterior lobe of the cerebellum: the child's hand is steady at rest but develops a tremor of increasing amplitude as it approaches the target.

### Heel–shin test (see Figure 4.28)
With the child lying on their back, ask them to run the heel of one foot down the front of the shin, and see how accurately this is done.

### Dysdiadochokinesis
Ask the child to pronate and supinate their forearms quickly and repeatedly slap one hand with the front and back of the other hand. Impairment of rapid alternating movements is called dysdiadochokinesia.

### Gait
Observe the gait with heel-toe walking along a line. In ataxia, movements will be clumsy and jerky.

### Romberg's sign
Ask the child to stand with feet together and eyes open and then closed. Romberg's sign is loss of postural sensation with unsteadiness when the eyes are closed (Figure 4.29).

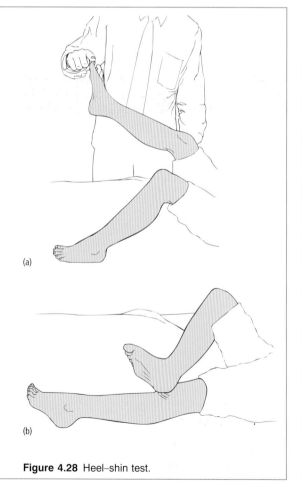

(a)

(b)

**Figure 4.28** Heel–shin test.

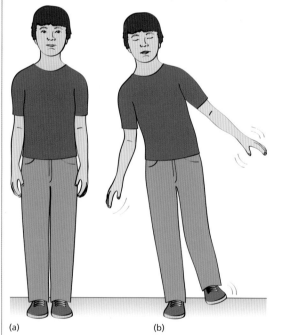

(a)                    (b)

**Figure 4.29** Romberg's test: (a) child standing with feet together and eyes open; (b) same child unbalanced with eyes closed (positive for Romberg's sign).

**Speech**

Note the quality of the child's speech. A child with a cerebellar lesion may have a halting, jerking dysarthria.

*Cranial nerves*

In older children the cranial nerves are tested in exactly the same way as they are in adults. Some information about cranial nerve function in young children can be obtained by observation (see below), but it is not always possible to formally examine the cranial nerves in uncooperative children.

| | |
|---|---|
| **I**<br>Olfactory nerve | Ask the child if he/she has a sense of smell, and test with a familiar non-irritant substance |
| **II**<br>Optic nerve | Fundi and vision (see p. 81) |
| **III, IV, VI**<br>Occulomotor trochlear and abducens nerves | Eye movements (see p. 81) |
| **V**<br>Trigeminal nerve | The motor component of the Vth nerve supplies the jaw muscles. Ask the child to open his/her mouth and bite hard. Palpate the masseter muscle. The Vth nerve also provides sensation to much of the face and is divided into the ophthalmic, maxillary and mandibular divisions. Test sensation to light touch in each of these areas. The corneal reflex is not routinely examined in children |
| **VII**<br>Facial nerve | Ask the child to screw up his/her eyes as tightly as possible and to show his/her teeth. Inability to bury the eyelashes on one side or close the eye, and drooping of the corner of the mouth, may indicate facial nerve palsy |
| **VIII**<br>Auditory nerve | Ask about hearing. If there is any doubt, or speech delay, you should obtain a hearing test |

| | |
|---|---|
| **IX, X, XII**<br>Glosso-pharyngeal, vagus and hypoglossal nerves | Ask the child to stick out his/her tongue, and look for tongue and uvula deviation. The gag reflex is not routinely examined in children |
| **XI**<br>Accessory nerve | Ask the child to turn his/her head to the sides against the resistance of your hand, and to shrug his/her shoulders |

# Neurological examination in babies

The neurological examination of babies (Box 4.10) is rather different from that of older children. Much is gained by observation and handling the baby, and a good developmental assessment is always required (see Chapter 5).

---

**Box 4.10 How to examine the nervous system in a baby**

**Observation**
Irritability/alertness
Position at rest
- frog position in hypotonia
- opisthotonos, scissoring in extreme hypertonia
Reduced spontaneous movement
Base of the spine
**Palpation**
Fontanelle
Head circumference
**Tone**
Prone
Supine
Pull to sit
Axillary suspension and weight bearing
Ventral suspension
Passive movements – assess popliteal angle
**Reflexes**
Deep tendon jerks
Primitive reflexes
**Vision**
**Hearing**
**Developmental assessment**

## Observation

Particular points to look for include:

- *Irritability.* Can the baby be consoled by cuddling?
- *Spontaneous movement.* Reduced movement suggests muscle weakness.
- *Position at rest.* See below.
- *Base of the spine.* Examine the base of the spine. A sacral dimple or tuft of hair can be an indication of a spinal abnormality.

## Palpation

The anterior fontanelle usually closes by 18 months. A bulging fontanelle suggests raised intracranial pressure and is a late sign in meningitis (p. 208).

## Tone

You assess tone by picking up and handling the baby. With experience you can identify hypo- and hypertonia. A floppy baby tends to slip through your hands, whereas a hypertonic baby feels stiffer. You can best assess tone by looking at the baby in a number of positions:

- *Supine position.* A hypotonic baby lies in a frog's leg position (see Figure 4.30). A hypertonic baby may have a retracted neck (opisthotonos) with scissoring of the legs.
- *Prone position.* Are the head and shoulders raised (depending on the baby's age)?
- *Pull to sit.* Pull the baby lying on its back into the sitting position. Head control is gradually achieved by 4 months of age. Head lag persists in a hypotonic baby. Look at the back to see how straight it is held.
- *Ventral suspension.* This is useful in a baby less than 3 months old. Put your hand under the baby's abdomen and lift him off the couch. A hypotonic baby will droop over your hand.
- *Axillary suspension.* Pick up the baby under the arms and test weight bearing. A floppy baby tends to slip through your hands like a rag doll. The hypertonic baby may demonstrate scissoring (see Figure 4.31). Babies generally start weight bearing when they are 5 months old.
- *Passive movements.* If tone is low, there is little resistance to passive movements. You can assess this by assessing the popliteal angle. If tone is high, the leg resists extension (Figure 4.32).

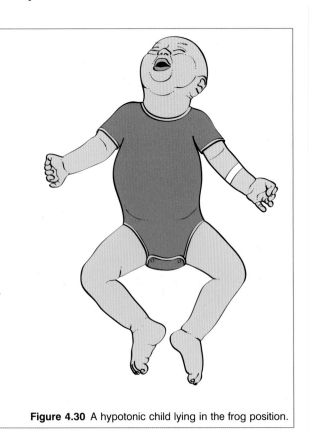

**Figure 4.30** A hypotonic child lying in the frog position.

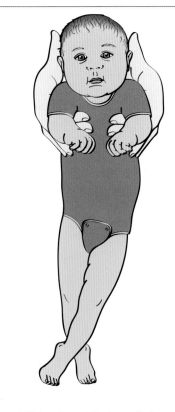

**Figure 4.31** Scissoring of the lower limbs.

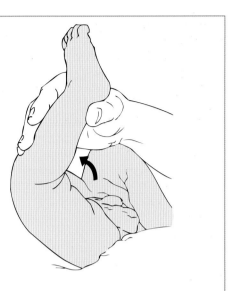

**Figure 4.32** The popliteal angle.

### Reflexes

#### Deep tendon reflexes

Check for these as described for older children. The ankle jerk may be more easily elicited by tapping your thumb over the ball of the foot (see Figure 4.27).

#### Primitive reflexes

Primitive reflexes (Figure 4.33) appear and disappear at different times, as shown in Table 4.6. If they are absent or persist beyond a given period, this suggests neurological dysfunction. The parachute reflex appears at 9 months of age and is elicited by pitching the baby forward. It comprises extension of both arms with extension of the hands (Figure 4.34). Asymmetry of this reflex may be an early sign of a unilateral upper motor neurone lesion (spastic hemiplegia).

### Vision

Check that the baby can fix and follow a silent moving object.

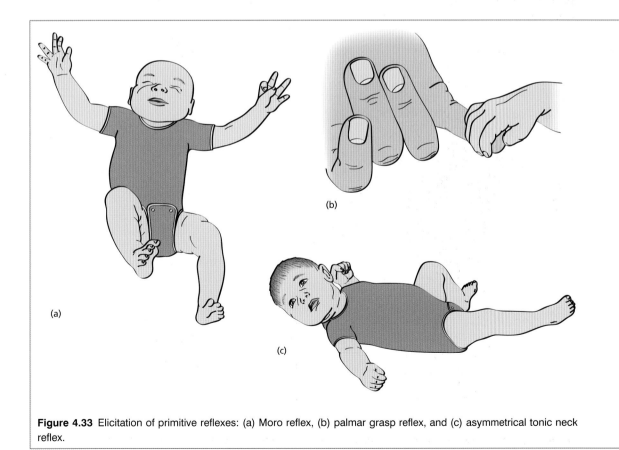

**Figure 4.33** Elicitation of primitive reflexes: (a) Moro reflex, (b) palmar grasp reflex, and (c) asymmetrical tonic neck reflex.

**Table 4.6** Age at which primitive reflexes appear and the latest age by which they should have disappeared. Persistence after this time is definitely abnormal

| Reflex | Description | Appearance | Disappearance |
|---|---|---|---|
| Stepping | The baby will step up when the dorsum of the foot touches the surface | Birth | 1 month |
| Moro | Symmetrical abduction and then adduction with extension of the arms when the baby's head is dropped back quickly into your hand (Figure 4.33a) | Birth | 3 months |
| Palmar grasp | Touching the palm with an object causes the baby to grip it (Figure 4.33b) | Birth | 3 months |
| Plantar reflex | Pressing on the ball of the foot causes the toes to curl | Birth | 8 months |
| Asymmetric tonic neck reflex (ATNR) | Turn the baby's head. The arm extends on the side the baby is facing and flexes on the opposite side (Figure 4.33c) | Birth | 6 months |
| Parachute reflex | Develops from 9 months and persists; elicit by pitching the baby forward suddenly (Figure 4.34) | 9 months | Persists |

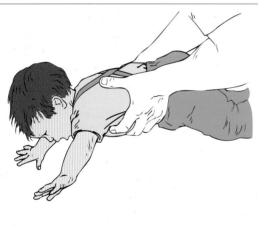

**Figure 4.34** The parachute reflex.

### Hearing

Screening for hearing is carried out neonatally on all babies (p. 24).

## The musculoskeletal system

Examination of the musculoskeletal system is very specialized. As an undergraduate you are only expected to examine a major joint such as the knee and to assess clinically for the presence of scoliosis.

### *Examination of a large joint*

#### Observation

• Observe the joint for swelling or redness. An effusion causes loss of definition of the joint. In the knee, the outline of the patella is lost, and if the effusion is mild, the normal concavity is lost first along its medial side.
• Observe the muscle bulk above and below the joint for wasting.

#### Palpation

• Palpate the joint for an effusion. This is most likely to be apparent in the knee. First look for the 'bulge sign' by milking fluid in the medial aspect of the knee into the lateral recess. Then firmly stroke the lateral side of the knee downwards to push the fluid back into the medial compartment. You will see a 'bulge' of fluid.
• If the effusion is large, use the 'patella tap' sign. Press firmly on the suprapatellar pouch with one hand to empty any fluid from there, then with the other hand push firmly downwards on the patella. If fluid is present in the knee, the patella will 'bounce'.

#### Range of movements

Move the joint through its normal range of movements to assess any limitation or contractures.

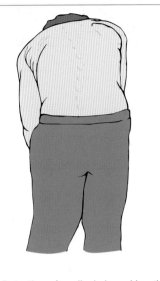

**Figure 4.35** Detection of scoliosis by asking the child to bend forward.

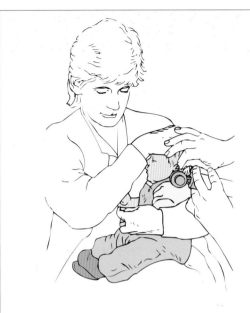

**Figure 4.36** Position to hold a baby for otoscopic examination.

### Scoliosis

Scoliosis is common in teenage girls, is usually idiopathic, and if severe can produce life-threatening cardiorespiratory compromise. It may be obvious by inspection of the back while the child is standing upright. The shoulders should be level, and note symmetrical prominence of a scapula.

The best way to examine a subtle scoliosis is to stand behind the child and ask him or her to bend forward at the waist and straighten up slowly. A fixed scoliosis causes prominence of the posterior ribs on the convex side of the bend (Figure 4.35).

## The ear, nose and throat

### Examination of the ear

Every doctor involved in the care of children should be able to examine ears competently. This is usually left to the end along with examination of the throat, as it is most likely to upset the young child. Ask the mother to hold the child on her lap with the child's head against her chest. To prevent a struggle, the mother's other hand should restrain the arms, and the legs be gripped gently between the mother's legs (Figure 4.36).

Hold the auroscope with your hand resting against the child's temple so that the instrument can move with the child. With your other hand, pull the pinna up to straighten the ear canal, or, in a baby, pull the earlobe down. Choose the largest possible speculum that will comfortably enter the meatus and do not advance it more than 0.5 cm in infants and 1 cm in older children. If wax is present, try to remove it gently.

Look at the tympanic membrane. The normal appearance is shown in Figure 4.37a. The membrane should be pale grey, shiny and translucent, with a light reflex at its anterior lower pole. Some middle ear structures can be seen through the membrane, including the handle of the malleus and the umbo. The normal drum lies in a neutral position. If there is increased pressure in the middle ear, as in otitis media, the drum bulges forward and is inflamed (Figure 4.37b). In glue ear (secretory otitis media), the drum may be retracted and dull and both the malleus and the umbo are very obvious (Figure 4.37c). The light reflex is also lost. In some cases, a fluid level can be seen through the membrane and air bubbles may also be present. Assessment of drum mobility is a specialized examination technique not carried out routinely.

### Examination of the nose

For a young child, sit the child as for examining the throat (see below). Examine the nostrils for inflammation, obstruction and polyps.

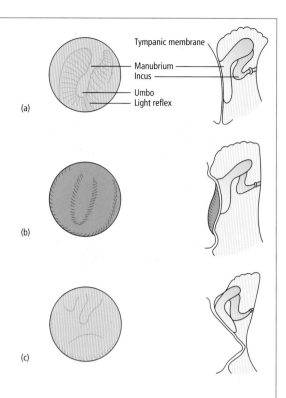

**Figure 4.37** Tympanic membrane appearances: (a) normal, (b) otitis media with a bulging drum, and (c) glue ear with a retracted drum.

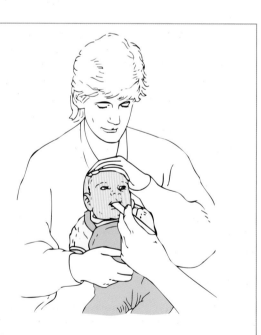

**Figure 4.38** Position for holding a child to examine the throat.

## Examination of the throat

Young children do not like to have their throats examined and this is best done with the child sitting on the mother's lap as shown in Figure 4.38. If the child is uncooperative and will not open his or her mouth, part the lips and teeth gently with the wooden spatula and depress the tongue. If the child cries, this facilitates the examination.

Examine the tonsils for size, redness and exudate. Normal tonsillar size varies enormously. The tonsils are lymphoid tissue and are very small at birth and grow to maximal size by 4–5 years, getting smaller in the early teens. Normal tonsils can appear very large in preschool children. If they meet in the midline, they are probably abnormally large. The signs of tonsillitis are discussed on p. 118.

In addition, examine the oropharynx, mucosa, teeth, tongue and palate. Feel for cervical lymphadenopathy.

## The visual system

> **Box 4.11 How to examine the eye**
>
> Assess each eye separately
> **Observation**
> **Visual acuity**
> **Eye movements**
> **Visual fields**
> **Reflexes**
>   Corneal light reflex
>   Pupillary reflex
>   Red reflex
> **Fundoscopy**
> **Cover test**

Look for any gross abnormality of the eyes. Note the size, shape and orientation, and examine the sclera, conjunctiva and iris. Look for a squint. Assess each eye separately: a child who has no vision in one eye may appear to have normal visual function if both eyes are assessed together (Box 4.11).

### Visual acuity

Gain visual attention in a newborn using a visually interesting object and move it to see if the baby's gaze follows. See if a toddler is able to see small blocks and tiny beads such as hundreds and thousands. Older children can be asked to count fingers, although it is obviously more accurate to use a Snellen chart. There

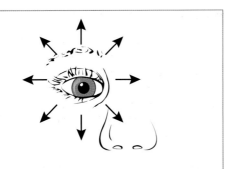

**Figure 4.39** The eight positions of gaze.

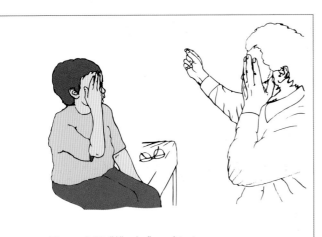

**Figure 4.40** 'Wiggly finger' test.

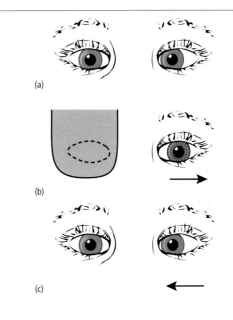

**Figure 4.41** Cover test to assess a squint.

are formal vision testing kits for young children: the Stycar rolling ball test uses small white balls of different sizes rolled across the floor.

## Eye movements

Ask the child to follow your finger through the full range of movement (see Figure 4.39). Note if there is limited movement in any direction. Bring your finger close to assess accommodation.

## Visual fields

The 'wiggly finger' test is used to assess children over 5 years, and compares the child's visual field with your own as a normal control. Sit one metre away from the child. Ask the child to look at your nose and hold his hand over his right eye. Cover your own left eye with your hand. Then gradually bring your finger into the child's range of vision and wiggle it at each of the eight sectors in turn (Figure 4.40). Ask the child to say when he first sees it. He should see the finger at the same point as you do. Repeat with the other eye.

## Reflexes

- *Corneal light reflex.* This is a misnomer as it is not really a reflex. The corneal light reflex is the reflection of a light source shone from about half a metre. The reflection should be symmetrically positioned in the centre of both corneas. If it is asymmetric, it indicates a squint.
- *Pupillary reflex.* Shine a bright light into the eye from 10 cm distance. You should see the pupil react and also consensual constriction in the other eye.
- *Red reflex.* This is also not a reflex. It is a test usually performed in the newborn period. Look through an ophthalmoscope 45 cm from the child's eye. A red reflection is normally seen. A white reflection suggests a cataract or other pathology.

## Fundoscopy

Fundoscopy is difficult in children. Ask the child to focus on a distant point. Approach the eye from the side and adjust the lens setting so that the retina comes into focus.

## *Cover test*

The cover test (Figure 4.41) is used to identify subtle and latent squints. Ask the child to look at an interesting object. Cover the normal eye without touching the face. The squinting eye rapidly flicks to fix on the object. Remove the cover and the squinting eye flicks

**Box 4.12 Examination for a squint**

Includes
- Corneal light reflex
- Ocular movements
- Visual acuity
- Cover test
- Fundoscopy

away again as the covered eye again becomes dominant. In a latent squint the squinting eye moves away when it is covered and flicks back again when the cover is removed.

If you suspect a squint your examination should include the features shown in Box 4.12.

# CHAPTER 5

# Developmental assessment

When I was One,
I had just begun.
When I was Two,
I was nearly new.
When I was Three,
I was hardly me.

*Now We Are Six,*
*AA Milne*

## COMPETENCES

### You must . . .

| Know | Be able to | Appreciate |
|---|---|---|
| • The key developmental milestones and at what age they are usually achieved<br>• At what age to be concerned if a milestone has not been achieved<br>• How to measure and weigh children accurately | • Engage the child and establish a rapport<br>• Carry out a developmental evaluation on a toddler by taking a history and observing the child | • That there is variability in the age when developmental milestones are achieved<br>• That you may need to repeat an evaluation before you can conclude that a child's development is concerning |

*Paediatrics and Child Health*, Third Edition. Mary Rudolf, Tim Lee, Malcolm Levene.
© 2011 Mary Rudolf, Tim Lee and Malcolm Levene. Published 2011 by Blackwell Publishing Ltd.

Developmental assessment (see Figure 5.1) is an integral part of the paediatric examination and carrying out a good assessment requires practice and skill. You need to be systematic in your approach to make sure that you have covered all areas of development and gained a good picture of the child's abilities. As a student you are expected to be able to competently assess preschool children, especially babies and toddlers. Figure 5.2 summarizes the key components.

It is helpful if you divide your developmental assessment into the four major areas:

- gross motor
- fine motor
- speech and language
- social

and attempt to work through each in turn (child permitting).

It is always hard to remember developmental milestones, but if you make sure that you learn the key landmarks indicated in Table 5.1, you will have a framework for assessing the child's skills. When you are with the child, concentrate on the tasks at hand and record carefully what you see. You can always check later to see the age at which a task is normally achieved.

Look to see whether the child can carry out the task, and also how it is carried out, as this can tell you whether there is a discrepancy between the child's understanding and performance. For example, a child with clumsiness or mild cerebral palsy may not be able to perform a motor task well, but may understand what is wanted, indicating that intellectual capacity is normal.

It is helpful to have a simple kit of tools to test development. A rattle, coloured one-inch blocks, a ball, and a formboard and crayons and paper will usually suffice, along with a few dolls or cars and simple pictures of common objects.

Major milestones of development for the first 2 years in each of the four developmental areas are summarized in Figures 5.3–5.6. You may find delay or abnormal development in one or more areas, and it is

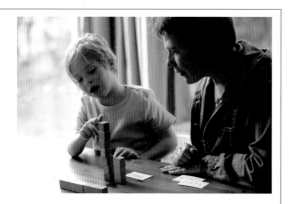

**Figure 5.1** Carrying out a developmental assessment. The most useful tools are small wooden bricks, a ball, a formboard and crayons and paper.

**Table 5.1** Milestones that are essential to memorize

| Age | Milestone |
| --- | --- |
| 4–6 weeks | Smiles responsively |
| 6–7 months | Sits unsupported |
| 9 months | Gets to a sitting position |
| 10 months | Start of pincer grasp |
| 12 months | Walks unsupported<br>Two or three words<br>Tower of two cubes |
| 18 months | Tower of three of four cubes |
| 24 months | Two- to three-word sentences |

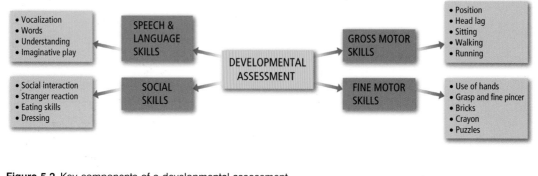

**Figure 5.2** Key components of a developmental assessment.

important that you carry out a thorough neurological examination to sort out whether there are neurological findings in addition.

Delay in all four areas usually indicates intellectual disability (p. 233), but an isolated delay in any one area is often not abnormal. Delay in walking alone (p. 231) is common and may have occurred in siblings or parents. Acquisition of speech is another common isolated delay; in all children with speech delay, deafness must be excluded. The interpretation of developmental delay is covered in detail in Chapter 12.

## Gross motor development

You should get an idea of gross motor skills (Figure 5.3) from a combination of informal observation and

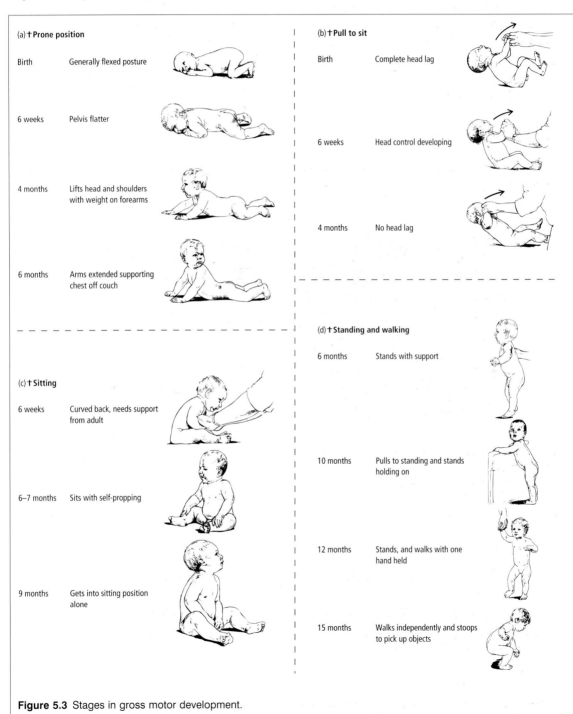

(a) † **Prone position**

| Birth | Generally flexed posture |
| 6 weeks | Pelvis flatter |
| 4 months | Lifts head and shoulders with weight on forearms |
| 6 months | Arms extended supporting chest off couch |

(b) † **Pull to sit**

| Birth | Complete head lag |
| 6 weeks | Head control developing |
| 4 months | No head lag |

(c) † **Sitting**

| 6 weeks | Curved back, needs support from adult |
| 6–7 months | Sits with self-propping |
| 9 months | Gets into sitting position alone |

(d) † **Standing and walking**

| 6 months | Stands with support |
| 10 months | Pulls to standing and stands holding on |
| 12 months | Stands, and walks with one hand held |
| 15 months | Walks independently and stoops to pick up objects |

**Figure 5.3** Stages in gross motor development.

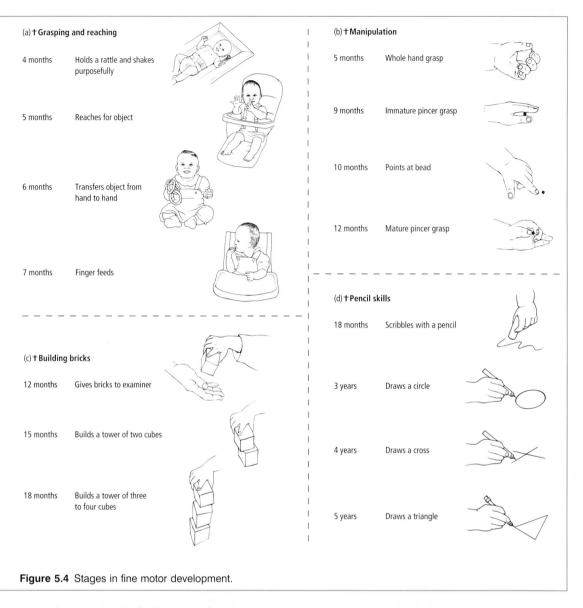

**(a) † Grasping and reaching**

| | |
|---|---|
| 4 months | Holds a rattle and shakes purposefully |
| 5 months | Reaches for object |
| 6 months | Transfers object from hand to hand |
| 7 months | Finger feeds |

**(b) † Manipulation**

| | |
|---|---|
| 5 months | Whole hand grasp |
| 9 months | Immature pincer grasp |
| 10 months | Points at bead |
| 12 months | Mature pincer grasp |

**(c) † Building bricks**

| | |
|---|---|
| 12 months | Gives bricks to examiner |
| 15 months | Builds a tower of two cubes |
| 18 months | Builds a tower of three to four cubes |

**(d) † Pencil skills**

| | |
|---|---|
| 18 months | Scribbles with a pencil |
| 3 years | Draws a circle |
| 4 years | Draws a cross |
| 5 years | Draws a triangle |

**Figure 5.4** Stages in fine motor development.

parental report. Start by looking at the baby's position. At birth an infant assumes a flexed posture, with the hips flexed and bottom tucked up when prone. By 6 weeks the pelvis is flatter on the table, and by 4 months the infant can lift head and shoulders off the couch. At 5 months he or she can roll over. By 6 months the arms are held extended, supporting the chest off the couch (Figure 5.3a).

Now get an idea of head control. Pull the baby to a sitting position and see the extent of head lag (Figure 5.3b). Good head control is achieved by 4 months. Then see how well the baby can sit. Sitting is achieved gradually as neck and trunk tone strengthen. The average age for sitting unsupported is 6–7 months, although at this stage the arms are still used for support. By 9 months the baby can get into the sitting position alone. By 11 months the child can pivot while sitting to reach toys (Figure 5.3c).

The next stage is mobility. A baby can move from sitting to crawling at 7–9 months, but some babies never pass through the crawling phase. Others bottom-shuffle. Pulling up to standing occurs at 10 months, and cruising (walking around while holding onto the furniture) occurs by 11 months (Figure 5.3d).

At around 12 months the baby walks with one hand held and can stand unsupported. Independent walking is achieved on average at 12–13 months, but this is very variable. At 15 months the baby can stand from crouching and can clamber up stairs.

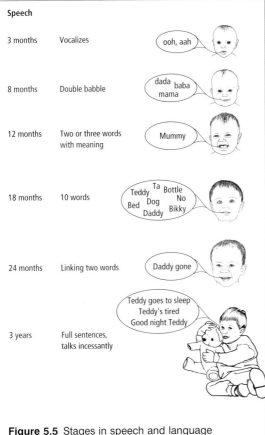

**Speech**

| 3 months | Vocalizes | ooh, aah |
| 8 months | Double babble | dada baba mama |
| 12 months | Two or three words with meaning | Mummy |
| 18 months | 10 words | Ta Bottle Teddy No Bed Dog Bikky Daddy |
| 24 months | Linking two words | Daddy gone |
| 3 years | Full sentences, talks incessantly | Teddy goes to sleep Teddy's tired Good night Teddy |

**Figure 5.5** Stages in speech and language development.

By 18 months the child can walk upstairs holding the banister and is very steady on the feet. He or she should be able to throw a ball without falling over. Failure to walk independently at 18 months requires investigation (p. 231).

## Fine motor development

Fine motor skills (Figure 4.2) require dexterity and cognitive ability. A child who lacks understanding of what he or she is being asked to do will not be able to demonstrate a task; you need to differentiate whether the problem is cognitive or motor.

Start by looking at how the baby uses his or her hands. At 1 month the hands are closed most of the time, but by 2 months they are held open. By 3 months the baby can hold a rattle and shake it. At 5 months he or she can reach out for a toy, and at 6 months can transfer it from one hand to the other. By 7 months the hands are used in play and exploration. The baby can grasp an object and bring it to the

mouth. This is the age where finger feeding is a natural development (Figure 5.4a).

By 9 months the finger movements become refined. At first there is a raking grasp using the whole palm, which by 10 months has developed into a scissor grasp using the thumb and first finger and, by 12 months, into finger–thumb apposition, also known as a pincer grasp (Figure 5.4b).

By 1 year, a baby will give a 2-cm square wooden block to you and release it. A child of 15 months can build a tower of two wooden cubes, and on of 18 months a tower of three to four cubes (Figure 5.4c). At this age a child scribbles with a crayon and can turn the pages of a book. Fine motor development advances rapidly after this. By the age of 3 children can draw a circle, at 4 years a cross and at 5 years a triangle (Figure 5.4d).

In the fourth year a child can draw a circle for a face and then progressively add limbs directly from the face, with one or two facial features such as eyes and mouth. It is not until 5 years that the child draws a body to which arms and hands are attached.

## Speech and language development

Speech and language development are summarized in Figure 5.5. You can expect young children to be too shy to talk to you directly and you will probably have to rely on a parent's report. In assessing language you need to try and assess:

- the child's understanding of receptive language
- the child's expressive language (speech)
- the child's play, which reflects their understanding of the world around them

A baby begins to vocalize at about 3 months and starts to enjoy playing with his or her voice. By 6 months he or she can make consonant sounds such as 'da', 'ba', 'ma' and 'ka'. By 8 months these are being combined into 'double babble' (dada, baba, mama).

The first recognizable word is spoken by 12 months, and two or three words are used with meaning. These words may be indistinct to any one other than the mother. Jargon (unintelligible but highly expressive 'language') develops at about 15 months of age. By 18 months the average child has 10–20 recognizable words, and by 24 months these are linked into two-word sentences. From then speech develops rapidly, so that by the age of 3 years the child can form full sentences and talks incessantly.

First get a grasp of how many words the child has. Then try to assess their understanding of language.

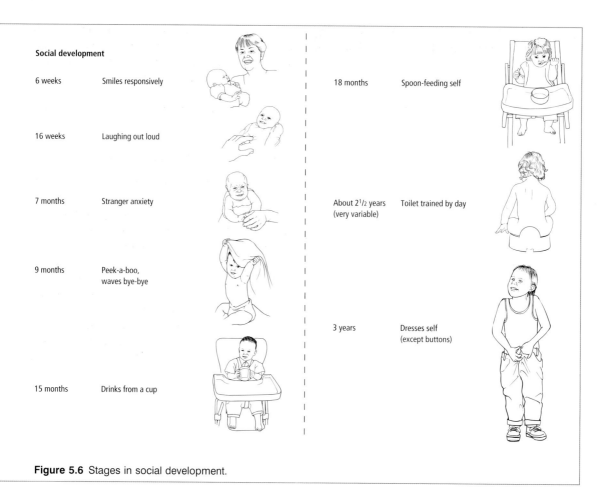

**Figure 5.6** Stages in social development.

Do they respond to 'where is daddy'? Can they carry out simple commands such as 'give' and 'take' or 'bring me'? Can they point to their nose or eyes? Lastly, explore their imaginative (or symbolic) play. Are they babying a doll, can they move a toy car forward? If a child hasn't yet started to talk but has rich imaginative play, it is a sign that their intellectual ability is less delayed.

If there is a delay in acquiring language it is essential to test hearing, as if this is not corrected language development can be irreversibly affected. Language delay is covered on p. 229.

## Social skills

Social development (summarized in Figure 5.6) refers to how a child interacts with people, and the acquisition of everyday skills such as eating and dressing. You will gain an idea of social skills by observing the child, and also from the parent. Sights and sounds are the most important stimuli that elicit reactions in a baby.

By 4 weeks babies quieten to speech, or open their eyes widely in response to the spoken word. At 6 weeks a baby smiles responsively, and this is a major milestone. For this to be considered a social reaction the child must smile in response to your (or a parent's) smile. Failure to smile by 8 weeks is definitely abnormal. By 12 weeks a baby squeals with pleasure, and by 16 weeks laughs out loud. By 20 weeks an infant smiles at him- or herself in a mirror.

At 7 months a baby begins to show 'stranger anxiety' and may get upset when you approach him. 'Permanence of objects' develops on average by 9 months – prior to this age, a baby shows no reaction when an object is dropped from view, but at 9 months will search for it. At this time a baby enjoys 'peek-a-boo' and by 10 months can appreciate that when a parent says 'no', he or she is displeased. Other important social features include waving bye-bye (9 months) and playing pat-a-cake (12 months).

At 15 months a child can drink from a cup, and use a spoon to eat with. At 24 months he or she may

| **Table 5.2** Developmental warning signs |
| --- |
| *At any age*<br>Maternal concern<br>Discordance in different developmental areas<br>Regression in previously acquired skills |
| *At 10 weeks*<br>No smile |
| *At 6 months*<br>Persistent primitive reflexes<br>Persistent squint<br>Hand preference<br>Little interest in people, toys, noises |
| *At 10–12 months*<br>No sitting<br>No double-syllable babble<br>No pincer grip |
| *At 18 months*<br>Not walking independently<br>Fewer than six words<br>Persistent mouthing and drooling |
| *At 2½ years*<br>No two- to three-word sentences |
| *At 4 years*<br>Unintelligible speech |

indicate toilet needs, with toilet training by day usually achieved by 2½ years (although night wetting is usual for some time beyond this). A baby starts to help with dressing by holding out an arm or leg at 1 year, and by 3 years should be able to dress and undress independently except for buttons and laces.

## Essential milestones and when to worry

It is impossible to remember all the milestones that children acquire in the course of development, but you do need to know the sequence of the stages for each of the developmental areas. This will help you carry out a developmental assessment thoroughly, and you can check whether the child's development is appropriate for age when you have completed your evaluation. There are some milestones that are essential to know, and these are shown in Table 5.1.

In addition, it is also important that you know when the lack of certain skills becomes abnormal and requires further investigation. These are summarized in Table 5.2.

# CHAPTER 6

# Investigations and their interpretation

We should use investigations like a drunk man uses a lamp post: for support rather than illumination.

*Anon.*

## COMPETENCES

### You must . . .

| Know | Be able to | Appreciate |
|---|---|---|
| • When common haematological and biochemical investigations are indicated and how to interpret abnormal results<br>• The criteria for diagnosing a urinary tract infection<br>• How to interpret CSF findings<br>• How to interpret the results of a sweat test<br>• When imaging is helpful, and the advantages and disadvantages of different types of scan | • Diagnose children presenting with an anaemic blood film<br>• Recognize biochemical test results indicative of dehydration, DKA and pyloric stenosis<br>• Interpret blood gases<br>• Read a chest X-ray<br>• Dipstick urine | • That investigations should only be requested to confirm a clinical diagnosis, and that 'fishing' for a diagnosis by ordering tests is poor medicine<br>• That the normal range of some biochemical tests differs in childhood<br>• That blood tests can be traumatic for children, and EMLA cream may help reduce the pain of blood taking |

*Paediatrics and Child Health*, Third Edition. Mary Rudolf, Tim Lee, Malcolm Levene.
© 2011 Mary Rudolf, Tim Lee and Malcolm Levene. Published 2011 by Blackwell Publishing Ltd.

## Introduction

Investigations should only be requested to confirm a clinical diagnosis or, if indicated, after taking a careful history and performing a physical examination. 'Fishing for a diagnosis by ordering a battery of tests is poor medicine, an unacceptable use of resources and not in the best interests of the child.

It is important to be able to interpret a number of investigations performed on children. In order to do this, you need to know the normal ranges for certain basic investigations. The importance of investigations is not simply to recognize if any value falls outside the normal range, but also to interpret the significance of the abnormality and how it influences diagnosis/management. The normal ranges in childhood for common investigations are listed in the tables below, together with the significance of abnormalities.

## Full blood count (FBC)

Normal values for the major haematological indices are shown in Table 6.1.

### Haemoglobin

At birth the haemoglobin concentration is high, with a mean of 18 g/dL, but falls rapidly to reach its lowest point at 2 months of age (range 9.5–14.5 g/dL) before increasing to a stable value at about 6 months. A low haemoglobin concentration indicates anaemia (p. 343). Figure 6.1 shows how it should be investigated.

### Mean cell volume

Mean cell volume (MCV) is a measurement of size (volume) of the red blood cell. In paediatrics, microcytic anaemia (MCV <76 fL) is the most common abnormality and is a result of iron deficiency anaemia (p. 345), thalassaemia trait (p. 346) or lead toxicity. An abnormally large red cell is rare and is most likely to be a result of folate deficiency. The MCV is normally high in the newborn for the first few weeks. A low MCV may precede a fall in haemoglobin level.

### Mean cell haemoglobin

Mean cell haemoglobin (MCH) refers to the amount of haemoglobin in the red cell. In iron deficiency anaemia it is usually low (hypochromic) in conjunction with microcytic anaemia.

### Examples of pathology

The two most important types of anaemia occurring in paediatrics are discussed below. Table 6.2 shows the important differences in distinguishing the two conditions.

### Microcytic hypochromic anaemia

The commonest causes of microcytic, hypochromic anaemia are iron deficiency (see Figure 6.2) and thalassaemia trait, although lead toxicity may also be responsible. To distinguish iron deficiency anaemia from thallassaemia trait, it is necessary to measure serum ferritin (low in iron deficiency anaemia) and

| Table 6.1 Normal range for the major haematological indices for children of 6 months and older | |
| --- | --- |
| | **Normal range** |
| Haemoglobin | 11–14 g/dL |
| Haematocrit | 30–45% |
| White cell count | 6.0–15.0 × 10⁹/L |
| Reticulocytes | 0–2% |
| Platelets | 150–450 × 10⁹/L |
| Mean cell volume | 76–88 (fL) |
| Mean cell haemoglobin | 24–30 pg |
| Erythrocyte sedimentation rate (ESR) | 10–20 mm in 1 hour |

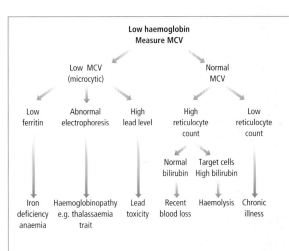
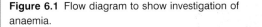

**Figure 6.1** Flow diagram to show investigation of anaemia.

**Table 6.2** Distinction between microcytic anaemia and anaemia resulting from haemolysis or blood loss (normal range)

|  | Microcytic hypochromic anaemia | Anaemia resulting from haemolysis or blood loss |
| --- | --- | --- |
| Haemoglobin | Low | Low |
| Haematocrit | Low | Low |
| White cell count | Normal | Normal |
| Reticulocytes | Low | High |
| Platelets | Normal | Low |
| Mean cell volume | Low | Normal |
| Mean cell haemoglobin | Low | Normal |

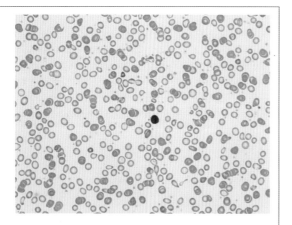

**Figure 6.2** A peripheral blood film in severe iron deficiency anemia. The red blood cells are microcytic and hypochromic with occasional target cells.

perform haemoglobin electrophoresis (abnormal in thalassaemia trait). However, as iron deficiency is so common, it is usual to give a therapeutic trial of iron supplementation first, and only investigate further if the response is inadequate. Lead poisoning is rare; if it is considered, a serum lead level is required.

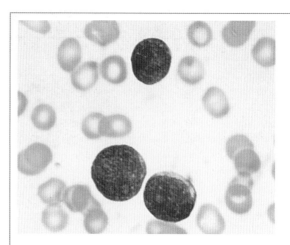

**Figure 6.3** Peripheral blood film of a child with acute lymphoblastic leukaemia.

**Anaemia with reticulocytosis**

This picture occurs as the result of haemorrhage or haemolysis. The reticulocyte count is increased, indicating an effort by the bone marrow to replenish the destroyed red cells. In haemolysis there may also be evidence of jaundice (p. 174), either clinically or on finding an elevated unconjugated bilirubin (Figure 6.1).

**Increased white cell count (leucocytosis)**

The white cell count is raised in three circumstances:

- *Viral infection* usually causes only a modest leucocytosis, with a preponderance of lymphocytes. In infectious mononucleosis, characteristic atypical lymphocytes are seen in the peripheral blood film.
- *Systemic bacterial infection* usually causes a higher white cell count ($15–30 \times 10^9$/L). The blood film shows that this is comprised mainly of excess polymorphonuclear granulocytes (neutrophils) with a preponderance of immature white cells (a left shift). These changes also can occur as the result of severe stress or administration of corticosteroids.
- In *leukaemia* the white cell count is very high, or occasionally very low, and blast cells are usually seen in the peripheral blood film (Figure 6.3). Platelet numbers are often also reduced.

## Blood chemistry

Modern analytical blood chemistry investigations can be done rapidly on small volumes of blood by an

**Table 6.3** Normal ranges for basic clinical chemistry variables

|  | Normal range |
|---|---|
| Sodium | 133–145 mmol/L |
| Potassium | 3.5–4.7 mmol/L |
| Chloride | 96–110 mmol/L |
| Bicarbonate | 20–27 mmol/L |
| Creatinine | 20–80 μmol/L |
| Urea | 2.5–6.5 mmol/L |
| Glucose | 3.0–6.0 mmol/L |
| Alkaline phophatase | Infant, 150–1000 unit/L |
|  | Child, 250–800 unit/L |

**Table 6.4** Causes of hyper- and hyponatraemia

| Causes | |
|---|---|
| *Hypernatraemia (Na⁺ >150 mmol/L)* | |
| Dehydration | Diarrhoea |
|  | Fluid deprivation |
| Excess sodium intake | Inappropriate milk feed preparation |
| *Hyponatraemia (Na⁺ <130 mmol/L)* | |
| Sodium loss | Gastroenteritis with hypotonic fluid replacement |
|  | Renal loss (renal failure) |
|  | Cystic fibrosis (p. 149) |
| Water excess | Excessive IV fluid administration |

automated process. One disadvantage of this is that the clinician receives results on all the variables that the machine is programmed to analyse, so the results printout may contain 12–20 different values. It is not necessary to memorize the normal ranges for all these, but it is important to be familiar with a limited number of them as shown in Table 6.3.

### Blood urea and serum creatinine

Urea and creatinine are widely used as an index of renal function and/or vascular hydration.

Urea is a major metabolite of protein breakdown and is both filtered and reabsorbed by the kidneys. Its concentration in the plasma is dependent on protein intake, state of catabolism and renal function. Because its value is dependent on so many variables, it is not a good measure of renal function. The commonest cause of an elevated urea concentration is dehydration.

Creatinine is produced by muscles at a constant rate and is influenced far less by catabolism than urea. It is filtered by the glomerulus, but a proportion is also secreted by the proximal tubules. Nevertheless, creatinine clearance is a reliable measure of glomerular filtration rate, and an isolated serum creatinine measurement is a much better index of renal function than urea.

### Sodium

In disease states sodium may be normal, increased (hypernatraemic; Na⁺ >150 mmol/L), or low (hyponat-

raemic; Na⁺ <130 mmol/L). These abnormalities are described under dehydration (p. 387). Causes of hypo- and hypernatraemia are shown in Table 6.4.

### Potassium

Potassium is the major intracellular cation and is in relatively low concentration in the extracellular spaces. Artefactually high serum potassium levels may be found as the result of red cell haemolysis caused by keeping blood for too long in the container before analysis. If the blood is seen to be haemolysed when it is analysed, the serum potassium level measured will be unreliable.

Hypokalaemia most often occurs as the result of gastroenteritis or pyloric stenosis (see below). Hyperkalaemia results from renal failure and increases as a result of metabolic acidosis. In diabetic ketoacidosis (DKA) the serum potassium is high, but drops rapidly after the DKA is treated.

### Alkaline phosphatase

Alkaline phosphatase represents a group of isoenzymes arising from bone and liver. It increases as a result of bone growth and is therefore higher in childhood; in neonates the normal range may be up to four times that of the adult.

A very high alkaline phosphatase concentration may represent bone disease (particularly rickets) or, less commonly in children, cholestatic liver disease.

# Blood gases and acid–base balance

Normal acid–base and blood gas values are shown in Table 6.5.

Disturbances in acid–base chemistry occur as the result of either respiratory or metabolic disorders. Table 6.6 lists the causes of acidosis and alkalosis.

## Blood pH

The acidity of blood is measured by pH. Normal pH range is 7.35–7.42; measurements above this refer to alkalosis and values below it indicate acidosis. In order to decide if the acidosis or alkalosis is metabolic or respiratory, you need to look at the $P_{CO_2}$ and bicarbonate levels (see below).

## $P_{O_2}$

The partial pressure of oxygen ($P_{O_2}$) in arterial blood indicates whether the child is hypoxic (low $P_{O_2}$) or hyperoxic (high $P_{O_2}$). If the $P_{O_2}$ is low, it is generally possible to increase it by using a mask or head box and adjusting the inspired oxygen to keep the $P_{O_2}$ in the normal range (normoxic). Transcutaneous oxygen saturation monitoring is now widely used for continuous oxygen assessment.

## $P_{CO_2}$

A high partial pressure of carbon dioxide ($P_{CO_2}$) indicates underventilation. This may occur in coma or be caused by intrinsic respiratory disease such as respiratory distress syndrome (p. 420). A high $P_{CO_2}$ causes respiratory acidosis (see Table 6.7).

A low $P_{CO_2}$ in a mechanically ventilated child indicates that the machine's settings are too high for the state of the child's lungs. It also occurs when a child hyperventilates and excessively 'blows off' carbon dioxide, as can sometimes occur with anxiety. A low $P_{CO_2}$ causes respiratory alkalosis (see Table 6.7).

## Bicarbonate

This anion varies with acid–base status. In metabolic acidosis the serum bicarbonate is low. Examples of situations where this occurs are neonatal asphyxia (p. 401) and diabetic ketoacidosis (p. 278).

In acute respiratory acidosis the bicarbonate may initially be normal, but then rises in an attempt to compensate and normalize the pH.

**Table 6.6** Causes of acidosis and alkalosis

|  | **Causes** |
|---|---|
| Metabolic acidosis | Severe gastroenteritis |
|  | Neonatal asphyxia |
|  | Shock |
|  | Diabetic ketoacidosis |
| Metabolic alkalosis | Pyloric stenosis |
| Respiratory acidosis | Respiratory failure of any cause |
| Respiratory alkalosis | Overventilation |
|  | Overbreathing |

**Table 6.5** Normal ranges for acid–base and blood gas measurements

| | |
|---|---|
| Arterial pH | 7.35–7.42 |
| Arterial $P_{CO_2}$ | 4.0–5.5 kPa |
| Arterial $P_{O_2}$ | 11–14 kPa (lower values in neonates, 8–10 kPa) |
| Arterial or venous bicarbonate | 17–27 mmol/L |

**Table 6.7** Changes in acid–base and blood gas values according to type of alkalosis or acidosis

|  | **Metabolic acidosis** | **Metabolic alkalosis** | **Respiratory acidosis** | **Respiratory alkalosis** |
|---|---|---|---|---|
| pH | Low | High | Low | High |
| $P_{O_2}$ | Normal | Normal | Normal or low | Normal or high |
| $P_{CO_2}$ | Normal or low* | Normal or high* | High | Low |
| Bicarbonate | Low | High | Normal or high* | Normal or low* |

* Compensated state.

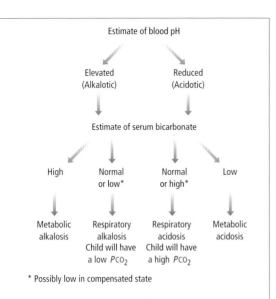

Estimate of blood pH

Elevated (Alkalotic) — Reduced (Acidotic)

Estimate of serum bicarbonate

High — Normal or low* — Normal or high* — Low

Metabolic alkalosis — Respiratory alkalosis Child will have a low $P_{CO_2}$ — Respiratory acidosis Child will have a high $P_{CO_2}$ — Metabolic acidosis

* Possibly low in compensated state

**Figure 6.4** Flow diagram to guide the interpretation of blood gas results.

The only cause of a high bicarbonate in paediatrics is excessive vomiting due to pyloric stenosis (see below and p. 176).

## A simple approach to interpreting blood gases

Blood gases are not difficult to interpret if you take a systematic approach (see Figure 6.4).

First look at the pH and decide if the child is acidotic (pH < 7.35) or alkalotic (pH > 7.42).

- *If the child is acidotic*, decide if the cause is respiratory or metabolic. To do this, you need to look at the $P_{CO_2}$ and the serum bicarbonate. If the $P_{CO_2}$ is high, it means the child is in respiratory distress and is not able to blow off carbon dioxide adequately, thus causing a respiratory acidosis. Confirm this by looking at the serum bicarbonate. It is likely to be high, as the body tries to compensate for the acidosis by retaining bicarbonate. The $P_{O_2}$ may be low if the respiratory condition means that the child is unable to take in enough oxygen.

If the child is acidotic but the $P_{CO_2}$ is normal or low, retention of carbon dioxide is obviously not the cause of the acidosis – so now turn to the bicarbonate. It will be low, indicating that the acidosis is metabolic. This occurs in neonatal asphyxia, gastroenteritis, diabetic ketoacidosis or shock, when the body tissues accumulate acid due to poor tissue perfusion. The

$P_{CO_2}$ may also be low in an attempt to raise the pH by blowing off carbon dioxide.

- *If the child is alkalotic*, the cause again will be respiratory or metabolic. Once again, look at the $P_{CO_2}$. If it is low, it means the child is hyperventilating (or being overventilated) and is blowing off too much carbon dioxide, thus making the pH rise and causing a respiratory alkalosis. You may find a low bicarbonate level as the body tries to compensate metabolically.

If the $P_{CO_2}$ is normal or high, the alkalosis is not respiratory and you will find the source is a high bicarbonate causing a metabolic alkalosis. Since the body is naturally an acid-producing machine, this situation is rare and essentially only occurs in pyloric stenosis when $H^+$ ions are lost through vomiting.

### *Examples of pathology*

#### Dehydration

Three types of dehydration occur: hyper-, iso- and hyponatraemic.

- *Isotonic dehydration.* In this form of dehydration, there are equal losses of sodium and water, so the serum sodium is normal. This is the commonest form, and children show physical signs commensurate with the degree of fluid loss.
- *Hyponatraemic dehydration.* In this type of dehydration, the serum sodium is less than 130 mmol/L. This is a result of $Na^+$ loss in excess of fluid loss. The cause is usually replacement of fluid losses, such as diarrhoea, with hypotonic solutions such as water or fizzy drinks. The child is lethargic and the skin is dry and inelastic.
- *Hypernatraemic dehydration.* In this type of dehydration the serum $Na^+$ is above 150 mmol/L. It may be caused by severe and acute water loss, but more commonly occurs when a parent gives overconcentrated formula feeds by incorrectly measuring out scoops of powdered milk. Metabolic acidosis is a common feature of this condition. The child characteristically appears to be very hungry, but has fewer clinical signs of dehydration. The skin feels doughy.

#### Diabetic ketoacidosis (p. 278)

The major metabolic and electrolyte abnormalities in DKA occur as a result of hyperglycaemia and ketoacidosis. The blood pH falls as a result of accumulation of ketoacids. As a consequence of the metabolic acidosis, the child attempts to compensate by hyperventilation (Kussmaul breathing, p. 380) which reduces the $P_{CO_2}$. The high blood sugar causes an osmotic diuresis which leads to progressive dehydration with increased creatinine/urea levels. The main biochemical abnormalities are therefore summarized as:

- pH                 low
- $P_{CO_2}$         low
- bicarbonate        low
- sodium             normal
- potassium          high
- creatinine/urea    high
- glucose            high

### Pyloric stenosis (p. 176)

In this condition vomiting causes excessive loss of hydrogen and chloride ions with increasing alkalosis. Because of the obstruction between stomach and duodenum, there is little sodium and potassium loss in the vomitus. Bicarbonate is increased and potassium is lost through the kidney in exchange for conserving hydrogen ions. The abnormalities seen in pyloric stenosis are:

- pH                 high
- bicarbonate        low
- chloride           low
- potassium          low
- sodium             normal or low
- creatinine/urea    normal or high

## Cerebrospinal fluid

Meningitis can only be diagnosed by examining the cerebrospinal fluid (CSF) at lumbar puncture. This should not be performed if there are signs of raised intracranial pressure as coning may occur (p. 209).

- The *pressure* of the CSF can be measured as the first drop of CSF emerges. This is most easily done by connecting a calibrated plastic tube to the needle and waiting for the fluid level to stabilize. The child must be quiet when the pressure is measured as crying causes an artefactually high pressure. Normal CSF pressure is <5 cm$H_2O$.
- The *colour* of the CSF should be described. It is normally absolutely clear, and cloudiness suggests infection. Bloodstained CSF may occur as a result of intracranial bleeding or as the result of a traumatic tap. A traumatic tap occurs if a blood vessel is penetrated by the needle on passage into the subarachnoid space. Intracranial bleeding can be differentiated from a traumatic tap by allowing the bloodstained fluid to drip into three successive containers. If the blood staining becomes less in successive containers, the tap was traumatic, but if the blood staining remains uniform throughout the three containers, it is likely to be because of intracranial haemorrhage. Old blood from a previous haemorrhage gives a yellow 'xanthochromic' appearance.

The CSF should be sent to the laboratory for the following analyses:

- *Microscopy.* No cells should be seen; more than five white cells in a non-bloody tap is indicative of meningitis. In bacterial meningitis there are a large number of polymorphs, whereas in viral meningitis there are smaller numbers of lymphocytes. Organisms may be seen on Gram's stain.
- *Chemistry.* A blood sugar should be taken at the same time as the lumbar puncture to compare the plasma with the CSF glucose concentration (the normal ratio is 2–3:1). In bacterial meningitis the CSF glucose is generally reduced to <50% of the plasma glucose. The chemistry results obtained from CSF contaminated by blood reflect serum rather than CSF levels and are therefore unreliable.
- *Culture.*
- *PCR.* If meningococcal or herpes infection are considered, the sample can be sent for polymerase chain reaction analysis.

Normal CSF findings and abnormalities found as a result of viral and bacterial meningitis are shown in Table 6.8.

## Urinalysis

It is important that you are able to examine urine, carry out urinalysis using commercially available dipsticks and interpret laboratory results. Fresh urine should be collected into a sterile container from a midstream specimen if possible. A urine bag applied over the genitalia can be used in babies, or sterile cotton balls placed in a clean nappy, but beware of contamination. If the child is ill, and cannot produce urine, the specimen needs to be obtained by suprapubic aspiration or catheterization.

### Observation

Look at the specimen in a clear test tube or equivalent container and comment on its colour and odour. In particular note the following:

- *Clarity.* Is the urine cloudy? (suggests infection).
- *Colour.* Red or brown urine suggests the presence of blood. A red or pink colour suggests the bleeding

**Table 6.8** Interpretation of CSF analysis

|  | Normal | Bacterial meningitis | Viral meningitis |
|---|---|---|---|
| Appearance | Clear | Turbid | Clear |
| Gram's stain | No organisms | Organisms identified | No organisms |
| White cells | <5/mm$^3$ | +++Polymorphs (in early stages cells may be absent) | + Lymphocytes (in early stages cells may be absent) |
| Protein | 0.15–0.4 g/L | High | Normal |
| Glucose | <50% of blood glucose | Low | Normal |
| Culture | No growth | Positive growth (unless partially treated) | No growth |

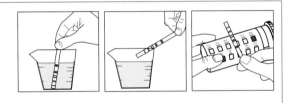

**Figure 6.5** Testing urine using dipsticks.

is from the lower urinary tract. Cola-coloured urine suggests the blood has come from the kidneys.
- *Odour.* A smell of acetone indicates the presence of ketone bodies.

## Dipstick testing

Dipsticks contain a number of reagent blocks, each one about 5 mm$^2$. Depending on the type of stick, there may be up to 10 reagent squares on the stick. The tests are all at best semiquantitative (expressed as +, ++, etc.), so if quantitative information is required, the urine should be sent to the laboratory for analysis.

The procedure for dipsticking is illustrated in Figure 6.5.

**1** Immerse the entire dipstick area (all the reagent squares) in the urine and remove the stick immediately.
**2** Shake off excess urine from the stick.
**3** Hold the strip in a horizontal position and compare the test areas with the colour chart label on the container.

Many of the reagent squares require the result to be read at an exact time after the exposure to urine.

This information is on the colour chart and is summarized in Table 6.9. Colour changes that occur after 2 minutes are of no reliability and should be discarded. Increasingly these dipsticks are placed into a point-of-care automated analyser which produces a printed report of the dipstick result.

## Urinalysis and culture

The only way to diagnose a urinary tract infection is on microscopy and culture. A pure growth of >10$^5$ colony-forming units (cfu) of a single organism is indicative of a urinary tract infection. There will also be >50 white cells. Except when a specimen has been obtained by catheter or suprapubic aspiration, contamination is often a problem. You should suspect contamination if more than one type of organism is grown, and if bacteria are found but unaccompanied by large numbers of white cells on microscopy. The laboratory will provide information on the sensitivity of the organism to a number of antibiotics.

If significant haematuria, proteinuria, nitrites or leucocytes (more than +) are found on the dipstick, the sample should be sent for microscopy in the laboratory.

### *Examples of pathology*

#### Haematuria

Haematuria can result from a urinary tract infection, acute glomerulonephritis, stone, tumour or a congenital malformation. The approach to diagnosing the cause of haematuria is discussed in detail on p. 301.

#### Proteinuria

Proteinuria is an important sign of renal disease. The standard way of quantifying it is through analysis of

**Table 6.9** Timing and interpretation of dipstick urinalysis

| Substance in urine | Time for block to be read | Comments |
| --- | --- | --- |
| Glucose | 30 s | This test is specific for glucose, not other reducing substances. Glycosuria is indicative of diabetes mellitus |
| Bilirubin | 30 s | Any bilirubin in the urine must be further investigated |
| Ketones | 40 s | Reagent block only reacts to acetoacetic acid, which occurs on fasting and is always present in DKA |
| Specific gravity | 45 s | Assesses how concentrated or dilute the urine is, particularly useful in the diagnosis of diabetes insipidus or the syndrome of inappropriate anti-diuretic hormone (SIADH) |
| Blood | 60 s | This is a very sensitive test and may be positive in clear urine. Quantification of haematuria by urine microscopy should be carried out if positive. For diagnosis of haematuria see p. 301 |
| pH | 60 s | pH correlates with the best colour match on card |
| Protein | 60 s | This is very sensitive and a trace or a '+' is usually not significant. If there is significant proteinuria, obtain a 24-hour urine collection for analysis in the lab |
| Urobilinogen | 60 s | High levels may be seen in jaundice |
| Nitrites | 60 s | A positive result suggests bacterial infection |
| Leucocytes | 120 s | A positive result suggests bacterial infection, especially if nitrites also positive. Confirm by sending urine for microscopy and culture |

DKA, diabetic ketoacidosis.

a 24-hour collection of urine. An important paediatric cause is nephrotic syndrome, where the child presents with generalized oedema (see p. 308).

### Urinary tract infection

A typical example of urine findings is as follows:

| | |
| --- | --- |
| Dipstick | Positive for blood, protein, nitrite and leucocytes (+, ++, etc.) |
| Urinalysis | White cells >50 × $10^6$<br>Red cells 1–10 × $10^6$ |
| Urine culture | >$10^5$ cfu/mL coliform species<br>Trimethoprim sensitive<br>Nitrofurantoin sensitive<br>Cefradine sensitive |

## Reading a chest X-ray

In most cooperative children a posterior–anterior (PA) film is taken in inspiration. This means that the child stands with his or her chest against the X-ray plate and the X-ray beam is directed from the back through the chest to the plate. In sick children or neonates the film is usually anterior–posterior (AP), when the baby lies supine on the plate with the X-ray beam above. If the X-ray is AP this should be written on the film. Assume the film to be PA unless you are told otherwise.

For a complete radiological examination of the chest a lateral X-ray is necessary (see below). Normal appearances and the anatomical landmarks are shown in Figure 6.6, and abnormal findings in Figures 6.7 and 6.8.

It is important to approach reading a chest X-ray in a systematic manner (see Box 6.1). You are not necessarily expected to make a correct diagnosis, but you are expected to describe your findings clearly. The following approach is recommended.

- *Identification.* Check the patient's name on the X-ray, the date that the X-ray was taken and the orientation (right and left).

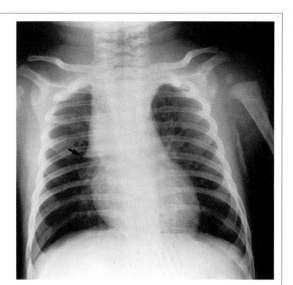

(a)

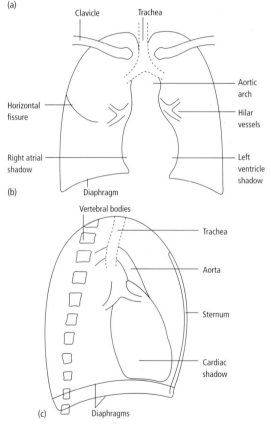

(b)

(c)

**Figure 6.6** (a) A normal PA chest X-ray. The thymus gland is seen as a 'sail-shaped' shadow (indicated by the arrow); (b) anatomical landmarks of a PA chest X-ray; (c) anatomical landmarks of a lateral chest X-ray.

- *Quality of the film.* Check that important anatomical landmarks have not been excluded, including the costophrenic angles, the ribs and soft tissues into the root of the neck. Comment on attached lines, endotracheal tube, drains, etc.
- Look at whether the *penetration* is good, under- or overexposed. An underexposed film will appear more white with less contrast and an overexposed film will be blacker with the bones clear but little distinction between the heart and the lung fields. Penetration is ideal if the vertebrae can just be seen through the heart shadow.
- Check the *positioning.* Is the patient standing square to the plane of the X-ray beam? You can see this by checking if the vertebral bodies and transverse processes are symmetrical. The clavicles and ribs should also be symmetrical. If there is rotation, the clavicles look asymmetrical. Estimating heart size or lung fields is unreliable in a rotated film.
- *Bony structures.* Look at the ribs, clavicles and vertebral bodies, and comment on any asymmetry or congenital abnormality. Count the ribs on both sides (12 pairs should be apparent). Missing ribs may occur as the result of cardiothoracic surgery or represent a congenital abnormality.
- *Diaphragms.* Both diaphragms should be clear, and the right is normally higher than the left because of the liver position. Examine the costophrenic angles, which should be clear and sharply defined. If they are not, a small pleural effusion is the cause. Look for air below the diaphragm, which is always abnormal.
- *Cardiac outline.* Measure the cardiac outline at its widest point and compare it to the widest diameter of the ribs to determine if there is cardiomegaly. In infants the normal ratio of cardiac to widest chest wall diameter is 0.6, and in older children a ratio of up to 0.5 is normal. Comment on the clarity of the cardiac outline. If the right border of the heart is obscured, this suggests right middle lobe collapse/consolidation (Figures 6.7 and 6.8b).
- *Lung fields.* The lung fields should be symmetrical and of uniform radiolucency. The only markings within the lung fields should be pulmonary blood vessels. Comment on the hilar shadows. It requires considerable experience to decide whether there is excessive hilar shadowing or whether this represents a normal chest X-ray appearance. Identify the horizontal fissure on the PA film (see Figure 6.6b).
- *Lateral chest X-ray.* A lateral film should be included as part of a full radiological assessment of the chest. Interpretation of lateral chest X-rays requires some experience, but the various normal landmarks should be recognized (see Figure 6.6c).

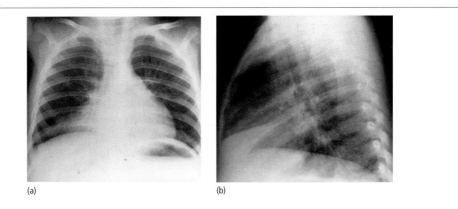

(a)     (b)

**Figure 6.7** Chest X-ray. (a) PA film showing collapse of right middle lobe with loss of definition of the right heart border; (b) the collapsed right middle lobe is seen as a wedge-shaped shadow on the lateral film.

**Box 6.1 Approach to reading a chest X-ray**

• Identify the film with name, date and laterality
• Comment on quality of the film (penetration and rotation)
• Examine bony landmarks and count ribs
• Examine the diaphragms
• Examine heart border. Comment on cardiomegaly and any lack of clarity of the heart outline
• Examine lung fields. Comment on symmetry, clarity and any opacity. Comment on hilar regions
• Examine lateral film

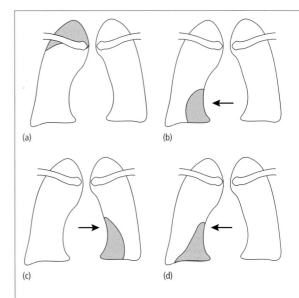

(a)     (b)

(c)     (d)

**Figure 6.8** Some commonly seen abnormal features of a chest X-ray film. The arrow represents possible deviation of the heart shadow which occurs with collapse rather than consolidation. (a) Right upper lobe collapse; (b) right middle lobe collapse with loss of the right cardiac outline; (c) left lower lobe collapse; (d) right lower lobe collapse with loss of right diaphragm shadow.

### Examples of pathology (see Figures 6.7 and 6.8)

#### Collapse and consolidation

Collapse and/or consolidation of a lung lobe can usually be seen by a focal opacity on the PA film (see Figures 6.7a and 6.8). A lateral chest X-ray film is necessary to define precisely the area of lung involved. The right middle lobe is a common site, which causes loss of definition of the right heart border. It is also seen as a wedge-shaped shadow on the lateral film. Right lower lobe collapse causes loss of the right diaphragm shadow.

If there is deviation of the mediastinal shadow with lung field opacity, this suggests collapse rather than consolidation.

#### Pleural effusion

Small pleural effusions blunt the costophrenic angles and large effusions cause extensive radio-opacity in the affected lung field, often with the mediastinal shadow pushed to the opposite side.

### Ultrasound

Ultrasound is a frequently used investigation in children. It is generally well tolerated and safe, and unlike

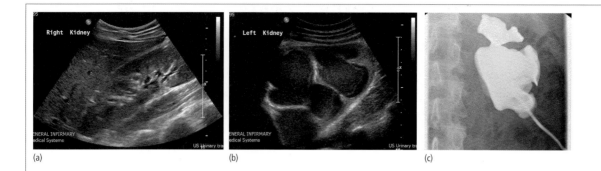

**Figure 6.9** (a) Ultrasound of normal right kidney. (b) Ultrasound of hydronephrotic left kidney, with dilated renal pelvis showing up as echo-poor area: contrast with normal right kidney seen in (a).
(c) Contrast study via nephrostomy, showing massive dilation of hydronephrotic renal pelvis and obstructed ureter (same patient as a and b). Images courtesy of Dr Rosemary Arthur.

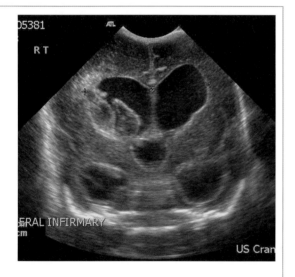

**Figure 6.10** Cranial ultrasound of a preterm neonate, showing a coronal view of dilated lateral ventricles. Intraventricular haemorrhage is visible on the right, with some surrounding venous infarction.

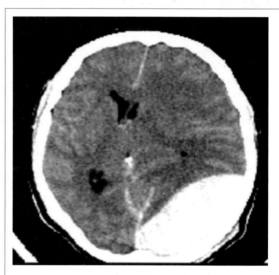

**Figure 6.11** Head CT scan showing a severe extradural haematoma on the left with compression of the left lateral ventricle and midline shift towards the right.

X-rays it does not involve exposure to ionizing radiation. Common indications for ultrasound include assessing the size and texture of abdominal and pelvic organs (Figure 6.9), assessing fluid collections within the chest, and imaging the brain via the anterior fontanelle (Figure 6.10).

## CT scan

Computed tomography (CT) scans generate detailed views of any region of the body as apparent 'slices'.

The technique is particularly useful for detecting large masses or bleeds within the head (Figure 6.11), and for detecting bronchiectasis and other lung disease (Figure 6.12). The child needs to lie still for 1–2 minutes, so toddlers usually require a general anaesthetic. Unfortunately, CT scans involve a relatively high dose of ionizing radiation, and this needs to be balanced against the value of the information the scan may provide.

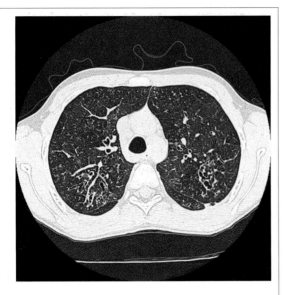

**Figure 6.12** High-resolution CT scan of the lungs, showing bronchiectasis affecting both upper lobes. This child has cystic fibrosis.

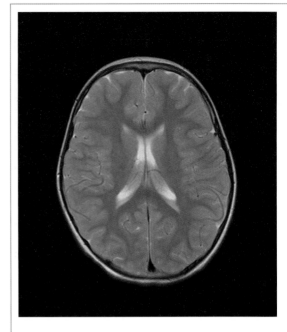

**Figure 6.13** MRI scan of a normal 6-year-old. On this $T_2$-weighted image, cerebrospinal fluid in the lateral ventricles appears white. The dark grey areas show areas rich in myelin.

## MRI scan

Magnetic resonance imaging (MRI) uses electromagnetic fields, rather than ionizing radiation, to produce very detailed 'slice' images. MRI is particularly good at imaging the brain and spinal cord, giving much more detail than CT scanning, particularly in terms of differentiating between white matter and grey matter (Figures 6.13, 6.14, 6.15). To get clear images the child needs to lie still for several minutes, and the scanner can be noisy, so general anaesthetic is usually required.

## Sweat test

The sweat test is the definitive test for cystic fibrosis (p. 149). It is performed by stimulating a small part of the arm to sweat by pilocarpine iontophoresis (Figure 6.16).

### Collection of sweat

Two padded electrodes are applied either side of the child's forearm. The pad is soaked with pilocarpine, which stimulates sweating locally. The pilocarpine is iontophoresed into the skin by passing a small electric current across the electrodes. Once this is carried out, the electrodes are removed and sweat is collected by

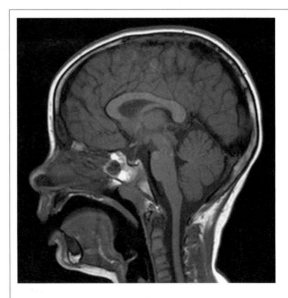

**Figure 6.14** Sagittal $T_1$-weighted MRI scan of a normal 6-year-old. Note the midline structures, including corpus callosum, brainstem and cerebellum. Note that cerebrospinal fluid appears black on $T_1$-weighted images.

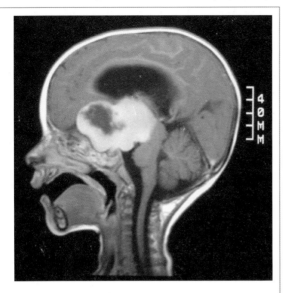

**Figure 6.15** Sagittal $T_1$-weighted MRI scan showing large white optic glioma, with some darker cystic change within it.

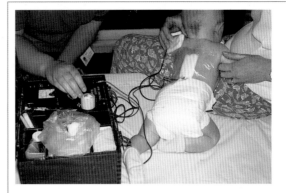

**Figure 6.16** A sweat test being performed. Pilocarpine is carried into the skin by low-voltage electric current. The sweat is collected by filter paper and analysed for sodium and chloride concentration.

placing a clean, preweighed filter paper square over the skin into which pilocarpine has penetrated. The filter paper should be taped to the skin with a plastic covering, to prevent evaporation of sweat, and then the entire area bandaged with a crepe bandage while sweat is collected over a period of at least 20 minutes. The filter paper is carefully removed. Clean plastic gloves must be worn during the entire procedure to avoid contamination of the filter paper with the examiner's own sweat. The filter paper is sent to the laboratory in an airtight plastic bag to prevent the sweat from evaporating. In the laboratory the filter paper is reweighed and both sodium and chloride measurements made.

### The sweat analysis

On arrival in the laboratory the filter paper is weighed again, and the difference between the pretest weight and the final weight represents the amount of sweat collected. For the test to be valid, at least 100 mg of sweat must be collected. If the difference in weight is less than this, the test is invalid and should be repeated.

Measurement of both sweat sodium and chloride is necessary to exclude or confirm cystic fibrosis.

### Diagnostic criteria for cystic fibrosis

- >100 mg of sweat
- Sweat sodium >60 mmol/L
- Sweat chloride >60 mmol/L

In cystic fibrosis the sweat chloride is usually higher than the sweat sodium value. In normal subjects the chloride is usually less than the sodium.

## Genetic testing

Over the last three decades, the genetic mutations associated with many inherited diseases have been identified. This is particularly the case for many metabolic conditions, neuro-degenerative diseases, and renal and respiratory conditions. These tests are generally used to confirm clinical suspicions regarding a diagnosis, as the relevant genetic mutation test has to be specifically requested. Genetic testing should only be performed if it is in the child's best interests and if the result will alter the management of that particular child during childhood. Otherwise, genetic testing should be deferred until the child becomes an adult and can make up his or her own mind whether or not to be tested. For example, children should not be tested for Huntington's chorea in childhood, even if the parents request it.

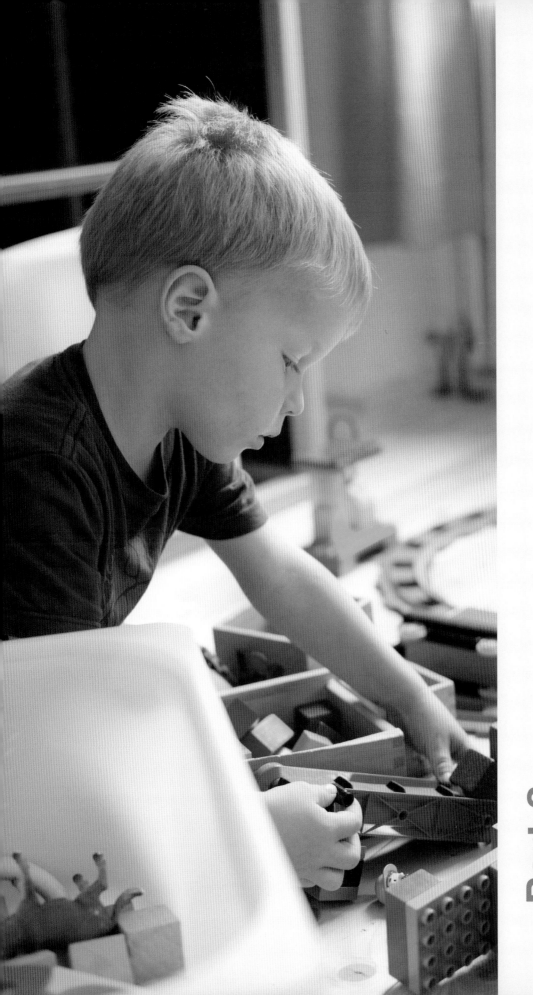

**Part 3**
**An approach to problem-based paediatrics**

# CHAPTER 7

# The febrile child

*The Doctor came round and examined his chest,*
*And ordered him Nourishment, Tonics, and Rest,*
*'How very effective,' he said as he shook*
*The thermometer . . . . . .*
*The Doctor next morning was rubbing his hands,*
*And saying, 'There's nobody quite understands*
*These cases as I do. ....'*
*The Dormouse and the Doctor, AA Milne*

## COMPETENCES

### You must . . .

| Know | Be able to | Appreciate |
| --- | --- | --- |
| • How to diagnose and manage the common and serious infections of childhood<br>• How to recognize and manage the common infectious exanthems<br>• How to bring down a temperature<br>• How to define PUO<br>• Features in a blood count that suggest bacterial infection | • Take a temperature accurately<br>• Recognize when a child has a serious infection<br>• Identify the common childhood exanthems<br>• Distinguish clinically between the different types of swellings in the neck | • That fever can be a very worrying symptom for parents<br>• That fever can be a serious sign in very young babies<br>• That it is mandatory to look for generalized lymphadenopathy and hepatosplenomegaly if you find enlargement of any lymph node |

*Paediatrics and Child Health*, Third Edition. Mary Rudolf, Tim Lee, Malcolm Levene.
© 2011 Mary Rudolf, Tim Lee and Malcolm Levene. Published 2011 by Blackwell Publishing Ltd.

# Fever as symptom and sign

## Finding your way around . . .

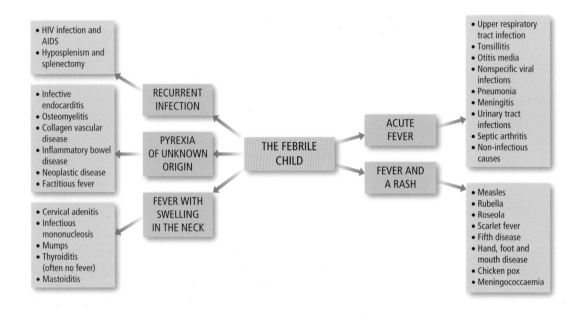

## Acute fever

| Common causes of acute fever in childhood | | |
|---|---|---|
| **Upper respiratory tract** | **Other infections** | **Other causes of fever** |
| Upper respiratory tract infection | Non-specific viral infections | Factitious: taking temperature |
| Otitis media | Viral exanthems—measles, | after a hot drink; deliberate |
| Tonsillitis | rubella, chicken pox, etc. | manipulation of the thermom- |
| Cervical adenitis | Influenza | eter (see p. 117) |
| Mastoiditis | Pneumonia | Excessive crying or exertion |
| Mumps | Urinary tract infection | Overheating due to excessive |
| Infectious mononucleosis | Meningitis | swaddling, etc. |
| | Septic arthritis | |

Fever is a very common symptom in children. High fever occurs in many non-serious conditions and is the body's response to pyrogens, which have an effect on the nuclei of the brain responsible for temperature control. Fever usually occurs as a result of infection, but may result from chronic inflammation or an immune response. The body's response to fever is to lose heat by skin vasodilatation, which causes the flush that is often seen in feverish children.

A fever is a temperature above 37.0 °C orally. One of the most important skills you will require as a doctor is to assess the child with a fever, decide on the likely cause, and treat appropriately. Babies under the age of 8 weeks are particularly difficult to assess, and may deteriorate rapidly. They need to be admitted. For the older baby and child your clinical evaluation should lead you to the likely focus of infection and a decision as to how ill the child is. Contrary to common belief, the height of the fever does not correlate either with serious infection or the presence of a bacterial infection.

The temperature should generally be taken using an electronic or chemical dot thermometer placed in the axilla, or an infrared tympanic thermometer in the ear. Rectal temperatures may be needed in unconscious children. Disposable plastic strip chemical thermometers are widely available but have been shown to register slightly higher temperatures than the mercury in glass thermometers. The commercially available plastic strip thermometer that is placed on the child's forehead is not reliable. The correct technique for taking a temperature is described in Box 7.1.

### History – must ask!

- *Character of fever.* Ask how long the fever has been present and whether it occurs at particular times of the day.
- *General features.* Poor appetite and malaise are non-specific features in any febrile child. Headache, diarrhoea and vomiting may also be non-specific.
- *Pain.* Has there been earache, headache, difficulty swallowing (dysphagia), dysuria which give clues to the cause? Excessive crying in a baby may be a feature of pain.
- *Specific symptoms.* Vomiting, diarrhea, coryza, cough, rash may all suggest a diagnosis.

### Box 7.1 Taking the temperature

Place the thermometer in the axilla and hold the arm down by the child's side for 3–5 minutes. Axillary temperatures are 0.5 °C lower than oral or rectal temperatures. If using an infrared tympanic thermometer, place the tip in the external auditory meatus, pointing anteromedially towards the tympanic membrane. Press the measurement button, and after a few seconds a reading will be obtained. Core body temperature is normally 37.5 °C and is measured by inserting a thermometer in the rectum. This is the most convenient method in infants or unconscious children

### Physical examination – must check!

- *General.* Does the child look seriously ill? Is the child dehydrated? Is there tachycardia or tachypnoea?
- *Skin.* Is there a rash? Petechial or purpuric lesions that do not blanch on pressure are hallmarks of meningococcaemia. (See Chapter 17 for how to diagnose exanthematous diseases.)
- *Chest.* Are there signs of respiratory distress? Examine carefully for signs of bronchiolitis or pneumonia.
- *Central nervous system.* Is the child orientated? Is the child floppy? In older children assess for the presence of neck stiffness or Kernig's sign.
- *Ears.* Examine the tympanic membranes. Are they red and/or bulging?
- *Throat.* Are the tonsils inflamed or is there an exudate? Is there lymphadenopathy?

*Note:* Leave the examination of throat and ears to the end as this often upsets young children.

### Investigations

In general, if the child does not look toxic, and a focus of infection is evident, the child does not need to be investigated. The investigations in Table 7.1 are only

**Table 7.1** Investigations that may be indicated in a child with fever (these are always required in an infant <8 weeks old)

| Investigation | What you are looking for |
| --- | --- |
| Full blood count | Elevated white cell count with increased neutrophil count suggests a bacterial infection |
| Throat swab | Culture of beta-haemolytic streptococcus requires treatment with penicillin |
| Blood cultures | Culture of a single organism indicates probable septicaemia Multiple organisms suggest contamination |
| Lumbar puncture | See Table 6.8, p. 97 |
| Chest X-ray | Consolidation (generalized or focal) indicates pneumonia |
| Urine analysis and culture | Pure growth of $>10^5$ cell colonies with >50 white cells, red cells and protein present, indicates infection (p. 304) |

required in ill-appearing children. In young babies there may be few or no localizing signs of infection and so they must be investigated. At any age urinary tract infection (UTI) should be suspected as the cause of fever. The only way to confirm or exclude this is by microbiological culture of the urine, and this needs to be considered if no other focus of infection can be found.

## Managing fever as a symptom

Fever is often an unpleasant symptom, and should be treated when the temperature is above 38.5 °C or below that level if the child is uncomfortable. It can be brought down by a number of methods:

• Undress the child. Many parents' reaction to a fever is to wrap the child with blankets. This must be discouraged.
• Antipyretics, of which paracetamol suspension (Calpol) and ibuprofen are most widely used. Aspirin should not be given to children because of its association with the development of severe liver disease (Reye's syndrome).
• Sponging or tepid baths. Heat loss is encouraged by sponging with lukewarm water to allow vasodilatation and evaporative heat loss. Cold water causes vasoconstriction and may increase body temperature.

Early and effective treatment of fever is particularly important in children prone to febrile convulsions (p. 393).

> **Key points: The child presenting with fever**
>
> • Confirm the presence of fever by recording the temperature
> • Assess whether the child requires hospital admission, but remember that the height of the fever does not relate to severity of illness
> • In babies less than 6 months old localizing signs may not be present
> • Take measures to reduce temperature
> • Examine for focal signs of infection
> • If a child looks ill, re-evaluate when the fever settles
> • Admit and investigate babies below 8 weeks of age
> • Start antibiotics only where clinically indicated
> • In a child who appears seriously unwell intravenous broad spectrum antibiotics are given early, before results of investigations become available

## Clues to the differential diagnosis of acute fever in children

| | Symptoms | Signs | Investigations |
|---|---|---|---|
| **Tonsillitis** | Sore throat | Tonsillar redness ± exudate<br>Cervical lymphadenopathy | Throat swab |
| **Otitis media** | Ear pain, irritability | Bulging and red tympanic membrane | |
| **Pneumonia** | Cough<br>Difficulty breathing | Respiratory distress<br>Dullness to percussion<br>Crepitations | Chest X-ray |
| **Meningitis** | Headache, irritability<br>Drowsiness | Neck stiffness* ± change in conscious level | Lumbar puncture |
| **Urinary tract infection** | Dysuria, frequency | | Urine microscopy and culture |
| **Meningococcal disease** | Malaise | Shock, purpura | Blood cultures |
| **Septic arthritis** | Joint pain, limp, refusal to walk | Swollen joint, limited movement of joint | Aspiration of joint |

*This sign is usually not present in young infants.

# Fever with a rash

| Common causes of fever and a rash | |
|---|---|
| Macular and maculopapular | Measles |
| | Rubella |
| | Roseola |
| | Scarlet fever |
| | Fifth disease |
| | Non-specific viral illnesses |
| Vesicular | Chicken pox |
| | Hand, foot and mouth disease |
| Purpuric | Meningococcaemia |

Most children presenting with fever and a rash have one of the common infectious diseases of childhood. Most of these exanthematous conditions require only supportive treatment and so a specific diagnosis is often not critical. However, the exception is meningococcaemia, which presents with a purpuric rash. It is life-threatening and must be identified promptly. The other reason for accurately diagnosing exanthematous conditions is for public health purposes so that epidemics can be recognized. A description of the characteristics of different rashes is given on p. 320.

## History – must ask!

- *Is the child ill?* Most of the exanthematous diseases are accompanied by fever and malaise. In measles and meningococcaemia the child is often very ill; in rubella, fifth disease and non-specific viral exanthems the child often appears remarkably well; measles is suspected if the three 'C's (coryza, cough and conjunctivitis) are present; in roseola the rash appears once the fever falls after 3–5 days; scarlet fever is preceded by tonsillitis.
- *Is the rash itchy?* Itchiness suggests chicken pox (if the rash is vesicular) or an allergic response (possibly due to antibiotics given for the underlying illness).
- *Past medical history.* A history of a previous attack of an infectious disease makes a further attack unlikely, but there is a high incidence of inaccurate diagnoses, particularly with maculopapular rashes. It is obviously relevant to ask about the child's immunization history. An atypical rash commonly follows some 10 days after measles, mumps and rubella (MMR) vaccination.
- *Contact with anyone ill.* Enquire whether anyone else in the family, or at school or nursery has been diagnosed as having an infectious disease.

## Physical examination – must check!

### The rash

You need to describe the rash carefully, focusing on the following:

- *Characteristics.* Is the rash macular, papular, maculopapular, vesicular, purpuric or petechial? An important part of the examination is to test the rash for blanching, as purpuric and petechial rashes do not blanch on pressure whereas maculopapular rashes do. Note that fever is usually absent in purpuric rash from other causes, namely Henoch–Schönlein purpura and idiopathic thrombocytopenic purpura).
- *Distribution.* Measles and rubella both start on the face and work their way down the body. Roseola and chicken pox are mostly on the trunk. Fifth disease is confined to the cheeks.
- *The presence of an enanthem.* Look in the mouth for an enanthem. In chicken pox the vesicles rapidly break down so that shallow ulcers are seen. In measles Koplik spots (appearing like grains of salt on a red background) are seen during the prodromal period only.

### General examination

Carry out a complete physical examination, although other than finding fever and possibly lymphadenopathy it rarely contributes to the diagnostic process.

## Investigations

In general, the viral exanthems do not need a serological confirmation of the diagnosis, unless for public health reasons. The exception, of course, is the development of a maculopapular rash in a pregnant girl, when rubella titres should be measured. If a sample is taken for viral titres, a second convalescent sample is required 10 days later, without which a diagnosis cannot be confidently made.

Blood sampling for culture and meningococcal polymerase chain reaction (PCR) are required in meningococcaemia. Cultures may prove negative as most children should have been given intramuscular penicillin prior to admission to hospital.

If the rash is petechial, a platelet count is required, as fever could be an incidental symptom in a child who was thrombocytopaenic.

## Management

Before the advent of immunization, childhood infectious diseases were common and regular epidemics occurred. There was little difficulty in recognizing these diseases then, but these clinical skills have now diminished. It is, however, still important to recognize

**Table 7.2** The course of childhood infectious diseases

| Disease | Incubation | Duration of rash | Recommended isolation |
|---|---|---|---|
| Measles* | 10–14 days | 5 days | From onset of catarrhal stage to day 5 of rash |
| Rubella* | 14–21 days | 2–3 days | None, except from non-immune women in first trimester of pregnancy |
| Roseola | Probably 10 days | 1 day | None |
| Scarlet fever | 2–4 days | 5 days | 1 day after start of treatment |
| Fifth disease | 4–14 days | Weeks | None |
| Chicken pox | 14–17 days | 6–10 days | Until all lesions are crusted (usually 5–6 days) |
| Mumps*† | 16–21 days | None | Until swelling subsides (usually 5–10 days) |
| Pertussis*† | 7 days | None | 4 weeks or until cough has ceased |

*Immunizations against these disease are routinely given (see p. 27).
†Mumps and pertussis are included for completeness although there is no associated rash.

the various diseases so that appropriate advice about incubation periods and recommendations for isolation can be made (Table 7.2). in general, children are infective during much of the incubation period and before the specific rash emerges.

Maculopapular rashes are often overdiagnosed clinically as being caused by measles or rubella. As these diagnoses are difficult to make unless in the midst of an epidemic, it is preferable to make the diagnosis of viral exanthem rather than a wrong diagnosis. If accurate diagnosis is required, confirmation by serological testing is necessary.

If meningococcaemia (see p. 128) is suspected, the child should immediately be given intramuscular penicillin, as rapid deterioration can occur, and urgent admission to hospital arranged.

## Clues to diagnosing a febrile illness with a rash

| | Type of rash | Characteristics of the rash | Other features |
|---|---|---|---|
| **Measles** | Maculopapular | Begins on the face and spreads downwards | Koplik spots, coryza, cough and conjunctivitis, ill child |
| **Rubella** | Macular | Tiny pink macules on the face and trunk, works downwards | Well child, lymphadenopathy sometimes |
| **Roseola** | Macular | Faint pink rash on the trunk | Rash occurs after fever defervesces |
| **Scarlet fever** | Maculopapular | Fine punctate red rash with sandpapery feel, followed by peeling | Strawberry tongue, perioral pallor, tonsillitis |
| **Fifth disease** | Maculopapular | 'Slapped cheek' appearance; lace-like rash on the arms, trunk and thighs | Well child, lasts up to weeks |
| **Chicken pox** | Vesicular | Occurs in crops on face and trunk. Papules, vesicles and crusts are present | Shallow ulcers of the mucous membranes |
| **Meningococcaemia** | Purpuric | Morbilliform (resembling measles), petechial or purpuric | May progress rapidly to shock and coma |

### Key points: Fever with a rash

- Decide if the rash is macular, maculopapular, vesicular or purpuric
- Determine if the child is ill
- If the rash is petechial or purpuric and the child is unwell, treat with penicillin IM and admit for investigation
- Beware of making a specific diagnosis of measles or rubella clinically. Without serological confirmation, 'viral exanthem' should be diagnosed

## Fever with a swelling in the neck

### Causes of fever and a swelling in the neck

| | |
|---|---|
| Cervical lymph nodes | Upper respiratory tract infection<br>Cervical adenitis<br>Infectious mononucleosis<br>Neoplastic processes (Table 3.3, p. 40) |
| Parotid gland | Mumps |
| Thyroid gland | Thyroiditis (generally no fever) |
| Mastoid | Mastoiditis |

The commonest glands to enlarge in the neck are the anterior cervical nodes, which drain the tonsils and pharynx. This may occur with any upper respiratory tract infection (URTI) and, if the child is not ill and the glands not obviously tender, is of little significance. Acute enlargement with fever is usually a result of streptococcal infection, with the differential diagnosis including infectious mononucleosis. Cytomegalovirus, toxoplasmosis and rubella are also causes which are often accompanied by generalized lymphadenopathy. Leukaemia and lymphoma are sometimes accompanied by striking degrees of lymph node enlargement, and other malignant tumours occasionally metastasize to lymph nodes.

Mumps is the commonest cause of parotid swelling, which can be unilateral or bilateral. Swelling of the mastoid process is included here, although it is not strictly part of the neck. Infection can spread from the adjacent ear and cause serious morbidity.

Goitre (swelling of the thyroid gland) is not usually accompanied by fever, although occasionally sore throat and fever can occur at the onset of autoimmune thyroiditis. Late-onset congenital hypothyroidism is sometimes identified when the child presents with an unrelated febrile illness. Since the iodization of salt, goitre secondary to iodine deficiency no longer exists in children brought up in Britain.

The first aspect of the clinical evaluation is to identify the site of origin of the enlarged gland(s). You can usually achieve this on your clinical examination.

### Clues to diagnosing enlarged glands in the neck

| | Features of the gland | Conditions causing enlargement of the gland |
|---|---|---|
| Cervical lymph nodes | May swell unilaterally or bilaterally along the anterior cervical chain | Upper respiratory tract infection |
| Parotid glands | Overlie the angle of the jaw. When enlarged they may be distinguished from the cervical lymph glands as they obscure the bony angle of the jaw and displace the ear upwards and outwards | Mumps |

(Continued)

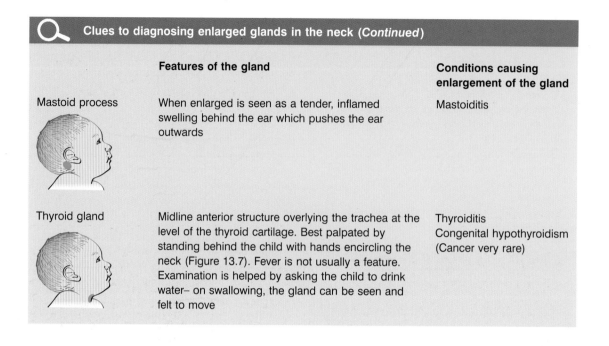

**Clues to diagnosing enlarged glands in the neck (*Continued*)**

| | Features of the gland | Conditions causing enlargement of the gland |
|---|---|---|
| Mastoid process | When enlarged is seen as a tender, inflamed swelling behind the ear which pushes the ear outwards | Mastoiditis |
| Thyroid gland | Midline anterior structure overlying the trachea at the level of the thyroid cartilage. Best palpated by standing behind the child with hands encircling the neck (Figure 13.7). Fever is not usually a feature. Examination is helped by asking the child to drink water– on swallowing, the gland can be seen and felt to move | Thyroiditis Congenital hypothyroidism (Cancer very rare) |

### History and physical examination – must ask and check!

The history and physical examination depend on the gland involved. Ask about malaise and fluid intake if you suspect infection of the lymph glands, parotids or mastoid. Focus your physical examination on identifying other sites of infection such as tonsillitis and otitis media, and an assessment of the child's hydration, as fluid intake is likely to be reduced. If you find cervical lymphadenopathy, you must examine the axillae, groins, liver and spleen to see if the lymphadenopathy is generalized.

If you diagnose a goitre you need to decide if the child is euthyroid, hypothyroid or hyperthyroid (see p. 270).

### Investigations (see Table 7.3)

In the primary care setting it is usually acceptable to treat cervical adenitis without laboratory confirmation of an organism. If you suspect infectious mononucleosis, a full blood count and Epstein–Barr virus screen are advisable. Mumps does not require investigation, but a serum or urine amylase is helpful if it is not clear if the swelling is sited in the parotid or lymph glands. Thyroid function tests and antibodies are indicated in a child with goitre.

**Table 7.3** Investigations which may be indicated for a swelling in the neck

| | Investigation | Significance |
|---|---|---|
| Cervical lymph nodes | Full blood count | Elevated white cell count and shift to the left in bacterial infection, atypical lymphocytes in infectious mononucleosis |
| | Epstein–Barr virus screen | Positive in infectious mononucleosis |
| | Throat culture | Group A haemolytic streptococcal infection needs antibiotics |
| Parotid glands | Serum or urine amylase | Elevated in mumps, and therefore distinguishes the parotid from the lymph glands |
| Mastoid process | Tympanocentesis | To identify responsible organism and drain infection |
| Thyroid gland | Thyroxine, thyroid-stimulating hormone | To confirm whether the child is hypo-, hyper- or euthyroid |
| | Thyroid antibodies | Often positive in thyroiditis |

> ### 🔧 Key points: Fever and swelling in the neck
>
> - Identify the gland involved
> - If the process is thought to be infective, assess how sick the child is and the state of hydration
> - If cervical lymphadenopathy is identified, look for generalized lymphadenopathy and hepatosplenomegaly
> - If a goitre is found, assess if the child is clinically hypothyroid, hyperthyroid or euthyroid
> - If mastoiditis is found, admit the child as a surgical emergency

## Pyrexia of unknown origin

### Causes of pyrexia of unknown origin

| Bacterial infection | Viral infection | Other causes |
| --- | --- | --- |
| Urinary tract infection | Infectious mononucleosis | Collagen vascular disease |
| Pneumonia | Hepatitis | Inflammatory bowel disease |
| Endocarditis | HIV infection | Neoplastic disease |
| Occult abscesses (NB dental) | | Factitious fever |
| Tuberculosis | | |
| Osteomyelitis | | |

In most children presenting initially with fever and no apparent site of infection, the diagnosis becomes apparent or the fever resolves within a short period of time. Pyrexia of unknown origin (PUO) refers to prolonged fever, which is defined as more than 1 week in young children and 2–3 weeks in the adolescent.

The underlying cause in most cases of PUO is infection. Usually it is an atypical presentation of one of the common illnesses such as UTI or pneumonia, although endocarditis is an important consideration in a child with congenital heart disease. Other significant causes include the collagen vascular diseases, malignancy, and inflammatory bowel disease in the adolescent. The disease that is most responsible for being a diagnostic puzzle is systemic juvenile chronic arthritis (Still's disease), which often presents as a remitting fever (see p. 292). Both Crohn's disease and ulcerative colitis may present as PUO alone, although often a careful history reveals abnormalities in bowel patterns, which have been accepted by the child as being normal. Leukaemia may present as PUO, but it is less usual for other malignancies to do so.

A thorough history and repeated physical examinations are particularly important as clues may emerge which can lead to a diagnosis.

### History – must ask!

- *Review of systems.* A thorough review of all organ systems is imperative as symptoms may be elicited which provide a lead to the aetiology.
- *Contact with infectious diseases.* Clues may be found on identifying someone in the family or school who is ill.
- *Travel.* Ask about any history of travel reaching back to birth, as re-emergence of disease may occur years after visiting an endemic area.
- *Exposure to animals.* Zoonotic infections can be acquired from pets or wild animals.
- *Genetic origin.* Tuberculosis is still prevalent in Asian communities. Some rare genetic disorders can cause PUO.

### Physical examination – must check!

A meticulous physical examination, including all organ systems, may lead to diagnostic clues and so save the child from a battery of investigations. The physical examination may need to be repeated a number of times to look for the emergence of new signs.

- *Temperature chart* (see Figure 7.9). Repetitive chills and temperature spikes are common in children with septicaemia from any cause, but particularly suggest an abscess, pyelonephritis or endocarditis. Factitious fever should be suspected if there is an absence of tachycardia and sweating associated with peaks of fever.
- *The mouth and sinuses.* Look for tenderness to tapping over the sinuses and teeth and transilluminate the sinuses. Finding candida in the mouth may be a clue to a disorder of the immune system. Hyperaemia of the pharynx may suggest infectious mononucleosis.
- *Muscles and bones.* Palpate the muscles and bones. Point tenderness suggests either osteomyelitis or bone marrow invasion from neoplastic disease. Generalized muscle tenderness occurs in collagen vascular disease.

- *Heart.* If you find a pathological murmur (see p. 192) or a change in character of a murmur you should be concerned that infective endocarditis has developed.

### Investigations (Table 7.4)

The number of investigations that can and often are performed are legion. You should only order investigations, beyond those commonly available, cautiously. It is important to obtain blood cultures at fever peaks as the yield at that time is much higher, and at least three specimens should be taken. In general, radiological tests should be guided by clues obtained on the clinical evaluation. Ultrasound, CT or MRI can be used to guide aspiration or biopsy of suspicious lesions.

**Table 7.4** Investigations and their relevance in pyrexia of unknown origin

| Investigation | Relevance |
|---|---|
| Full blood count | Elevated white cell count and shift to the left in bacterial infection. Very high white cell count in leukaemia |
| Urine analysis and culture | Occult urinary tract infection |
| Examination of blood smear | Parasitic infections, e.g. malaria |
| ESR or plasma viscosity | Elevated in bacterial infection. Highly elevated in collagen vascular disease and malignancy |
| Blood cultures (aerobic and anaerobic) | Bacterial infection. Repeated samples needed to diagnose endocarditis, osteomyelitis and occult abscesses |
| Liver function tests | Hepatitis |
| TB skin test | Tuberculosis |
| X-rays: chest, bones, sinuses, gastrointestinal tract | Characteristic findings with bacterial infection |
| Bone marrow aspirate | Leukaemia, metastatic neoplasms, rare infections |
| Serological tests | Infectious mononucleosis, other infections, rarely helpful in collagen vascular disease |
| Radioactive scans | Helpful in detecting osteomyelitis and abdominal masses, tumours, abscesses |
| Echocardiography | In endocarditis vegetations can be seen on the leaflets of heart valves |
| Ultrasonography | Identification of intra-abdominal abscesses |
| Total body CT or MRI scanning | Detection of neoplasms and abscesses |

ESR, erythrocyte sedimentation rate.

## Managing the child with a PUO

In general, the child should be hospitalized for careful observation as much as for investigation. This may also provide relief of parental anxiety. Antipyretics should not at first be given as they obscure the pattern of fever. Antibiotics should never be used as antipyretics, and empirical trials should in general be avoided, as they are dangerous and can obscure the diagnosis of infections such as endocarditis and osteomyelitis.

It is helpful to know that the child with PUO has a better prognosis than that reported for adults, and that the cause is usually an atypical presentation of a common childhood illness. In many cases no diagnosis is established but the fever abates spontaneously.

Vary rarely, factitious fever – caused by the patient (often adolescent) or parent manipulating the thermometer – is the cause of a PUO. If this is in any way suspected, temperatures must be documented in hospital by an individual who stays with the patient while the temperature is being taken.

---

**⚙ Key points: Pyrexia of unknown origin**

- A thorough history and repeated physical examinations are required and may save the child from multiple, unpleasant investigations
- Hospitalization is needed to confirm and observe the pattern of the fever
- The characteristics of the fever may give a clue to diagnosis
- Samples for blood culture should be taken at the peak of fever

---

## Recurrent infections

**Causes of recurrent serious infections**

Defective white cell function
Immunoglobulin deficiency
    Congenital deficiency
    HIV
Splenectomy
Chest
    Foreign bodies
    Cystic fibrosis
Urinary tract
    Reflux
Meningitis
    Congenital dermal sinus

Most children experience recurrent minor infections. These are commonly respiratory infections, colds and tonsillitis, which peak when the child starts school or nursery or when an older sibling brings infections home. Poor nutrition, poverty, poor housing and inadequate hygiene may be contributing factors. Breast-feeding provides some protection during infancy, at least from otitis media and gastroenteritis.

The common recurrent minor infections of childhood may cause great parental concern, but should not initiate a diagnostic exploration. However, the child who experiences recurrent infections of a serious nature needs to be thoroughly evaluated for the underlying cause. Details of the investigation of immune deficiency states are beyond the scope of this book.

# Febrile illnesses

## Upper respiratory tract infection

Upper respiratory tract infection (URTI) is very common in young children, particularly when they first start playgroup and school, as they become exposed to a number of viral organisms for the first time to which they have no immunity. The mother often describes her child as having 'one cold after another', but mothers (and doctors) need to understand that frequent mild infections in these young children are common and benign.

**Clinical features.** The child often has coryza (runny nose) and sneezing or acute pharyngitis associated with fever. After a few days the child's nose becomes blocked, with consequent mouth breathing. A cough is often present, for which the child may unnecessarily receive repeated courses of antibiotics. On physical examination purulent mucus is visible in the nares or running down the upper lip. The tympanic membranes may be inflamed, and in acute pharyngitis the pharynx, the soft palate and the tonsillar fauces are red and swollen, often accompanied by cervical lymphadenopathy. Investigation is unnecessary unless the child has a tonsillar exudate, when a throat swab for culture may be taken.

**Management.** Treatment is symptomatic. In infants, nasal obstruction may be a particular problem as young babies are obligate nose breathers and cannot breathe through their mouths, and saline nasal drops immediately before feeds may be helpful. Fever in older children is treated with antipyretics and nasal obstruction may be relieved by a decongestant, but ephedrine should not be used for more than a few days because of the risk of mucosal hypertrophy. Antibiotics are *not* indicated for uncomplicated URTI.

## Tonsillitis

Tonsillitis is usually caused by a viral infection, particularly in young children. In children over 5 years, the commonest bacterial organism is the group A beta-haemolytic streptococcus.

**Clinical features.** The child is feverish and usually complains of a sore throat, although younger children may experience abdominal pain due to mesenteric

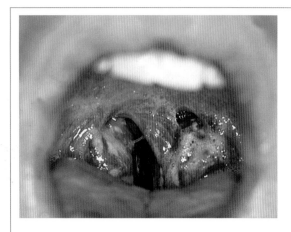

**Figure 7.1** Acute tonsillitis in an 8-year-old child presenting with fever and a sore throat.

adenitis. On examination the tonsils are enlarged and inflamed (Figure 7.1), although it is important to remember that tonsils normally enlarge to a maximum size by 4–5 years. This normal enlargement should not be confused with infection. A white exudate and tender enlarged cervical lymph glands suggest bacterial infection. Exudates can also occur in infectious mononucleosis and diphtheria (now very rare due to immunization). A throat swab should be taken where bacterial infection is suspected (exudate, systemic illness, frequent recurrences and tender cervical lymphadenopathy).

**Management.** Symptomatic treatment with saline gargles and paracetamol is helpful. Most cases of tonsillitis in young children do not require antibiotics. Streptococcal tonsillitis should be treated with penicillin for 10 days. Tonsillectomy is only rarely indicated even in recurrent tonsillitis.

**Prognosis.** The prognosis is good. Complications include:

- Otitis media.
- Chronic tonsillitis. Upper airway obstruction and sleep apnoea is an important complication of chronically enlarged tonsils and this requires tonsillectomy.
- Peritonsillar abscess (quinsy).
- Post-streptococcal allergic disorders, e.g. acute glomerulonephritis (p. 307).

## 👁 Tonsillitis at a glance

**Epidemiology**
Common, except under 24
  months

**Aetiology**
Beta-haemolytic strep, group A
Viral

**History**
Sore throat, dysphagia
Fever
Abdominal pain

**Physical examination**
Large inflamed tonsils with
  exudate
Cervical lymphadenopathy

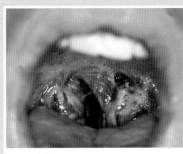
Exudate in acute follicular tonsillitis.

**Confirmatory investigations**
Throat swab grows beta-
  haemolytic strep, group A

**Differential diagnosis**
Viral pharyngitis
Infectious mononucleosis

**Management**
Antipyretics for fever
Gargles
Penicillin for 10 days

**Prognosis/complications**
Recurrent tonsillitis ⎤ Most
Otitis media          ⎦ common
Peritonsillar abscess (rare but
  serious)
Acute glomerulonephritis
  (certain strains of strep only)

## Otitis media

This is an extremely common childhood disorder and occurs most frequently in the first 7 years of life. It may also occur in the neonate. The commonest infecting organisms are viruses, *Streptococcus pneumoniae* and *Haemophilus influenzae*. Otitis media is especially common in conditions associated with eustachian tube dysfunction because fluid cannot drain from the middle ear. Eustachian tube dysfunction commonly occurs following the common cold, in adenoidal hypertrophy, cleft palate and in children with Down's syndrome.

**Clinical features.** Otitis media usually presents with fever, a painful ear and hearing loss, and is often preceded by an URTI. In younger children, anorexia, vomiting and diarrhoea may be the presenting features and there may be no obvious symptoms pointing to the ear as the source of infection. For this reason it is important to examine the ears (p. 79) in all febrile children. In otitis media the tympanic membrane is inflamed and bulging, with loss of the light reflex (Figure 7.2). Perforation of the tympanic membrane may occur spontaneously, in which case the ear canal will be obscured by pus. The diagnosis is made on

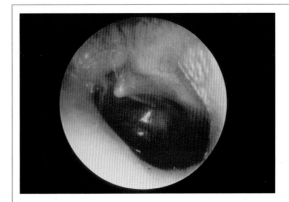

**Figure 7.2** Bulging tympanic membrane seen on otoscopy of a child with otitis media. Note the inflammation and loss of landmarks.

otoscopic findings, and culture of pus is generally unhelpful.

**Management.** Many cases are caused by viruses and resolve spontaneously, and hence in children over 6 months of age antibiotics are only given for symptoms that have persisted for at least 48 hours. Amoxicillin is a suitable choice.

**Prognosis.** Most cases of otitis media resolve satisfactorily even if perforation has occurred. Complications may occur and include secretory otitis media, conductive deafness (p. 248) and mastoiditis (p. 123).

### Secretory otitis media and glue ear

In secretory otitis media, recurrent acute infections lead to a thick glue-like exudate building up in the middle ear, and conductive hearing impairment (p. 248). On examination the tympanic membrane appears thickened and retracted with an absent light reflex. If there is significant hearing loss, ventilation tubes (grommets) may be inserted through the tympanic membrane to allow aeration of the middle ear. These are particularly indicated if there is language delay due to the conductive deafness associated with glue ear.

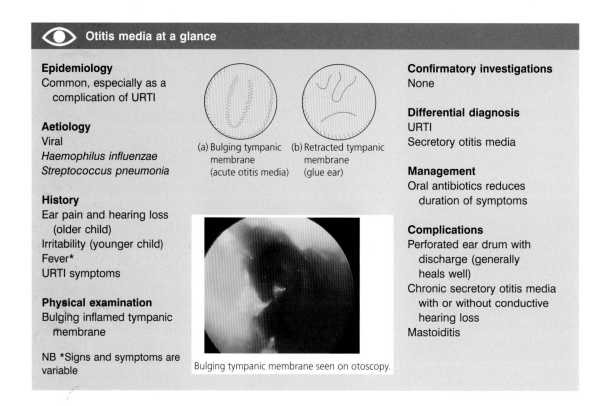

## Otitis media at a glance

**Epidemiology**
Common, especially as a complication of URTI

**Aetiology**
Viral
*Haemophilus influenzae*
*Streptococcus pneumonia*

**History**
Ear pain and hearing loss (older child)
Irritability (younger child)
Fever*
URTI symptoms

**Physical examination**
Bulging inflamed tympanic membrane

NB *Signs and symptoms are variable

(a) Bulging tympanic membrane (acute otitis media)
(b) Retracted tympanic membrane (glue ear)

Bulging tympanic membrane seen on otoscopy.

**Confirmatory investigations**
None

**Differential diagnosis**
URTI
Secretory otitis media

**Management**
Oral antibiotics reduces duration of symptoms

**Complications**
Perforated ear drum with discharge (generally heals well)
Chronic secretory otitis media with or without conductive hearing loss
Mastoiditis

## Non-specific viral infections

Febrile illnesses of a non-specific nature are caused by a number of viruses of which the influenza virus is one. These viruses are spread by droplet from the upper respiratory tract of affected children and adults.

**Clinical features.** Children usually present with a brief but acute illness with fever, malaise, chills, headache, cough and myalgia. A non-specific erythematous rash is a relatively common symptom. The term 'flu' is often used to describe these symptoms. There are no specific physical signs on examination, and it is unnecessary to do a viral screen to identify the causative agent.

**Management.** Treatment is symptomatic with antipyretics. Antibiotics are only necessary if there is evidence of secondary bacterial infection.

**Prognosis.** Some children are particularly susceptible to viral infections, such as those who have cystic fibrosis or congenital heart disease or those who are immunosuppressed. These children should receive regular influenza immunization.

## Cervical adenitis

Cervical adenitis results from infection by the group A beta-haemolytic streptococcus. The child presents as acutely unwell with tender swollen cervical lymph glands, with or without signs of tonsillitis. Bacterial infection is indicated by an elevated white cell count with a shift to the left, and the organism confirmed by positive throat or blood culture. In the primary care setting it is acceptable to prescribe penicillin on a clinical basis without laboratory confirmation.

# Infectious mononucleosis (glandular fever)

The Epstein–Barr virus is the cause of this infection. When tonsillitis is prominent the differential diagnosis includes streptococcal infection and diphtheria.

**Clinical features.** Infectious mononucleosis usually presents in the child, as in the adult, with marked cervical lymphadenopathy, fever, sore throat and enlarged purulent tonsils. Generalized lymphadenopathy and splenomegaly are commonly found, and a macular rash occurs in 10–20% of cases, especially if ampicillin is inadvertently given. Hepatitis often occurs with jaundice.

**Investigations.** The diagnosis is supported by the presence of atypical lymphocytes in the blood film which may account for 10–25% of the total white cell count. The test for heterophile antibodies is positive in 60% of cases in the first week of the illness and Epstein–Barr virus IgM is present in the early stages. Liver function tests may be abnormal.

**Management and prognosis.** Infectious mononucleosis is a self-limiting disease. The course of the condition is variable. The throat may be so inflamed as to preclude drinking, and if so the young child particularly must be examined repeatedly to ensure that dehydration is not developing. Children often recover from infectious mononucleosis without the prolonged fatigue and depression which characterize adolescent and adult infection.

## Infectious mononucleosis at a glance

**Aetiology**
Epstein–Barr virus

**History**
Fever (a)
Sore throat

**Physical examination**
Large purulent tonsils (b)
Generalized lymphadenopathy,
    particularly cervical (c)
Splenomegaly (d)
Hepatomegaly*
Macular rash*

**Confirmatory investigations**
Atypical lymphocytes (10–25%
    of white cell count) on blood
    smear
Positive heterophile antibody
    test in 60%
Epstein–Barr virus IgM-positive
    early
Abnormal liver function tests

NB *Signs and symptoms are variable

**Differential diagnosis**
Streptococcal tonsillitis
(Diphtheria now rare)
Leukaemia
Lymphoma
Toxoplasmosis
Cytomegalovirus
Hepatitis

**Management**
Supportive
Consider steroids if symptoms
    very severe

**Prognosis/complications**
Self-limiting disease
Dehydration may develop in the
    young child
Fatigue/depression are rare in
    children

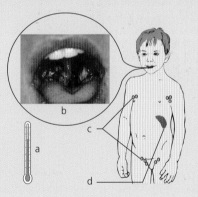

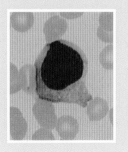

# Mumps

Mumps remains the commonest cause of parotitis despite the introduction of immunization (see p. 30). It is, in general, a mild illness in childhood. The child is contagious until the swelling has resolved.

**Clinical features.** After a long incubation period of 16–21 days, the child presents with fever and malaise, and enlargement of the parotid glands, which may be bilateral or unilateral (Figure 7.3). The child can usually drink but may experience pain on swallowing particularly sweet or sour liquids. The swelling lasts for 5–10 days.

**Management.** The diagnosis is usually obvious clinically, particularly during an epidemic. However, if in doubt as to whether the swelling is parotid, confirmation can be obtained by measuring serum or urinary amylase, which will be raised.

**Complications.** The importance of mumps lies in its complications, principally deafness and meningoencephalitis. The incidence of post-mumps deafness is one in 15 000. The virus attacks the eighth nerve, causing sensorineural deafness which is usually severe and unilateral. Meningoencephalitis is very common, but is usually mild and characterized by headache, neck stiffness and photophobia. The cerebrospinal

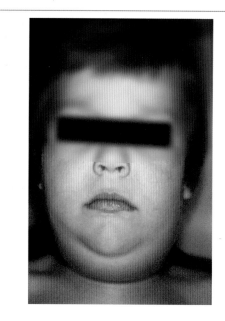

**Figure 7.3** An 11-year-old child with mumps. Note the swelling of the parotid gland obscuring the angle of the jaw. CDC/Patricia Smith; Barbara Rice.

fluid contains an increased number of lymphocytes and raised protein. Orchitis does occur, but very rarely in the prepubertal boy. Mumps has been implicated in the development of diabetes.

---

### 👁 Mumps at a glance

**Immunization**
Live attenuated virus given at
  12–18 months

**Aetiology**
Mumps virus

**History**
Fever (**a**)
Malaise
Neck swelling
Pain on swallowing sweet/
  sour liquids

**Physical examination**
Unilateral or bilateral parotid
  swelling (**b**)
10% Meningoencephalitis (**c**)

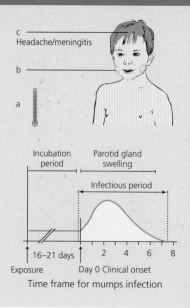

c ——— Headache/meningitis

b ———

a

Incubation period    Parotid gland swelling

Infectious period

16–21 days    2  4  6  8
Exposure    Day 0 Clinical onset
Time frame for mumps infection

**Confirmatory investigations**
None required
(Serum/urinary amylase raised)

**Differential diagnosis**
Cervical lymphadenopathy

**Management**
Supportive

**Course**
Incubation period 16–21 days
Contagious until swelling
  subsides

**Complications**
Sensorineural deafness
Meningoencephalitis
Orchitis rare in prepubertal boy

## Mastoiditis

Mastoiditis is now a rare but serious infection of childhood which demands emergency treatment. The infection usually extends from otitis media, and the responsible bacteria is *Haemophilus influenzae*. Treatment is by surgical drainage and intravenous antibiotics.

## Measles

Despite the widespread use of MMR immunization, measles is still occasionally seen. It is a miserable and very infectious viral illness characterized by a distinctive maculopapular rash (see Figure 7.4a) in conjunction with the three 'Cs' (cough, coryza and conjunctivitis). Immunization with a live attenuated vaccine is given at about 13 months and 3–5 years (see p. 29).

**Clinical features.** After an incubation period of 10–14 days there is a prodromal illness with fever and upper respiratory symptoms, followed by onset of the rash on the 3rd or 4th day. The rash begins on the face and behind the ears and spreads downwards to cover the whole body. In contrast to some of the other childhood infectious diseases the child is ill and irritable. The rash begins to fade after 3 or 4 days and becomes blotchy. During the prodromal period a distinctive exanthem can be visualized. Koplik spots (see Figure 7.4b), looking like grains of salt on a red background, appear on the buccal mucosa of the cheeks. In developing countries there is a high morbidity and mortality and diarrhoea is a common feature.

**Complications.** Acute otitis media and bronchopneumonia are common complications. The serious complication of post-measles encephalitis occurs in one in 5000 cases and causes drowsiness, vomiting, headache and convulsions. The prognosis for normal neurological survival is poor. It generally occurs a week after the measles is diagnosed and is probably caused by an immunological cross-reactivity between measles virus and neural tisue. Subacute sclerosing encephalitis (SSPE) is a very rare complication which occurs some 4–10 years after an attack and is characterized by slow progressive neurological degeneration.

**Management.** Treatment of measles is supportive. Antibiotics are required if otitis media or bronchopneumonia develop. The child is contagious from before the onset of the rash to the 5th day of the rash.

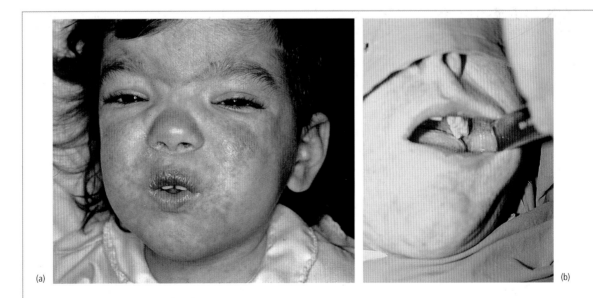

(a)   (b)

**Figure 7.4** (a) A 2-year-old child with measles, demonstrating the typical maculopapular rash, conjunctivitis and miserable appearance. (b) Koplik spots.

## Measles at a glance

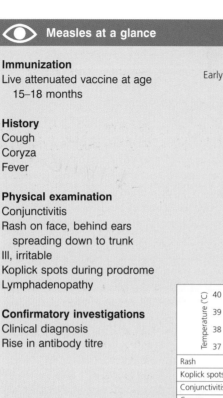

**Immunization**
Live attenuated vaccine at age
   15–18 months

**History**
Cough
Coryza
Fever

**Physical examination**
Conjunctivitis
Rash on face, behind ears
   spreading down to trunk
Ill, irritable
Koplick spots during prodrome
Lymphadenopathy

**Confirmatory investigations**
Clinical diagnosis
Rise in antibody titre

Early          Late

**Differential diagnosis**
Non-specific viral exanthem
Rubella
Scarlet fever

**Management**
Supportive
Antibiotics for otitis media and
   pneumonia
Child is contagious until day 5

**Course**
Incubation period 10–14 days
Rash lasts 5 days

**Complications**
Otitis media and pneumonia
   common
Post-measles encephalitis rare
   but serious
Subacute sclerosing
   encephalitis (SSPE) very rare
High morbidity and mortality in
   developing countries

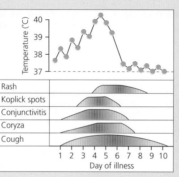

## Rubella (German measles)

Rubella is usually a mild illness and the rash may not even be noticed. The importance of the condition does not lie with the effect on the child, but on the devastating effects on the fetus if rubella is contracted by a mother during the first trimester of pregnancy. The fetus may die or develop congenital heart disease, mental retardation, deafness and cataracts. In order to reduce exposure of young mothers to the virus, and to protect girls before they reach childbearing age, rubella immunization is given in early childhood (p. 53). If a rash occurs during pregnancy, rubella titres should be measured immediately and again after 10 days to determine whether recent infection has occurred.

**Clinical features.** After an incubation period of 14–21 days, the rash appears as tiny pink macules on the face and trunk and works its way down

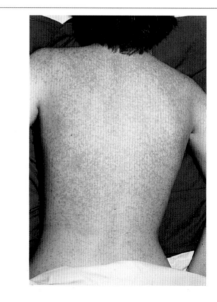

**Figure 7.5** Rubella. A 10-year-old girl with rubella – small pink macules shown on the back.

the body (Figure 7.5). The suboccipital lymph nodes are enlarged and there may be generalized lymphadenopathy. Thrombocytopenia, encephalitis and arthritis are rare complications. The rash is quite non-specific, and the diagnosis of rubella is often made erroneously and overconfidently on clinical grounds.

**Management.** No specific management is required.

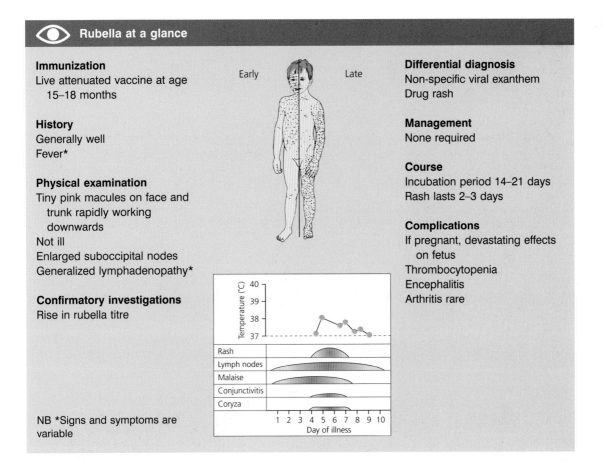

**Rubella at a glance**

**Immunization**
Live attenuated vaccine at age 15–18 months

**History**
Generally well
Fever*

**Physical examination**
Tiny pink macules on face and trunk rapidly working downwards
Not ill
Enlarged suboccipital nodes
Generalized lymphadenopathy*

**Confirmatory investigations**
Rise in rubella titre

Early     Late

**Differential diagnosis**
Non-specific viral exanthem
Drug rash

**Management**
None required

**Course**
Incubation period 14–21 days
Rash lasts 2–3 days

**Complications**
If pregnant, devastating effects on fetus
Thrombocytopenia
Encephalitis
Arthritis rare

NB *Signs and symptoms are variable

| | 1 2 3 4 5 6 7 8 9 10 |
|---|---|
| Rash | |
| Lymph nodes | |
| Malaise | |
| Conjunctivitis | |
| Coryza | |
| | Day of illness |

## Roseola

Roseola affects children under the age of 2 years and has a very characteristic course.

**Clinical features.** The child has a pronounced fever reaching to 39 or 40°C lasting for 3–4 days. In general, despite the height of the temperature the child does not seem to be particularly unwell, although febrile convulsions may occur on the first day. Occipital lymph nodes are often enlarged. On the 4th day the temperature drops and a faint pink macular rash appears on the trunk, lasting for only a few hours or a day or so. The child then makes an uneventful recovery.

**Management.** The fever needs to be controlled. There are no recommendations to isolate the child.

## Scarlet fever

Scarlet fever, which is now uncommon, is the only childhood maculopapular exanthem caused by a bacterium and therefore requiring antibiotic treatment (although children with measles may need antibiotics for complications). It is caused by a strain of group A haemolytic streptococci.

**Clinical features.** After an incubation period of 2–4 days fever, headache and tonsillitis appear. The rash (Figure 7.6) develops within 12 hours and spreads

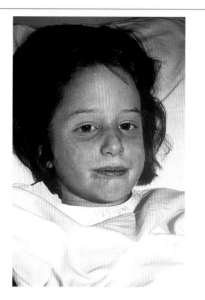

**Figure 7.6** Scarlet fever. Note the fine punctate maculopapular rash and perioral pallor.

rapidly over the trunk and neck, with increased density in the neck, axillae and groins. It has a fine punctate erythematous appearance, a 'sandpapery' feel and blanches on pressure. The tongue initially has a white coating, which desquamates leaving a sore 'red strawberry' appearance. The rash lasts about 6 days and is followed by peeling, which is useful in making a retrospective diagnosis.

**Investigations.** Throat swab may show group A streptococcus, and anti-streptolysin O (ASO) titre is usually elevated.

**Management.** A 10-day course of penicillin or erythromycin eradicates the organism and may prevent other children from being infected.

**Complications.** Sequelae such as rheumatic fever and acute glomerulonephritis (see p. 307) are now rare in developed societies.

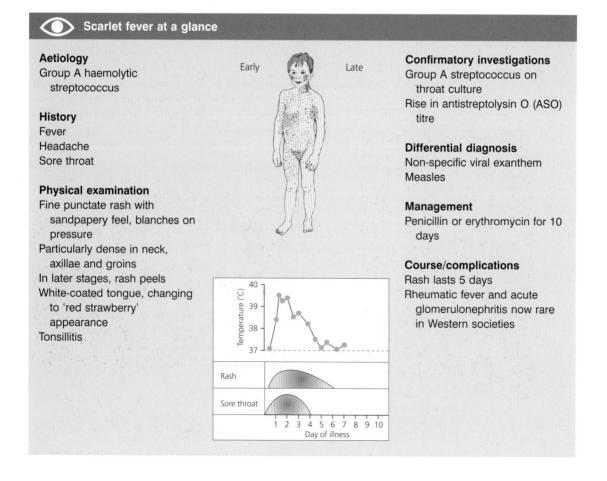

**Scarlet fever at a glance**

**Aetiology**
Group A haemolytic
    streptococcus

**History**
Fever
Headache
Sore throat

**Physical examination**
Fine punctate rash with
    sandpapery feel, blanches on
    pressure
Particularly dense in neck,
    axillae and groins
In later stages, rash peels
White-coated tongue, changing
    to 'red strawberry'
    appearance
Tonsillitis

Early    Late

**Confirmatory investigations**
Group A streptococcus on
    throat culture
Rise in antistreptolysin O (ASO)
    titre

**Differential diagnosis**
Non-specific viral exanthem
Measles

**Management**
Penicillin or erythromycin for 10
    days

**Course/complications**
Rash lasts 5 days
Rheumatic fever and acute
    glomerulonephritis now rare
    in Western societies

# Fifth disease (erythema infectiosum)

This condition is caused by human parvovirus B19. It is called fifth disease because it was the fifth of five illnesses to be described with somewhat similar rashes. (The other four were rubella, measles, scarlet fever and Filatov–Dukes disease–a mild, atypical form of scarlet fever.)

**Clinical features.** The illness usually begins with the sudden appearance of livid erythema of the cheeks, giving the child a 'slapped cheek' appearance. There are usually no prodromal symptoms, and fever is absent or low grade. A symmetrical maculopapular lace-like rash (Figure 7.7) then appears on the arms, trunks, buttocks and thighs. The rash can last up to 6 weeks and may be pruritic. Recrudescences may appear with temperature, exercise and emotional upset. Arthralgia and arthritis occur infrequently.

**Management.** Isolation is not required, and as the illness is mild and the duration of the rash may be prolonged, children should be allowed to attend school.

# Chicken pox (varicella)

Chicken pox is a common and highly contagious disease of childhood which, luckily, is usually mild in this age group. It may be contracted from a patient with shingles. Children who are immunocompromised (such as those on corticosteroids or being treated for leukaemia) are at risk for severe, often fatal chicken pox. If such a child comes into contact with chicken pox, prophylaxis with zoster immunoglobulin should be considered. A vaccine against chicken pox is part of routine immunization in the United States, but currently is only given to those in high-risk groups in the United Kingdom.

**Clinical features.** After an incubation period of 14–17 days the rash (Figure 7.8) appears on the trunk and face. The spots appear in crops, passing rapidly through the stages of macule to papule and then vesicle. The appearance of the vesicles have been likened to 'dewdrops' on an erythematous base. The vesicles rapidly turn into pustules and then crust over. At the height of the illness the lesions simultaneously consist of papules, vesicles and crusts. Itching is constant and annoying. Vesicles in the mucous membranes, particularly in the mouth, rapidly become macerated and form shallow ulcers. The severity of the disease varies from a few lesions in a well child to many hundreds of lesions with severe toxicity.

**Complications.** The commonest complication is secondary infection of the lesions and scarring. A more severe complication is encephalitis, which produces cerebellar signs with ataxia. Thrombocytopenia with haemorrhage into the skin can occur. Varicella pneumonia is uncommon in children.

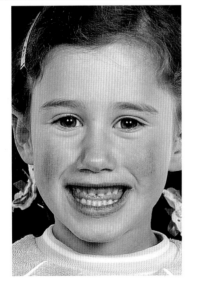

**Figure 7.7** Fifth disease. Note the 'slapped cheek' rash in a well looking child.

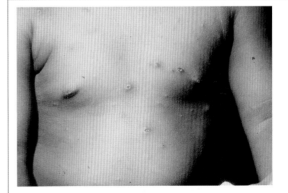

**Figure 7.8** Chicken pox. Note the characteristic vesicular rash at various stages of development, although few have reached the pustular or crusted stage.

**Management.** Itching can be alleviated to some extent by cool baths and application of calamine lotion. If the child is very distressed, promethazine syrup can be helpful. Cutting fingernails short and keeping them clean can reduce secondary infection.

The child is contagious until all the lesions have crusted over. If the disease develops in an immunocompromised child, urgent admission for intravenous acyclovir is indicated.

---

### 👁 Chicken pox at a glance

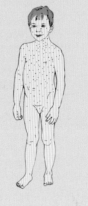

**Aetiology**
Herpes virus (contracted from chicken pox or shingles)

**Immunization**
Vaccine for high-risk groups
Immunoglobulin indicated for immunocompromised child exposed to chicken pox

**History**
Fever
Itching lesions
Irritability*

**Physical examination**
Lesions: a mixture of papules, vesicles, pustules and crusts over the trunk and face
Ulcers in mouth
May look toxic if severely affected*

**Confirmatory investigations**
Clinical diagnosis

NB *Signs and symptoms are variable

**Differential diagnosis**
Usually unequivocal

**Management**
Relieve itching by cool baths, calamine lotion ± promethazine syrup
Child contagious until all lesions crusted
If child is immunocompromised, give IV acyclovir

**Course**
Incubation period 14–17 days
Lesions last 6–10 days

**Complications**
Secondary infection of lesions
Encephalitis (cerebellar signs with ataxia)
Thrombocytopenia with skin haemorrhages
Chicken pox is severe or even fatal for the immunocompromised child

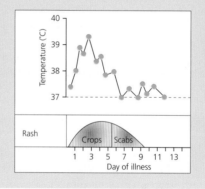

---

## Hand, foot and mouth disease

Hand, foot and mouth disease is caused by a Coxsackie virus. It occurs in epidemics affecting young children. Vesicular lesions appear on the palms of the hands and fingers, the soles of the feet, and in the mouth. The vesicles clear by absorption of the fluid in about a week. There may be a low-grade fever.

## Meningococcal septicaemia

Meningococcal septicaemia often starts insidiously and then may rapidly become severe and life-threatening. The underlying organism, *Neisseria meningitidis*, most commonly causes meningitis, but in some cases septicaemia is the predominant presenting condition.

**Clinical features.** There is often a short coryzal prodrome, followed by fever (Figure 7.9), malaise and the development of a petechial/purpuric rash. The hallmark of meningococcaemia is petechial or purpuric skin lesions that do not blanch on pressure. The purpura may enlarge rapidly as the child deteriorates (Figure 7.10). Signs of meningitis may be present. Meningococcal septicaemia is often fulminant with

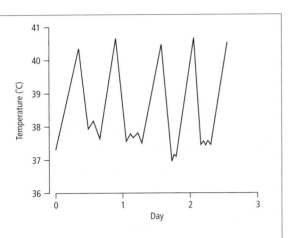

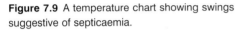

**Figure 7.9** A temperature chart showing swings suggestive of septicaemia.

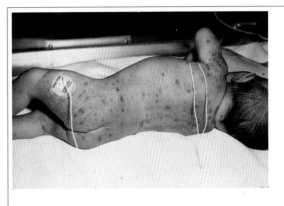

**Figure 7.10** Meningococcaemia. Note the typical purpuric lesions that do not blanch under pressure.

**Box 7.2 Managing the child with meningococcal septicaemia**

• Give IM or IV penicillin as soon as diagnosis suspected
• Arrange rapid admission to hospital and give regular IV cefotaxime
• Treat shock with intravenous fluids
• Treat all close contacts with rifampicin

rapid deterioration, disseminated intravascular coagulopathy and shock. Death may occur within a few hours of presentation, caused by shock and adrenal failure (Waterhouse–Friderichsen syndrome).

**Management (see Box 7.2).** As the course so often is fulminant, treatment must be started on the basis of strong clinical suspicion rather than awaiting the result of investigations. Any ill child seen at home with petechial or purpuric lesions should be given penicillin immediately by the family doctor. This should preferably be given intravenously, but intramuscular injection is acceptable. If it is possible to take blood cultures prior to giving antibiotics this is preferable, but it may not be feasible. The child must be rushed to hospital as quickly as possible.

Management in hospital consists of antibiotics (intravenous cefotaxime) and intensive care directed towards supporting the circulation. Shock is a common and severe feature, and massive volumes of plasma may be necessary to reverse this. Mortality is high.

The meningococcus colonizes the upper respiratory tract of asymptomatic children, and close contacts of children with meningococcal infection are at increased risk of infection. Such contacts should be given a 2-day course of prophylactic rifampicin.

**Prognosis.** Mortality is high in children who present with meningococcal septicaemia; some die before reaching hospital. Even with rapid antibiotic treatment, death may occur as a result of irreversible shock. If the child survives, the prognosis for intact recovery is good. Only a relatively small proportion of those who survive meningococcal septicaemia will have long-term sequelae.

## HIV infection and AIDS

Paediatric acquired immunodeficiency syndrome (AIDS) is caused by human immunodeficiency virus (HIV) type 1. The two paediatric populations at risk are:

1 infants born to infected mothers;
2 adolescents who acquire infection sexually or by the intravenous use of drugs.

There is essentially no risk of being infected by casual contact with an HIV-infected child in the family, at

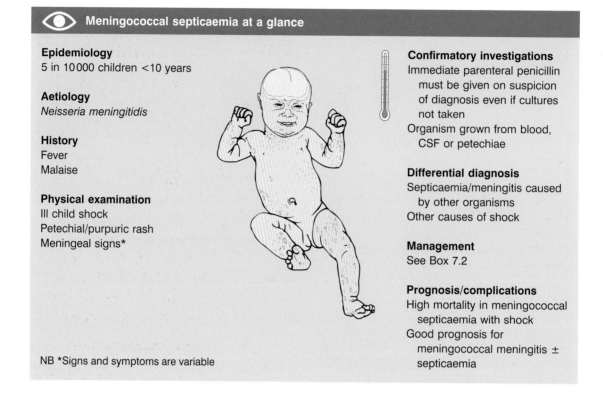

**Meningococcal septicaemia at a glance**

**Epidemiology**
5 in 10 000 children <10 years

**Aetiology**
*Neisseria meningitidis*

**History**
Fever
Malaise

**Physical examination**
Ill child shock
Petechial/purpuric rash
Meningeal signs*

**Confirmatory investigations**
Immediate parenteral penicillin
must be given on suspicion
of diagnosis even if cultures
not taken
Organism grown from blood,
CSF or petechiae

**Differential diagnosis**
Septicaemia/meningitis caused
by other organisms
Other causes of shock

**Management**
See Box 7.2

**Prognosis/complications**
High mortality in meningococcal
septicaemia with shock
Good prognosis for
meningococcal meningitis ±
septicaemia

NB *Signs and symptoms are variable

nursery or at school. Most children with HIV are diagnosed before the age of 3 years.

**Clinical features.** Infected infants are usually diagnosed because they have features of immunodeficiency – namely, failure to thrive, diarrhoea, candidiasis or hepatosplenomegaly – or because they develop severe bacterial infections. Severe life-threatening infections include pneumonia, septicaemia, persistent pulmonary infiltrates, *Pneumocystis jiroveci* pneumonia (PCP), tuberculosis and systemic candida.

**Diagnosis.** Diagnosis is made by the detection of HIV antibody, which is very specific and sensitive. However, passive maternal transplacental IgG obscures the diagnosis in young infants, as the antibody may still be measurable up to the age of 18 months in uninfected clinically well infants. Hence, in children under 2 years of age, detection of HIV antigen is required to confirm the diagnosis.

**Management.** At present the goals of intervention in HIV-infected patients focus on the use of antiviral drugs, prophylactic antibiotics, viral vaccines and, where necessary, immune serum globulin. The psy-

chosocial and emotional needs of the family must also be addressed.

**Prognosis.** Of babies born to HIV-positive mothers 20–30% become HIV positive themselves, although this rate can be dramatically reduced by preventive measures. In children with clinical HIV infection the prognosis is very variable, but in general, the earlier and more severe the presentation, the worse the prognosis.

**Prevention.** The administration of combination antiretroviral therapy including zidovudine to HIV-infected pregnant women, and delivery by caesarean section, reduces the transmission of the virus to infants. At birth the infant should also receive zidovudine for 4 weeks. In developed countries where the risks of bottle-feeding are low, HIV-positive mothers should not breast-feed, as the virus may be transmitted in breast milk. For the adolescent and adult, prevention of HIV includes precautions in coming into contact with bodily fluids and the practice of safe sex, with the use of condoms.

*To test your knowledge on this part of the book, please see Chapter 25.*

## 👁 HIV infection and AIDS at a glance

**Epidemiology**
Infants born to infected mothers
Adolescents: acquired sexually
    or by IV drug use

**Aetiology**
Human immunodeficiency virus
    type 1

**Prevention**
Perinatal management:
• zidovudine to HIV-positive
  pregnant women
• delivery by caesarean section
• zidovudine at birth
• avoidance of breast-feeding
  (Western countries)
Other ages:
• universal precautions for body
  fluids
• safe sex

**History**
Severe bacterial infections
Poor weight gain
Diarrhoea*
Loss of developmental
    milestones*

NB *Signs and symptoms are
variable

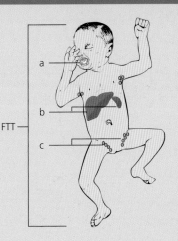

FTT

**Physical examination**
Failure to thrive (FTT)
Candidiasis (**a**)
Hepatosplenomegaly (**b**)
Lymphadenopathy (**c**)
Chest signs*
Other specific signs relating to
    organs involved*

**Confirmatory investigations**
HIV antibody detection (*but in*
    infants this may have been
    passively acquired and is not
    necessarily a sign of infection)
Immunological testing

**Differential diagnosis**
Depends on organ systems
    involved
Other immunodeficiency
    disorders

**Management**
Antiviral drugs
Prophylactic antibiotics
Viral vaccine
Immune serum globulin
Psychosocial/emotional support

**Prognosis/complications**
20–30% babies born to
    HIV-positive mothers become
    infected
High risk for pneumonia,
    septicaemia, persistent
    pulmonary infiltrates,
    *Pneumocystis jiroveci
    pneumonia*, tuberculosis,
    systemic candida
Variable prognosis: earlier and
    more severe presentations
    have worse prognosis

# CHAPTER 8

# Respiratory disorders

Christopher Robin
Had wheezles
And sneezles,
They bundled him
Into
His bed.
They gave him what goes
With a cold in the nose,
And some more for a cold
In the head.
*'Now We are Six', AA Milne*

## COMPETENCES

### You must . . .

| Know | Be able to | Appreciate |
|---|---|---|
| • How to diagnose and manage the common and serious respiratory conditions<br>• The key preventer and reliever medications used in asthma and how to administer them to children of different ages<br>• How to read a chest X-ray (p. 98) | • Examine the respiratory system competently<br>• Recognise the signs of respiratory distress<br>• Carry out peak flow measurements<br>• Carry out the Heimlich procedure<br>• Show a child how to use an inhaler<br>• Recognize when a child with asthma is in severe respiratory distress | • Appreciate the impact that asthma or cystic fibrosis has on the child and family<br>The principles involved in managing chronic respiratory disorders |

*Paediatrics and Child Health*, Third Edition. Mary Rudolf, Tim Lee, Malcolm Levene.
© 2011 Mary Rudolf, Tim Lee and Malcolm Levene. Published 2011 by Blackwell Publishing Ltd.

# Respiratory symptoms and signs

## Finding your way around . . .

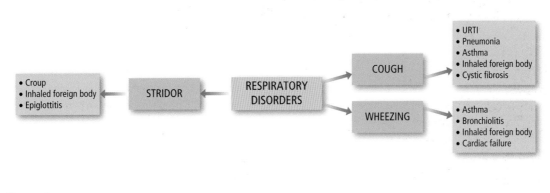

## Cough

| Causes of cough by age | | |
|---|---|---|
| **Infancy** | **Preschool** | **School-age to adolescence** |
| Infections | Infections | Asthma |
|   upper respiratory tract |   upper respiratory tract | Infections |
|   bronchiolitis |   croup |   upper respiratory tract |
|   pneumonia |   acute bronchitis | Cigarette smoking |
| Congenital malformations of the |   pneumonia | Postnasal drip |
|   airway | Foreign body | Psychogenic |
| Gastro-oesophageal reflux | Asthma | Cystic fibrosis |
| Cystic fibrosis | Cystic fibrosis | |
| | Passive smoking | |

Cough is a common symptom occurring with fever in an acutely ill child or as a troublesome and persistent problem. It generally results from a simple viral infection but may be an indicator of a serious infection or a chronic condition such as asthma (see Red Flag box).

### Evidence of serious chronic lower respiratory tract disease in children

- Productive cough which improves with antibiotics but quickly recurs
- Restriction of activity
- Failure to grow or gain weight
- Clubbing
- Persistent tachypnoea

Illnesses causing cough vary with age, although the commonest cause of cough for all ages is infection affecting the upper or lower respiratory tract. A cough may persist and perpetuate itself after any illness, as coughing can injure the tracheal mucosa, making it more susceptible to irritation. Passive exposure to smoking exacerbates coughing and respiratory disease.

In infancy, upper respiratory tract infections (URTIs) can be particularly troublesome as the infant's ability to feed can be affected. Bronchiolitis, which affects the small airways (see p. 153), is a disease specific to this age group. If cough is chronic in infancy, serious causes such as congenital anomalies of the airways or aspiration of stomach contents should be considered.

In the preschool years, exposure to respiratory illnesses increases and cough is very common. Bronchitis is a rather non-specific term used either in relation to a productive cough (acute bronchitis) or bronchospasm. It is important to appreciate, however, that chronic bronchitis is not a paediatric disease. Asthma (see p. 141) often presents for the first time in the preschool years, and may be manifested by cough as well as wheeze. Foreign bodies are also common, and the cough may occur some time after the episode of choking has been forgotten.

In older children, asthma and minor infections are the commonest causes of cough. Smoking must be considered as a possible cause of cough in adolescence.

### History – must ask!

- *What does the cough sound like?* The sound of the cough can give a clue to the aetiology (Table 8.1). The rattling sound of mucus in the tracheobronchial tree is quite distinctive from either a dry laryngeal cough or the wheezy cough of asthma.
- *What is the sputum like?* Young children swallow sputum, rather than expectorate, so asking about the sputum is of limited value. Older children, however, may be able to cooperate. Persistent purulent sputum suggests suppurative lung disease such as cystic fibrosis or bronchiectasis. In asthma sputum is clear and tenacious. Bloody sputum, if not from nasopharyngeal irritation, suggests a foreign body.

**Table 8.1** Characteristics of coughs

| | |
|---|---|
| Loose, productive | Bronchitis, wheezy bronchitis, cystic fibrosis, bronchiectasis |
| Wheezy | Asthma, wheezy bronchitis |
| Barking | Croup |
| Paroxysmal (with or without vomiting) | Cystic fibrosis, pertussis, foreign body, asthma |
| Nocturnal | Asthma, sinusitis |
| Most severe on waking | Cystic fibrosis, bronchiectasis |
| With vigorous exercise | Exercise-induced asthma, cystic fibrosis, bronchiectasis |
| Disappears with sleep | Habit cough |

- *When is the coughing worst?* A non-productive nocturnal cough suggests bronchospasm, postnasal secretions, or gastro-oesophageal reflux. A productive cough on getting up suggests bronchiectasis or cystic fibrosis. Paroxysms of coughing suggest either a foreign body or pertussis, and coughing related to eating points to aspiration.
- *Is the cough acute, persistent or recurrent?* Coughing may persist for weeks even after a mild respiratory infection. However, persistent cough in conjunction with other signs may indicate a chronic lung condition. Recurrent coughing, particularly at night, suggests asthma. Diaries kept by parents are valuable if the cough is persistent or chronic.
- *Is the child ill?* Fever indicates infection, but does not differentiate between upper and lower respiratory tract infection. If the child is ill, lower respiratory tract infection must be considered (see pneumonia, p. 151).
- *Are there associated symptoms or precipitating factors?* Coughing with wheezing strongly points to asthma, and other atopic manifestations in the child or the family helps in the diagnosis. Exacerbations during the spring and summer suggest an allergic aetiology. An episode of choking might be recalled, suggesting inhalation of a foreign body. Chronic symptoms of oily diarrhoea suggest cystic fibrosis.
- *Does anyone smoke in the family?* Passive smoking has an irritant effect on the young airway and can cause coughing in itself. It also predisposes to asthma and infections. Adolescents may not confess to smoking, particularly if accompanied by a parent.
- *Past medical history.* A history of previous chest infections, particularly if confirmed radiologically, should suggest chronic lung disease.

### Physical examination – must check!

- *Growth.* Measure height and weight in all children, as poor growth occurs in chronic conditions such as cystic fibrosis, bronchiectasis, immunodeficiency or severe asthma.
- *Signs of respiratory distress.* Tachypnoea, subcostal and intercostal retractions (Fig. 4.14, p. 64) and alar flaring indicate respiratory distress and in childhood are often more significant than auscultation findings. In an infant an expiratory grunting sound suggests severe respiratory distress. Tachypnoea may be the only sign of serious respiratory pathology.
- *Examination of the chest.* Examination of the chest is obviously important. However, interpret your findings on auscultation cautiously. Transmitted sounds from the upper airways are commonly heard in the

child with a cold, and must be differentiated from crepitations. Focal chest signs are less reliable than in adults in indicating the site of infection. Expiratory wheezing suggests the diagnosis of asthma, but may not be present between attacks unless the asthma is severe. Decreased air entry indicates bronchial obstruction from any cause.

• *Other signs.* Clubbing in a child with a cough suggests the possibility of suppurative lung disease or associated cardiac pathology. Signs of atopy such as eczema or allergic-appearing eyes point towards a diagnosis of asthma.

### Investigations (see Table 8.2)

Investigations are required if a child has evidence of pneumonia or chronic lung disease (see Red Flag box). The interpretation of chest X-rays is covered on p. 98. X-rays are too often repeatedly obtained in children with asthma.

**Table 8.2** Investigations and their relevance in a coughing child

| Investigation | What you are looking for |
|---|---|
| Full blood count | Raised white count and shift to the left with bacterial infection |
| | Possible eosinophilia in asthma |
| Blood culture | Lower respiratory tract infection |
| Pernasal swab | To identify pertussis |
| Chest X-ray* | Lower respiratory tract infection |
| Chest X-ray and barium swallow | Congenital anomalies of the airway, gastrointestinal reflux |
| Sweat test | Cystic fibrosis |
| Videofluoroscopy and bronchoscopy | Aspirated foreign body |
| Trial of bronchodilators ± peak flow measurements | Asthma |

* See 'Reading a chest X-ray', p. 98.

If a foreign body is suspected, chest fluoroscopy is required to look for mediastinal shift on inspiration. Bronchoscopy is needed to confirm the diagnosis and remove the foreign body.

A sweat test for cystic fibrosis is indicated for recurrent productive cough, particularly if accompanied by poor growth or abnormal stools. As asthma is a common cause of recurrent cough, diagnosis using tests of peak flow are desirable when the child is old enough to cooperate.

### Managing cough as a symptom

Antibiotics have no place in the management of URTIs, and should only be given if there is good evidence of infection of the lower tract. A good trial of bronchodilators, delivered by a technique appropriate for age, is required when asthma is suspected or diagnosed (see p. 141).

Psychogenic cough is a diagnosis of exclusion. Characteristically, an early-school-age child will have a recurrent loud "brassy" barking dry cough that never occurs when the child is asleep. The family are often very anxious about the cough. If there is no suggestion of serious pathology in the history or examination, the child and family should be reassured. The cough will often resolve if ignored by the family for several weeks; if it persists, futher investigation may be necessary.

Smoking is an important cause and exacerbator of cough. Every effort must be made to discourage exposure, whether passive or active.

> **Key points: A coughing child**
>
> • Transmitted sounds from the upper airways are commonly heard and should not be confused with crepitations or wheeze
> • Observation of tachypnoea, intercostal or subcostal retractions and alar flaring are often more important signs than findings on auscultation
> • Asthma commonly presents with cough in young children as well as wheezing
> • High fever in itself does not indicate lower respiratory tract infection
> • In a child with chronic or persistent cough, look for evidence of chronic lung disease

## Clues to the differential diagnosis of the coughing child

| | Fever | Features of cough | Respiratory signs |
|---|---|---|---|
| **Upper respiratory tract infection (URTI)** | +/− | Non-productive | None, other than transmitted sounds |
| **Pneumonia** | + | Productive | Alar flaring, intercostal, subcostal retractions, +/−/? dullness to percussion, diminished breath sounds |
| **Asthma** | − or +/− if URTI present | Wheezy, often nocturnal or on exercise | Alar flaring, intercostal, subcostal retractions, expiratory wheeze (but may be absent at time of examination) |
| **Foreign body** | − (until infection develops) | Often preceded by choking episode | Wheeze, diminished breath sounds on right |

## Wheezing

### Commoner causes of wheezing

Asthma
Bronchiolitis and other viral agents
Aspiration of food or a foreign body
Sequelae of neonatal lung disease
    (bronchopulmonary dysplasia)
Cardiac failure

Noisy breathing is a common symptom in children which may be caused by partial obstruction of either the upper or lower airway. The upper airway comprises the nose, pharynx, larynx and extrathoracic portion of the trachea. The lower airway comprises intrathoracic trachea, bronchi and bronchioles. Partial obstruction of the upper airway causes an inspiratory noise (*stridor*) and partial obstruction of the lower airway an expiratory *wheeze*. In many cases noises can be heard on both inspiration and expiration, and it requires concentration to determine the phase of breathing in which the predominant noise occurs.

A wheeze is a prolonged musical note heard mainly on expiration and is very common in childhood. It may also be referred to as a *rhonchus* on auscultation. It is fairly easily distinguished from stridor (p. 139), which is an inspiratory upper airway noise. Transmitted noises from the upper airway are often heard when auscultating the young child's chest. This may make interpretation of intrathoracic noises

more difficult. It may be helpful to hold the bell of the stethoscope to the child's throat and listen to the upper airway noise. These noises can then be mentally subtracted from the noises heard when listening for lower airway signs.

Wheezing is caused by partial obstruction of the intrathoracic airways and is a result of intrinsic or extrinsic factors (Figure 8.1). Bronchi have a layer of smooth muscle within the wall of the tube. Various factors may cause the muscle to spasm thereby narrowing the tube. Intrinsic factors are mediated through histamine release as part of the inflammatory response which causes acute narrowing of the bronchi and bronchioles. The commonest causes are allergy and infection. Extrinsic causes of airway narrowing include

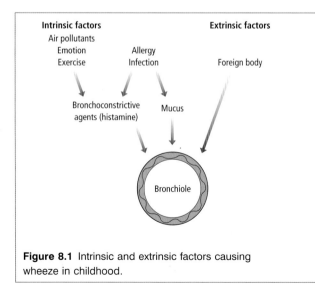

**Figure 8.1** Intrinsic and extrinsic factors causing wheeze in childhood.

the presence of a foreign body and mucus oversecretion as a result of infection. Therefore viral infection may cause wheeze from both constriction of the tube's muscle wall as the result of intrinsic release of vaso-constrictive substances and from the production of mucus as a result of the infectious agent.

It is estimated that 20% of all children will wheeze at some time in the first 5 years of life. Children (particularly under 3 years of age) are prone to wheezing with viral infections, as bronchospasm, mucosal oedema and secretions have a greater impact in narrowing their relatively smaller airways. The first episode of wheezing may cause great parental anxiety and, if there is a family history of asthma, the first episode of viral-induced wheeze may cause the parents to jump to the conclusion that their child also has asthma.

The clinical evaluation is important to determine the degree to which wheezing is affecting the child and to identify conditions other than asthma which may present with wheezing. It is important to remember that asthma is by definition a recurring condition and should be diagnosed with caution in toddlers. In any wheezing child you must look for respiratory distress.

### History – must ask!

Take the history from the parents if the child is young or acutely distressed.

- *The acute episode.* Was there a triggering event? Asthma is often triggered by exposure to allergens such as house-dust mite, pet hair, grass pollens and irritants such as tobacco smoke. It is also precipitated by acute emotion, physical exercise or going out on a cold morning. Viral infection can be an important trigger for asthma, but may be a cause of wheezing in its own right, for example in bronchiolitis.
- *Severity of the episode.* Find out how incapacitated the child is. Ask if he or she is able to feed normally and if the wheezing interferes with play and activity. Severe wheeze and breathlessness may affect the child's ability to talk.
- *Family history.* Asthma is suggested by a family history of *atopy*, including asthma, eczema or hay fever.
- *History of choking.* Aspiration of food or a foreign body is most likely in toddlers who are mobile and put everything they find into their mouth.
- *Apnoea.* Bronchiolitis and other viral infections cause wheezing in infants and may be associated with apnoea and quite severe respiratory distress.

### Physical examination – must check!

- *Assessment of growth.* Plot the child's height and weight on a growth chart. Growth failure does not occur unless the asthma is very severe; poor growth suggests a condition such as cystic fibrosis.
- *Signs of respiratory distress.* Signs of respiratory distress include shortness of breath (dyspnoea), tachypnoea, alar flaring, intercostal and subcostal recession (see p. 376) and the use of accessory muscles for breathing. Features of severe respiratory distress include an inability to talk (in the older child), cyanosis, confusion, restlessness and drowsiness, and any of these symptoms demands rapid assessment and investigation.
- *Chest signs.* In contrast to adults, chest signs in young children are often not localized and may not relate to X-ray findings. Listen for hyper-resonance and dullness on percussion. On auscultation, widespread crepitations with wheezing suggest infection, particularly bronchiolitis in infants, whereas unilateral wheeze suggests aspiration of a foreign body. Wheezing may also be a sign of cardiac failure in a child with congenital heart disease, in which case listen for murmurs, assess the heart size and examine the upper abdomen for hepatomegaly.
- *Other signs.* Look for signs of chronic lung disease such as barrel chest and clubbing. Clubbing is suggestive of chronic suppurative lung disease and rarely occurs in chronic asthma.
- *Peak flow.* This should be part of the assessment of any wheezing or breathless child who is old enough to cooperate (see p. 145)

### Investigations

Most children with acute wheeze require only a careful history and examination. However, an acute onset of wheeze in a very young child, asymmetrical signs on examination or failure to thrive demand investigation. The acutely ill child needs a full blood count and chest X-ray. Repeated chest X-rays in a child with recurrent episodes of acute wheeze are not warranted, particularly where this is thought to be caused by asthma.

The child who shows severe signs of respiratory distress will also need careful assessment for respiratory failure. Oxygen therapy is monitored by transcutaneous oxygen measurement and oxygen titrated against oxygen saturation. Arterial blood gas measurement may help determine the need for respiratory support (see p. 94).

## Managing wheezing

Children with acute onset of wheeze and their parents may be very frightened by the symptom, and reassurance is necessary after appropriate assessment. Immediate management is directed towards assessing whether the child is in actual or incipient respiratory failure, when respiratory support may be required. The need for oxygen therapy is assessed by transcutaneous pulse oximetry.

Asthma is the commonest cause of recurrent wheezing, and provided there is no indication of other conditions on history or physical examination, you should give a trial of a bronchodilator to confirm the diagnosis. Clinical improvement in wheezing indicates that the bronchospasm is reversible and a diagnosis of asthma can be made. In the older, cooperative child, peak flow measurements before and after the trial are useful.

Some babies wheeze very persistently. If the wheeze is not affecting eating, temperament and growth, this need not arouse too much concern. Such children have been called 'happy wheezers' and the symptoms subside as they grow. Milk allergy is often implicated, but withdrawal of cow's milk protein is only rarely effective. A more important intervention is to stop exposure to cigarette smoke.

---

### Key points: The wheezing child

- Asthma is by definition *recurrent* wheezing
- Diagnose asthma with caution below the age of 2 years
- Tachypnoea, alar flaring and intercostal/subcostal recessions are signs of respiratory distress
- Unilateral wheeze in a toddler is suggestive of a foreign body
- Children with asthma in general do not need a chest X-ray at each attack
- Localized chest findings often do not correlate with those on the X-ray

---

### Clues to the differential diagnosis of wheezing in children

| | Age | Percussion | Auscultation | Chest X-ray | Specific features |
|---|---|---|---|---|---|
| **Asthma** | Any age but diagnosed with caution in a child <2 years | Increased percussion note | Widespread wheeze. Variable crepitations | Overinflated | Recurrent wheezing. Triggered by URTI or allergens. Responsive to bronchodilators. Family history of atopy |
| **Foreign body** | Toddlers | Focal dullness with increased resonance if compensatory emphysema | Unilateral wheezing and crepitations, or focal reduced air entry | Segmental collapse or emphysema | Unilateral wheezing. May be preceded by choking episode |
| **Bronchiolitis** | Babies | Variable | Widespread wheeze and crepitations | Overinflation, consolidation | Apnoea may be a feature in infants. Often RSV+. Increased lymphocytes on FBC. Wheeze is often unresponsive to bronchodilators |
| **Viral-induced wheeze/ wheezy bronchitis** | Toddlers | Normal | Wheeze and crepitations | Normal | Wheezing with URTI |
| **Cardiac failure** | Any age | Normal | Wheeze | Enlarged heart | Child with congenital heart disease. Hepatomegaly also a feature |

RSV, respiratory syncytial virus; FBC, full blood count.

# Stridor

### Causes of stridor

*Acute causes*
Croup
Acute epiglottitis
Foreign body

*Chronic causes*
Laryngomalacia
Subglottic stenosis

Stridor is a noise heard on inspiration and is caused by narrowing of the extrathoracic upper airway. Stridor is most likely to arise from the larynx and is usually a sign of croup, a non-severe, self-limiting viral illness which is very common in young children, particularly in the winter. The challenge of the condition is to recognize those children with an acute but non-severe self-limiting illness who can be observed at home and those who, if untreated, may develop life-threatening upper airway obstruction.

### History – must ask!

- *Coryza and fever.* The commonest cause of stridor is croup (acute laryngotracheobronchitis), when the stridor coincides with a barking cough. It is often preceded by coryzal symptoms and fever. The main differential diagnosis is epiglottitis (a life-threatening illness which was not uncommon prior to the introduction of *Haemophilus influenza* B (HiB) immunization). In epiglottitis the child is severely ill.
- *Nature of the stridor.* The degree of stridor depends on the effort of the inspiratory breath. The stridulous noise is usually louder when the child cries and is softer during sleep.
- *Aspiration.* Aspiration of a foreign body should always be considered in acute stridor. If a foreign body is a cause of upper airway obstruction the stridor is usually very severe and the child is dramatically ill.
- *Features of onset.* Laryngomalacia (floppy larynx) is a congenital condition which resolves with age. Subglottic stenosis can develop after a previous intubation.

### Physical examination – must check!

- *Chest signs.* Signs in the chest including crepitations and wheeze are strongly suggestive of croup and are very uncommon with acute epiglottitis or upper airway foreign body obstruction.

- *Airway obstruction.* Stridor is an important sign because it may proceed to acute airway obstruction, a potentially fatal condition. Never examine the throat of a child with severe stridor, as acute airway obstruction may occur; this examination should only be undertaken in the presence of an anaesthetist who can intubate the child if necessary. Signs of increasing airway obstruction include:
  - cyanosis;
  - confusion;
  - reduction in stridor with exhaustion;
  - drooling with increasing dysphagia.

### Investigations

If the child is suspected of having impending respiratory failure or acute epiglottitis, a full blood count and blood culture should be done and blood gases measured. Care must be taken to avoid precipitating acute airway obstruction, and if this is considered to be a risk, prior intubation is necessary.

### Managing stridor

Stridor caused by croup is usually a self-limiting condition, but in a few cases progressive airway obstruction occurs. Mild stridor is best managed at home with no specific treatment, although sitting in a steamy room may be suggested to relieve the symptom. If the condition worsens, hospital assessment is necessary. Intubation by an experienced doctor is needed if there are signs of impending airway obstruction.

If acute epiglottitis is suspected, urgent transfer to hospital for assessment, antibiotic treatment and intubation is essential as airway obstruction is very likely to develop.

Complete upper airway obstruction caused by a foreign body is a medical emergency and if untreated will rapidly lead to death. The Heimlich manoeuvre is used as emergency treatment to relieve the obstruction (p. 377).

### Key points: The child with stridor

- Assess how severe the airway obstruction is and observe any progression
- Assess the likelihood of foreign body aspiration
- Look for the systemic features of acute epiglottitis, and hospitalize as an emergency
- Do not examine the throat if epiglottitis is suspected

| | Age | Clinical features |
|---|---|---|
| **Croup** | 6–24 months | Coryzal prodrome<br>Barking cough |
| **Epiglottitis** | 2–7 year | Toxicity and high fever<br>Drooling |
| **Foreign body** | 9–18 months | History and sudden onset |
| **Laryngomalacia** | Newborn | Presents at birth and persists<br>Worse on crying<br>Improves with age |
| **Subglottic stenosis** | 0–6 months | Previous history of intubation<br>Exacerbations with URTI |

*Clues to the differential diagnosis of stridor*

# Chest pain

**Causes of chest pain**

Idiopathic
Psychogenic
Stitch
Musculoskeletal
Oesophagitis/gastro-oesophageal reflux
Cardiovascular (very rare)

Chest pain is a relatively common complaint which is usually benign and self-limited, but generates a lot of anxiety because of the connotations that chest pain has for adults. Musculoskeletal pain can occur as a result of muscle strain, cough, trauma and stress fracture. Pain at the costochondral junctions due to costochondritis is not uncommon and is often preceded by an URTI or exercise. A stitch is a familiar type of pain thought to be caused by peritoneal ligament stress occurring when exercising in the upright posture. Oesophagitis (see p. 175) can present as pain in older children.

## History – must ask!

The history is important as there are rarely any physical signs. Ask about the duration, frequency, quality and location of the pain, and whether there is any exacerbation or relief with position, exertion, eating, coughing or stress.

## Physical examination – must check!

Your examination should focus on the presence of fever or weight loss, signs of trauma and altered breathing patterns, as well as inspection of the chest and spine and a good respiratory and cardiac assessment.

## Investigations

Investigations such as blood counts, sedimentation rate, chest X-ray and electrocardiogram (ECG) are rarely required but may provide extra reassurance.

## Managing chest pain

You should acknowledge the pain, provide relief for the symptoms in terms of rest and simple analgesics, and reassure the family of the benign nature of the problem.

# Respiratory disorders

## Asthma

### Definition and pathophysiology

The definition of asthma is episodic, reversible, intrathoracic airway obstruction. Reversibility may occur spontaneously or as a result of therapy. The symptoms of asthma, cough and wheeze, are caused by narrowing of the bronchi and bronchioles as a result of bronchoconstriction, mucosal swelling and viscid secretion obstructing the lumen. Various allergic and non-specific stimuli may initiate this process in the susceptible individual by triggering the release of histamine and other mediators. These stimuli include dust mites, air pollutants, cigarette smoke, cold air, viral infections, stress and exercise.

### Prevalence

Asthma is the commonest chronic condition of childhood, affecting up to 20% of children. There is clustering of cases in children living near motorways or in urban environments.

### *Initial presentation of asthma*

Most children with asthma become symptomatic in infancy or the preschool years. The diagnosis is made clinically on the basis of a persistent or recurrent cough or wheeze, which is responsive to medication. A family or past medical history of atopy contributes to the diagnosis.

### Diagnosis in infancy

Many babies have episodes of wheezing, in part as a result of their relatively narrow airways, which readily become obstructed. These episodes may be related to infection by the respiratory syncytial virus (RSV). The majority of wheezing babies do not persist in having troublesome symptoms, and there is therefore no advantage to labelling them as having a chronic medical condition, particularly as the treatment of the wheezy baby is the same whether he or she has a diagnosis of asthma or not (see p. 136). However, if the baby has another atopic condition or there is a family history of atopy and asthma, the wheezing is more likely to be a manifestation of asthma. In infancy, as the airways are so narrow, the contribution of secretions and mucosal oedema to the obstruction is greater, and there is often a poor response to bronchodilator treatment.

### Diagnosis in childhood

Recurrent episodes of coughing and wheezing, especially if aggravated or triggered by exercise, viral infection or inhaled antigens, are highly suggestive of asthma. The diagnosis is made on the basis of the response to bronchodilator treatment. In the younger child this response is judged clinically by the reduction in respiratory distress and wheeze. In the older child, reversibility of airway obstruction can be demonstrated by peak flow measurements. Although X-rays are not often indicated in the child with asthma, a chest X-ray should be considered at the first episode to exclude a foreign body in the lung or oesophagus.

### Allergy testing

Allergy tests are not usually carried out unless the diagnosis is in doubt. Skin testing is not usually helpful, as false positives and false negatives are common and a skin response may not reflect airway hypersensitivity. Radioallergosorbent tests (RAST) may identify allergens to be avoided.

### *Management of asthma*

The goals of management include those for any chronic condition of childhood (see p. 38). The principal goal is the prevention and relief of symptoms of wheeze and cough, both night and day (see Box 8.1). The child and the parents must be educated so that they can manage a large part of the disease themselves. Good management should promote normal growth and development and allow the child to become involved and participate in all types of exercise and sport.

> ### Box 8.1 Goals in managing asthma
>
> - Rapid relief of symptoms
> - Prevention of symptoms both night and day
> - Normal levels of activity, including sport
> - Normal growth and development
> - Self-management

## Medication

The principles of management are shown in Box 8.2. Most asthma medications are delivered by inhalation, where possible, as this ensures delivery of the drug direct to the target organ, the bronchioles, causing a more immediate effect and at a lower dose than if the drug is taken orally. The recommended step-by-step plan to control symptoms is shown in Table 8.3. The child needs to be regularly reviewed to see if gradual step-down is possible, or if step-up is required. If long-term oral or high-dose inhaled steroids are needed, the side effects of adrenal suppression and poor growth may occur.

The drugs used for treating asthma may be classified into 'relievers' and 'preventers'. All children require 'relievers', which are usually beta-agonists such as salbutamol or terbutaline, although the antimuscarinic ipratropium bromide is sometimes used. If the child needs to use 'reliever' treatment frequently, the condition warrants prophylactic management with 'preventer' medication in the form of inhaled steroids or leukotriene receptor antagonist.

Medications need to be inhaled to be most effective. The delivery system chosen must be appropriate for the child's age and capability, which will be affected by the severity of the symptoms (Table 8.4).

### Spacer device

Infants and toddlers can usually be given inhaled medication by using a spacer device with a valve

---

**Box 8.2 Management of asthma**

- Medications must be delivered by inhalation whenever possible
- Use beta-agonists to relieve symptoms
- If used frequently, introduce inhaled steroids
- Treat acute attacks promptly with high-dose inhaled bronchodilator; consider short course of prednisone
- If attack persists, admit for nebulizer treatment, intravenous steroids +/– aminophylline.
- In severe cases ventilation may be required
- In poorly controlled asthma, refer to a respiratory paediatrician; consider alternate-day oral steroids

---

**Table 8.3** The medical management of asthma in children*

| <5 years | 5-12 years |
| --- | --- |
| *Step 1 Mild intermittent asthma* | |
| Inhaled short-acting $\beta_2$-agonist prn | Inhaled short-acting $\beta_2$-agonist as required |
| *Step 2 Regular preventative therapy* | |
| Add inhaled steroids 200–400 µg/day | Add inhaled steroids 200–400 µg/day |
| *Step 3 Add-on therapy* | |
| 6 months – 5 years | 1. Add inhaled long-acting $\beta_2$-agonist (LABA) |
| Add leukotriene receptor antagonist | 2. Consider leukotriene receptor antagonist or oral theophylline |
| <6 months | |
| Proceed to step 4 | |
| *Step 4 Persistent poor control* | |
| Refer to respiratory paediatrician | Increase dose of inhaled steroids (800 µg/day) |
| *Step 5 Continuous or frequent use of steroids* | |
| Not used | Add oral low-dose daily steroids |
| | Refer to respiratory paediatrician |

* Adapted from the Asthma Guidelines of the British Thoracic Society and the Scottish Intercollegiate Guidelines, May 2008.

**Table 8.4** Delivery of medication for asthma at different ages

| Age (years) | Delivery system |
| --- | --- |
| 0–4 | Metered dose inhaler and valved spacer with face mask<br>Nebulizer for acute episodes |
| 5–8 | Metered dose inhaler with valved spacer with mouthpiece (use for preventer and for reliever for significant attacks).<br>Dry powder inhaler for reliever for mild symptoms |
| 8–12 | Consider dry powder inhalers for preventer and reliever inhalers |
| >12 | As above. Consider breath-activated metered dose inhaler |

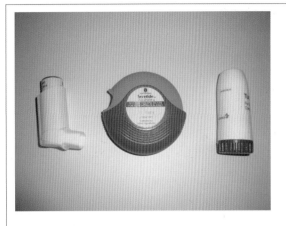

**Figure 8.3** Metered dose inhaler, a dry powder Accuhaler, and dry powder Turbohaler.

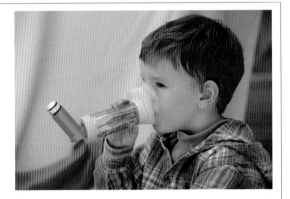

**Figure 8.2** Child using a spacer device.

system (Figure 8.2). A metered dose inhaler dispenses the dose into the chamber and the child inhales the medication over six or seven inhalations. The device ensures that the medication reaches the lungs rather than landing in the mouth or throat. Even young infants can use a spacer device if a closely fitting mask is attached. It is useful for the older child too in an acute attack, when he or she may not be able to use a dry powder system or metered dose inhaler directly. In this circumstance up to ten puffs can be delivered one at a time into the chamber to provide a therapeutic effect.

**Dry powder systems (Figure 8.3)**
These are suitable for many school-age children. A good inspiratory effort is needed to trigger the system,

and so in a severe attack the child may need to resort to a spacer device.

**Breath-activated metered dose inhaler**
This device requires a good degree of coordination, and it has been shown that many adults do not use it effectively. It should only be prescribed in children over the age of 12 years, and only after thorough instruction and checking of technique.

**Nebulizer**
For severe asthma attacks, and some children who cannot cooperate with inhalers via spacers, a mains pump and nebulizer are needed to provide an aerosol which is then delivered by a face mask held close to the child's face (Figure 8.4).

Management of an acute attack
An acute episode of asthma may be precipitated by allergens, viral infection or exercise. The child experiences cough, wheeze and breathlessness, and on examination the chest is generally hyper-resonant and widespread rhonchi are heard. Signs of severe respiratory distress include dyspnoea, cyanosis and recession of the subcostal and intercostal muscles. A chest X-ray is not usually required but may show an overinflated chest with no other abnormalities. Peak flow is reduced.

If the attack does not respond quickly to the child's usual treatment at home, he or she will need urgent treatment by multiple puffs of bronchodilator via spacer or nebulizer attached to an air compressor or compressed oxygen supply. This may be given by the GP, but if a doctor is not immediately available

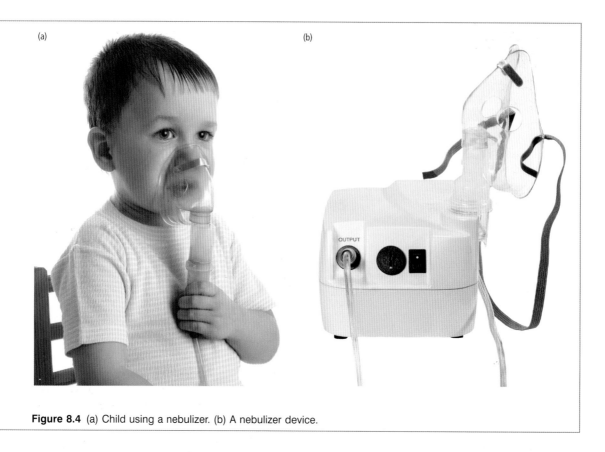

**Figure 8.4** (a) Child using a nebulizer. (b) A nebulizer device.

the child must be taken to hospital for treatment. If there is a good response, the child is sent home after a period of observation. If the episode is severe or recurrent, a short course of oral steroids may be required. Prednisone given for only 3–4 days does not require tapering off and will not cause adrenal suppression or affect growth.

If there is inadequate improvement from the high-dose bronchodilator, the child must be admitted for further high-dose inhaled or nebulized bronchodilator and, if required, intravenous steroid, aminophylline or beta-agonist infusion. Most severe attacks respond rapidly to this treatment, but occasionally intubation and ventilation is required.

In general, children with asthma are often subjected to a large number of unnecessary chest X-rays. Beyond the initial episode at diagnosis, X-rays are only indicated if another problem such as pneumonia, pneumothorax or foreign body is suspected. This is best assessed after the bronchospasm has been relieved.

### Environmental control
Symptoms and drug requirements may be minimized by reducing exposure to allergens and irritants. Particularly critical is protection from exposure to cigarette smoke. Smoking in the home, at least in the child's presence or bedroom, must be avoided. The teenager must be warned about the undesirability of smoking.

House dust, house-dust mites, grass pollens and pets are the commonest allergens. Complete avoidance of house dust is impossible, but feather pillows, duvets and fitted carpets can be avoided. Mattresses should be covered with plastic and the child's room cleaned regularly. Pets, especially cats, may present a problem, and while it is hard to remove a family pet, acquiring new pets can be discouraged.

It is commonly believed that certain foods can cause asthma. Exclusion diets are not generally indicated, but occasionally certain foods or fizzy drinks are identified as causing attacks. It seems reasonable to avoid these, but care must be taken to make sure the diet remains balanced.

### Monitoring the condition
Asthma is monitored by keeping a diary of symptoms, where wheezing, cough and activity levels are recorded along with medications given. In the child old enough to cooperate, peak flow monitoring can form part of the record.

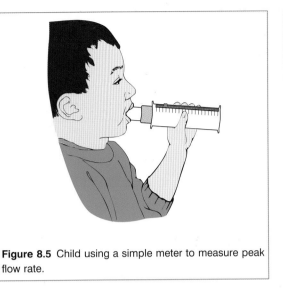

**Figure 8.5** Child using a simple meter to measure peak flow rate.

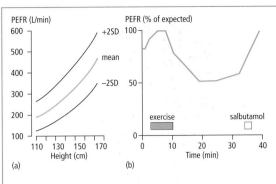

**Figure 8.6** Peak flow chart: how exercise can affect peak flow. (a) The peak flow rate must be related to the child's height to interpret whether it is low. (b) Fall in peak flow rate with exercise in an asthmatic child. Peak flow rate recovers on administration of salbutamol.

## Peak flow monitoring (Figure 8.5)

The majority of children do not need sophisticated lung function tests; however, the peak flow rate is a useful measure of asthmatic control. In the surgery or hospital, a Wright's peak flow meter is used, though it is also useful for the family to have a simple meter for home use.

Peak flow rate (PFR) measures the volume of air moved in a forced expiration. The child is instructed to inhale, place the mouth piece in his or her mouth and to blow out as hard as he or she can. The needle records the peak flow of that exhalation. The procedure should be repeated three times, and the highest reading recorded. Measurements can be taken before and after treating an attack, and in children on high doses of preventive medication measurements should be recorded daily, before morning and evening medications.

Peak flow rate is measured in litres per minute. Values must be related to the size of the child. The standardized chart is shown in Figure 8.6, with an example of how PFR changes with exercise in an asthmatic child.

### The diary

An example is shown in Figure 8.7. The diary serves two functions. It allows the physician to review the child's course and in conjunction with regular clinical reviews to advise on changes in medication requirements. It also may alert the physician to other factors affecting the child, such as stress, compliance or environmental triggers. The diary's second function is to help the family follow the course of the condition, make sensible decisions about the need for medication and alert them when to obtain medical advice.

### Routine follow-up of the child with asthma

Regular follow-up (see Checklist) is required for all children with asthma. The frequency of visits depends on the severity of the condition and how capable and confident the family is on managing symptoms.

---

### ✓ Checklist for review of a child with asthma

**If the child is new to you or the clinic, check:**
- ☐ The family's understanding of asthma and their ability to make adjustments in medications
- ☐ Inhaler technique
- ☐ Environmental control, especially smoking
- ☐ Accessibility of inhaler at school

**At routine follow-up, review:**
*History*
- ☐ Diary, or if unavailable ask about symptoms of cough and wheeze
- ☐ Frequency of reliever treatment
- ☐ Number of severe attacks
- ☐ Number of absences from school as a result of asthma
- ☐ Any activities restricted because of asthma

*(Continued)*

✓ **Checklist for review of a child with asthma** (*Continued*)

*Physical examination*
☐ Height and weight
☐ Examination of chest
☐ Consider checking inhaler technique

*Investigations*
☐ Peak flow measurement

**Action:**
☐ Advise on increasing or decreasing preventer treatment
☐ Consider changing device as child matures
☐ Counsel about particular issues such as life-style and independence

| Date this card was started: **26th March** | 1 | 2 | 3 | 4 | 5 | 6 | 7 | 8 | 9 | 10 |
|---|---|---|---|---|---|---|---|---|---|---|
| **1 WHEEZE LAST NIGHT** — Good night ...0 / Slept well but slightly wheezy ...1 / Woke x 2–3 because of wheeze ...2 / Bad night, awake most of time ...3 | 0 | 0 | 1 | 0 | 0 | 3 | 2 | 1 | 0 | 0 |
| **2 COUGH LAST NIGHT** — None ...0 / Little ...1 / Moderately bad ...2 / Severe ...3 | 0 | 0 | 0 | 0 | 1 | 2 | 2 | 0 | 0 | 0 |
| **3 WHEEZE TODAY** — None ...0 / Little ...1 / Moderately bad ...2 / Severe ...3 | 0 | 0 | 0 | 1 | 2 | 2 | 2 | 1 | 0 | 0 |
| **4 ACTIVITY TODAY** — Quite normal ...0 / Can only run short distance ...1 / Limited to walking because of chest ...2 / Too breathless to walk ...3 | 0 | 0 | 0 | 1 | 1 | 2 | 2 | 1 | 0 | 0 |
| **5 NASAL SYMPTOMS** — None ...0 / Little ...1 / Moderately bad ...2 / Severe ...3 | 0 | 0 | 0 | 0 | 0 | 0 | 0 | 0 | 0 | 0 |
| **6 METER (best of 3 blows)** — Before breakfast medicines | 200 | 200 | 200 | 150 | 150 | 150 | 100 | 200 | 200 | 200 |
| Before bedtime medicines | 200 | 200 | 200 | 125 | 125 | 100 | 150 | 200 | 200 | 200 |
| **7 DRUGS** (number of doses actually taken during the past 24 hours) — Name of drug: *Salbutamol*, Dose prescribed: *2 puff prn* | — | — | — | 1 | 2 | 4 | 4 | 2 | — | — |

**8 COMMENTS**

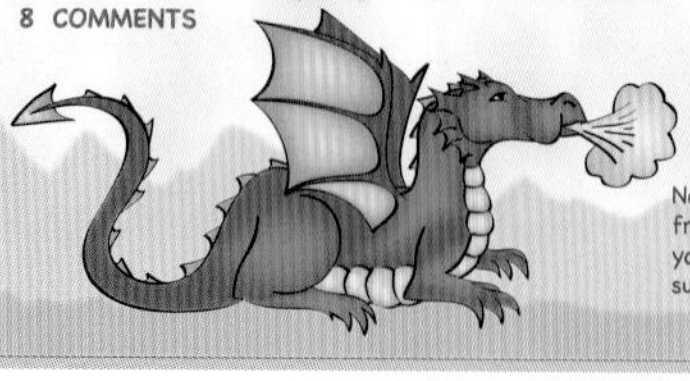

Note if you see a doctor (D) or stay away from school (S) or work (W) because of your chest and anything else important such as an infection (I)

**Figure 8.7** Diary kept by a 9-year-old boy showing good control of his asthma until day 6 and 7.

**History.** It is important to find out how often the child is coughing or wheezing, and the degree to which everyday activities are affected. It is also important to ascertain whether there have been any severe attacks in the interim or absences from school, and whether the child is experiencing any psychosocial difficulties as a result. A diary can be helpful in monitoring asthma (see Figure 8.7).

**Physical examination.** At routine appointments, more often than not there is no evidence of asthma on physical examination. In the child with chronic severe asthma the chest may take on a barrel shape and Harrison's sulcus (an anterolateral depression of the thorax at the insertion of the diaphragm) may be present (Figure 4.15). Clubbing of the fingers is rare even in severe asthma and suggests other causes of chronic obstructive lung disease.

**Investigations.** Pulmonary function tests other than peak flow measurements are rarely indicated. The long-term management of asthma is essentially clinically based.

### Issues for the family

#### Education

The family has to be taught how to recognize the symptoms and signs of asthma, and how the medications differ in their action. They need to know how to use the various inhalation devices and to identify when the child is too distressed to take the medication by the usual route. They must also learn the technicalities of peak flow monitoring and, if the child is severely affected, the importance of keeping an effective diary and utilizing it to make changes in treatment. Parents may need to adapt the home environment, and smoking is likely to be the most important and difficult issue to tackle. As the child grows he or she needs to take responsibility, and must learn how and when to use an inhaler independently, particularly at school.

It does not seem that there is any particular advice to give the family regarding the prognosis for subsequent children being affected other than avoiding smoking antenatally as well as postnatally. Although breast-feeding protects against the development of eczema in susceptible infants, no such clear connection has been established for asthma.

#### Psychosocial

Asthma too often is responsible for absences from school and interferes in full participation in both school and extracurricular activities. Even when symptoms are controlled during the day, children perform poorly following disturbed nights. A particularly difficult period may be during adolescence, when poor compliance or smoking may complicate the picture.

Asthma is a condition which can be frightening for the child and the family. This may lead to a tendency to overprotect the child. As emotional factors can trigger symptoms, this too can affect the functioning of the family. The role of the health professional is important not only in managing the physical symptoms of asthma, but also in addressing these issues and maximizing the child's chance of leading a full and normal life.

### Issues at school

Given the prevalence of asthma, there are likely to be two or three children with asthma in any class. It is important, therefore, that all teachers have an understanding of the condition. In the young child the teacher must be able to recognize symptoms and help the child in administering his or her therapy.

It is critical that all asthmatic children have ready access to their inhalers. Older primary school children should be allowed to carry the inhaler around at all times, and certainly should have it with them for sports activities. Younger children should have the inhaler accessible in their tray–it will do no good locked in the teacher's drawer or the school office. Teaching staff need to understand that inadvertent use by the child or friends will cause no harm. A spare inhaler should be prescribed to be kept in school.

Staff at school can also be helpful in reporting symptoms to the parents or school nurse. This may be of particular value at secondary school, when poor compliance can be a particular issue.

### Prognosis

Most children with asthma improve as they grow older. Preschool children who wheeze only with colds are likely to grow out of it in the early school years. The prognosis varies with the severity of the condition. Only 5% of those with mild asthma progress to develop severe disease. In contrast, 95% of those with severe disease continue to suffer as adults. After remission, asthma may recur in adulthood.

## Asthma at a glance

### Epidemiology
Commonest chronic respiratory condition. Some 10% of children are affected

### Aetiology/pathophysiology
Environmental factors cause bronchoconstriction, mucosal oedema and excessive mucus production in a genetically predisposed child

### How the diagnosis is made
Diagnosis is clinical, based on recurrent or persistent cough/wheeze which is reversed by bronchodilators

### Clinical features
*History*
- Recurrent episodes of cough/wheeze
- Nocturnal cough
- Dyspnoea
- History of atopy*
- Family history of atopic disease*

*Physical examination*
- Expiratory wheeze
- Normal chest exam between attacks
- Acute, often severe respiratory distress during attack
- Barrel-shaped chest if long-standing asthma*
- Poor growth, delayed puberty if severe disease*

*Investigations*
- Reduced peak flow rate, improved by bronchodilators
- Hyperinflation on chest X-ray

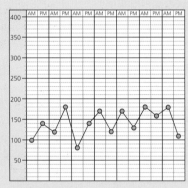

Peak flow chart

### General management
*Medication*
involves 'preventers' and 'relievers' by delivery system appropriate for age

*Environmental control*
- No smoking in child's presence
- Dust/mite-free environment

*Monitoring of asthma*
- Home diary of symptoms and treatment
- Peak flow meter

*Education*
- Understanding asthma
- Competent use of inhalers
- Environmental control
- Self-management

*School*
- Education of staff
- Inhalers must be accessible
- Monitoring of school performance, absences and compliance

### Management of acute problems
Acute attacks need prompt treatment, often by nebulizer and short course of steroids

### Points for routine follow-up
*Monitor*
- symptoms of cough/wheeze
- activity levels
- school absence
- acute attacks
- growth
- chest exam
- peak flow rate

### Prognosis
Asthma resolves over time for most children unless severe. Deaths still occur from asthma in the UK

NB *Signs and symptoms are variable

# Cystic fibrosis

## Prevalence and pathophysiology

Cystic fibrosis is the commonest cause of suppurative lung disease in children in the UK. It is inherited as an autosomal recessive condition, one in 25 of the population being carriers. In northern Europe the commonest mutant gene is $\Delta F508$.

This gene codes for a protein which controls sodium and chloride transport across the membrane of secretory epithelial cells. The mutation leads to a high salt content of sweat, and thick secretions produced by the epithelial cells of some organs. Clinically, in the lungs, the thick mucus obstructs the small airways and predisposes to infection. In the pancreas, the ducts become obstructed and fibrosis develops. Similarly, biliary cirrhosis and obstruction of the vas deferens with male infertility may occur.

## Initial presentation of the child with cystic fibrosis

Approximately 20% of patients present with meconium ileus (obstruction of the bowel by thick meconium, p. 420) at birth. Most of the remainder will present through newborn screening performed on the Guthrie card, performed throughout the United Kingdom since 2007 (see p. 23). Some older children may still present with chronic and persistent respiratory symptoms.

The diagnosis is made by sweat test (see Figure 6.16). Sweat is collected by pilocarpine iontophoresis. A low-voltage electric current is used to carry pilocarpine into the skin of the forearm and to locally stimulate the sweat glands. Sweat is collected by filter paper and then analysed for sodium and chloride concentrations. Elevated levels (>60 mmol/L Na and Cl in a minimum sample of 100 mg sweat) are diagnostic of cystic fibrosis.

## Clinical features of cystic fibrosis

### Respiratory tract

The lungs are normal at birth, but the child later develops a tendency to frequent and prolonged infections. Unless treatment is rigorous, the cough becomes chronic and productive. In severe cases there may be digital clubbing, chest deformity and growth retardation (see Figure 8.8). The rate of progression of lung disease is very dependent on the intensity of treatment.

The chest X-ray in advanced cystic fibrosis shows patchy collapse, consolidation, cystic and linear shadows and overinflation (Figure 8.9). Sputum

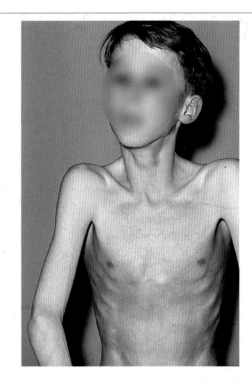

**Figure 8.8** A boy severely affected by cystic fibrosis, with barrel chest and reduced muscle mass.

typically cultures *Haemophilus* species, *Staphylococcus aureus* or *Pseudomonas aeruginosa*. *Bronchiectasis is best evaluated by performing a CT scan of the chest (Fig. 8.10).*

### Intestinal tract

Most children show evidence of malabsorption caused by exocrine pancreatic insufficiency. Symptoms include frequent, bulky, greasy stools and failure to gain weight even when food intake appears large. A protuberant abdomen, decreased muscle mass and poor growth are typical signs.

Fat globules and a low chymotrypsin level are found in the stool. A sweat test is required to make the diagnosis (see p. 102). A chest X-ray is usually normal in the early stages.

## Management of the child with cystic fibrosis

The principles involved in the follow-up of any child with a chronic medical condition (p. 38) are important for the child with cystic fibrosis. Medical management must focus on both the respiratory and gastrointestinal tracts.

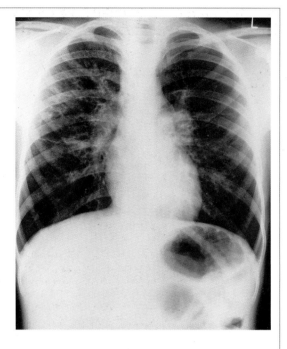

**Figure 8.9** Chest X-ray of a boy with cystic fibrosis. There is gross overinflation of the lungs with hilar enlargement and ring shadows caused by bronchial wall thickening and bronchiectatic change.

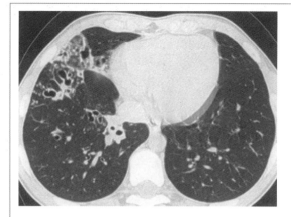

**Figure 8.10** High-resolution chest CT scan image of a child with severe bronchiectasis caused by cystic fibrosis.

### Respiratory tract

The aim of treatment is to clear secretions, prevent infections and treat them promptly and effectively when they occur. Parents are taught how to carry out regular chest physiotherapy. Antibiotic therapy is often required, intravenously or orally, at high dosage for prolonged periods.

### Malabsorption and diet

Children require dietary adjustment, pancreatic enzyme replacement and supplementary vitamins to correct their loss of pancreatic function and inadequate digestion of fat and protein. Pancreatic enzyme supplements have to be taken with all meals and snacks.

The diet needs to be high in energy and protein, and there is no need to restrict fat. Dietary supplements are often needed at times of illness or if there is anorexia, and all patients require supplements of the fat-soluble vitamins A, D and E. Extra salt is also needed in hot weather or if the child is febrile to replace losses in sweat.

### *Prognosis*

Cystic fibrosis remains a life-limiting condition although the outlook has improved greatly in recent years so that average life expectancy is now 30–40 years. In general, with good treatment, most individuals can lead relatively normal lives in the childhood years. Growth may slow down in later childhood and puberty may be delayed. In adulthood, the slow progression of lung disease may eventually become disabling. Lung transplantation is considered in severe cases.

Cystic fibrosis may affect other systems. Diabetes develops in some children during adolescence. Most males are azospermic, but have unimpaired sexual function.

## 👁 Cystic fibrosis at a glance

### Epidemiology
Commonest cause of
   suppurative lung disease in
   UK children
One in 25 individuals are carriers

### Aetiology
Gene mutation affects sodium
   and chloride transport across
   secretory epithelial cells →
   airway obstruction and
   pancreatic insufficiency

### History
Chronic cough +/− wheezing (**a**)
Frequent chest infections
Failure to thrive (FTT)
Frequent, bulky, greasy stools (**b**)
History of meconium ileus*
Family history of cystic fibrosis*

### Physical examination
Poor growth (**1**)
Chest deformity
Wheezing and crepitations (**2**)
Clubbing (**3**)
Protuberant abdomen (**4**)

NB *Signs and symptoms are
variable

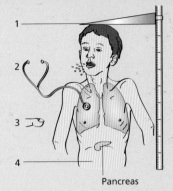

Pancreas

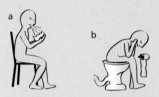

### Confirmatory investigations
Elevated sodium (>60 mmol/L)
   and chloride on sweat test
Screening of stool samples at
   birth in some centres
Chronic changes on chest X-ray
Decreased stool chymotrypsin

### Differential diagnosis
Other causes of chronic lung
   disease
Other causes of malabsorption

### Management
Lungs:
• physiotherapy
• frequent and prolonged
   courses of antibiotics, often
   needed IV
Nutrition:
• pancreatic enzyme
   supplements
• high protein, high calorie diet
• fat soluble vitamins and salt
• dietary supplements at times

### Prognosis/complications
Chronic deteriorating lung
   disease
Life expectancy now 30–40 years
Usually reasonable quality of life
   in childhood

### Non-respiratory problems:
• diabetes
• delayed puberty
• biliary atresia
• male infertility

## Pneumonia

Pneumonia is caused by a wide range of viral and bacterial organisms as shown in Table 8.5. *Streptococcus pneumoniae* often causes lobar pneumonia.

Predisposing factors to acute pneumonia should always be considered in children who present with pneumonia. These include:

• congenital abnormality of the tracheo-bronchial tree;
• inhaled foreign body;
• persistent lobar collapse;
• chronic aspiration;
• large left to right intracardiac shunt;
• immunocompromise.

**Clinical features.** The child with acute pneumonia presents with a short history of fever, cough and respiratory distress. Meningismus may be present, and shoulder tip or abdominal pain can divert attention

**Table 8.5** The commoner organisms causing pneumonia

*Bacterial*
*Streptococcus pneumoniae* (especially in younger children)
*Mycoplasma pneumoniae* (more insidious onset)
*Haemophilus influenzae* (uncommon in Britain)
Group B beta-haemolytic streptococcus (only in the newborn)

*Viral*
Respiratory syncytial virus
Influenza viruses
Parainfluenza
Adenovirus
Coxsackie viruses

from the correct diagnosis. Signs of respiratory distress include tachypnoea, nasal flaring, and intercostal and subcostal recession (Fig. 4.14, p. 64). Grunting is also a common feature in severely affected infants. Dullness to percussion indicates underlying consolidation, and crepitations are commonly heard. Focal signs in young children (in contrast to adults) may not correlate with the anatomical site of infection seen on the X-ray. Diagnosis is made by X-ray and may show focal (confined to a lobe) or diffuse changes (Figure 8.11). Sputum (obtained in older, cooperative children) and blood cultures should be taken, which may isolate the infecting organism. Cold agglutinins are present in the serum in cases of *Mycoplasma pneumoniae*.

**Management.** Antibiotics should be used in all cases of pneumonia. If the child is acutely ill, intravenous penicillin is given, but oral amoxycillin is appropriate in a less ill child.

**Prognosis.** Complications of pneumonia include:

- lung abscess (rare, but may follow staphylococcus infection);
- empyema (infected pleural effusion);
- pneumothorax;
- septicaemia with infective foci elsewhere;
- bronchiectasis (following pertussis or measles in malnourished children);
- pleural effusion.

---

## 👁 Pneumonia at a glance

### Aetiology
Viral (particularly respiratory
   syncytial virus in infants)
*Strep. pneumoniae* at all ages
*Mycoplasma pneumoniae* at
   school age
*Staphylococcus aureus* and
   *Haemophilus influenzae*
   uncommon

### History
Fever
Cough
Respiratory distress
Shoulder tip/abdominal pain*
Sputum production in older
   child*

### Physical examination
Tachypnoea
Nasal flaring
Intercostal/subcostal regression
Grunting in infants
Meningism*

### Confirmatory investigations
Chest X-ray: focal consolidation
   suggests bacterial cause;
   diffuse consolidation suggests
   viral
Blood count: leucocytosis and
   shift to left if bacterial
Blood culture
Cold agglutinins in older child
   for mycoplasma

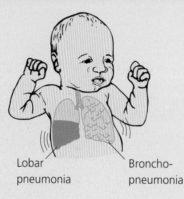

Lobar
pneumonia

Broncho-
pneumonia

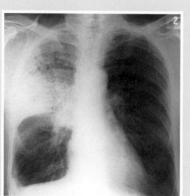

### Differential diagnosis
URTI
Bronchiolitis
Acute bronchitis
Asthma
Non-specific viral infection
Inhaled foreign body

### Management
Appropriate antibiotic (based on
   appearance of chest X-ray);
   often amoxicillin or IV
   penicillin if acutely ill
Antipyretics
Repeat chest X-ray 1 month
   post-treatment
Cough syrup unnecessary

### Prognosis/complications
Complete recovery usual
Rare complications include:
- lung abscess
- empyema
- pneumothorax
- septicaemia
- bronchiectasis

NB *Signs and symptoms are variable

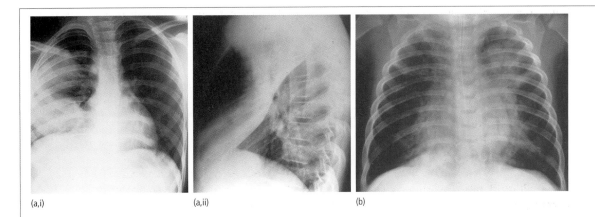

(a,i) (a,ii) (b)

**Figure 8.11** (a,i) Chest X-ray of a boy presenting with fever and cough. Consolidation of the right upper and middle lobes are seen. (a,ii) The lateral film shows the consolidation clearly delineated posteriorly by the oblique fissure. (b) X-ray of a child with viral pneumonia. Diffuse shadowing is seen throughout the lung fields.

## Bronchiolitis

Bronchiolitis is an acute viral infection which causes respiratory distress and wheezing in infants less than 18 months, due to obstruction of the small airways. It is usually caused by respiratory syncytial virus (RSV), and occurs in epidemics in the winter months. Parainfluenza virus and adenovirus can also cause bronchiolitis. Infants with congenital heart disease or underlying chronic lung disease may be very severely affected by bronchiolitis.

**Clinical features.** The illness starts with coryza, followed by signs of respiratory distress, including wheeze and cough. Some babies have difficulty feeding and may develop apnoea. On examination there is overexpansion of the chest, and wheeze and crepitations on auscultation.

**Diagnosis.** Chest X-ray shows overinflated lungs, and collapse or consolidation may be seen (Figure 8.12). A nasopharyngeal aspirate (NPA) can be taken to look for RSV in the respiratory secretions using immunofluorescence.

**Management.** Most babies are not ill and, provided they take feeds well, they can be managed at home. Admission is required if there is cyanosis, increasing respiratory distress, apnoea or poor feeding. Treatment is largely supportive, with oxygen given to maintain adequate saturations. Ventilatory support may be necessary in severely affected babies.

**Prognosis.** Most babies recover uneventfully from this condition within 7–10 days. Immunity is short-

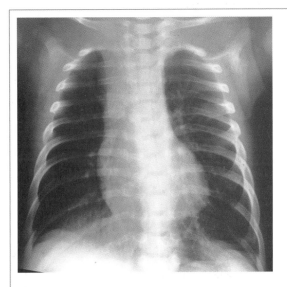

**Figure 8.12** Chest X-ray of an 8-week-old baby with bronchiolitis. The X-ray shows gross overinflation of the lungs, clearly seen by the level of the diaphragm and the intercostal spaces. There is also some bronchial wall thickening.

lived and recurrent bronchiolitis is not uncommon. Many babies who suffer from bronchiolitis show a predisposition to recurrence of wheeze through infancy. Death is rare, but can occur in babies who have severe underlying chronic lung disease. A monoclonal antibody (palivizumab) against RSV can be given prophylactically to high-risk infants throughout the winter months to provide passive immunity against infection.

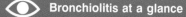

**Bronchiolitis at a glance**

**Aetiology**
Respiratory syncytial virus
 (RSV), occasionally other
 viruses
Only infants and babies affected

**History**
Coryza
Difficulty breathing
Feeding difficulty
Fever*

**Physical examination**
Widespread wheezing and
 crepitations
Tachypnoea
Subcostal/intercostal retractions
Nasal flaring
Overinflated chest

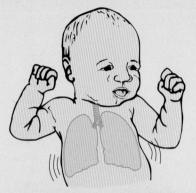

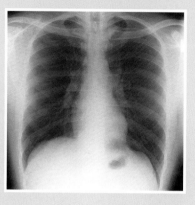

NB *Signs and symptoms are
variable

**Confirmatory investigations**
RSV confirmed by
 immunofluorescence of
 nasopharyngeal secretions
Chest X-ray shows overinflation
 of lungs and patchy areas of
 collapse

**Differential diagnosis**
Asthma (see text)
Pneumonia

**Management**
Supportive

**Prognosis/complications**
Usually good, but mortality
 1–2%
High proportion go on to have
 recurrent wheeze through
 infancy

## Aspirated foreign body (see also p. 377)

Foreign bodies are usually aspirated by toddlers who are mobile and put small objects into their mouths. Small plastic or wooden beads and peanuts are most likely to be aspirated. Peanuts are particularly danger-ous as they swell in the airway, become firmly lodged and are difficult to remove because they tend to frag-ment. Children, particularly toddlers, may aspirate a foreign body without the parent realizing that this has occurred.

**Clinical features.** Usually there is an immediate episode of coughing or choking, or a history of such an episode days or weeks earlier, but the child may present with cough alone. The main symptoms are respiratory distress and wheeze, with cough as a prom-inent feature. The chest may appear asymmetrical, with a localized dull percussion note if collapse has occurred distal to the obstruction. As the commonest place for a foreign body to lodge is the right main bronchus (Figure 8.13), there may be signs of right

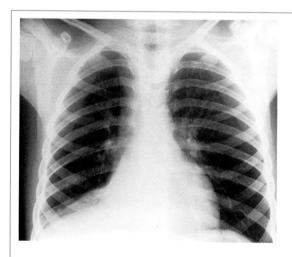

**Figure 8.13** X-ray of a child admitted with fever and cough which failed to respond to treatment. At bron-choscopy a Dinky car steering wheel was found in the right intermediate bronchus. The chest X-ray shows collapse of the right middle and lower lobe with loss of definition of the right hemidiaphragm and right heart border.

lung collapse and unilateral wheezing. Compensatory emphysema may occur around the collapsed lobe, producing a percussion note of increased resonance. Ideally an inspiratory and expiratory chest X-ray is required, where segmental collapse or hyperinflation is seen.

**Management.** If aspiration of a foreign body is suspected, bronchoscopy should be performed. Removal of the foreign body is curative. Complete airway obstruction is a medical emergency and should be treated with the Heimlich manoeuvre (p. 377).

**Prognosis.** If there is delay in diagnosis, bronchiectasis may occur in the lung distal to the obstruction, causing destruction of bronchial architecture. This leaves dilated air sacs which become chronically infected and eventually require surgical removal.

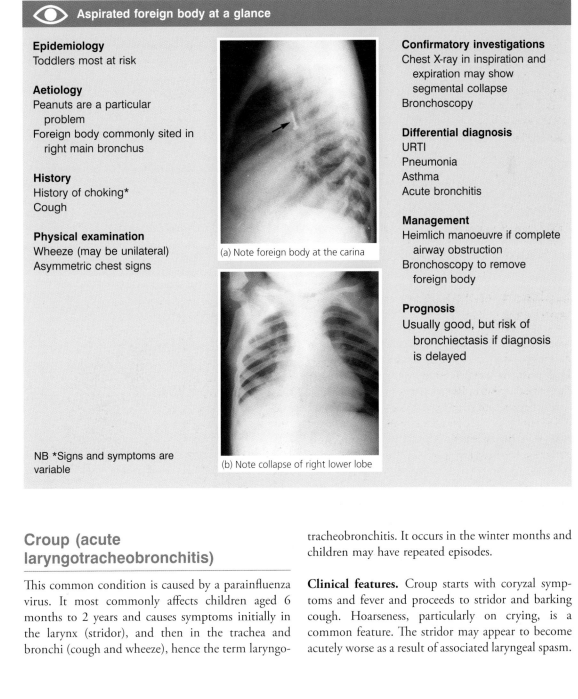

**Aspirated foreign body at a glance**

**Epidemiology**
Toddlers most at risk

**Aetiology**
Peanuts are a particular problem
Foreign body commonly sited in right main bronchus

**History**
History of choking*
Cough

**Physical examination**
Wheeze (may be unilateral)
Asymmetric chest signs

(a) Note foreign body at the carina

**Confirmatory investigations**
Chest X-ray in inspiration and expiration may show segmental collapse
Bronchoscopy

**Differential diagnosis**
URTI
Pneumonia
Asthma
Acute bronchitis

**Management**
Heimlich manoeuvre if complete airway obstruction
Bronchoscopy to remove foreign body

**Prognosis**
Usually good, but risk of bronchiectasis if diagnosis is delayed

NB *Signs and symptoms are variable

(b) Note collapse of right lower lobe

# Croup (acute laryngotracheobronchitis)

This common condition is caused by a parainfluenza virus. It most commonly affects children aged 6 months to 2 years and causes symptoms initially in the larynx (stridor), and then in the trachea and bronchi (cough and wheeze), hence the term laryngo-tracheobronchitis. It occurs in the winter months and children may have repeated episodes.

**Clinical features.** Croup starts with coryzal symptoms and fever and proceeds to stridor and barking cough. Hoarseness, particularly on crying, is a common feature. The stridor may appear to become acutely worse as a result of associated laryngeal spasm.

Further progression down the respiratory tract may cause wheezing and tachypnoea. Although usually mild, it may progress rapidly in young children to become very severe. Signs of deterioration include increased work of breathing, cyanosis and restlessness. Severe deterioration is often accompanied by a reduction in the stridulous noise.

**Management.** Most cases resolve spontaneously. There is no evidence that humidity shortens the duration or severity of the stridor. However, adequate fluids are essential to prevent dehydration. If the child worsens, hospital assessment is required. Oral dexamethasone is used to reduce the airway inflammation and often results in a dramatic clinical improvement. In cases that remain severe, hospital admission is required, and, rarely, nebulized therapy such as adrenaline or even early intubation by an experienced anaesthetist may be needed.

---

### Croup at a glance

**Epidemiology**
Commonly affects children
    aged 6 months to 2 years

**Aetiology**
Parainfluenza virus

**History**
Stridor and barking cough
Coryza
Fever
Hoarseness*

**Physical examination**
Stridor
Wheezing*
Tachypnoea*
Cyanosis if severe

**Confirmatory investigations**
Nil

**Differential diagnosis**
Acute epiglottitis
Foreign body

**Management**
Humidity and oral fluids
Intubation if exhaustion or
    imminent obstruction

**Prognosis**
Good

NB *Signs and symptoms are variable

---

## Acute epiglottitis

Acute epiglottitis is a lifethreatening condition caused by infection with *Haemophilus influenzae*. It is now very rare since *Haemophilus influenzae* B (HiB) immunization was introduced. It presents with signs of toxicity, fever, drooling and inability to swallow. If the condition is suspected, examination of the mouth must not be attempted as acute and total airway obstruction may occur. Protection of the airway is the first aim, and investigations need to be done after intubation. Blood cultures grow *Haemophilus influenzae* and treatment is with intravenous cefotaxime. With airway protection and appropriate antibiotics the prognosis is excellent, but death or severe brain injury were seen when acute airway obstruction occurred.

*To test your knowledge on this part of the book, please see Chapter 25.*

# CHAPTER 9

# Gastrointestinal disorders

*The churning inside me never stops; Days of suffering confront me.*

*Job 30: 27*

## COMPETENCES

### You must . . .

| Know | Be able to | Appreciate |
|---|---|---|
| • The normal stool pattern for babies<br>• How to assess hydration in infants and toddlers<br>• How to manage fluids and diet in a baby or child with acute gastroenteritis<br>• The signs and symptoms that suggest a chronic disease in a child with diarrhoea<br>• How to manage a child who is constipated<br>• How to investigate a child who is jaundiced<br>• The characteristic features of colic | • Interpret results of a sweat test<br>• Advise a parent about oral rehydration and diet for a child with gastroenteritis<br>• Differentiate non-organic from organic recurrent abdominal pain<br>• Develop an approach to managing recurrent abdominal pain | • The difference between vomiting and posseting<br>• That constipation is not diagnosed on infrequent stools alone<br>• That antiemetics and antidiarrhoeal agents are generally inappropriate for children<br>• That encopresis is a sign of severe behavioural problems<br>• That most recurrent abdominal pain is non-organic but children still benefit from medical attention |

*Paediatrics and Child Health*, Third Edition. Mary Rudolf, Tim Lee, Malcolm Levene.
© 2011 Mary Rudolf, Tim Lee and Malcolm Levene. Published 2011 by Blackwell Publishing Ltd.

# Gastrointestinal symptoms and signs

## Finding your way around . . .

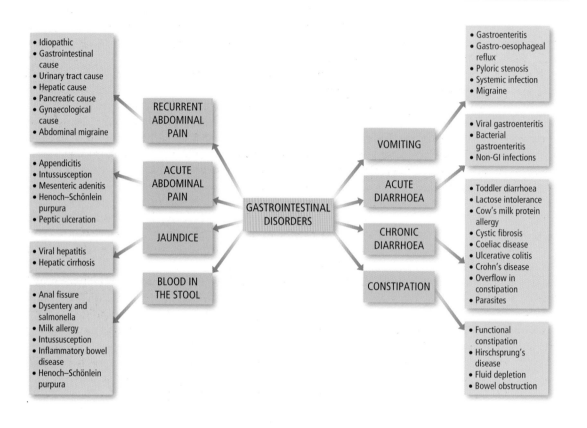

- Idiopathic
- Gastrointestinal cause
- Urinary tract cause
- Hepatic cause
- Pancreatic cause
- Gynaecological cause
- Abdominal migraine

RECURRENT ABDOMINAL PAIN

- Appendicitis
- Intussusception
- Mesenteric adenitis
- Henoch–Schönlein purpura
- Peptic ulceration

ACUTE ABDOMINAL PAIN

- Viral hepatitis
- Hepatic cirrhosis

JAUNDICE

- Anal fissure
- Dysentery and salmonella
- Milk allergy
- Intussusception
- Inflammatory bowel disease
- Henoch–Schönlein purpura

BLOOD IN THE STOOL

GASTROINTESTINAL DISORDERS

VOMITING

- Gastroenteritis
- Gastro-oesophageal reflux
- Pyloric stenosis
- Systemic infection
- Migraine

- Viral gastroenteritis
- Bacterial gastroenteritis
- Non-GI infections

ACUTE DIARRHOEA

CHRONIC DIARRHOEA

- Toddler diarrhoea
- Lactose intolerance
- Cow's milk protein allergy
- Cystic fibrosis
- Coeliac disease
- Ulcerative colitis
- Crohn's disease
- Overflow in constipation
- Parasites

CONSTIPATION

- Functional constipation
- Hirschsprung's disease
- Fluid depletion
- Bowel obstruction

## Vomiting

**Common causes of vomiting**

*Infancy*
Gastroenteritis (p. 178)
Gastro-oesophageal reflux
Overfeeding
Anatomic obstruction
  pyloric stenosis
  intussusception (p. 184)
  bowel obstruction
Systemic infection, particularly meningitis,
pyelonephritis

*Childhood*
Gastroenteritis (p. 178)
Systemic infection
Toxic ingestion or medications (p. 390)
Whooping cough (p. 27)

*Adolescence*
Gastroenteritis (p. 178)
Systemic infection
Migraine (p. 217)
Pregnancy
Bulimia (p. 441)

The return of small amounts of food during or shortly after eating is called *regurgitation*. When this occurs in a baby at or after a milk feed it is known as *posseting* and is seen as effortless, low-volume, frequent 'spills' from the mouth. More complete emptying of the stomach is called *vomiting*. Within limits, regurgitation is normal, especially during the first 6 months or so of life. It can be reduced by winding the baby during and after a feed, by gentle handling, by preventing the baby from becoming upset and swallowing air before feeding, and by propping the baby after a feed. A common cause of apparent vomiting in the bottle-fed infant is overfeeding, as the infant will often continue to suck on a bottle even after the comfortable capacity of the stomach has been achieved. A surprisingly large volume of excess milk can then be regurgitated back as the parent tries to wind the baby. Provided the child is gaining weight and generally contented, the family can be reassured that it is simply a laundry problem, and that the baby will grow out of it by the time he or she is walking at about 1 year. If very troublesome, and the baby is not breast-fed, food thickeners can be added to the milk. 'Rumination' refers to chronic regurgitation, which is often self-induced by the baby. If it occurs with growth failure, psychological factors should be suspected.

Vomiting is one of the commonest symptoms of infancy, if not of childhood. Vomiting may be associated with a variety of disturbances, both trivial and serious. It is most commonly associated with gastro-enteritis (p. 178), but may accompany any infection, from minor ailments such as otitis media to more serious illnesses such as pyelonephritis. Vomiting may also be the first symptom of a potentially lethal disease such as meningitis or pyloric stenosis. In infants, the first step is to differentiate simple regurgitation from vomiting. If vomiting is truly the problem, the underlying diagnosis can usually be suspected by a thorough history and physical examination. Worrying features are shown in the Red Flag box.

---

**Worrying features in a vomiting child**

- Bile-stained vomitus*
- Blood in the vomitus
- Drowsiness
- Refusal to feed
- Malnutrition
- Dehydration

*This suggests intestinal obstruction and is always a serious sign which must be investigated urgently.

---

### History – must ask!

- *How well is the child?* The general health of the child, and particularly appetite, is a guide to the severity of the problem. Significant vomiting is likely to be accompanied by weight loss and, if long term, poor weight gain. Fever suggests an infective cause.
- *What is the vomiting like?* Decide whether a baby is vomiting, posseting or regurgitating. Vomiting from infectious causes tends to be non-projectile, whereas in pyloric stenosis it can be dramatically projected over a distance. Paroxysms of coughing (as occur in whooping cough) can precipitate vomiting. Blood-stained vomiting indicates inflammation in the upper gastrointestinal tract. Bile-stained vomitus is a serious sign, suggesting intestinal obstruction; it must be investigated urgently.
- *Are there associated symptoms?* Gastroenteritis and other infections are usually accompanied by diarrhoea. Constipation suggests intestinal obstruction. Irritability or pain may accompany infection or reflux. Aspiration and apnoea are worrying signs of gastro-oesophageal reflux.
- *Bottle-fed babies.* Ask how much milk the baby is taking. If the baby is taking in excess of 200 mL of milk per kilogram body weight in 24 hours, and is well with no weight loss, then regurgitation secondary to overfeeding is likely.
- *Adolescents.* You need to focus your questions to adolescents differently. Ask about symptoms of migraine, and consider gynaecological causes. Bulimia rarely presents as vomiting as the adolescent is careful to hide this symptom.

### Physical examination – must check!

- *General examination.* Carry out a full examination to exclude infection in sites other than the gastrointestinal tract, particularly if there is fever. Severe infection such as meningitis or pyelonephritis can present with vomiting. Poor weight gain indicates dehydration in the short term, and malnutrition in the longer term. Exclude hypertension.
- *Signs of dehydration.* Persistent vomiting leads to dehydration. The signs of dehydration are described on pp. 385–90.
- *The abdomen.* The abdomen may be tender in gastroenteritis, with increased bowel sounds. In the rare event of intestinal obstruction, the bowel sounds are tinkling or absent. In the vomiting infant, palpation of an 'olive' (Figure 9.1) is diagnostic of pyloric stenosis. Severe tenderness may suggest appendicitis, particularly if the onset of the pain preceded the vomiting.

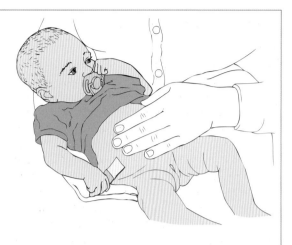

**Figure 9.1** Palpation of the abdomen for pyloric stenosis.

## Investigations

Investigations are usually only required if significant reflux is suspected, in which case pH monitoring and a barium meal may be indicated. In suspected pyloric stenosis an ultrasound scan is definitive if the pyloric tumour is seen.

## Management of the vomiting

Antiemetics have no place in the management of vomiting in young children (other than rare specific circumstances such as during chemotherapy for childhood cancer). The child needs to be maintained in a well-hydrated state, by offering water or oral hydration fluids in small amounts frequently. If the child develops signs of significant dehydration, intravenous fluids are required (see p. 388).

> ### 🔑 Key points: The vomiting child
>
> - In infants – differentiate posseting from vomiting
> - Look for evidence of infection, whether gastroenteritis or extra-gastrointestinal
> - Determine whether the child is dehydrated
> - In the infant with projectile vomiting, palpate the abdomen carefully for pyloric stenosis
> - Suspect reflux in the infant or child with physical disability, failure to thrive, blood-stained vomitus, irritability, aspiration or apnoea
> - Bright green bile-stained vomiting should be referred straight to the surgeons as the child may need an emergency laparotomy for bowel obstruction
> - Exclude hypertension as a cause

## Acute diarrhoea

> ### Causes of acute diarrhoea
>
> Viral gastroenteritis
> Bacterial gastroenteritis
>   shigella
>   *Escherichia coli*
>   salmonella
>   campylobacter
> Infections outside the gastrointestinal tract
> Antibiotic-induced

Diarrhoea is defined as an increase in the frequency, fluidity and volume of faeces. Children are likely to experience as many as three acute severe episodes in the first 3 years of life. These episodes are almost invariably infectious in aetiology, although the infection may be outside the gastrointestinal tract.

When you assess a child with diarrhoea, you need to focus on whether the child requires treatment for dehydration or has an infection outside the gastrointestinal tract that has precipitated the diarrhoea. A search for an underlying organism is generally unimportant unless you suspect dysentery.

Any form of infection can cause acute diarrhoea, particularly in the young child. These commonly include URTIs, chest infections, otitis media and urinary tract infection (UTI). If otitis media, UTI or pneumonia is detected, the appropriate antibiotic should be given. Non-infective causes of diarrhoea include intussusception, a serious condition that may present with bloody (characteristically 'redcurrant jelly') stools (see p. 184). Antibiotic therapy in itself commonly causes diarrhoea.

## History – must ask!

- *What is the illness like?* Get a good description of the illness, and whether the increase is in frequency, volume or liquidity of the stools. This provides a guide to whether the child is likely to be dehydrated. Blood, mucus, abdominal pain and fever suggest a bacterial cause – important to recognize for public health reasons.
- *Is the child likely to be dehydrated?* Apart from frequency of stools, there are other clues as to whether the child is dehydrated. If he or she is urinating

infrequently (less than three times in 24 hours is a guide) some degree of dehydration is likely. A history of weight loss is also important.

• *Are there other symptoms?* Symptoms such as earache, dysuria or coryza suggest an infection outside the gastrointestinal tract. Convulsions and pain are characteristic of shigella.

• *Is anyone else affected?* If others in the family or at child care are affected, consider a cause such as food contamination – useful epidemiological information.

### Physical examination – must check!

• *Assessment of hydration.* This is covered in detail on p. 387. You need to assess the state of alertness, moistness of mucous membranes, presence of tears, skin turgor, sunken fontanelle and eyes, and pulse rate.

• *Signs of any extra-gastrointestinal infection.* Otitis media, tonsillitis and chest infections commonly cause diarrhoea.

• *Weight.* Always weigh the child. If a recent weight is available, weight loss provides important evidence of dehydration. In any event, the weight is a valuable baseline if the child deteriorates.

### Investigations

If the child is not dehydrated, nor the stools bloody, investigations are not generally necessary unless the child is hospitalized or has been exposed to others with proven bacterial gastroenteritis. Stool microscopy and culture is needed if there is blood and mucus in the diarrhoea. Rotavirus can be detected by stool immunoassay. If extra-gastrointestinal infection is suspected, confirmation may be required from blood and urine cultures or X-ray. Investigations to be considered are shown in Table 9.1.

### Managing acute diarrhoea

#### Fluids

The management of dehydration is covered on p. 388. If signs of dehydration are mild or absent, the child can be managed at home. Cow's milk is usually stopped but breast-feeding is continued. If the baby is on a bottle, it is traditional to give clear fluids for the first day. The toddler and older child can be offered dilute apple juice or a flat cola drink, but babies should be given oral rehydration fluids which provide electrolytes and calories in the appropriate balance. Gradually solids are introduced – bananas, rice, apple sauce and toast (the 'BRAT' diet) are foods that are generally recommended. Milk is sometimes reintroduced in diluted form, but there is no evidence that this gradual introduction is beneficial, and may result in the child receiving inadequate calories. If diarrhoea persists, you need to recheck the state of hydration to see if more aggressive management is required.

#### Use of antiemetics and antidiarrhoeal agents

These agents have no place in the management of diarrhoea in young children. They are ineffective and have a high incidence of side effects.

---

**Key points: Acute diarrhoea**

• Assess the degree of hydration (see Table 21.8)
• Look for evidence of infection outside the gastrointestinal tract
• Identify features suggestive of bacterial gastroenteritis

---

**Table 9.1** Investigations to be considered in acute diarrhoea

| Investigation | Indication | What you are looking for |
| --- | --- | --- |
| Stool microscopy and culture | Blood and mucus in the stool | Bacterial gastroenteritis |
| Stool immunoassay | Hospitalized child | Rotavirus |
| Blood count | High fever | Possible bacterial infection |
| Blood and urine culture, chest X-ray | Suggestion of extra-gastrointestinal infection in clinical evaluation | Bacterial infection |

## Clues to the differential diagnosis of acute diarrhoea

| | Rotavirus | Shigella | Escherichia coli | Salmonella | Campylobacter |
|---|---|---|---|---|---|
| Age | <2 years | 1–5 years | <2 years | Any | Any |
| Stool | Watery | Watery, blood, mucus, pus | Loose | Loose and slimy | Watery, blood, mucus |
| Pain | Occasional | Common | Common | Common | Common |
| Fits | Rare | 10% | Rare | Rare | Rare |
| Vomiting | Common | Common | Common | Common | Rare |
| High fever | Common | Common | Rare | Common | Common |
| Season | Winter | Usually late summer | Usually late summer | Usually late summer | Usually late summer |

## Chronic diarrhoea

### Common causes of chronic or recurrent diarrhoea

*Watery*
Nonspecific diarrhoea
Toddler diarrhoea
Lactose intolerance
Parasites – *Giardia lamblia*
Cow's milk protein allergy
Overflow diarrhoea in constipation

*Fatty*
Cystic fibrosis
Coeliac disease

*Bloody*
Ulcerative colitis
Crohn's disease

**Table 9.2** Normal stool patterns

| 0–4 months | Breast-fed | 2–4 per day (range 1–7), yellow to golden, porridgy consistency, pH 5. Infrequency of stools is also normal (up to once per week) |
|---|---|---|
| 0–4 months | Bottle-fed | 2–3 per day, pale yellow to light brown, firm, pH 7 |
| 4 months–1 year | | 1–3 per day, darker yellow, firmer |
| After 1 year | | Formed, like adult stool in odour and colour |

Chronic diarrhoea is a common complaint, particularly in infants and young children. However, there is a large variation in normal bowel patterns (Table 9.2) at this age and, before launching into any form of assessment, a good description of the stool pattern should be obtained in order to be sure that diarrhoea is really a problem. Broadly speaking, the diarrhoeal illnesses of childhood can be divided into malabsorption, inflammation and infections. However, when working through a differential diagnosis it may be more helpful to think in terms of the characteristics of the stool.

In your clinical evaluation, you must differentiate the healthy child who has loose frequent stools from the child with a medical problem. You should identify any worrying features suggesting a pathological process, and request appropriate investigations so that a definitive diagnosis can be made.

Infants with cystic fibrosis (see p. 149) often present with diarrhoea and failure to thrive as a result of pancreatic insufficiency, rather than with the respiratory symptoms seen in older children. Inflammatory bowel disease is a cause of chronic diarrhoea in late childhood and adolescence; both Crohn's disease (p. 182) and ulcerative colitis (p. 182) are characterized by unpredictable exacerbations and remissions. The soiling that results from constipation is sometimes interpreted as being diarrhoea. A careful bowel history is required along with evidence of constipation on examination.

### History – must ask!

- *What are the stools like?* You should ask about the bowel pattern, including any increase in frequency, volume and fluidity of the stools, so you can decide whether the pattern is abnormal or not. The stools' appearance, consistency and presence of blood or mucus are helpful in coming to a diagnosis, but odour and 'flushability' are usually not.
- *What precipitated the diarrhoea?* The problem may have been precipitated by an episode of acute infective diarrhoea, or you may identify troublesome foods. There may be other affected individuals in the family or at child care.
- *Are there associated symptoms?* It is important to determine whether the diarrhoea is an isolated problem in an otherwise healthy child or whether there are concomitant symptoms. Weight loss or abdominal pain are particularly significant.
- *Review of symptoms.* As many diseases can cause failure to thrive with rather non-specific bowel symptoms, a complete review of symptoms is required.
- *A symptom diary.* As for most recurrent and chronic problems, asking the family to keep a diary is helpful to assess the severity and pattern of the symptom.

### Physical examination – must check!

- *Growth measures.* Height, weight and head circumference must be recorded and compared with earlier measurements (if available). Poor weight gain suggests a process that needs further evaluation. Height and weight also serve as a critical baseline if the diarrhoea persists for any length of time.
- *Other features.* Your examination should include an evaluation of hydration, pallor, abdominal distension, tenderness and finger clubbing.
- *General examination.* As diseases of many different organ systems can cause failure to thrive, a complete examination is required.
- *Anorectal examination.* Any significant degree of diarrhoea causes perianal irritation, particularly if the child is still in nappies. Rectal examination is not routinely indicated, but consider it to rule out impaction (if soiling is considered as the diagnosis) and to obtain a sample of the stool.

### Laboratory investigations (Table 9.3)

If a child is thriving and there are no accompanying symptoms or signs, laboratory investigations are rarely necessary. However, if you are concerned that a pathological process is present, investigations are required and should help you differentiate the three types of chronic and persistent diarrhoea – malabsorption, inflammatory and infection.

#### Malabsorption

The commonest causes of malabsorption in childhood result from pancreatic insufficiency, protein intolerance and lactose intolerance.

- *Pancreatic insufficiency.* In pancreatic insufficiency (as occurs in cystic fibrosis), low faecal elastase levels are found in the stool, and on microscopic inspection fat globules are seen.
- *Protein intolerance.* The commonest form of protein intolerance is coeliac disease. Coeliac antibodies are useful as a screening test. If positive, or there are other concerns that malabsorption is present, jejunal biopsy is needed to confirm the diagnosis.
- *Sugar malabsorption.* Sugar malabsorption (secondary lactose intolerance is the commonest) is suggested by the presence of reducing substances in the stool and a low pH. The low pH results from bacterial production of organic acids from the unabsorbed sugar. The breath hydrogen test is another indirect measure of carbohydrate malabsorption. An oral dose of the sugar being tested is given, and if there is malabsorption, the enteric bacteria act on it to produce hydrogen gas, which is measured in the expired air.

#### Inflammation

Faecal blood loss suggests inflammatory bowel disease or food sensitivity. A very high plasma viscosity or ESR level supports inflammatory bowel disease. The diagnosis is made by barium studies and endoscopy.

#### Infection

Repeated examination of at least three stool specimens should identify parasitic infection, of which *Giardia lamblia* is the commonest. Urine culture excludes chronic UTI as a cause for diarrhoea.

### Managing diarrhoea as a symptom

Many children have episodes of loose, frequent stools for which no cause is found. These may follow on

**Table 9.3** Laboratory investigations in the assessment of chronic diarrhoea

| Investigation | Finding | Significance |
| --- | --- | --- |
| *Blood* | | |
| Full blood count | Anaemia | Blood loss, malabsorption or poor diet |
| | Eosinophilia | Parasites or atopy |
| Plasma viscosity or sedimentation rate | High | Nonspecific finding. If very high, suggestive of inflammatory bowel disease |
| Coeliac antibodies | Present | Screening test for coeliac disease |
| *Stool* | | |
| Occult blood | Positive | Cow's milk intolerance, inflammatory bowel disease |
| Ova and parasites | Positive | Parasite identified |
| Reducing substances and pH* | Positive and low pH | Sugar intolerance (usually lactose) |
| Chymotrypsin | Low | Pancreatic insufficiency |
| Microscopy for fat globules | Globules seen | Fat malabsorption (usually pancreatic insufficiency) |
| *Other* | | |
| Urine culture and sensitivity | Positive | Urinary tract infection |
| Sweat test | Elevated sweat $Na^+$ and Cl-concentration | Cystic fibrosis |
| Breath hydrogen test | High $H_2$ | Sugar intolerance |
| Jejunal biopsy | Flattened villi | Coeliac disease |
| Barium meal and enema | Characteristic lesions | Inflammatory bowel disease |
| Endoscopy | Characteristic lesions | Inflammatory bowel disease |

* This is performed by mixing stool with water and testing it with Clinitest tablets (as for urinary glucose).

from an acute episode of gastroenteritis. If the child is well and thriving, reassurance is all that is required, with monitoring of growth for the duration of symptoms.

Antidiarrhoeal medication has no place in the management of diarrhoea in children. Food intolerance is often a concern, and omission of suspected foods may be tried, although care must be taken to ensure that the child's nutritional intake is not compromised.

> **Key points: Chronic diarrhoea**
>
> • Check that the stool pattern is really abnormal for age
> • Attempt to classify the character of the stool – watery, fatty or bloody
> • Identify any features suggestive of significant pathology, e.g. weight loss or poor weight gain, abdominal pain

## Clues to the differential diagnosis of chronic diarrhoea

| | Characteristics of diarrhoea | Associated features | Age of child |
|---|---|---|---|
| Non-specific diarrhoea | Loose watery stools | Thriving child, may follow episode of acute gastroenteritis | Any age |
| Toddler diarrhoea | Loose with undigested food in stool | Thriving child, may have large fluid intake | Toddler |
| Lactose intolerance | Watery, low pH, reducing substances in stool | Follows acute gastroenteritis | Baby and toddler |
| Giardiasis | Watery | Weight loss and abdominal pain variable | Any age, common in nurseries |
| Cow's milk protein allergy | Watery, may be bloody | May have urticaria, stridor or bronchospasm | Babies |
| Functional constipation | Soiling rather than diarrhoea | Constipated stool palpable per abdomen or per rectum | Any age |
| Cystic fibrosis | Fatty | Failure to thrive, respiratory symptoms | Usually infancy |
| Coeliac disease | Fatty | Failure to thrive, irritability, muscle wasting, abdominal distension | Usually late infancy, but can be any age |
| Inflammatory bowel disease | Bloody in ulcerative colitis | Weight loss, exacerbations and remissions, abdominal pain and anorexia in Crohn's disease | Late childhood and adolescence |

## Recurrent abdominal pain

### The more common causes of recurrent abdominal pain

*Idiopathic*
*Psychogenic*
*Gastrointestinal*
  Irritable bowel syndrome
  Oesophagitis
  Peptic ulcer
  Inflammatory bowel disease
  Constipation
  Malabsorption
  Giardiasis

*Urinary tract*
  Infections

*Hepatic*
  Hepatitis

*Pancreas*
  Pancreatitis

*Gynaecological*
  Dysmenorrhoea
  Pelvic inflammatory disease
  Haematocolpos
  Ovarian cyst

*Other*
  Abdominal migraine
  Lead poisoning

Recurrent abdominal pain is one of the commonest symptoms presenting in children, with 10–15% of school-age children at some point experiencing it. Of these, only 1 in 10 are found to have an organic problem, the majority having no identifiable cause for the pain. Rarely, abdominal pain can be a manifestation of a more serious chronic childhood disorder relating to the gastrointestinal, urinary or gynaecological systems.

The purpose of your clinical evaluation is to decide as rapidly as possible whether there is an organic or non-organic cause for the pain. Table 9.4 summarizes the features that will help you come to that decision. If there is no indication of an organic cause then appropriate reassurance and support is needed, rather than letting anxiety linger that there might be a serious problem that you have not identified.

### History – must ask!

Take a complete history, reviewing the child's lifestyle and habits as well as focusing on symptoms related to each organ system.

- *What is the pain like?* The character of the pain can help you identify the cause. The child may be able to describe whether the pain is colicky or constant, and how it is related to daily activities, bowel habit or diet. Even if the child cannot describe the pain, the site can often be located. Non-organic pain is classically periumbilical, and it has been said that the further the pain is from the umbilicus, the greater the chances that an aetiology can be identified. A diary kept by the family can be quite helpful in clarifying the frequency of episodes and their relation to other events.
- *What is the timing?* Is there a temporal relationship between the onset of abdominal pain and school. Is it less at weekends?
- *Are there other abdominal symptoms?* Symptoms related to specific organ systems may give clues to an organic cause. Constipation, diarrhoea or vomiting suggest a gastrointestinal cause, and frequency and dysuria suggest a cause in the urinary tract. Do not forget to enquire about gynaecological symptoms in teenage girls.
- *Are there general constitutional symptoms?* General constitutional symptoms such as anorexia, weight loss and fever are important indicators that there is a serious underlying cause.
- *Are there emotional or family difficulties?* You should always enquire about emotional and family problems, as they are commonly associated with abdominal

**Table 9.4** Features differentiating organic and non-organic causes of abdominal pain

| | Organic | Non-organic |
|---|---|---|
| Characteristics | Day and night | Periodic pain with intervening good health |
| | Character depends on underlying cause | Often periumbilical |
| | | If psychosomatic, may be related to school hours |
| History | Weight loss and/or reduced appetite | Otherwise healthy child |
| | Lack of energy | |
| | Recurrent fever | |
| | Organ-specific symptoms, e.g. change in bowel habit, polyuria, menstrual problems, vomiting | |
| | Occult or frank bleeding from any orifice | |
| | Family history of gastrointestinal problems | |
| Physical exam | Ill appearance, growth failure, swollen joint | |
| Preliminary investigations | Anaemia leucocytosis, raised sedimentation rate or eosinophilia on blood count | Normal, thriving child |
| | Abnormal urinalysis and/or culture | Normal |

pain. Try to establish how much the symptoms interfere with life at home and at school.

• *Family history.* A family history of gastrointestinal disease, especially peptic ulcers, may be relevant.

### Physical examination – must check!

You should always carry out a complete physical examination. Don't limit it to the region below the diaphragm and above the pelvis!

• *Growth.* Height and weight measurements are particularly important, as weight loss indicates serious pathology. If the problem is long-standing, fall-off in growth may also occur.

• *General examination.* Look for signs of pallor, jaundice and clubbing.

• *Abdominal examination.* Examine the abdomen for hepatomegaly, splenomegaly, enlarged kidneys or a distended bladder.

• *Anorectal examination.* Inspection of the anus and a rectal examination are not routine in children, but need to be carried out if there is any suspicion of sexual abuse, and at times for constipation.

### Investigations (Table 9.5)

The diagnosis of non-organic pain can be made in many children on the basis of the history and examination. If in doubt, a full blood count, sedimentation rate, stools for ova and parasites, and urinalysis and culture can be helpful as inflammatory bowel disease, chronic UTI and gastrointestinal parasites may present

**Table 9.5** Useful investigations in assessing the child with recurrent abdominal pain

| Investigation | What are you looking for? |
| --- | --- |
| *Blood tests* | |
| Full blood count | Anaemia, eosinophilia, infection |
| Sedimentation rate or plasma viscosity | Elevated in inflammatory bowel disease |
| Liver function tests | Liver dysfunction |
| Urea and electrolytes | Renal failure |
| Amylase | Pancreatitis |
| *Urine test* | |
| Urinalysis and culture | Urine infection |
| *Stool* | |
| Ova and parasites (x3 samples) | Gastrointestinal parasites, e.g. giardiasis |
| Occult blood | Gastrointestinal blood loss, e.g. inflammatory bowel disease or peptic ulcer |
| *Ultrasound* | |
| Abdominal and pelvic | Urinary obstruction at all levels, organomegaly, abscesses, pregnancy, ovarian cyst and torsion |
| *X-ray* | |
| Plain abdominal | Constipation, renal calculi if radiopaque, lead poisoning |
| Barium swallow and follow-through | Oesophagitis and reflux, peptic ulcer, Crohn's disease, congenital malformations of the gut |
| | Ulcerative colitis |
| Barium enema | Oesophagitis and reflux |
| *Endoscopy* | Peptic ulceration |
| | Colitis |

with abdominal pain alone. You should only consider further investigations if there are findings suggestive of a particular disease process.

## Managing abdominal pain

The management of abdominal pain obviously depends on the aetiology. Analgesics are often prescribed, but are in fact usually unhelpful in relieving the pain. If you have come to the conclusion that an organic cause is unlikely, the family still require care. The approach described in Box 9.1 may be helpful.

---

**Key points: Recurrent abdominal pain**

• Obtain a full picture of the pattern of episodes of pain
• Identify symptoms related to the various abdominal organs
• Determine whether there are any constitutional symptoms
• Decide if the pain is likely to be organic or functional in origin
• Obtain a picture of the psychosocial circumstances and the effect the pain has on the child's activities

---

**Box 9.1 Managing the child with non-organic recurrent pain**

• Assure the parents and child that no major illness appears to be present. In particular, rule out and focus on diagnoses which concern the family
• A diagnosis of psychosomatic pain should not be made simply by exclusion of pathology. Positive emotional and psychological causes must be identified
• In the child where neither an organic nor a psychosomatic cause is found, it can be helpful to label the diagnosis, such as 'tension headache', or 'growing pains', while qualifying this with an explanation that the aetiology is unknown
• Identify those symptoms and signs which the parents should watch for and which would suggest the need for a re-evaluation
• Do not communicate to the parents that the child is malingering
• Develop a system of return visits to monitor the symptom. Having the family keep a diary of pain episodes and related symptoms can be helpful
• During return visits, allow time for both the child and parent to uncover stresses and concerns
• Make every effort to normalize the life of the child, encouraging attendance at school and participation in regular activities

---

**Clues to the diagnosis of recurrent abdominal pain**

| | Features of the pain | Associated symptoms |
|---|---|---|
| **Idiopathic recurrent abdominal pain** | Periodic<br>Periumbilical | Well between episodes |
| **Psychogenic pain** | Periodic | Psychosomatic symptoms |
| **Irritable bowel syndrome** | Non-specific | Flatus and variable bowel pattern |
| **Peptic ulcer** | Epigastric<br>Relieved by food and antacids | In children <6 years pain is often exacerbated by food (opposite to adult pattern) |
| **Gastro-oesophageal reflux** | May be chest pain | Vomiting<br>Failure to thrive |
| **Inflammatory bowel disease** | Colicky (Crohn's) | Anorexia<br>Diarrhoea +/− blood and mucus<br>Weight loss |
| **Constipation** | Colicky | Hard, infrequent stools |
| **Parasitic infection (e.g. giardiasis)** | Variable | Variable |
| **Urinary tract infection** | Back or loin pain | Dysuria, frequency, enuresis |
| **Dysmenorrhoea** | Varies with menstrual cycle | |
| **Pelvic inflammatory disease** | Low abdominal pain | Vaginal discharge |
| **Lead poisoning** | Variable, generalized | Anorexia and irritability<br>Pica<br>Hypochromic microcytic anaemia |
| **Abdominal migraine** | Recurrent, may be severe | Nausea and vomiting<br>Family history of migraine |

# Acute abdominal pain

**Commoner causes of acute abdominal pain in children**

| Bowel | Renal | Other | |
|---|---|---|---|
| Acute appendicitis | Urinary tract pneumonia | Lower lobe | infection |
| Intussusception | Hydronephrosis | | |
| Mesenteric adenitis | Renal calculus | | |
| Henoch–Schönlein purpura | | | |
| Peptic ulceration | | | |
| Inflammatory bowel disease | | | |
| Intestinal obstruction | | | |
| Constipation | | | |
| Gastroenteritis | | | |

Abdominal pain in children is a very common symptom. Acute and chronic or recurrent abdominal pain are discussed separately, as the presentation and causes are quite different.

When a child presents with acute and severe abdominal pain, the differential diagnosis includes a number of important conditions which require surgical intervention.

In some children, pain presents acutely and settles spontaneously, only to recur some time later. There may be a gradual merging of episodes of acute abdominal pain with more chronic pain, and this can make the categorization of acute and chronic abdominal pain difficult. Acute intra-abdominal pathology may occur in very small babies when a clear history of pain cannot be given by the patient.

### History – must ask!

It is often hard to elicit a good description of the intensity, duration and position of the pain, as this will depend on the child's age and verbal skills. In younger children, there is very often no clear history of pain.

- *Pain.* The features of pain in young children include intermittent spasms of screaming for no obvious cause. In older children, the child may be able to point to the area of pain or rub the affected part of the abdomen. Children are not good at localizing the point of maximum pain and often refer to pain all over the abdomen. Ask specifically whether the pain wakes the child at night and whether it is related to eating particular foods. Pallor during a bout of screaming is an important feature. In older children, a description of the pain migrating from the perium-

bilical area to the right iliac fossa is very suggestive of acute appendicitis.

- *Blood in stool.* A history of blood in the stool should always be treated seriously. In children with intussusception, the classical description is 'redcurrent jelly' stools consisting of blood and mucus.
- *Associated features.* Ask about any other features such as anorexia (a particular feature of acute appendicitis); vomiting and diarrhoea; whether there has been any joint pain or swelling.

### Physical examination – must check!

The physical examination must be undertaken very carefully and with great sensitivity, as the child may anticipate additional pain when the examiner's hand is placed on the abdomen. It may be most appropriate to examine young children while they are lying on their mother's lap, and sometimes the child's confidence can be gained by placing the examiner's hand on the child's and lightly palpating the abdomen in that manner. This makes the child feel more in control. It is most important to watch the child's face during palpation of the abdomen because this will give a very useful clue as to whether palpation elicits pain. It is obvious that as little additional pain should be inflicted on the child as possible.

- *General observation.* If the pain is a result of a condition causing peritoneal irritation (peritonism), the child lies very still and movement causes severe pain. Spontaneous movement of the child is an important feature in elucidating the severity of the pain.
- *General examination.* Conditions remote from the abdomen may cause abdominal pain, including tonsillitis and mesenteric adenitis, or basal pneumonia

causing pain referred to the abdomen. The child may have tachycardia and an increase in blood pressure in association with pain.

• *Abdomen.* Examination of the acute abdomen may cause extreme agitation in a child who anticipates that the examining doctor will make the pain worse. It is extremely important to reassure the child first, but not to say that 'it will not hurt', as this may be untrue. It is best to precede the examination with an explanation of what will be done and a promise to be as gentle as possible.

The signs of peritonism include great reluctance to move spontaneously, rebound tenderness, guarding and rigidity.

• *Rectal examination.* Although rectal examination may be a considerable intrusion on the child's person, it is an important part of the physical examination in the child who may have an acute appendicitis. It should not, however, be a routine part of all abdominal examinations.

### Investigations

If the child has been vomiting, assessment of serum electrolytes and urea is essential to assess the state of hydration. Important investigations in the child with acute abdominal pain are shown in Table 9.6.

### Managing acute abdominal pain

The most important question to ask yourself when assessing a child with an acute abdomen is whether the child requires a laparotomy. If the child has signs of peritonism (guarding or rigidity, rebound tenderness or severe tenderness on rectal examination), the answer is likely to be 'yes' and a surgical opinion is urgently required. Bowel rupture will rapidly progress to peritonitis and shock. Although acute appendicitis is by far the most likely cause of peritonism, there are other rare conditions that can cause this condition. The precise diagnosis is not important because this will be discovered at operation.

Expectant management is appropriate if the child does not have signs of peritonism. Repeated, regular examination of the child's abdomen will determine whether the condition is resolving or getting worse. If there is any doubt as to whether the child has peritonism, a surgical opinion may be very valuable.

For non-operative causes of abdominal pain, treatment depends on the underlying condition.

---

**Key points: Abdominal pain**

• The child with peritonitis lies very still, reluctant to move
• Signs of peritonism include rebound tenderness, guarding and rigidity
• Pallor and intermittent bouts of screaming suggest intussusception

---

**Table 9.6** Basic investigations in children with acute abdominal pain and their significance

| Investigation | Significance |
| --- | --- |
| Full blood count | Leucocytosis found in acute appendicitis and urinary tract infection |
| Urine microscopy and culture | Pyuria and organisms indicate infection |
| Plain abdominal X-ray | Intussusception (Figure 9.8) Obstruction |
| Ultrasound scan | May be particularly helpful in intussusception, and to exclude renal pathology |
| Contrast enema | For diagnosis and treatment of intussusception, see p. 185 |

---

**Clues to the diagnosis of acute abdominal pain**

| Diagnosis | Clinical features |
| --- | --- |
| Acute appendicitis | Tachycardia |
| | Anorexia |
| | Peritonism |
| Intussusception | Intermittent screaming |
| | Pallor |
| | 'Redcurrant jelly' stool |
| Mesenteric adenitis | Recent viral infection |
| | No peritonism |
| Henoch–Schönlein purpura | Joint pain or swelling |
| | Blood in stool |
| | Purpura on extensor surfaces |
| Urinary tract infection | Dysuria |
| | Frequency |
| | Enuresis |
| Peptic ulceration | Night pain |
| | Relief by food |

# Constipation

---

**Causes of constipation**

*Acute*
Fluid depletion
Bowel obstruction

*Chronic*
Functional constipation
Hirschsprung's disease
(Breast-fed babies)

---

In normal children, there is a wide range in frequency of bowel movements. In the past, children were trained to open their bowels each morning and this regularity is still seen in elderly patients. With less rigid ideas of child-rearing, most children have no set pattern to their toilet habits. Some will have more than two movements per day and others go several days with none. You should therefore base your diagnosis of constipation on hardness of stools and painful defecation rather than infrequency of bowel movements alone. This rule of thumb is particularly relevant in the exclusively breast-fed infant, where it can be normal for the baby to pass only one stool in 7 days. Inexperienced parents may become alarmed by this, but the stools are soft and semi-liquid, and reassurance is all that is required.

Constipation is common, and is nearly always functional in nature. It may occur if fluid depletion occurs during hot weather or following a febrile illness, particularly if vomiting has occurred. The problem can usually be resolved by increasing the fluid intake, but a simple episode of constipation can be responsible for the development of more chronic constipation.

Organic causes of constipation are rare, the most important being Hirschsprung's disease (see p. 426). This should be considered if the constipation goes back to infancy, and particularly if the child is failing to thrive and has marked abdominal distension. Bowel obstruction is also very rare and results from congenital malformations of the gut. The presentation is usually an acute abdomen (see p. 169) rather than constipation.

The principal purpose of your evaluation is to assess the severity of the complaint in order to evaluate the need for treatment. You can rule out rare organic causes on the basis of your history and physical examination.

## History – must ask!

- *What are the symptoms?* Is the child truly constipated or are the stools infrequent but normal? The hardness of the stool, painful defecation, crampy abdominal pain and the presence of blood on the stool or toilet paper indicate the former, although long-standing constipation can be painless.
- *Constipation history.* Constipation is often precipitated by a period of fluid depletion, as in hot weather, or during a febrile illness or one where vomiting has occurred. When constipation is chronic, it is often not possible to recall the onset. Mismanagement of toilet training can be a factor. Constipation starting during early infancy suggests Hirschsprung's disease, whereas functional constipation usually has a later onset. Previous history of an anal fissure is significant.
- *Are there associated symptoms?* Bowel obstruction results in constipation, but vomiting and abdominal pain are usually present.
- *What is the diet like?* A dietary history is important in order to base subsequent advice on dietary management of constipation.

## Physical examination – must check!

- *Growth.* Review the growth chart, as failure to thrive occurs with Hirschsprung's disease.
- *General examination.* Hard, indentable faeces are often palpable in the left lower quadrant of the abdomen and above.
- *Anorectal examination.* Rectal examination is not usually indicated for constipation, but if it is carried out, hard stools are found. Inspection of the anus is important as fissures may be seen, and, in addition, signs of sexual abuse could indicate a less benign reason for pain on defecation.

## Investigations

A plain X-ray of the abdomen may show enormous quantities of faeces in the colon (Figure 9.2). However, this investigation is not usually required. The diagnostic test for Hirschsprung's disease is rectal biopsy, and is indicated if the history goes back to infancy and the child has shown poor growth.

---

**Key points: Constipation**

- Assess the severity of the constipation
- Attempt to identify a precipitating cause
- Constipation from infancy, in conjunction with failure to thrive, suggests Hirschsprung's disease

---

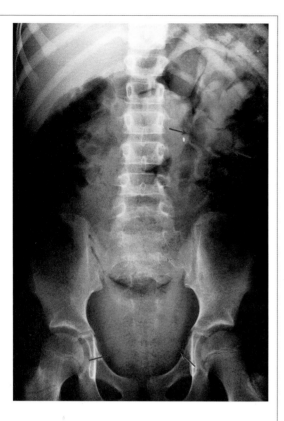

**Figure 9.2** X-ray of the abdomen of a 12-year-old boy with chronic constipation. The rectum and sigmoid colon are grossly distended by faeces, as indicated by the arrows.

## Blood in the stool

### Causes of blood in the stool

*Infancy*
Anal fissure
Dysentery and salmonella
Milk allergy
Intussusception
Swallowed maternal blood at birth

*Older children*
Anal fissure
Dysentery and salmonella
Inflammatory bowel disease
Intussusception
Henoch–Schönlein purpura
Intestinal polyp

The appearance of blood in the stool is usually alarming. The commonest cause is an anal fissure, which may or may not be visualized. This results from the passage of a large hard stool which tears the delicate rectal mucosa. Bloody diarrhoea is a rare manifestation of cow's milk allergy in babies.

### History – must ask!

- *What is the stool like?* Constipation and dysentery are easily differentiated on history. The parent or child should be able to describe whether the blood is outside the stool, indicating that the site of bleeding is in the lower bowel (usually constipation), or whether it is mixed in with the stool, which suggests pathology higher up. In intussusception, the blood is characteristically described as being 'like redcurrant jelly'. Blood from the upper intestinal tract is usually digested and appears as melaena, and has a black, tarry consistency, and a characteristic odour.
- *Is there pain?* Pain is a useful symptom. Constipation severe enough to cause bleeding is usually associated with significant pain on defecation. In intussusception (p. 184), the baby has rhythmical attacks of screaming from pain. A description of pain in the older child may suggest peptic ulcer or inflammatory bowel disease.
- *Is there bleeding from other sites?* Bleeding from other sites indicates a more generalized bleeding disorder.

### Physical examination – must check!

- *General examination.* High fever occurs with dysentery. If significant blood has been lost, the child may appear anaemic. The rash of Henoch–Schönlein purpura is usually characteristic ,with purpura on the extensor surfaces (see Figure 17.14a).
- *The abdomen.* In any of the conditions resulting in rectal bleeding the abdomen may be tender. In constipation, you may palpate faecal loading in the left lower quadrant and above.
- *Anal and rectal examination.* Inspect the anus. The commonest finding is an anal fissure (see Figure 9.9), which results from passage of a large hard stool. Signs of more gross trauma indicate abuse. If there is no fissure, a rectal examination may be needed to confirm constipation or to obtain a stool sample for culture or occult blood.

### Investigations

Investigations are not required if a diagnosis of constipation is made. Bloody diarrhoea requires stool culture to confirm dysentery. If intussusception is suspected, an urgent barium enema is required for diagnosis and treatment (see p. 185). Inflammatory bowel disease requires confirmation, radiologically and endoscopically.

| The commoner causes of jaundice in childhood | |
| --- | --- |
| **Predominantly unconjugated** | **Predominantly conjugated** |
| *Haemolysis* | *Hepatic* |
| Haemolytic disease of the newborn (p. 425) | Hepatitis |
| Sickle cell disease (p. 346) | Cystic fibrosis |
| Spherocytosis | Cirrhosis |
| *Hepatic* | *Obstructive* |
| Rare | Hepatitis |
| | Biliary atresia |

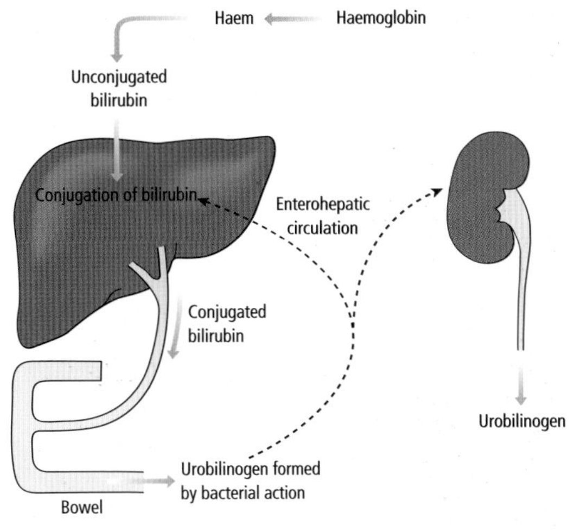

**Figure 9.3** Bilirubin metabolism.

## Jaundice

Jaundice outside the neonatal period is always a significant sign, and the child must be investigated rapidly and fully so that a definite diagnosis can be made. It is the commonest sign of liver disease, but may also occur as the result of non-liver pathology, notably haemolysis. Neonatal jaundice is discussed in Chapter 22.

Jaundice is caused by accumulation in the skin of the yellow pigment bilirubin. Bilirubin metabolism is summarized in Figure 9.3. Bilirubin is produced as a result of the breakdown of haem from haemoglobin. This is insoluble and referred to as unconjugated bilirubin. Unconjugated bilirubin is metabolized by the liver cells to a soluble conjugated form and is excreted via the hepatic and bile ducts into the duodenum. Bilirubin and bile salts in the bowel aid the absorption of fats and fat-soluble vitamins. Approximately one half of the conjugated bilirubin is reabsorbed from the bowel as urobilinogen in the enterohepatic circulation. Urobilinogen may be excreted in the urine or remetabolized through the liver. In jaundice, excessive conjugated (soluble) bilirubin may be excreted in the urine, which causes the urine to be a dark 'tea' colour.

The causes of jaundice can be divided into those that cause either predominantly unconjugated or conjugated hyperbilirubinaemia. Outside the neonatal period, unconjugated hyperbilirubinaemia is usually caused by haemolysis. Conjugated hyperbilirubinaemia can be divided into either hepatic or obstructive causes.

### History – must ask!

- *Features of jaundice.* Ask about the duration of the jaundice. The first sign of a more insidious onset is a yellow appearance to the sclerae of the eyes. Onset is rapid in haemolysis.
- *Malaise.* Ask about the duration of malaise, abdominal pain and presence of anorexia.
- *Symptoms of anaemia.* Anaemia occurs as the result of haemolysis. Symptoms such as breathlessness and pallor may be present.
- *Pruritus.* Pruritus refers to intense skin irritation and occurs as a result of deposition of bile salts in the skin.
- *Urine.* Ask about the colour of the urine (and observe it). Very dark-coloured ('coca-cola') urine strongly suggests a conjugated cause of the jaundice.
- *Steatorrhoea.* This refers to frothy, foul-smelling stool which floats in the toilet pan and is commonly seen in children with long-standing cirrhotic liver disease.

### Physical examination – must check!

- *Growth.* Failure to thrive or poor growth may occur as the result of any long-standing cause of liver disease.

- *Skin signs.* Scratch marks may be seen on the skin. Signs of long-standing liver disease include spider naevi, clubbing and ascites.
- *Hepatosplenomegaly.* Carefully palpate the liver for enlargement and firmness. A hard liver suggests cirrhosis. Splenomegaly, if large, may suggest haemolysis, but splenomegaly may also occur as a result of cirrhosis.

## Investigations

The investigations that are indicated in the child with jaundice are shown in Table 9.7.

---

**Key points: Jaundice**

- Jaundice is first seen in the sclerae
- Dark urine and pale faeces indicate conjugated jaundice
- Presence of anaemia and splenomegaly are suggestive of haemolysis
- As part of an initial assessment of jaundice, measure both conjugated and unconjugated components of serum bilirubin

---

**Table 9.7** Basic investigations indicated for the child with jaundice

| Investigation | What you are looking for |
|---|---|
| Haemoglobin (Hb) | Low Hb with increased reticulocytes indicates haemolysis |
| Bilirubin | Unconjugated excess suggests haemolysis |
| | Conjugated excess suggests hepatic or post-hepatic disease |
| Liver enzymes | Elevated in hepatitis |
| Alkaline phosphatase | Elevated in cirrhosis or in cases of long-standing jaundice |
| Serology | Identification of hepatitis virus |

---

**Clues to the differential diagnosis of jaundice**

| | Haemolysis | Infectious hepatitis | Cirrhosis |
|---|---|---|---|
| **Onset of jaundice** | Acute | Acute | Insidious |
| **Dark urine** | – | + | +++ |
| **Anorexia** | – | +++ | + |
| **Pruritus** | – | – | +++ |
| **Anaemia** | +++ | – | + |
| **Hepatosplenomegaly** | +++ | – | ++ |
| **Liver tenderness** | + | ++ | – |

# Gastrointestinal disorders

## Dental caries

Dental caries, or tooth decay, is one of the commonest chronic diseases worldwide. The prevalence has decreased markedly in developed countries since the 1970s, in association with increased fluoridation of drinking water and improved oral hygiene.

**Clinical features.** Dark spots or pits may be seen on the surface of the teeth; there may be associated areas of yellowish dental plaque. 'Baby-bottle tooth decay' classically presents in infants or young toddlers with the upper front teeth severely decayed (Figure 9.4), there is often a history of the child being frequently pacified in their cot for long periods with a sugary drink in a bottle with teat.

**Investigations.** In developed countries dental caries can be an early marker of neglect, and the child should be clinically assessed for other markers such as failure to thrive. A dietary history should be taken, particularly focusing on intake of sugary drinks and food.

**Management.** The child should be referred to a dentist, and dietary advice given to the parents. Children with congenital heart disease or who are immunosuppressed are at particular risk from dental caries as the infection may become disseminated, and thus should undergo regular dental surveillance.

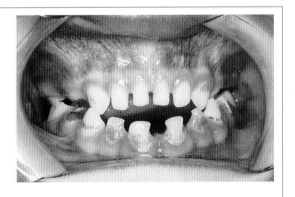

**Figure 9.4** Severe dental caries in a 2- year-old child who was given milk and juice by propping the bottle in the cot during night feeds.

## Gastro-oesophageal reflux

Gastro-oesophageal reflux is very common in babies and also in children with developmental disabilities, such as severe cerebral palsy. It results from a chronically lax gastro-oesophageal sphincter, or frequent spontaneous decreases in sphincter tone, which allows reflux of stomach contents back up the oesophagus.

**Clinical features.** The symptoms range from trivial posseting to life-threatening episodes. Common problems are vomiting, oesophagitis, aspiration and, to a lesser extent, apnoea. Vomiting is the commonest complaint and may cause failure to thrive. Oesophagitis causes irritability and anorexia, and should be particularly suspected if there is blood in the vomitus or occult blood in the stools. Opisthotonos (arching of the back) and other head posturing may occur and is possibly an attempt to reduce the pain associated with acid reflux. Aspiration can manifest as episodes of choking and must be suspected in the baby with recurrent episodes of pneumonia. Reflux can also cause reflex apnoea and bradycardia. The relationship to acute life-threatening events (see p. 396) is controversial.

**Investigations.** In mild cases, a careful clinical assessment is sufficient, and the diagnosis is confirmed by the response to treatment. In more severe or complex cases, a barium swallow can be helpful, although results must be interpreted with caution as reflux, which is episodic, may not be demonstrated during the X-ray, and also because it can be seen in normal asymptomatic children. The severity and frequency of reflux can be documented by continuous pH and/or impedance monitoring (usually 24 hours) with a probe placed in the lower third of the oesophagus. Oesophagoscopy with biopsy is the best technique for demonstrating oesophagitis, which may also be suspected if a ragged mucosal outline is seen on the barium meal.

**Management.** In mild uncomplicated cases, propping the child, thickening the feeds and attending to burping may resolve the problem. In infancy a prokinetic such as erythromycin may be helpful in increasing gastric emptying. If oesophagitis is present, drugs may be prescribed to reduce gastric acid production (ranitidine, omeprazole). If symptoms do not respond to a good trial of medical agents, or if recurrent aspiration and apnoea are major problems, surgery is indicated, the commonest procedure being Nissen fundoplication.

---

### 👁 Gastro-oesophageal reflux at a glance

**Epidemiology**
Common in babies, and children with
Down's syndrome and severe cerebral palsy

**Aetiology**
Lax gastro-oesophageal sphincter

**History**
May be asymptomatic
Vomiting*
Irritability and anorexia*
Choking*
Apnoea*
History of pneumonia*

**Physical examination**
Normal
Chest signs if aspirating*
Failure to thrive*
Opisthotonos*

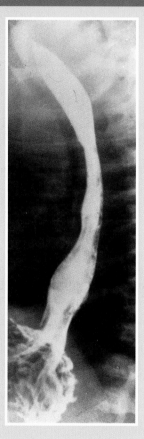

**Confirmatory investigations**
Response to trial of antireflux medication
Barium swallow: reflux visualized
pH monitoring: increased acidity in oesophagus
Oesophagoscopy: oesophagitis

**Differential diagnosis**
Normal posseting
Colic in young babies
Other causes of vomiting (p. 158)
Other causes of recurrent pneumonia
Other causes of apnoea (p. 415)

**Management**
Thickened feeds and propping
Medication: drugs to reduce gastric acid production (ranitidine, omeprazole)
Surgery: Nissen fundoplication required if aspirating, apnoea or poor response to medication (rare)

**Prognosis/complications**
Reflux resolves in most normal children by the time they are eating solids/walking

NB *Signs and symptoms are variable

---

## Pyloric stenosis

Pyloric stenosis is caused by hypertrophy and hyperplasia of the pylorus muscle. It usually develops in the first 4–6 weeks of life, and is commonest in firstborn male children.

**Clinical features.** The vomiting is characteristically projectile and generally occurs during or immediately after feeding (although not necessarily at every feed). The vomit may be blood-tinged but is not bile-stained. The infant is hungry and is prepared to take another feed immediately. Weight loss is seen on examination, with varying degrees of dehydration. In advanced cases, the infant may be moribund. Visible peristalsis from the left upper quadrant to the right is most prominent immediately after a feed or just prior to vomiting. Careful palpation (Figure 9.1) should reveal a hard mobile tumour (the pylorus), which feels like an acorn or an olive just to the right of the epigastrium. Once the tumour has been palpated there is no need for barium studies or ultrasound. However, if the diagnosis is suspected, but the tumour not palpable, the diagnosis can be confirmed by ultrasound (Figure 9.5). If vomiting is protracted, the loss of acidity from the stomach results in hypochloraemic alkalosis and reduced sodium and potassium levels in the serum (see p. 94).

**Management.** Treatment is surgical. The Ramstedt procedure consists of splitting the pylorus muscle, without penetrating the mucosa. If the infant is dehydrated, rehydration must take place prior to surgery with replacement of sodium, chloride and potassium (see p. 388). Oral feeds can be gradually given within hours postoperatively.

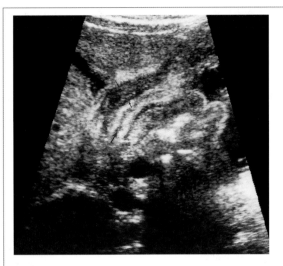

**Figure 9.5** Ultrasound of a baby with pyloric stenosis. Arrows indicate the elongated pyloric canal (thick arrow) and thickened pyloric muscle (thinner arrow).

## 👁 Pyloric stenosis at a glance

**Epidemiology**
Age 4–6 weeks
Mainly boys
7 boys : 1 girl
Age 1–10 weeks

**Aetiology**
Hypertrophy and hyperplasia of
the pylorus muscle

**History**
Projectile vomiting during or just
after feed (**a**)
Infant hungry immediately after
vomit
Constipated

**Physical examination**
Weight loss +/– dehydration
Visible peristalsis from left
upper quadrant to right upper
quadrant (**b**)
Mobile olive-sized tumour
palpable to right of
epigastrium during feed (**c**)

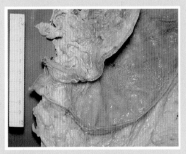

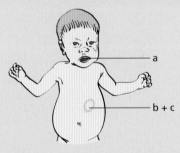

**Confirmatory investigations**
Abdominal ultrasound (not
needed if 'olive' felt)
Hypochloraemic alkalosis
(see p. 94)
Low serum sodium and
potassium

**Differential diagnosis**
Posseting
Gastro-oesophageal reflux
Gastritis
Systemic infection

**Management**
Rehydration
Surgical correction: Ramstedt
procedure

**Prognosis/complications**
Excellent following surgery

# Colic

The term 'colic' describes a common symptom of paroxysmal crying which occurs in babies principally under 3 months of age, and which is presumed to be of intestinal origin. Certain infants are particularly susceptible to colic. It may be associated with hunger and swallowed air, or discomfort and distension caused by overfeeding.

**Clinical features.** The clinical pattern is characteristic. The attack usually begins suddenly, with crying which often lasts more or less continuously for several hours. The face may be flushed, the abdomen distended and tense, the legs drawn up and the hands clenched. The attack may end when the infant is completely exhausted, but often there is relief when faeces or flatus are passed. Attacks commonly occur late in the afternoon or evening. Careful physical examination is important to eliminate the possibility of intussusception, strangulated hernia or other disorders.

**Management.** Holding the baby, or carrying him or her in a sling close to the parent, can soothe, and secure swaddling occasionally helps. No effective remedies have been found, although recent research suggests that sucrose may be effective. Changes of infant formula, although commonly tried, are rarely helpful. Support and sympathy are important in successful management of the problem, which resolves spontaneously over a few months.

## Colic at a glance

**Epidemiology**
Babies under 3 months old

**Aetiology**
Presumed to be intestinal in origin

**History**
Crying for several hours, often late in the day
Face flushed, legs drawn up*
Abdomen distended*
Relief on passing flatus or faeces*

**Physical examination**
Normal

**Confirmatory investigations**
None

**Differential diagnosis**
Discomfort and stress
Reflux oesophagitis
Acute onset:
• intussusception
• otitis media

**Management**
Reassurance and support

**Prognosis/complications**
Usually resolves by 3 months old

NB *Signs and symptoms are variable

# Viral gastroenteritis

Viral infection is the commonest cause of gastroenteritis in young children, and rotavirus is the main agent responsible for winter epidemics.

**Clinical features.** Diarrhoea usually begins after 1–2 days of low-grade fever, vomiting and anorexia, although in the younger child the onset is often more rapid.

**Management and prognosis.** Management is discussed on p. 161. Antibiotics should not be given as they encourage gut superinfection with other organisms. The diarrhoea usually resolves within a week.

# Bacterial gastroenteritis

Bacterial gastroenteritis presents a similar picture to viral gastroenteritis. The commonest pathogens are *Escherichia coli*, shigella, salmonella and campylobacter.

**Clinical features.** The clinical features are described in the *Clues to the differential diagnosis of acute diarrhoea* (above). Particularly noteworthy is the fact that meningismus and febrile fits occur with shigella infection, and that bloody stools are characteristic of shigella or campylobacter.

**Management and prognosis.** Antibiotics should not be used in uncomplicated gastroenteritis caused by salmonella, shigella or *E. coli* as they tend to prolong the carrier state. Campylobacter infections are also often self-limiting but can be treated with oral erythromycin. If there is a clinical suspicion of septicaemia in association with gastroenteritis, the child should be admitted to hospital and treated with appropriate antibiotics intravenously. About 10% of children with E. coli 0157 gastroenteritis will develop renal failure (haemolytic uraemic syndrome, HUS).

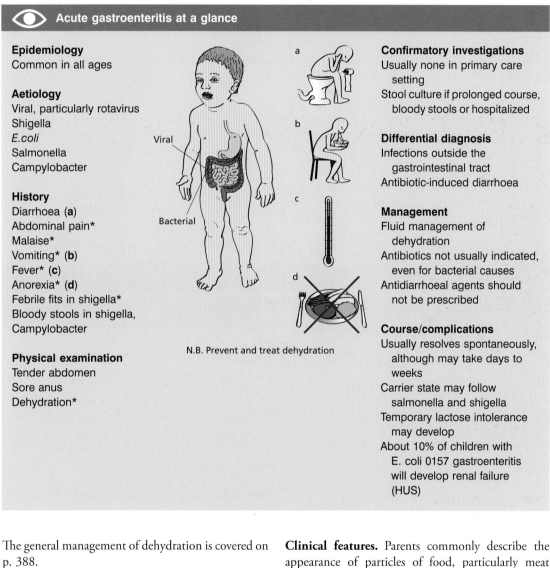

## Acute gastroenteritis at a glance

**Epidemiology**
Common in all ages

**Aetiology**
Viral, particularly rotavirus
Shigella
*E.coli*
Salmonella
Campylobacter

**History**
Diarrhoea (**a**)
Abdominal pain*
Malaise*
Vomiting* (**b**)
Fever* (**c**)
Anorexia* (**d**)
Febrile fits in shigella*
Bloody stools in shigella,
Campylobacter

**Physical examination**
Tender abdomen
Sore anus
Dehydration*

Viral

Bacterial

N.B. Prevent and treat dehydration

**Confirmatory investigations**
Usually none in primary care
setting
Stool culture if prolonged course,
bloody stools or hospitalized

**Differential diagnosis**
Infections outside the
gastrointestinal tract
Antibiotic-induced diarrhoea

**Management**
Fluid management of
dehydration
Antibiotics not usually indicated,
even for bacterial causes
Antidiarrhoeal agents should
not be prescribed

**Course/complications**
Usually resolves spontaneously,
although may take days to
weeks
Carrier state may follow
salmonella and shigella
Temporary lactose intolerance
may develop
About 10% of children with
E. coli 0157 gastroenteritis
will develop renal failure
(HUS)

The general management of dehydration is covered on p. 388.

## Toddler diarrhoea

Nonspecific diarrhoea is very common in the toddler age group. It is likely to be caused by a rapid gastro-colic reflex.

**Clinical features.** Parents commonly describe the appearance of particles of food, particularly meat fibres, peas and beans, in the stool. The child may have a large fluid intake, particularly of fruit juices. The diagnosis should only be made if the child is thriving.

**Management and prognosis.** In some instances, a reduction in fluid intake can be helpful, but usually,

...he toddler is thriving, reassurance is all that is ...quired. In some cases of frequent stooling with severe parental anxiety, loperamide may be used to slow bowel transit time. As the child matures the symptoms resolve.

## Lactose intolerance

Secondary lactose intolerance is common in the baby and young child. During an acute episode of gastro-enteritis, the superficial mucosal cells containing lactase are stripped off, resulting in high levels of poorly absorbed lactose in the bowel, which prolongs the diarrhoea. Congenital lactose intolerance is extremely rare.

**Clinical features.** The diarrhoea, which is watery in nature, follows an acute episode of gastroenteritis. The diagnosis is suspected if the gastroenteritis persists for several days, particularly if the temperature has resolved. Laboratory evidence is found in a low stool pH (<6.0) and the presence of reducing substances (lactose) in the stool (>0.5%). It is rarely necessary to perform lactose challenge or breath hydrogen tests.

**Management and prognosis.** In the bottle-fed baby, an empirical change of infant formula to a lactose-free milk can be tried. Soy milk formulas can be used in infants greater than 6 months of age, but contain oestrogens, and thus in younger infants specially for-mulated lactose-free milks should be used. The baby should revert to cow's milk formula once symptoms are resolved. The breast-fed baby needs no change of milk, and symptoms should eventually resolve.

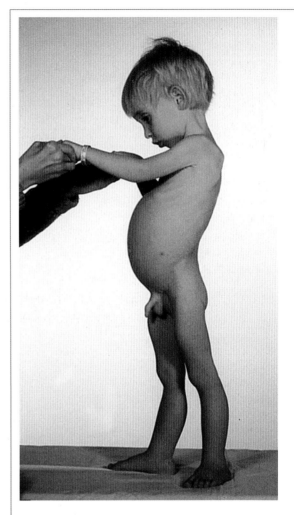

**Figure 9.6** A 2-year-old child with coeliac disease, showing marked abdominal distension and wasted buttocks.

## Coeliac disease (Figure 9.6)

Coeliac disease results from a permanent inability to tolerate gluten, a substance found in wheat and rye.

**Clinical features.** Most children present before the age of 2 years with failure to thrive, irritability, ano-rexia, vomiting and diarrhoea, although some have few symptoms. Examination classically shows abdom-inal distension, wasted buttocks, irritability and pallor. The stools are pale and foul. Additional physi-cal signs may include mouth sores, a smooth tongue, excessive bruising, finger clubbing and peripheral oedema.

The range of clinical features is very wide, and some persons affected have such mild symptoms that the diagnosis is only made in adulthood. The most constant features are decrease in weight gain and linear growth.

**Investigations.** Anaemia is common, usually with an iron-deficient picture, but folate too may be low. Most children eating significant amounts of fat will have steatorrhoea and the faecal smear will demonstrate fat globules. Detection of coeliac antibodies can be used as a screening test, but a definitive diagnosis must be made by jejunal biopsy. The characteristic finding is subtotal villous atrophy (Figure 9.7).

**Management.** Response to a gluten-free diet, which consists of eliminating all wheat and rye products, is

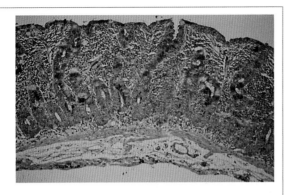

**Figure 9.7** Histology of a jejunal biopsy taken from a child with coeliac disease, showing atrophy of the villi.

usually prompt, with an improvement in mood, resolution of diarrhoea and good growth. The diet is quite constricting, but special gluten-free products are now widely available. As the intolerance to gluten is permanent, the diet has to be continued indefinitely. Before consigning the child to this life-long dietary restriction, he or she should be rechallenged with gluten after at least 2 years of the diet (to allow for full villi regeneration) and the biopsy repeated.

**Prognosis.** The prognosis is excellent provided the child adheres to the diet.

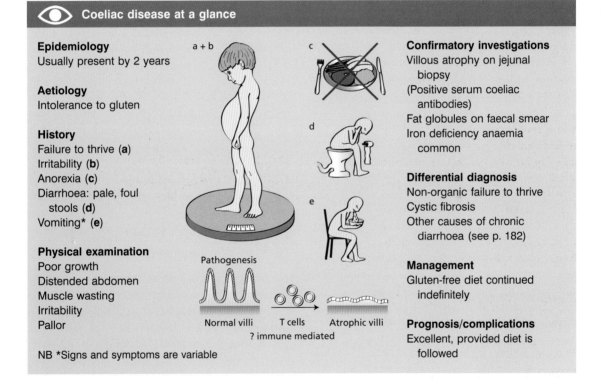

## Coeliac disease at a glance

**Epidemiology**
Usually present by 2 years

**Aetiology**
Intolerance to gluten

**History**
Failure to thrive (**a**)
Irritability (**b**)
Anorexia (**c**)
Diarrhoea: pale, foul stools (**d**)
Vomiting* (**e**)

**Physical examination**
Poor growth
Distended abdomen
Muscle wasting
Irritability
Pallor

NB *Signs and symptoms are variable

a + b
c
d
e

Pathogenesis

Normal villi    T cells    Atrophic villi
? immune mediated

**Confirmatory investigations**
Villous atrophy on jejunal biopsy
(Positive serum coeliac antibodies)
Fat globules on faecal smear
Iron deficiency anaemia common

**Differential diagnosis**
Non-organic failure to thrive
Cystic fibrosis
Other causes of chronic diarrhoea (see p. 182)

**Management**
Gluten-free diet continued indefinitely

**Prognosis/complications**
Excellent, provided diet is followed

## Cow's milk protein intolerance

Allergy to cow's milk protein is rare and often overdiagnosed.

**Clinical features.** Cow's milk protein intolerance is a cause of chronic diarrhoea and vomiting. Classically,

the diarrhoea is bloody, and urticaria, stridor and bronchospasm may occur. Very rarely, the sensitivity can be life-threatening. The condition is less common in babies who have been breast-fed.

The diagnosis is clinical. Symptoms should subside within 1 week of withdrawing cow's milk from the diet. The child should be rechallenged after a period of time (in hospital if the original symptoms were severe), and observed for recurrence of symptoms.

**Management and prognosis.** Treatment consists of removing cow's milk from the diet. Soy milk infant formulas provide adequate nutrition from 6 months of age. Younger infants require a special cow's milk protein free formula. In most cases, the intolerance is transitory, usually resolving in 1–2 years. Prolonged breast-feeding reduces the likelihood of cow's milk intolerance.

## Crohn's disease

Crohn's disease is a cause of chronic diarrhoea in late childhood and adolescence. The underlying cause of this chronic inflammatory condition is unknown. Both Crohn's disease and ulcerative colitis are characterized by unpredictable exacerbations and remissions.

**Clinical features.** Crohn's disease presents with recurrent abdominal pain, anorexia, growth failure, fever, diarrhoea, oral and perianal ulcers and arthritis.

**Investigations.** Inflammatory markers such as (C-reactive protein) CRP and ESR are persistently elevated. The diagnosis is confirmed by barium studies and endoscopy.

**Management.** Remission can be induced by nutritional programmes based on elemental diets. This approach is as effective as steroids and avoids the hazard of growth impairment. Surgical resection may be indicated in localized disease.

**Prognosis.** The inflammatory activity continues to remit and exacerbate throughout life.

## Ulcerative colitis

Like Crohn's disease, ulcerative colitis is a chronic inflammatory condition with unpredictable exacerbations and remissions.

**Clinical features.** Ulcerative colitis presents with diarrhoea containing blood and mucus. Early on,

these episodes may be short-lived and thought to be simply infective in nature. Systemic upset in terms of pain, weight loss, arthritis and liver disturbance may occur.

**Management.** Treatment is by corticosteroid enemas or suppositories. Sulphasalazine may be given orally, and steroids, immunosuppressive therapy and even colectomy may be required in severe cases.

**Prognosis.** Most cases starting in childhood are severe in terms of activity and extent of involvement. There is a high risk of colonic cancer developing later in life.

## Idiopathic recurrent abdominal pain

There is no identifiable organic cause for the majority of children presenting with recurrent abdominal pain. In this circumstance, the expression 'recurrent abdominal pain' is often used as a diagnostic term, in itself implying that the pain is functional rather than organic. In some children, the abdominal pain is truly psychosomatic and related to stress at home or at school.

**Clinical features.** Children with recurrent abdominal pain suffer very real pain, which can be severe. The periodicity of the complaint and intervening good health are characteristic of the syndrome. The children are often described as being sensitive, highly strung and high-achieving individuals, although this is by no means always true.

**Management and prognosis.** Management must be directed towards reassurance, maximizing a normal lifestyle and minimizing school absence. The approach described for children with any form of nonorganic pain in Box 9.2 is generally helpful. If there are psychosocial causes, these need to be addressed. In most cases, simply indicating the link and explaining that children tend to experience tummy aches in a similar way to which adults experience headache is enough to reassure the parents and child. Some children utilize the pain, whether real or fictitious, to their own ends, so missing school or unpleasant events. In this circumstance, confrontation is not usually helpful. An understanding attitude, while maintaining that absence from school is unnecessary, is a good approach. In the majority of children the pain resolves over time.

## Idiopathic recurrent abdominal pain at a glance

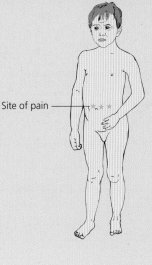

**Epidemiology**
10–15% of school children

**Aetiology**
None identified
May be psychosomatic

**History**
Periodic pain, healthy between
   attacks
Often periumbilical site
Stress at home or at school*
Stools may vary from pellets to
   unformed*
Colic as a baby*

Site of pain

**Physical examination**
Normal

**Confirmatory investigations**
None

**Differential diagnosis**
See p. 168

**Management**
Reassurance
Minimizing school absence

**Prognosis/complications**
Resolves over time in the
   majority of cases

NB *Signs and symptoms are variable

## Irritable bowel syndrome

The term 'irritable bowel syndrome' is sometimes used instead of 'recurrent abdominal pain', particularly if there are minor gastrointestinal symptoms and no psychological stresses identified. It has been suggested that the discomfort results from a dysfunction of the autonomic system of the gut.

**Clinical features.** The bowel pattern may be described as varying from pellets to unformed stool. Flatus can also be a feature, and many of these children have a history of colic as babies.

**Management and prognosis.** Using the term 'irritable bowel syndrome' often gives families the reassurance that a diagnosis has been made. The symptoms usually resolve over time, but relapses are common.

## Peptic ulcer

Peptic ulcer is now being recognized as an important cause of abdominal pain in childhood. As in the adult, the organism *Helicobacter pylori* is implicated as a cause of gastritis and ulcers in childhood.

**Clinical features.** The pain may have the classic features of adult peptic ulcer, being epigastric in site and relieved by food. In contrast, in young children under 6 years of age the pain often appears to occur immediately after eating. There may be a family history of peptic ulceration.

**Management.** If the diagnosis is suspected, a trial of antacids, $H_2$-receptor antagonists or proton-pump inhibitors may be used empirically; but if symptoms are persistent, confirmation of the diagnosis is required by barium studies or gastroscopy and biopsy followed by institution of appropriate therapy in the form of $H_2$-receptor antagonists or proton-pump inhibitors and eradication of *H. pylori* with antibiotics.

## Acute appendicitis

Appendicitis is the commonest cause of an acute abdomen in childhood and occurs in three to four per 1000 children. It can occur at any age including very young infants, but is most common over 5 years of age. It presents most difficulties in diagnosis when it occurs in very young children.

There is no such condition as the 'grumbling appendix'. The child either does have an acute appendicitis or does not.

**Clinical features.** In older children, the presentation may be classical, with the description of pain initially in the periumbilical area, moving after a few hours into the right iliac fossa. In young children, a history of pain will not be given, although the mother will often report that she thinks her baby is in pain. The features of abdominal pain in babies are described above, but the two most important features of acute appendicitis are anorexia and great reluctance to move. Rectal examination must be performed on all children where acute appendicitis is suspected. If there is doubt as to whether the child has acute appendicitis, regular re-examination is very important to determine whether the symptoms and signs are getting better or worse.

**Investigations.** Full blood count, electrolytes and urea are essential. Abdominal X-ray is not usually very helpful.

**Management.** Management is always surgical in acute appendicitis. A surgical opinion should be obtained when the diagnosis is suspected.

**Prognosis.** This is very good with skilled surgery. Peritonitis may cause severe illness, requiring many weeks for full recovery. If intraperitoneal adhesions occur as a result of peritonitis, later bowel obstruction may occur.

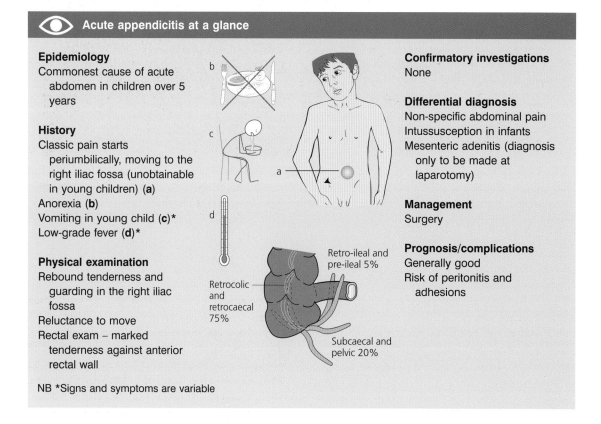

## Acute appendicitis at a glance

**Epidemiology**
Commonest cause of acute abdomen in children over 5 years

**History**
Classic pain starts periumbilically, moving to the right iliac fossa (unobtainable in young children) (a)
Anorexia (b)
Vomiting in young child (c)*
Low-grade fever (d)*

**Physical examination**
Rebound tenderness and guarding in the right iliac fossa
Reluctance to move
Rectal exam – marked tenderness against anterior rectal wall

NB *Signs and symptoms are variable

**Confirmatory investigations**
None

**Differential diagnosis**
Non-specific abdominal pain
Intussusception in infants
Mesenteric adenitis (diagnosis only to be made at laparotomy)

**Management**
Surgery

**Prognosis/complications**
Generally good
Risk of peritonitis and adhesions

Retro-ileal and pre-ileal 5%
Retrocolic and retrocaecal 75%
Subcaecal and pelvic 20%

## Mesenteric adenitis

This condition is often diagnosed where no other cause for acute abdominal pain can be found. It is caused by acute enlargement of intra-abdominal lymph nodes as the result of infection in the upper respiratory tract, chest or abdomen (gastroenteritis). The acutely enlarged lymph nodes cause pain which may be severe.

**Clinical features.** Children with mesenteric adenitis usually have a recent history of infection and signs may still be present in throat or chest. Peritonism and

guarding never occur in this condition. It is a diagnosis of exclusion.

**Management.** After other conditions have been excluded, the management is expectant.

**Prognosis.** The prognosis is excellent.

## Intussusception

Intussusception is caused by invagination of one part of the bowel into another (Figure 9.8). The common-

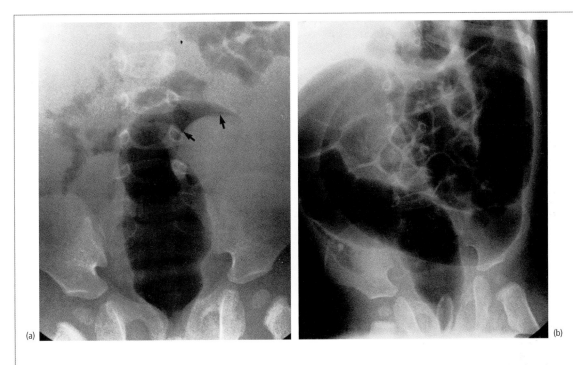

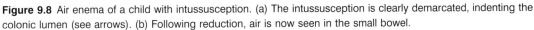

**Figure 9.8** Air enema of a child with intussusception. (a) The intussusception is clearly demarcated, indenting the colonic lumen (see arrows). (b) Following reduction, air is now seen in the small bowel.

est site is the terminal ileum into the caecum. It occurs most frequently between 3 months and 2 years of age. Enlarged lymphatic tissue in the bowel walls (Peyer's patch) may form the leading edge of the intussusception, and this may occur following a recent viral URTI or gastroenteritis.

**Clinical features.** Classically, the child presents with episodes of severe screaming associated with pallor. The pain is episodic and the child may appear well between colicky episodes. Passage of a 'redcurrant jelly' stool occurs in about 75% of cases, and this is an important specific finding. In a proportion of children with intussusception, the symptoms and signs may be very non-specific.

Abdominal examination often reveals a sausage-shaped mass in the right side of the abdomen. A plain abdominal X-ray may show signs of bowel obstruction, with the typical rounded edge of the intussusception contrasted against the radiolucent lumen of the normal bowel. Ultrasound examination may also be useful in making the diagnosis.

**Management.** In most children, the intussusception can be relieved by contrast enema examination. This is both diagnostic and curative, as the pressure when the contrast is inserted can be gradually increased to force back the intussuscepting bowel, which can be seen on fluoroscopy. Care must be taken not to use too high a pressure for fear of bowel perforation. Reduction by contrast enema should only be used if the history is less than 24 hours and there is no evidence of peritonism or severe dehydration. Surgical reduction is used if enema reduction fails or if the child is unsuitable for contrast treatment.

**Prognosis.** Intussusception may be very non-specific in its presentation and is a condition that must always be considered in a child who is acutely but intermittently unwell. Unfortunately, children still die of this condition because the diagnosis is not considered.

Recurrence of the intussusception is uncommon, but if it occurs the presence of a polyp should be considered as the cause of the repeated bowel invagination.

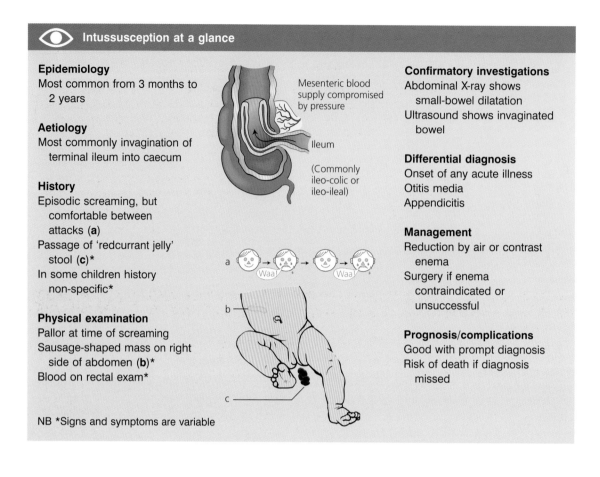

**Intussusception at a glance**

**Epidemiology**
Most common from 3 months to 2 years

**Aetiology**
Most commonly invagination of terminal ileum into caecum

**History**
Episodic screaming, but comfortable between attacks (**a**)
Passage of 'redcurrant jelly' stool (**c**)*
In some children history non-specific*

**Physical examination**
Pallor at time of screaming
Sausage-shaped mass on right side of abdomen (**b**)*
Blood on rectal exam*

NB *Signs and symptoms are variable

Mesenteric blood supply compromised by pressure

Ileum

(Commonly ileo-colic or ileo-ileal)

**Confirmatory investigations**
Abdominal X-ray shows small-bowel dilatation
Ultrasound shows invaginated bowel

**Differential diagnosis**
Onset of any acute illness
Otitis media
Appendicitis

**Management**
Reduction by air or contrast enema
Surgery if enema contraindicated or unsuccessful

**Prognosis/complications**
Good with prompt diagnosis
Risk of death if diagnosis missed

## Constipation

Chronic constipation often stems from an episode when passage of a large hard stool is painful or causes an anal fissure. The child responds by withholding further stools in order to avoid pain. The stools remain in the colo-rectum where water is reabsorbed, and the stools become harder and even more painful to pass. Constipation is exacerbated further as the child withholds stool to prevent the severe pain that is experienced on defecation. Eventually, the cycle becomes self-perpetuating and the rectum so stretched that dilatation of the colon may occur, resulting in megacolon (Figure 9.2). Constipation is a particular problem in immobile children with physical disabilities.

Constipation may be accompanied by the passage of blood due to an anal fissure caused by hard stool damaging the delicate rectal mucosa (see Figure 9.9). The fissure may or may not be visible.

**Clinical features.** It is often not possible to recall the start of the cycle of constipation, and the parent and doctor are simply faced with the chronically constipated child, who may also be soiling (see below).

**Management.** Management can be divided into three stages (Table 9.8):

**1** evacuation of the constipated stools and retraining of the bowel;
**2** maintenance to prevent relapse;
**3** vigilance that the cycle does not recommence.

If there is an anal fissure the underlying constipation must be treated aggressively to the point of very soft stools, so that the anal fissure is not reopened at each bowel movement. Application of anaesthetic jelly may allow some relief of pain at defecation.

**Prognosis.** Constipation often recurs. However, provided active management is started early, the problem is usually controllable. Foods that can promote good bowel habits are shown in Box 9.2.

## Table 9.8 Management of constipation

| | |
|---|---|
| Stage 1:<br>Evacuation<br>of the bowel | *Diet:* in simple cases this alone is effective (see adjacent box)<br><br>*Laxatives:* stool softeners such as lactulose can be prescribed. The dose can safely be increased on a daily basis until the stools become liquid, when it should be reduced. The aim should be to attain soft stools almost to the point of diarrhoea and to sustain this for at least 2 weeks. Bowel stimulants such as Senokot may also be prescribed<br><br>*Enemas:* rarely required |
| Stage 2:<br>Maintenance | Stools should be kept soft either by diet or laxatives for 3–6 months Children should be encouraged to have daily bowel movements by sitting on the toilet at a fixed time once or twice each day for 5–10 minutes |
| Stage 3:<br>Vigilance | Treatment should be started at the first indication of recurrence of hard stools |

## Box 9.2 Foods that can promote good bowel habits

High-fibre foods
Wholewheat bread and flour
Bran
High-fibre breakfast cereals
Fruit (particularly the peel)
Vegetables
Beans

Nuts
Stool softeners
Fluids of any sort
Orange juice
Prune juice
Fruit

## Constipation at a glance

**Epidemiology**
Any age, but particularly
   problematic in immobile
   disabled children

**Aetiology**
Cycle of painful defaecation and
   withholding

**History**
Infrequent hard stools
Painful defaecation
Abdominal pain*
Soiling*

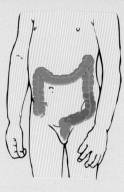

**Physical examination**
Indentable mass in left lower
   quadrant
Hard stool on rectal examination
   (PR not often indicated)
Anal fissure*

**Confirmatory investigations**
Faecal loading +/– megacolon
   on plain abdominal X-ray
   (investigation not usually
   indicated)

**Differential diagnosis**
Hirschsprung's disease

**Management**
Dietary advice
Laxatives

**Prognosis/complications**
Problem may recur periodically

NB *Signs and symptoms are variable

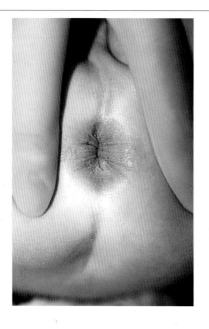

**Figure 9.9** An anal fissure (at 6 o'clock) in a child suffering from constipation with rectal bleeding.

## Anal fissure

The underlying cause of an anal fissure is the passage of a large hard stool which tears the delicate rectal mucosa. Constipation is exacerbated further as the child withholds stool to prevent the severe pain that is experienced on defaecation. Treatment consists of aggressively treating the underlying constipation (see p. 187), to the point of very soft stools, so that the anal fissure is not reopened at each bowel movement. Application of anaesthetic jelly may allow some relief of pain at defecation.

## Encopresis and soiling

Encopresis refers to the voluntary passage of formed stool in inappropriate places (including underwear) by a child who is mature enough to have acquired bowel continence. The term is also sometimes confusingly and inappropriately used in reference to soiling. Encopresis is indicative of behavioural difficulties, often of a severe nature. Simple behavioural management in terms of understanding and encouragement, and the use of positive reinforcement can be attempted, but more intense psychiatric or psychological help is usually necessary.

The term 'soiling' differs from encopresis and is used in two contexts. The first is when a child is not toilet trained by the usual age of about 2 years, and it is certainly seen to be a problem if this has not been achieved by the age of 4 years. Immaturity in acquiring bowel continence may result from inappropriate toilet training. A programme of regular toilet training needs to be instituted, with much positive reinforcement for successes.

The second situation where the term is used is where there is faecal staining of underwear from leakage of liquid stool around impacted faeces when a child is constipated. This is sometimes mistaken for diarrhoea. The problem must be approached by addressing the underlying constipation (see above). Resolution of the soiling will then result. Soiling in both circumstances is a problem, causing social inconvenience and embarrassment for both the child and the family.

## Viral hepatitis

Hepatitis is mainly caused by viral infections, including hepatitis A, hepatitis B, hepatitis C (rare), Epstein–Barr virus and cytomegalovirus. The commonest is hepatitis A, which is spread by faecal contamination of food and water. It is associated with poor hygiene and limited sanitation. The highest incidence for hepatitis A infection in children is 5–15 years of age and the incubation period is 2–6 weeks.

Hepatitis B is rare in children and is acquired by contamination with blood products, with an incubation period of 2–6 months. The infection is most commonly acquired by vertical transmission from mother to baby, although if the mother has hepatitis B antibodies her baby is protected. Immunization of the newborn infant is possible if the infected mother is recognized antenatally (p. 425).

**Clinical features.** The onset of hepatitis A infection is usually insidious. The child is unwell, with anorexia and nausea, and jaundice appears 5 days later. The liver is tender on palpation, but not enlarged. The urine is dark and the stools may be pale. Investigations show high liver enzymes (transaminases) with conjugated hyperbilirubinaemia. The virus can be identified serologically, and in the case of hepatitis B the presence of surface and core antigens must be identified.

**Management.** There is no specific treatment for viral hepatitis. Hepatitis A infection is highly infectious during the prodromal phase, but by the time jaundice is apparent the patient is no longer excreting the virus. Hospital treatment is only required for complications of the condition. Control of cross-infection is essential as a public health measure. Hepatitis B is highly infectious and great care must be taken with handling blood products of infected mothers or children. Immunization of at-risk babies is essential (p. 425),

and an immunoglobulin injection is also given to these babies at birth.

**Prognosis.** The prognosis is good following hepatitis A infection, and development of chronic hepatitis is rare. Chronic hepatitis is commoner following hepatitis B, with an increased risk of subsequent hepatocellular carcinoma in adult life for carriers.

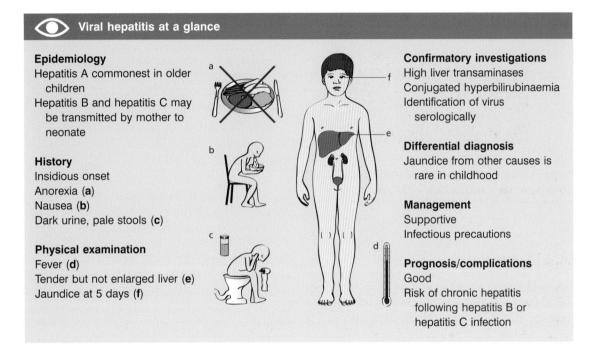

## Viral hepatitis at a glance

**Epidemiology**
Hepatitis A commonest in older children
Hepatitis B and hepatitis C may be transmitted by mother to neonate

**History**
Insidious onset
Anorexia (**a**)
Nausea (**b**)
Dark urine, pale stools (**c**)

**Physical examination**
Fever (**d**)
Tender but not enlarged liver (**e**)
Jaundice at 5 days (**f**)

**Confirmatory investigations**
High liver transaminases
Conjugated hyperbilirubinaemia
Identification of virus serologically

**Differential diagnosis**
Jaundice from other causes is rare in childhood

**Management**
Supportive
Infectious precautions

**Prognosis/complications**
Good
Risk of chronic hepatitis following hepatitis B or hepatitis C infection

## Hepatic cirrhosis

Hepatic cirrhosis represents the end stage of a number of chronic liver disorders, both infectious and metabolic. Cirrhosis in children most commonly follows biliary atresia (p. 426).

**Clinical features.** Jaundice may not be prominent. The presenting features may be failure to thrive as a result of steatorrhoea, and vitamin deficiency disorders, such as spontaneous haemorrhages caused by vitamin K deficiency. Clinical examination reveals an enlarged firm liver which may feel knobbly. Other features of chronic liver disease include spider naevi, ascites, palmar erythema and clubbing. Investigations must be pursued to identify the underlying cause.

**Management.** Management of cirrhosis is highly specialized and needs to be undertaken in a recog-

nized centre regularly dealing with chronic liver disease in children. Particular attention must be paid to appropriate nutrition and correction of fat-soluble vitamin deficiency disorders:

• *Malabsorption.* The lack of bile salts causes steatorrhoea and malabsorption, so the diet needs to be supplemented with medium-chain fatty acids which do not require bile salts for their absorption.
• *Vitamin deficiency.* Fat-soluble vitamin deficiency is common in long-standing conjugated jaundice. Vitamins A, D, E and K should be routinely supplemented to avoid deficiency states.
• *Pruritus.* Itching may be very severe, and may be reduced by cholestyramine.
• *Liver transplantation.* This is increasingly becoming a therapeutic resort in end-stage liver diseases. Surgery is limited to a few national centres.

## Parasites

The commonest parasite causing diarrhoea in Britain is *Giardia lamblia*, which commonly causes outbreaks in day-care nurseries. It is endemic in some overseas holiday destinations and infection may be related to travel abroad.

**Clinical features.** The infected child may either be asymptomatic or have a combination of diarrhoea, weight loss and abdominal pain. The diagnosis is made on microscopic examination of the stool. Three separate specimens are required as excretion of the cysts can be irregular. The blood count may show eosinophilia, and the parasite can be detected in duodenal aspirate (obtained when jejunal biopsy is undertaken for coeliac disease).

**Management and prognosis.** Treatment is with metronidazole, and in an outbreak asymptomatic carriers should be treated. Treatment failure is common.

## Threadworms (enterobiasis)

Threadworm infection causes intense itching of the anus and occasionally the vulval area. It is a common infestation particularly affecting preschool children. The threadworms reside in the gut, and the gravid females migrate by night to the perianal region to deposit their eggs. Scratching transmits the eggs to the fingers and the eggs become disseminated and ingested.

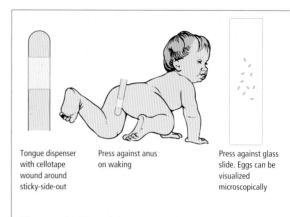

Tongue dispenser with cellotape wound around sticky-side-out

Press against anus on waking

Press against glass slide. Eggs can be visualized microscopically

**Figure 9.10** The sticky-tape test for threadworms.

**Clinical features.** The infestation may be asymptomatic or may be recognized if a child is seen to be scratching or complains of itching or anal pain.

**Management.** The diagnosis can sometimes be made by examining the anal area during itching, when a tiny (5 mm) white worm may be seen. Alternately, the sticky-tape test can be applied (Figure 9.10). Sticky-tape is applied around the end of a tongue depressor, with the sticky side outermost. This is placed against the child's anus on rising in the morning, and then applied to a glass slide. The threadworm eggs can then be visualized microscopically. Examination of stool specimens does not identify threadworms. Treatment consists of a single dose of mebendazole. The whole family may need to be treated. Reinfection is very common.

*To test your knowledge on this part of the book, please see Chapter 25.*

# CHAPTER 10

# Cardiac disorders

## COMPETENCES

### You must . . .

| Know | Be able to | Appreciate |
| --- | --- | --- |
| • How children with congenital heart defects present | • Carry out a good cardiac examination<br>• Differentiate clinically between innocent and pathological murmurs<br>• Take a good history to differentiate syncope from other fits, faints and funny turns | • That finding a murmur may induce parental anxiety |

*Paediatrics and Child Health*, Third Edition. Mary Rudolf, Tim Lee, Malcolm Levene.
© 2011 Mary Rudolf, Tim Lee and Malcolm Levene. Published 2011 by Blackwell Publishing Ltd.

# Cardiac symptoms and signs

## Finding your way around . . .

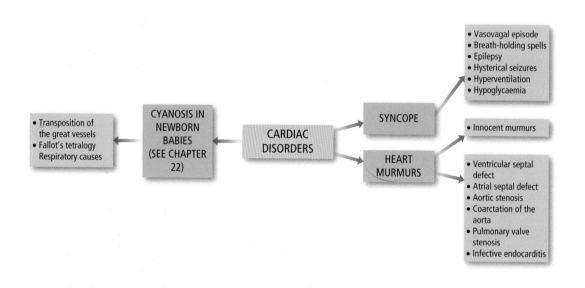

## Heart murmurs

Heart murmurs are very common in childhood, particularly between the ages of 3 and 7 years. The vast majority of these murmurs are not associated with significant haemodynamic abnormalities and are referred to as functional or innocent. It is important to learn to clinically distinguish an innocent murmur from a murmur caused by cardiac disease (Box 10.1). This can save the child from unnecessary investigations and the family from anxiety. If you suspect that a murmur might be pathological, you should look for signs and symptoms of cardiac failure.

---

**Box 10.1 Common cardiac murmurs**

| Innocent murmurs | Pathological murmurs |
| --- | --- |
| Systolic ejection murmur | Ventricular septal defect ✓ |
| Venous hum | Atrial septal defect ✓ |
| Vibratory murmur | Aortic stenosis ✓ |
| | Coarctation of the aorta ✓ |
| | Pulmonary valve stenosis ✓ |
| | *Patent ductus arteriosus |
| | *Fallot's tetralogy |
| | *These conditions do not usually present with cardiac murmurs |

## 👁 Ventricular septal defect (VSD) at a glance

### Epidemiology
Commonest congenital heart lesion

### Aetiology/pathophysiology
Clinical features depend on the size of the VSD
There is no correlation between loudness of murmur and size of shunt

### Presentation
Murmur usually detected at routine examination

### History
Most asymptomatic
Breathlessness on feeding and crying*
Failure to thrive*
Recurrent chest infections*

### Physical examination
- Harsh pansystolic murmur at lower left sternal border
- Clinically enlarged heart*
- Parasternal thrill*
- Radiation of murmur over whole chest*
- Signs of congestive heart failure*

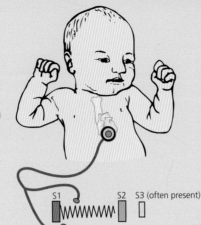

S1    S2    S3 (often present)

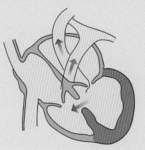

### Investigations
Small defect: normal chest X-ray and ECG
Large defect: cardiomegaly and large pulmonary arteries on X-ray, biventricular hypertrophy on ECG
Echocardiography confirms the diagnosis

### Differential diagnosis
See Clues box on p. 194
See Table 10.1

### Management
Reassurance for small defects
Treatment of cardiac failure if present
Surgery if medical management fails
Antibiotic prophylaxis for infective endocarditis

### Prognosis/complications
Small defects tend to close spontaneously
Excellent prognosis for larger defects after surgery
Increased pulmonary blood flow through an uncorrected large VSD causes pulmonary hypertension (cor pulmonale) with reduced life-span

NB *Signs and symptoms are variable

---

### History – must ask!

- **Does the baby or child have symptoms of heart failure?** Fatigue and breathlessness are the most important symptoms of cardiac failure. Ask about feeding, as a baby in heart failure can take only small volumes of milk, becomes short of breath on sucking and often perspires. An older child tires on walking and may become breathless too.
- **Have the parents noticed cyanosis?** This would be an unusual finding in most children identified as having a cardiac murmur.
- **Is there a family history of congenital heart disease?** There is a higher risk of heart defects in siblings of children with congenital heart disease.

Asking about the family history can help you appreciate the level of anxiety about the murmur.

### Physical examination – must check!

The cardiac examination is discussed in more detail on pp. 60–3, but the salient points are highlighted here:

- **The murmur.** Pathological and innocent murmurs have different characteristics (Table 10.1). Listen for radiation over the praecordium, the back and the neck, and with the child both sitting and lying, as some innocent murmurs lose their intensity in changing position.

**Table 10.1** Characteristics of innocent and pathological murmurs

| Innocent | Pathological |
|---|---|
| Systolic | Pansystolic or diastolic |
| Musical quality | Harsh or long |
| No radiation | A thrill, radiation or cardiac symptoms always indicate a pathological murmur |
| Varies in intensity with posture and respiration | |
| Asymptomatic | |
| Normal peripheral pulses | |

- **Growth.** Failure to thrive and poor growth are important signs of cardiac failure in childhood, and are also important in monitoring medical management.

- **Vital signs.** Tachycardia is a sign of cardiac failure. The character of the pulse can also give a clue to cardiac pathology. Palpate the femoral pulses, as in coarctation of the aorta they are absent or weak and delayed compared with the radial pulse. Take the blood pressure, and if you suspect coarctation you need to do this in both arms and legs.
- **Other signs of heart failure.** Tachypnoea, hepatomegaly and crepitations in the lungs are the major clinical manifestations of cardiac failure in childhood. Peripheral oedema is rare.
- **Cyanosis.** Cyanosis is unlikely in a child presenting with a cardiac murmur, but if present suggests urgent investigation is required.

---

**Key points: Cardiac murmurs**

- Describe the murmur
- Describe the heart sounds
- Look for signs and symptoms of heart failure, including failure to thrive

---

**Clues to the clinical diagnosis of pathological cardiac murmurs**

| | Characteristics of the murmur | Associated clinical features |
|---|---|---|
| Ventricular septal defect | Loud harsh pansystolic murmur at left sternal border, radiating all over the chest | If severe: heart failure, failure to thrive and recurrent chest infections |
| Atrial septal defect | Soft systolic murmur in second left intercostal space, wide fixed splitting of the second sound | |
| Aortic stenosis | Systolic ejection murmur at right upper sternal border, radiating to the neck and down the left sternal border | Exercise-induced dizziness and loss of consciousness in a minority of older children |
| Coarctation | Systolic murmur over the left side of the chest, especially at the back | Absent or delayed weak femoral pulses. Hypertension in arms |
| Pulmonary stenosis | Systolic ejection murmur over the upper part of left chest anteriorly and conducted to the back, usually preceded by an ejection click | May be associated with cyanosis if more than mild |
| Patent ductus arteriosus | Pansystolic murmur in neonates. Continuous murmur after 3 months of age | Collapsing pulse |

---

### Investigations

Investigations are only required if the murmur is thought to be pathological. A chest X-ray provides information about cardiac size and shape and pulmonary vascularity. The electrocardiograph (ECG) gives further information about ventricular and atrial hypertrophy. Echocardiography is important in evaluating cardiac structure and performance, gradients across stenotic valves and the direction of flow across a shunt. Cardiac catheterization is now rarely required for diagnosis.

### Management of the child with a murmur

If the murmur is thought to be innocent, discuss its lack of significance with the parents. Reassure them fully so that lingering doubts do not generate anxiety and overprotectiveness. It is helpful to describe that the murmur is simply a 'noise' and does not indicate the presence of a cardiac defect. In general no investigations are required. If a murmur is considered to be pathological, referral to a cardiologist is required.

## Cyanosis

All babies are cyanosed at birth before they take their first breath, but they should rapidly (within minutes) become a healthy pink colour. Routine saturation monitoring of all newborn babies is now recommended to screen for congenital cyanotic heart disease. Many older infants will present with concerns regarding a transient bluish discolouration of the lips, lasting just a few seconds, and often associated with feeding. If the infant is otherwise well, thriving on the centiles, and has a normal examination and oxygen saturations, the parents should be reassured.

Of greater concern is persistent cyanosis. This is usually most obviously noted in the lips and tongue, but can be difficult to spot, particularly in newborn babies or children with dark skin. Children who have had persistent cyanosis for some time may also have digital clubbing. It is not unusual for babies with congenital cyanotic heart disease to present with oxygen saturations of 60–70%. Administration of oxygen generally makes little or no difference to this saturation, in contrast to cyanosis caused by respiratory problems.

## Fainting / syncope

Fainting or syncope is quite a common symptom, particularly in teenage girls. It occurs when there is hypotension and decreased cerebral perfusion. Individuals with poor vasomotor reflexes can faint on standing up rapidly or during prolonged standing. It is distinguished from other fits, faints and funny turns (see p. 203) by preceding blurring of vision, lightheadedness, sweating and nausea. There are no tonic or clonic movements. Consciousness is rapidly regained on lying flat. As it can rarely be a symptom of cardiac arrhythmias or poor cardiac output, it is prudent to obtain standing and lying blood pressure and an ECG if there is any doubt as to the cause of the faint.

### Clues to the differential diagnosis of syncope

| | Characteristic features | Precipitating event | EEG |
|---|---|---|---|
| **Syncopal attacks** | Blurred vision, light-headedness, sweating and nausea, resolves on lying down | Painful or emotional stimulus, prolonged standing | Normal* |
| **Hyperventilation** | Excessive deep breathing, sometimes tetany. Resolves on breathing into a paper bag | Excitement | Normal* |
| **Hysterical seizures** | Gradual onset, asynchronous flailing movements, no incontinence or postictal state | Often an emotional stimulus | Normal unless the child has in addition genuine epilepsy |

*EEG not required to make the diagnosis.

# Cardiac conditions

## Innocent (functional) murmurs

These murmurs are commonly heard in children and have no clinical significance. Figure 10.1 shows the sites where they are best heard.

### Systolic ejection murmur

This is a short systolic murmur occurring during ejection and heard along the left sternal edge or at the apex. It is musical in character, frequently sounding like the vibration of a tuning fork. It varies in intensity when the child changes from lying to sitting and is intensified by fever, excitement or exercise.

### Pulmonary flow murmur

This murmur is caused by rapid flow of blood across a normal pulmonary valve. It is a brief, high-pitched, blowing murmur, best heard in the second left intercostal space with the child lying down.

### Venous hum

A venous hum is caused by flow through the systemic great veins. It is a blowing, continuous murmur heard at the base of the heart just below the clavicles, sounding like a soft hum during both systole and diastole. It varies with positioning of the head and disappears when the child lies down.

## Defects causing a left to right shunt

The commonest defects occur between the two sides of the heart at the level of the ventricles or atria. The hole allows shunting of blood from the left to the right side of the heart. If the hole is large and allows a considerable volume of blood to be shunted, an added burden is imposed on the heart, and hypertrophy, dilatation and failure result. A large heart with a prominent pulmonary artery and increased vascular markings are seen on chest X-ray and signs of ventricular hypertrophy on the ECG.

### Atrial septal defect (Figure 10.2)

As the murmur is soft, it may not be detected until the child starts school.

**Clinical features.** The systolic murmur, which is heard in the second left interspace, is caused by high flow across the normal pulmonary valve and not by flow across the defect. Characteristically the second heart sound is widely split and is 'fixed' (does not vary with respiration). Occasionally the child may experience breathlessness, tiredness on exertion, or recurrent chest infections.

**Management.** If the defect is moderate or large, closure is carried out using an occluding device placed by cardiac catheterization, or by open heart surgery.

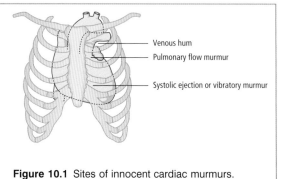

**Figure 10.1** Sites of innocent cardiac murmurs.

Venous hum
Pulmonary flow murmur
Systolic ejection or vibratory murmur

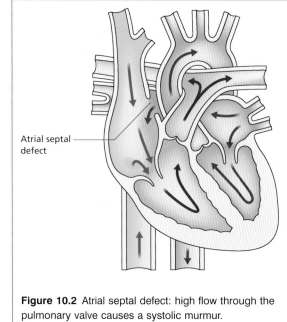

Atrial septal defect

**Figure 10.2** Atrial septal defect: high flow through the pulmonary valve causes a systolic murmur.

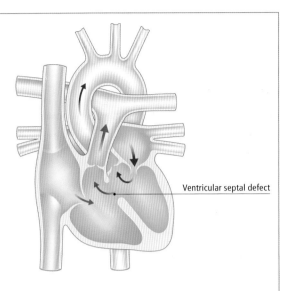

**Figure 10.3** Ventricular septal defect: blood flows through the defect to the right side of the heart leading to pulmonary hypertension, cardiomegaly and prominent pulmonary arteries. © British Heart Foundation 2008.

**Prognosis.** The prognosis following surgery is good. If untreated, cardiac symptoms usually develop in the 3rd decade of life or later.

### Ventricular septal defect (Figure 10.3)

This is the commonest of all congenital heart lesions.

**Clinical features.** The clinical features depend on the size of the defect. If it is small the child is asymptomatic. A larger defect causes breathlessness on feeding and crying, failure to thrive, and recurrent chest infections. On auscultation a harsh pansystolic murmur is heard at the lower left sternal border. Where there are large defects the heart is enlarged clinically, a thrill is present and the murmur radiates over the whole chest. The child may have signs of congestive heart failure and be severely ill. Cardiac failure does not occur immediately following birth as the pulmonary vascular resistance is initially high, inhibiting a left to right shunt. There is no correlation between the loudness of the murmur and the size of the shunt.

**Investigations.** If the defect is small, the chest X-ray and ECG are normal. The child with a large defect will have cardiomegaly and large pulmonary arteries on X-ray and demonstrate biventricular hypertrophy on ECG. Echocardiography confirms the diagnosis.

**Management.** Small defects usually close spontaneously and the parents can be reassured of their benign nature. Initial management of large defects is medical and aimed at control of the cardiac failure. If the child does not respond, surgical treatment is required. Antibiotic prophylaxis should be considered in any child with a ventricular septal defect undergoing dental and other procedures that can cause bacteraemia, as there is an increased risk of infective endocarditis (see p. 201).

**Prognosis and complications.** Small defects tend to close spontaneously, or may remain the same size but become insignificant as the child grows. For larger defects, the prognosis after surgery is excellent. If a large ventricular septal defect is uncorrected, pulmonary hypertension can result from the increased pulmonary blood flow, making the defect inoperable and reducing the child's life-span (cor pulmonale).

## Congenital heart disease at a glance

**Epidemiology**

7–8 infants per 1000 live births
Commonest lesion is a
ventricular septal defect (VSD)

**Aetiology/pathophysiology**

Genetic and environmental
factors are implicated

**How the diagnosis is made**

Most children are identified by
routine detection of a heart
murmur
Others present with heart
failure, cyanosis or on
antenatal screening
Diagnoses are confirmed by
CXR, ECG, echocardiography
and cardiac catheterization

**Clinical features**

**Heart murmur:** distinctive
features of pathological
murmurs are described in
Table 10.1 and box: Clues to
the clinical diagnosis of
pathological cardiac murmurs
• **Cyanosis:** central cyanosis is
seen on the tongue and lips.
Clubbing, polycythaemia,
reduced exercise tolerance
and failure to thrive are seen
with longstanding cyanosis
• **Heart failure:** breathlessness,
sweating, poor feeding,
recurrent chestiness, failure to
thrive, tachypnoea, tachycardia, enlarged heart,
hepatomegaly (not oedema in
childhood)

NB *Signs and symptoms are variable

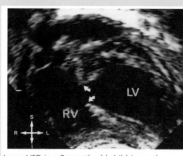

Large VSD in a 3-month-old child (curved arrows)

Apical four-chamber echocardiographic view

**General management**

• Most defects are amenable to
corrective or palliative surgery
• Heart failure is treated with
diuretics, ACE inhibitors or
digoxin
• Prophylaxis against infective
endocarditis is considered
• Nutritional supplements if
child is failing to thrive
• **Education:**
Advise regarding anxiety and
overprotection
Children with severe disease
self-restrict activity naturally
Contraceptive advice for
teenage girls
• **School:**
Need to be aware of any
limitations in activity
Special arrangements for
physical education when
necessary

**Points for routine follow-up**

• Growth
• Signs or symptoms of cardiac
failure
• Evidence of infective
endocarditis

**Prognosis**

Good after repair of simple
lesions (e.g. PDA, ASD, PS)
Restricted lifestyle following
palliative procedures for
complex heart disease

## Obstructive lesions

Obstructive lesions occasionally occur at the pulmonary and aortic valves and along the aorta, causing
hypertrophy in the chamber of the heart proximal to
the lesion. If the obstruction is severe, heart failure
may develop.

### Aortic stenosis (Figure 10.4)

Aortic stenosis may occur in isolation or in combination with other heart defects.

**Clinical features.** In most cases aortic stenosis is
identified by discovery of a heart murmur on routine

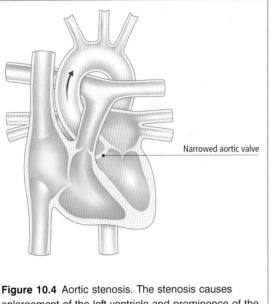

**Figure 10.4** Aortic stenosis. The stenosis causes enlargement of the left ventricle and prominence of the ascending aorta. © British Heart Foundation 2008.

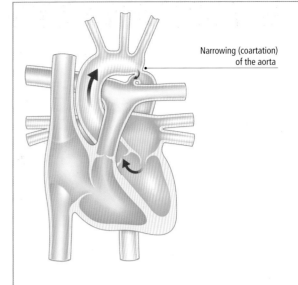

**Figure 10.5** Coarctation of the aorta. Blood flow to the lower limbs is maintained through a patent ductus arteriosus. © British Heart Foundation 2008.

examination, although in severe cases heart failure may develop in infancy. Some older children may become symptomatic, experiencing faintness or dizziness on exertion. The systolic ejection murmur is heard at the right upper sternal border and radiates to the neck and down the left sternal border. The murmur may be preceded by an ejection click and the aortic second sound is soft and delayed. The peripheral pulse is of small volume and the blood pressure may be low. A thrill may be palpable at the lower left sternal border and in the suprasternal notch over the carotid arteries.

**Investigations.** The chest X-ray may show a prominent left ventricle and prominence of the ascending aorta. Left ventricular hypertrophy is found on ECG. Echocardiography is useful in evaluating the exact site and severity of the obstruction.

**Management.** If the stenosis is severe it is relieved by balloon valvuloplasty – a catheter tip is passed through the aortic valve from the femoral artery and a balloon inflated to widen the stenosed valve. If this is unsuccessful, open heart surgery is required. Infective endocarditis is a risk and prophylaxis should be considered.

**Prognosis.** Children with aortic stenosis are at risk for sudden death, and so this is the one congenital heart lesion in which strenuous activity should be avoided. If surgery is carried out in childhood, reoperation is often required at a later date.

### Coarctation of the aorta (Figure 10.5)

This is a localized constriction of the aorta, usually occurring at the origin of the ductus arteriosus. Arterial blood bypasses the obstruction, reaching the lower half of the body through collateral vessels which enlarge. The left ventricle hypertrophies to overcome the obstruction, and heart failure may result. In severe cases the baby may present with collapse at the end of the 1st week of life when the ductus arteriosus (through which systemic blood flow has been maintained) closes (p. 426).

**Clinical features.** The systolic murmur is usually heard over the left side of the chest, especially at the back. The cardinal sign of coarctation is disparity in the pulses and blood pressure of the arms and legs. The right brachial and radial pulses are normal, but the femoral pulses are absent or weak and delayed. Hypertension is found in the right arm, but not when measured in the legs.

**Investigations.** The left ventricle may be prominent on X-ray, and rib notching may be seen where enlarged intercostal arteries have eroded the underside of the

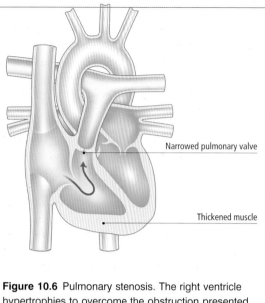

**Figure 10.6** Pulmonary stenosis. The right ventricle hypertrophies to overcome the obstruction presented by stenosis of the pulmonary valve. © British Heart Foundation 2008.

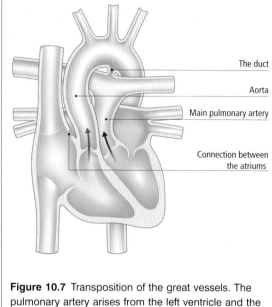

**Figure 10.7** Transposition of the great vessels. The pulmonary artery arises from the left ventricle and the aorta from the right. The open ductus allows mixing of the blood. © British Heart Foundation 2008.

ribs. An ECG may show left ventricular hypertrophy.

**Management.** Surgery to resect the narrowed section of the aorta is required as soon as the diagnosis is made.

**Prognosis and complications.** Following surgery, narrowing may recur at the resected site and surgery is then required again. If the coarctation is left untreated, serious complications related to hypertension develop.

### Pulmonary stenosis (Figure 10.6)

In this condition the pulmonary valve is thickened and stenosed, and the right ventricle hypertrophies to overcome the obstruction.

**Clinical features.** A short ejection systolic murmur is heard over the upper part of the left chest anteriorly and is conducted to the back. It is usually preceded by an ejection click. With mild or moderate stenosis there are usually no symptoms, and the heart is of a normal size. In more severe stenosis a systolic thrill is palpable in the pulmonary area.

**Investigations.** On chest X-ray, dilatation of the pulmonary artery is seen beyond the stenosis and, if

severe, an enlarged right atrium and ventricle. The ECG shows right axis deviation, and right atrial and ventricular hypertrophy.

**Management.** The extent of the stenosis can be demonstrated by echocardiography and cardiac catheterization. If it is severe, balloon valvuloplasty is performed.

**Prognosis.** Surgery is generally successful and further procedures are rarely required.

## Congenital cyanotic heart disease

### Transposition of the great vessels (Figure 10.7)

Transposition of the great vessels is the commonest cause of congenital cyanotic heart disease presenting in the neonatal period. In transposition of the great vessels, the aorta arises from the right ventricular outflow tract and the pulmonary artery from the left ventricle. Mixing of venous and arterial blood occurs through the ductus arteriosus and often through a septal defect which may accompany this condition. The less mixing of blood occurs between the two circulations, the more intensely cyanosed the baby appears.

**Clinical features.** The cyanosis may be difficult to spot, particularly in babies with dark skin, but affected infants often appear pale and there may be difficulty establishing feeds. Transcutaneous pulse oximetry should be performed to confirm the cyanosis, and the condition is diagnosed by X-ray (a narrow cardiac pedicle) and by echocardiography.

**Management.** Surgery offers the opportunity of cure by switching the origins of the pulmonary artery and aorta. Emergency treatment of a severely cyanosed child with poor systemic circulation is by an infusion of prostaglandin to maintain the ductus open, and many babies will also need an emergency balloon septostomy to improve mixing of blood within the heart.

### Fallot's tetralogy (Figure 10.8)

Fallot's tetralogy refers to a cardiac anomaly involving four characteristic features:

- ventricular septal defect;
- overriding of the aorta;
- infundibular pulmonary stenosis;
- right ventricular hypertrophy.

This condition, rarely diagnosed in the newborn, presents with cyanosis at about 3 months of age. The treatment is surgical and the prognosis is generally good.

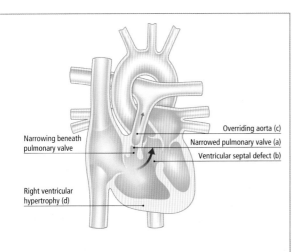

**Figure 10.8** Fallot's tetralogy. (a) Pulmonary stenosis; (b) ventricular septal defect with shunt; (c) overriding aorta; (d) right ventricular hypertrophy. © British Heart Foundation 2008.

Labels on figure:
Narrowing beneath pulmonary valve
Right ventricular hypertrophy (d)
Overriding aorta (c)
Narrowed pulmonary valve (a)
Ventricular septal defect (b)

## Infective endocarditis

Although rare in childhood, infective endocarditis is a serious condition that can have a poor outcome, particularly if the diagnosis is delayed. Children with congenital heart disease or an indwelling central venous catheter are at greatest risk. The usual organisms are streptococci and staphylococci.

**Clinical features.** There is often a gradual onset of malaise and temperatures over a few weeks, although presentation can occur more acutely. On examination fever, a new or changing murmur, petechiae, splinter haemorrhages, and hepatosplenomegaly may be seen. The most important investigation is to perform multiple blood cultures before commencing antibiotic treatment, as it is important to determine the causal organism and perform antibiotic susceptibility testing. Echocardiography may show vegetations.

**Management.** Complete eradication of the infection is required and appropriate intravenous antibiotics are given for 4–8 weeks.

## Syncope

Syncope, or fainting, occurs when there is hypotension and decreased cerebral perfusion. Syncope is quite common, particularly in teenage girls reacting to painful or emotional stimuli. It also occurs in the teenage years in individuals with poor vasomotor reflexes who faint on standing up rapidly or during prolonged standing.

**Clinical features.** Blurring of vision, light-headedness, sweating and nausea precede the loss of consciousness which is rapidly regained on lying flat. There may be a history of an unpleasant stimulus or prolonged standing.

**Management and prognosis.** Rarely, syncope is a symptom of cardiac arrhythmias or poor cardiac output in childhood. The evaluation should therefore include a clinical cardiac examination, standing and lying blood pressure and an ECG if there is any doubt as to the cause of the faint.

Simple syncope usually becomes less of a problem in adulthood. Syncope occurring with exercise or associated with chest pain is likely to have a cardiac cause and should be urgently referred to a cardiologist.

*To test your knowledge on this part of the book, please see Chapter 25.*

# CHAPTER 11
# Neurological disorders

It is thus with regard to the disease called Sacred: it appears to me to be nowise more divine nor more sacred than other diseases, but has a natural cause like other affections …

*Hippocrates, 400BC*

## COMPETENCES

### You must . . .

| Know | Be able to | Appreciate |
| --- | --- | --- |
| • How to distinguish fits, faints and funny turns clinically<br>• How epilepsy is diagnosed and managed<br>• The principle of a monotherapy approach to anticonvulsants<br>• The clinical features of migraine and tension headaches<br>• The signs of raised intracranial pressure<br>• How a child with hydrocephalus presents | • Take a history to differentiate fits, faints and funny turns<br>• Take a full history from a child with epilepsy, including the impact on family and school life<br>• Place a child who is fitting in the recovery position<br>• Differentiate the causes of headache by clinical assessment<br>• Develop an approach to the management of a child with recurrent functional headaches | • That fits, faints and funny turns, although usually benign, generate great anxiety<br>• The impact that epilepsy has on the child and family<br>• The stigma that epilepsy may still have<br>• That most recurrent headaches in childhood are non-organic<br>• That non-organic pain requires medical attention too |

*Paediatrics and Child Health*, Third Edition. Mary Rudolf, Tim Lee, Malcolm Levene.
© 2011 Mary Rudolf, Tim Lee and Malcolm Levene. Published 2011 by Blackwell Publishing Ltd.

# Neurological symptoms and signs

## Finding your way around . . .

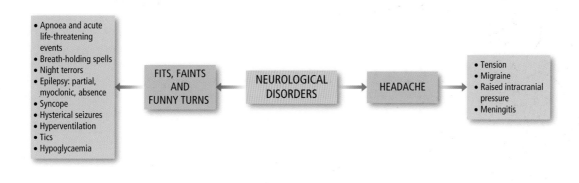

## Fits, faints and funny turns

| Box 11.1 Types of fits, faints and funny turns at different ages | | |
|---|---|---|
| *In infancy* | *Beyond infancy* | *School-age* |
| Apnoea and acute life-threatening episodes | Febrile convulsions | Epilepsy |
| Febrile convulsions | Breath-holding | Syncope |
| Breath-holding | • cyanotic spells | Hyperventilation |
| Infantile spasms | • pallid spells | Hysteria |
| Epilepsy | Night terrors | Tics |
| Hypoglycaemia and metabolic conditions | Epilepsy | |
| | Benign paroxysmal vertigo | |

Children can present with a variety of episodes associated with transient altered consciousness. The term 'fits, faints and funny turns' tends to refer to episodes which present after the event is over and may be recurrent, rather than generalized convulsions or coma presenting as a medical emergency (see pp. 380–5). As the presentation of these problems varies with different stages of childhood, it is best to consider them according to age (Box 11.1). Most of these attacks are benign, but they can arouse considerable concern.

Rarely metabolic disturbance, including hypoglycaemia, may cause loss of consciousness with seizures or a less dramatic alteration in consciousness. An underlying metabolic problem should be suspected in a child if there are features such as significant vomiting, developmental delay, dysmorphism, hepatosplenomegaly or micro- or macrocephaly. Hypoglycaemia may be suspected if the episode has a temporal relationship to food.

Young babies not uncommonly present for medical attention with episodes of having been found limp or twitching – this is labelled as an acute life-threatening event (ALTE). The concern lies in whether a cardiac arrhythmia, convulsion or choking episode has precipitated the event. More often than not, the babies are admitted to hospital for observation and discharged after an uneventful night. If these episodes recur, a serious cause needs to be excluded.

Most commonly, parents and teachers raise concerns over 'funny spells' that they have observed in children at home and in the classroom. As the child is rarely observed by the doctor, the history is of paramount importance. You should make every effort to obtain the history from a witness rather than a second-hand version.

### History – must ask!

• *What was the episode like?* When you take the history, it helps to visualize the episodes as they are described and then 'replay' the event back to the witness to make sure that you have obtained an accurate picture. It is important to establish what the child is doing at the onset, and whether there are any precipitating factors. Other important information includes:

  • the length of the episode;
  • loss of or alteration in consciousness;
  • a description and demonstration of any involuntary movements;
  • change in colour, whether pallor or cyanosis;
  • the reaction of the child to the event;
  • was there a postictal phase?

• *Developmental history.* A developmental evaluation is particularly important if you are considering infantile spasms or metabolic conditions.
• *Family history.* A history of epilepsy, developmental problems, febrile seizures and metabolic disorders in the family may be relevant.

### Physical examination – must check!

The physical examination is rarely helpful in between episodes, which is another reason why the history is so important. However, you do need to carry out a careful cardiac and neurological examination. Dysmorphic features, micro- or macrocephaly and hepatosplenomegaly are suggestive of a metabolic disorder.

### Investigations

The diagnosis of an episode is essentially clinical (see the two Clues boxes on the differential diagnosis of fits, faints and funny turns). Investigations are rarely helpful, although they must be considered if apnoea, cardiac arrhythmia, epilepsy or a metabolic problem is suspected. The appropriate investigations are discussed in the relevant sections.

---

**Key points: Diagnosing fits, faints and funny turns**

• Decide on the basis of the history what type of episode has occurred
• Only carry out investigations if merited by the nature of the episode

---

**Clues to the differential diagnosis of fits, faints and funny turns in infants and preschool children**

| | Characteristic features | Precipitating event | EEG |
|---|---|---|---|
| **Apnoea and ALTE** | Usually found limp or twitching | None apparent | Depends on cause |
| **Breath-holding spells (cyanotic)** | Stops breathing, becomes cyanotic and extends, may lose consciousness. Then becomes limp and breathes normally. No postictal state | Always precipitated by crying from pain or anger | Normal* |
| **Reflex anoxic spells (pallid)** | Turns pale and collapses. Rapid recovery | Bump on head or other minor injury | Normal* |
| **Night terrors** | Wakes from sleep disorientated and frightened. May be autonomic signs | Sleep | Normal* |
| **Benign paroxysmal vertigo** | Sudden unsteadiness. Frightened and clings to parent. No postictal state | None | Normal* |
| **Infantile spasms** | Jack-knife spasms occurring in clusters. Developmental regression | Often occur on waking | Hypsarrhythmia |
| **Epilepsy** | As for the school-age child | | |

*EEG not required to make the diagnosis. ALTE, acute life-threatening event.

## Clues to the differential diagnosis of fits, faints and funny turns in the school-age child

| | Characteristic features | Precipitating event | EEG |
|---|---|---|---|
| **Syncopal attacks** | Blurred vision, light-headedness, sweating and nausea, resolves on lying down | Painful or emotional stimulus, prolonged standing | Normal* |
| **Hyperventilation** | Excessive deep breathing, sometimes tetany. Resolves on breathing into a paper bag | Excitement | Normal* |
| **Hysterical seizures** | Gradual onset, asynchronous flailing movements, no incontinence or postictal state | Often an emotional stimulus | Normal unless the child has in addition genuine epilepsy |
| **Tics** | Rapid, repetitive, brief, involuntary movements which can be voluntarily controlled | Anxiety and fatigue | Normal* |
| **Absence seizures** | Fleeting vacant look | None | Characteristic 3-per-second spike and wave activity |
| **Myoclonic epilepsy** | Shock-like jerks causing sudden falls. Most common in children with known neurological condition | None | Abnormal |
| **Focal epilepsy** | Twitching or jerking of face, arm or leg | None | Abnormal |
| **Temporal lobe epilepsy** | Altered or impaired consciousness with strange sensations or semipurposeful movements such as chewing or sucking. May be a postictal phase | None | Discharges arising from the temporal lobe |

*EEG not required to make the diagnosis.

# Headaches

## Causes of headache

Tension headache
Migraine
Raised intracranial pressure
Hypertension
Dental caries
Infection
Meningitis (acute)
Haemorrhage (rare)
Tumour (rare)
(Eye strain)

Children may present with acute onset of severe headache or, more commonly, a history of recurrent headaches. If the headache is acute and severe and the child ill, the possibility of serious pathology must be considered and intracranial infection (p. 208), haemorrhage (p. 220) or tumour (p. 40) excluded. Meningitis presents with a severe acute headache in a febrile child. Bacterial and viral meningitis are described on p. 208.

An underlying cause for recurrent headaches is rarely found, and the diagnosis of tension headaches can generally be confidently diagnosed on clinical evaluation. They are distinguishable from migraine by their character and lack of associated features. Hypertension is usually asymptomatic in childhood, but headache can be a symptom, and measurement of blood pressure is mandatory in any child presenting with headache.

Headaches often accompany minor systemic infections. Dental caries, sinusitis and otitis media are all treatable causes of headache, and signs of these problems should be sought on clinical evaluation. Eye strain is often blamed for headaches, although there is little evidence for this. However, it does no harm to recommend an assessment of visual acuity.

Rarely headaches can be a sign of an intracranial lesion. Features that should arouse concern are shown in the Red Flag box.

---

### 🏳 Features of concern in a child with headache

- Acute onset of severe pain
- Fever
- Headache intensified by lying down
- Associated vomiting
- Fall-off in school performance or regression of developmental skills
- Consistently unilateral pain
- Cranial bruit
- Hypertension
- Papilloedema
- Fall-off in growth

---

### History – must ask!

Find out if the headache is acute, persistent or recurrent. Seek a detailed description of the pain in terms of the character, pattern of attacks and location, although this may be difficult in young children. Try to find out how much school has been lost through headaches. A diary of symptoms kept for a few weeks can be very helpful in demonstrating patterns of attacks and associated symptoms.

- *What are the headaches like?* A constricting or band-like pain suggests tension headache, whereas throbbing suggests migraine. Headaches caused by raised intracranial pressure are classically exacerbated by lying down.
- *Is there a pattern to the attacks?* The pattern of attacks is helpful in sorting out the severity of the problem as well as identifying particular events that precipitate an attack. Waking at night, or early morning headaches, suggest raised intracranial pressure, particularly if accompanied by vomiting. Tension headaches tend to occur towards the end of the day and psychogenic headaches may be linked to events such as particular lessons.
- *Where are the headaches located?* The location of the pain can be helpful. Tension headaches are rather

non-specific, migraine is classically unilateral and headaches caused by intracranial pathology are often localized to the site of the lesion.
- *Are there associated symptoms?* Associated symptoms such as nausea and vomiting, a preceding aura and photophobia support a diagnosis of migraine.
- *Are there emotional and behavioural problems?* Emotional and behavioural difficulties are a cause of headaches, can also exacerbate them and may affect academic performance. However, you must be wary of always attributing headaches to these difficulties, as intracranial lesions, although rare, can be the cause of headache and also affect behaviour and intellectual function.
- *Family history.* Ask if there is a family history of headaches and migraine. This can help in making a diagnosis, and is important in management, as children may be suggestible to developing symptoms if headaches are prevalent in the home.

### Physical examination – must check!

A careful physical examination is important in order to determine whether there is any evidence of serious pathology. In persistent or recurrent headaches there are usually no signs. Features of concern are shown in the Red Flag box.

It is important to exclude the following:

- *Is the child ill?* Fever, meningeal signs and reduced level of consciousness point to meningitis or meningoencephalitis.
- Hypertension.
- *Signs of raised intracranial pressure* – slow pulse, high blood pressure, papilloedema and, in the pre-school child, enlarging head circumference.
- *Focal neurological signs.* The presence of focal signs should always alert the clinician to the possibility of serious underlying pathology, and may help determine the site of a lesion. Cranial nerve palsies and cerebellar signs (nystagmus, ataxia and intention tremor) suggest an infratentorial tumour. Signs of focal spasticity indicate a cerebral lesion, while delayed growth and puberty and visual field defects suggest a pituitary tumour.

Look, too, for evidence of dental caries, sinus tenderness and carotid bruits.

### Investigations

Investigations are rarely indicated unless there is evidence of raised intracranial pressure or neurological signs. In this circumstance, a computed tomography (CT) scan or magnetic resonance imaging (MRI) is indicated.

### Managing headaches as a symptom

Simple analgesia with paracetamol is usually adequate. If the headaches persist, the approach described in Box 9.1 (p. 168) may be helpful.

---

**⚙ Key points: Headaches**

- A good history usually identifies the headache's aetiology
- Serious pathology can usually be excluded on physical examination
- Signs of raised intracranial pressure include headache exacerbated on lying down, vomiting, papilloedema, hypertension and bradycardia
- Investigations are only indicated if there are physical signs

---

**🔍 Clues to diagnosing headaches**

| | Character of the headache | Timing of the headache | Associated features | Physical examination |
|---|---|---|---|---|
| **Tension** | Constricting, band-like | Towards the end of the day | Nil | Normal |
| **Migraine** | Throbbing, unilateral | Not specific | Nausea, vomiting, aura, photophobia, family history | Normal |
| **Raised intracranial pressure (RICP)** | Worse on lying down, may be localized to site of lesion | Early morning Waking at night | Vomiting without nausea, other features depend on site of lesion | Slow pulse, high blood pressure, papilloedema, enlarging head circumference, focal signs |
| **Meningitis** | Severe, acute | Not specific | Fever, neck stiffness | Drowsiness, irritability, Kernig's sign |

---

## Squint (strabismus)

**Causes of squint**

*Non-paralytic strabismus*
Failure of binocular alignment
Refractive errors
Ocular abnormalities, e.g. cataracts
*Paralytic strabismus*

Squints are very common in childhood. They may be convergent, divergent or alternating. Some squints are manifest, but some may be latent and only appear with fatigue, illness and stress.

Most squints in childhood are caused by a failure of binocular alignment of the eyes, the reason for which is unknown. More rarely a squint may be caused by an underlying ocular or refractive problem. Rarely, squints are a result of paralysis of the extraocular muscles, in which case serious pathology may be the cause.

Irrespective of the cause, the image from the squinting eye is suppressed in the optical cortex so that diplopia is avoided. If the squint is left untreated, the visual pathways from the squinting eye become irreversibly suppressed and a permanent visual defect develops. This is known as amblyopia (see below).

### Physical examination – must check!

Evaluation involves simple observation, tests of vision and the application of two relatively simple clinical techniques: the corneal light reflex test and the cover test. The latter is particularly important if a squint is latent. These are described in detail on pp. 81–2.

### Management

It is important to confirm the presence of a squint and to refer the child for treatment early before irreversible suppression of visual acuity occurs. All fixed squints, and any squint persisting beyond 5 or 6 months of age, need to be referred for ophthalmological evaluation.

# Neurological disorders

## Meningitis

Meningitis is a common and serious illness in childhood caused by viral or bacterial infection invading the membranes overlying the brain and spinal cord. Bacterial infections usually remain confined to the meninges, but viruses may invade the underlying brain, causing meningoencephalitis. The causes of meningitis beyond the newborn period are shown in Table 11.1.

Meningitis is more common in the neonatal period than at any other time of life (see p. 424 in newborn chapter). The neonate shows no focal signs of meningitis in its early phases, so the paediatrician must have a high suspicion of this condition and perform a lumbar puncture if any doubt as to the diagnosis.

**Clinical features.** Viral meningitis is usually preceded by pharyngitis or gastrointestinal upset. The child then develops fever, headache and neck stiffness. The classical feature of head retraction as seen in adults is a late feature of meningitis in children. Neck stiffness is not a reliable sign in infants, and the diagnosis must be considered in any irritable febrile child.

In bacterial meningitis, drowsiness is an early feature; the infant has a vacant expression with staring eyes and, in severe cases, may present with coma. A reduction in the normal level of consciousness is always a serious sign, but this rarely occurs in viral meningitis. The cry is often high pitched ('meningeal'). Convulsions are common in infants and may be the presenting feature, although a history of the child being off colour and refusing feeds for a few hours is often obtained.

On examination the child looks ill and a squint of acute onset is common. Petechial haemorrhages may be present in the early stages of meningococcal disease (pp. 128, 322). Papilloedema is rarely seen in children, and Kernig's sign, although present in older children, is often absent or a late sign in infancy. A bulging fontanelle in infants is a late sign.

The differential diagnosis of meningitis includes:

- septicaemia and other forms of severe infection;
- other causes of raised intracranial pressure (p. 218);
- meningismus – neck stiffness as a result of tonsillitis, otitis media, pneumonia and pyelonephritis.

**Diagnosis.** Distinction between bacterial and viral meningitis cannot reliably be made clinically. If meningitis is suspected, a lumbar puncture must be carried out and the cerebrospinal fluid (CSF) examined (see p. 96). The one contraindication to lumbar puncture is the clinical suspicion of raised intracranial pressure (papilloedema is present), because of the risk of coning (see below).

The appearance of the CSF gives important clues as to the cause of the meningitis. In bacterial meningitis the fluid is often cloudy. Microscopy is essential to count and identify the cells. In some cases of fulminating bacterial meningitis there may be few, or no cells at all, but the fluid is teeming with bacteria. Organisms can be best identified by Gram's stain and this should be a routine part of the CSF examination. The fluid must be cultured to confirm the type of infecting organism.

The CSF findings usually allow the distinction between viral or bacterial meningitis (Table 6.8). If the child has been treated with antibiotics in the few days prior to admission no organisms may grow, despite the cell count suggesting a bacterial cause. This is referred to as partially treated meningitis, and these children should be treated as if they had bacterial meningitis.

**Table 11.1** Causes of meningitis outside of the neonatal period

| |
| --- |
| *Viral causes* |
| Mumps virus |
| Coxsackie viruses |
| ECHO virus |
| Herpes simplex |
| Poliomyelitis (only in developing countries) |
| *Bacterial causes* |
| *Neisseria meningitidis* (commonest cause in UK) |
| *Streptococcus pneumoniae* |
| *Haemophilus influenza* type B (now rare) |
| Tuberculous meningitis (rare in UK) |

**Coning.** 'Coning' refers to herniation of the brainstem and/or cerebellar structures through the foramen magnum. It follows a lumbar puncture when the release of spinal fluid results in a pressure differential between the intracranial structures and the intraspinal compartment. The contents of the posterior intracranial fossa are thus squeezed into the upper spinal canal, causing very acute and severe brainstem neurological signs with paralysis and respiratory inhibition which may be irreversible.

**Management (see Box 11.2).** Viral meningitis is usually self-limiting and requires no specific treatment. Herpes simplex meningoencephalitis, a very rare condition, is treated with the antiviral agent acyclovir.

Treatment of bacterial meningitis is directed towards antimicrobial sterilization of the CSF and

avoidance or treatment of complications. Intravenous cefotaxime should be used for 10–14 days depending on the organism, along with steroids (dexamethasone) to reduce meningeal inflammation. Meningococcal meningitis is associated with a high carrier rate of

**Box 11.2 Managing meningitis**

- For viral meningitis no specific treatment is required. Supportive care is required
- If lumbar puncture suggests a bacterial cause, use appropriate intravenous antibiotics
- If partially treated meningitis, give intravenous cefotaxime
- Steroids reduce complication rate in bacterial meningitis
- Give rifampicin to all close contacts of meningococcal meningitis cases

## Meningitis at a glance

**Epidemiology**
0.5% children <10 years
Neonates are particularly prone to meningitis

**Causal factors**
Bacterial and viral meningitis are equally common
After the neonatal period the following bacteria are responsible:
- *Neisseria meningitidis*
- *Streptococcus pneumoniae*

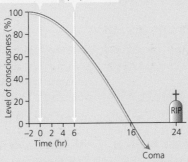

Rapid progression of bacterial meningitis in a baby

**Presentation***
Classical symptoms include fever, drowsiness, headaches, bulging fontanelle and convulsions Kernig's sign seen in older children In early stages and in infants symptoms and signs are often non-specific
Neck stiffness is a late sign in infants

**Differential diagnosis**
Lumbar puncture is essential to make diagnosis in any suspected cases
Viral and bacterial causes distinguished on CSF findings

**Management**
See Box 11.2

**Prognosis**
Excellent in viral cases
Deafness is the commonest sequela
In bacterial meningitis, 10% sustain severe neurological damage

NB *Signs and symptoms are variable

*Neisseria meningitidis* in the nasopharynx, and all household contacts should be given prophylactic rifampicin to reduce the risk of cross-infection, along with the infected child after completion of intravenous antibiotics. Meningococcal septicaemia is discussed on p. 128.

**Complications and prognosis.** The prognosis for bacterial meningitis depends on the delay between onset and the start of effective treatment. Important complications of bacterial meningitis include:

- hydrocephalus;
- subdural effusion;
- acute adrenal failure;
- deafness;
- major deficit (cerebral palsy and/or learning difficulties in 10%).

Neonatal meningitis (p. 424) carries a worse prognosis than bacterial meningitis in older children.

Viral meningitis carries a good prognosis in the majority of cases. Sensorineural hearing impairment (p. 247) is the commonest long-term complication of mumps meningitis. Herpes meningoencephalitis is very rare and is associated with high mortality and morbidity rates.

# Epilepsy

Before discussing the problem of epilepsy, it is important to clarify terms. 'Seizures', 'convulsions' or 'fits' are non-specific, interchangeable terms which describe an impairment or loss of consciousness, abnormal motor activity, sensory disturbances or autonomic dysfunction. 'Epilepsy' is defined as a condition of *recurrent* fits resulting from paroxysmal involuntary disturbances of brain function, which are unrelated to fever or an acute cerebral insult.

The classification of epilepsy was changed in 1981, and the International Classification of Epileptic Seizures is now generally accepted. It divides seizures into those that are *generalized* from the onset, and those that are *focal*, beginning in a localized or focal area of the brain, but may become generalized resulting in a tonic–clonic seizure. The classification of seizures according to the International League Against Epilepsy (ILEA) is shown in Table 11.2.

In the majority of children with epilepsy, the condition is idiopathic with no underlying detectable structural brain pathology. In some children, particularly those with neurological signs and/or learning difficulties, there is a demonstrable lesion which disrupts the electri-

**Table 11.2** International League Against Epilepsy (ILAE) classification of seizures

*Generalized*

Generalized tonic–clonic seizures
Tonic seizures
Absence seizures
Myoclonic seizures
Atonic seizures

*Focal*

Focal motor seizures
Focal sensory seizures

*Focal according to likely location*

Frontal lobe seizures
Temporal lobe seizures
Parietal lobe seizures
Occipital lobe seizures

cal activity of the brain. Epilepsy can also result from severe cerebral insult such as trauma or infection.

## Generalized seizures

### Generalized tonic–clonic seizures (GTCS)

Generalized tonic–clonic fits start with a sudden loss of consciousness when the child falls to the ground, the limbs extend, the back arches and breathing stops. The teeth are tightly clenched and the tongue may be bitten. This tonic stage is followed by a clonic phase when intermittent jerking movements of the limbs and face occur, with the onset of irregular breathing, and often micturition and salivation. This clonic phase may last only a few minutes, but if prolonged beyond 30 minutes is called status epilepticus (p. 213). At the end of the seizure, the child relaxes and normal respiration resumes. A period of postictal depression follows, where the child may remain sleepy and disorientated for some time.

### Absence seizures

These attacks consist of a fleeting (5–20 seconds) impairment of consciousness, which is unassociated with falling or involuntary movements. The child is often assumed to be daydreaming, being seen to stop what he or she is doing and look vacant before continuing as before. Academic progress can be affected if these episodes occur with any frequency. The diagnosis of absence seizures is confirmed by EEG, which shows characteristic bursts of 3-per-second spike and wave activity (Figure 11.1).

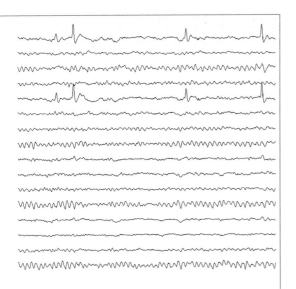

**Figure 11.1** EEG of an 8-year-old boy presenting with absence seizures. The EEG during hyperventilation shows 3-Hz spike and wave activity bilaterally.

## Myoclonic seizures

Myoclonic seizures take the form of shock-like jerks, often resulting in sudden falls. They most commonly occur in children who have evidence of a structural neurological disorder and, in particular, in some rare cerebral degenerative conditions.

## Infantile spasms (West syndrome)

Infantile spasms are a form of myoclonic epilepsy, but are usually considered separately, as they have a particularly poor prognosis. The age of onset is usually between 3 and 8 months of age. The majority of infants show typical flexion spasms ('jack-knife' or 'salaam' spasms) lasting a few seconds and occurring in clusters lasting up to half an hour. They often occur on waking from sleep, and there may be a history of perinatal complications such as asphyxia or meningitis. Development prior to the onset may have been normal or delayed, but following the onset there is generally a regression of developmental skills and the prognosis is poor. The EEG provides confirmation of the diagnosis, showing a characteristic 'hypsarrhythmic' (chaotic) pattern.

## Focal seizures

Focal seizures usually consist of twitching or jerking of one side of the face, an arm or a leg (focal motor

seizures). Sometimes these seizures can manifest as a strange sensation such as tingling in one part of the body (focal sensory seizures). Consciousness is usually retained or only slightly impaired. Sometimes the jerking can start in one part of the body and spread (the so-called Jacksonian march). The child may experience temporary weakness of the involved part of the body after an attack. Focal seizures sometimes progress to full blown tonic–clonic attacks, in which case they are called secondarily generalized seizures.

## Temporal lobe seizures

Attacks consist of altered or impaired consciousness associated with strange sensations, hallucinations or semipurposeful movements. Falling does not usually occur, but commonly there are chewing, sucking or swallowing movements during the attack, which usually lasts a few minutes. The child may appear unaware of the surroundings and not respond when spoken to. There may be a postictal phase, and on coming around the child has little recollection of what has happened. The diagnosis is very dependent on a careful description of the attack, but the EEG may be helpful if it shows discharges arising from the temporal lobe.

### Prevalence

The prevalence of epilepsy in school children is in the order of about 4–5 per 1000. However, the diagnosis is often made erroneously, and it has been estimated that as many as 25% of children referred to specialized clinics do not have epilepsy. Learning difficulties are very common (70% has been cited) in children with epilepsy.

### *Diagnosing epilepsy*

The diagnosis of epilepsy is a clinical one, often based entirely on the history, as the fits may never be observed by medical professionals. A good detailed history is therefore the key to accurate diagnosis and classification of the type of epilepsy. Given the number of children who are erroneously given the diagnosis of epilepsy, it is critical to review the description of the fits carefully to confirm the diagnosis. Other fits which can be mistaken for epilepsy are described in detail on pp. 203–5 with their differentiating features. The diagnosis of epilepsy is by definition one of recurrent fits and therefore can only be made if there has been more than one attack.

Physical examination is important. Although the majority of epilepsy is idiopathic, the finding of neurological signs indicates possible underlying pathology and needs investigation.

### Electroencephalography

The EEG is characteristic for absence seizures and infantile spasms, but otherwise is only diagnostic in the unlikely event of its being obtained during an attack. Outside of this eventuality, it must be interpreted with caution, as 5% of normal children show epileptiform activity on EEG, and 40–50% of children with established clear-cut epilepsy have normal EEGs on first testing.

Recordings taken over a 24-hour period can be helpful in patients experiencing daily or nightly episodes, and video EEG recordings are occasionally obtained in situations where the type of epilepsy is in question and clinical observation can be correlated with the electrical activity. An example of a generalized seizure on EEG is shown in Figure 11.2.

### Radiological investigations

A magnetic resonance brain scan is indicated in children with focal neurological deficits, focal EEG changes, and focal or intractable seizures, as in these children it is important to exclude a focal lesion such as a brain tumour or evidence of encephalitis. A general anaesthetic is generally needed. CT scans may be useful if an acute bleed is suspected.

> **Box 11.3 Goals in managing epilepsy**
>
> - Ensure the diagnosis is correct
> - Control fits
> - Minimize drug side effects
> - Ensure that any learning difficulties are addressed
> - Help the child live a normal life with full participation in activities at home and school

> **Box 11.4 Medical management of epilepsy**
>
> - Only treat if fits are epileptic and recurrent
> - Use monotherapy when possible, increasing the drug to maximum therapeutic levels before introducing a second drug
> - Check plasma levels if control is inadequate, and non-compliance is considered as a cause
> - For those with tonic–clonic epilepsy, training parents in the use of buccal midazolam or rectal diazepam to treat a prolonged seizure should be considered
> - Intravenous drugs should be reserved for hospital use

## Management of epilepsy

The goals when managing a child with epilepsy are shown in Box 11.3. First it is important to ensure that the diagnosis is correct, so that the child is not unnecessarily labelled as having a long-term debilitating condition. Beyond this, the aim is to control fits, while minimizing the unwanted side effects of anticonvulsant therapy. Management must also ensure that any learning difficulties are addressed and the child is encouraged to lead a normal life with full participation in activities at home and in school.

The principles involved in the medical management of epilepsy are shown in Box 11.4. Fits should only be treated if they are epileptic and recurrent.

### Medication

The goal of antiepileptic drug therapy is to achieve the greatest control of fits while producing the least degree of untoward side effects. This is best achieved through a monotherapy approach.

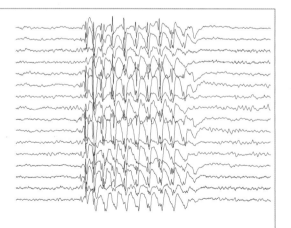

**Figure 11.2** EEG of a 10-year-old boy with generalized tonic–clonic seizures.

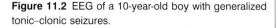

**Table 11.3** Seizure type and drug therapy

| Type of epilepsy | Drug of first choice |
|---|---|
| *Generalized* | |
| Tonic-clonic seizures | Carbamazepine, valproate, lamotrigine |
| Absence seizures | Ethosuxamide, lamotrigine, valproate |
| Myoclonic | Valproate |
| *Focal* | Carbamazepine, lamotrigine |
| Infantile spasms | Vigabatrin |

**Table 11.4** Side effects of anticonvulsants

| Anticonvulsant | Side effects |
|---|---|
| Valproate | Vomiting, anorexia, lethargy, hair loss, hepatotoxicity |
| Ethosuximide | Abdominal discomfort, skin rash, liver dysfunction, leucopenia |
| Clonazepam | Drowsiness, irritability, behavioural abnormalities, excessive salivation |
| Carbamazepine | Dizziness, drowsiness, diplopia, liver dysfunction, anaemia, leucopenia |

N.B. The teratogenic effects of valproate need to be considered in girls. These effects in newer antiepilepsy medications are not yet known.

- Therapy should be initiated with the most effective drug for the type of fit (Table 11.3), starting at the lowest limit of the therapeutic range.
- The dose should be gradually increased once the drug has reached a steady-state plasma level (about five times the drug half-life).
- A second drug should be added if the first is ineffective at a verified maximum therapeutic plasma level and the dose increased as before.
- The first drug should be gradually decreased unless it was partially effective, in which case it may be continued.
- Drugs should be given at intervals no longer than one half-life. Drugs with sedative effects should be given at bedtime and, if a seizure pattern exists, the peak level timed to coincide with time of seizures.

Unfortunately, all anticonvulsants have side effects, some of which may be transient or settle on reduction of the dose. Others are life-threatening (Table 11.4).

## Other management issues

If there is doubt about the diagnosis itself or whether it is a recurrent problem, and the neurological examination and EEG are normal, watchful waiting rather than anticonvulsant therapy is the optimal approach, as the true cause of the paroxysmal disorder eventually becomes evident.

The mainstay of treatment is medical, though a very few cases are amenable to surgery. This should be reserved for children with intractable focal fits who have clinical and electrographic evidence of a discrete epileptic focus and who have had well-documented trials of various antiepileptic medications.

For most children with epilepsy, restriction of physical activity is unnecessary, other than recommending that the child should be attended by a responsible adult while bathing and swimming. Avoiding cycling in traffic and climbing high gymnastic equipment is prudent. Application for a driving licence can only be made if the young person has been fit-free whilst awake for 12 months, whether on or off medication.

## Acute fits

The management of generalized convulsions is covered in detail in Chapter 21. A child having an acute generalized tonic–clonic fit should be positioned in the recovery position so that patency of the airway is ensured (see p. 382). The fit can be terminated by giving buccal midazolam or rectal diazepam, and parents may be instructed on how to do this (see Box 11.5). Intravenous drugs should only be given in the hospital setting where facilities are available in the event of a respiratory arrest. Children do not need to be hospitalized each time a fit occurs. Emergency treatment is not required for other types of epileptic fits.

## Status epilepticus

Status epilepticus is defined as a prolonged convulsion lasting 30 minutes or more, or a series of shorter convulsions with failure to regain consciousness

---

**Box 11.5 Instructions for the use of rectal diazepam or buccal midazolam**

*Rectal diazepam* comes in a dispenser that is easily inserted into the child's rectum.

• Put the child in the knee–chest position, lying on his or her side
• Remove the cap from the rectal diazepam dispenser
• Insert the nozzle gently through the anus up to the hilt of its spout
• Squeeze the contents of the tube slowly (over 2–3 minutes) into the child's rectum
• Remove the applicator, lie the child in the recovery position and stay with him or her
• The medication is likely to make the child sleepy for several hours

*Buccal midazolam* is increasingly being used instead of rectal diazepam for emergency treatment of seizures. It is more acceptable to most parents, and more appropriate should a seizure require treatment in a public place.

• Buccal midazolam is given as a liquid into the side of the mouth between the gums and cheek
• It is absorbed quickly into the bloodstream
• It should be given slowly using a plastic syringe, as the child might choke on it if given too quickly
• If possible the dose is divided, so half is given to the inside of one cheek, and half to the other
• Watch carefully for any signs of reduced breathing and check to see if seizure is terminated

---

between them. Rapid treatment of a prolonged convulsion is necessary. The airway must be maintained, oxygen given and blood glucose checked. If rectal diazepam has been given, intravenous lorazepam should also be given. Rectal paraldehyde or intravenous phenytoin may be tried. If all these have failed, an anaesthetist should be called and the child should undergo rapid sequence induction of anaesthesia with thiopental. Any child with prolonged seizures should be monitored carefully on an intensive care unit.

## Monitoring the condition

The family should be encouraged to keep a diary recording any fits along with medications received, side effects (see Table 11.4) and behavioural changes. This allows accurate review of the child's condition and the effect of drugs prescribed.

Routine monitoring of blood levels of anticonvulsants is not required. However, if the child's fits remain uncontrolled or drug toxicity is suspected, they should be determined. Blood levels below the therapeutic range can result from inadequate dosage, poor absorption, rapid drug metabolism, drug interactions and deliberate or accidental non-compliance.

## Routine follow-up of a child with epilepsy (see Checklist)

**History.** The diary should be reviewed for frequency and types of fits. Identifying periodicity may be helpful in adjusting drug therapy. If fits are persistent, a cause must be sought and the delicate issue of compliance addressed. Side effects of the drugs must be noted to help assess the suitability of the medication. The family need to be able to express any problems they may be having in coping. The child's progress at school is important, given the association of learning difficulties with epilepsy and the difficulties that may arise with peers.

**Physical examination.** A physical examination is not generally required if all is going well. If there is any deterioration in control, a full physical examination is required, focusing on the neurological system and developmental stages.

**Investigations.** Routine investigations are not generally required. Anticonvulsant levels are only required if the child's fits remain uncontrolled or drug toxicity is suspected. Blood levels below the therapeutic range can result from non-compliance, or poor absorption, rapid drug metabolism and drug interactions as well as inadequate dosage.

## Issues for the family
### Education

Most parents are initially frightened by the diagnosis of epilepsy and require support and accurate information about the condition. The family need to know about the duration of the seizure disorder, side effects of drugs and fits, the dangers of sudden withdrawal of medication, aetiology and social and academic repercussions. There are often concerns about genetic implications, and in the adolescent girl the

> ### ✓ Checklist for review of a child with epilepsy
>
> If the child is new to you or the clinic, check:
> - ☐ The diagnosis is substantiated
> - ☐ The family's understanding of epilepsy
> - ☐ The family's ability to cope with tonic–clonic seizures when relevant
> - ☐ Imaging studies have been carried out if seizures are partial
>
> **At routine follow-up, review:**
> *History*
> - ☐ Diary, or if unavailable ask about:
>   - frequency of fits
>   - side effects of drugs
>   - educational and social problems at school
> - ☐ Number of absences from school as a result of epilepsy
>
> - ☐ Any activities restricted because of epilepsy
>
> *Physical examination*
> - ☐ Height and weight plus signs of drug side effects – jaundice, hirsutism, etc.
> - ☐ Neurological examination if there has been a change in fits
>
> *Investigations*
> - ☐ Plasma levels of drugs if control is poor
>
> *Action*
> - ☐ Advise on adjusting medication
> - ☐ Counsel about psychosocial difficulties
> - ☐ Contact school if there are problems there

teratogenic effects of anticonvulsants and effects of the oral contraceptive pill must be discussed. It is important that the parents learn how to manage an acute fit safely.

## Psychosocial

Epilepsy still carries a stigma and fears may be expressed, not only in the family, but also among teachers and social contacts. Parents should be encouraged to treat the child as normally as possible and not to thwart the child's independence. Issues related to independence are likely to become particularly prevalent in adolescence, when compliance, too, may become a problem. In terms of career guidance, it is important that the adolescent is aware that certain occupations, such as nursing and certain branches of the armed forces, are closed to individuals with epilepsy.

## Issues at school

The majority of children with epilepsy attend mainstream schools and it is essential to harness the cooperation of the school staff, as their role can be very important. Their concerns naturally focus around the possibility of tonic–clonic seizures occurring at school. They must be taught the correct management of these fits, although unfortunately most schools will not take

the responsibility of administering buccal midazolam or rectal diazepam. It is also important that schools are aware of the manifestations of other types of fit such as absence spells that the child may experience, as well as side effects of drugs, and that these are reported to the parents or school nurse.

Physical exercise is another issue for school. Unless the child is prone to frequent fits, he or she should not be excluded from any activities including swimming, although a responsible adult must be in attendance and know of the child's epilepsy.

Further, it is important that the teaching staff are aware of the relationship of epilepsy to learning difficulties and that appropriate help is provided if the child's academic progress is affected. Lastly, children with epilepsy may suffer from stigmatization and social difficulties. The school may need to facilitate integration of the child socially.

## Prognosis

The prognosis for idiopathic generalized seizures is good. More than 70% of these children seem to 'grow out' of the condition during childhood. A very small minority continue to have frequent fits despite anticonvulsant therapy. Therapy can be discontinued gradually if a child has been free of fits for 2 years.

## The child with epilepsy at a glance

### Epidemiology
Approximately 4 per 1000 schoolchildren
Learning difficulties are a common association

### Aetiology/pathophysiology
Paroxysmal involuntary disturbances of brain function resulting in recurrent seizures

### How the diagnosis is made
The diagnosis is largely clinical, based on the description of the attacks. EEG has a limited value in the diagnostic process

### Clinical features

### Generalized tonic–clonic seizures (grand mal)
Tonic phase:
- Sudden loss of consciousness
- Limbs extend, back arches
- Teeth clench, breathing stops
- Tongue may be bitten*
  Clonic phase:
- Intermittent jerking movements
- Irregular breathing
- Micturition and salivation*
Postictal phase:
- Child sleepy and disorientated

### Absence seizures
Fleeting (5–20 seconds) impairment of consciousness (daydreaming)
No falling or involuntary movements
EEG: characteristic bursts of 3-per-second spike and wave activity

### Myoclonic seizures
Shock-like jerks, often causing sudden falls
Usually occur in children with a structural neurological/cerebral degenerative condition

*Signs and symptoms are variable

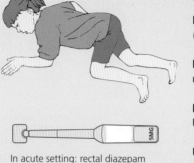

In acute setting: rectal diazepam

### Clinical features (cont.)

### Focal seizures
Twitching or jerking of face, arm or leg
Consciousness usually retained
Jacksonian pattern (starts focally and spreads)*
Temporary weakness of involved part of the body after attack*
May progress to full-blown tonic–clonic attacks*

### Temporal lobe seizures
Altered or impaired consciousness associated with strange sensations, hallucinations or semipurposeful movements
Chewing, sucking or swallowing movements*
Postictal phase with amnesia*
EEG may show discharges arising from the temporal lobe

### Infantile spasms
Onset usually at 3–8 months of age
Flexion spasms ('jack-knife' or 'salaam')
Lasts a few seconds, in clusters lasting up to half an hour
Regression of developmental skills
History of perinatal asphyxia or meningitis*
EEG – characteristic hypsarrhythmic Pattern

### General management

**Medication:**
(see Table 11.3 and Box 11.4)

**Restriction of activities:** none, unless fits are intractable

**Education:**
Understanding of epilepsy and drugs used
Use of rectal diazepam for tonic–clonic fits
Career guidance
Driving restrictions
Teratogenicity of anticonvulsants during pregnancy

**School:**
Education of staff
Addressing learning difficulties
Supervision in swimming and gymnastics
Monitoring of school performance, absences and compliance

### Management of acute problems
Tonic–clonic attacks – position child to ensure airway is patent, if >10 mins give diazepam rectally
Only give IV medications in hospital

### Points for routine follow-up
Monitor:
Frequency of fits
Side effects of drugs
Psychosocial and educational problems
Anticonvulsant levels if uncontrolled

### Prognosis
Generally good, with resolution of fits in >70% of children with idiopathic epilepsy. Poor prognosis for infantile spasms

# Migraine

Migraine is a common cause of headache in the school-age child, and is thought to result from constriction followed by vasodilatation of the intracranial arteries.

**Clinical features.** Onset is usually in late childhood or early adolescence. Classically, the attack is preceded by an aura (caused by constriction of the vessels), which is often visual in nature, but may consist of other fleeting neurological sensations. Within a few minutes, a throbbing unilateral headache occurs accompanied by nausea and vomiting. Sleep usually ends the attack. In younger children, the attack is often bilateral with no aura, nausea or vomiting. Rarely, complicated migraine occurs when focal neurological symptoms and signs are present. The migraine headache always causes some reduction in the child's ability to function normally.

There is often a history of repeated vomiting or travel sickness when the child was younger, and a positive family history is usually present. There is no confirmatory test for migraine and diagnosis is made on the presence of some of the following:

* episodic nature;
* aura;
* visual disturbance;
* nausea (in 90% of cases);
* unilateral headache;
* family history;
* impairment of normal function during an attack.

**Management.** First-line treatment is rest, with simple analgesia. In some children, attacks are precipitated by certain foods such as chocolate, cheese or nuts, and withdrawal of these items from the diet can be helpful. If attacks are frequent, prophylaxis with propranolol or pizotifen should be considered. Sumatriptan, a 5-hydroxy-tryptamine agonist, is useful in aborting acute migraine attacks in adolescents. It is not recommended for use in childhood.

**Prognosis.** Migraine headaches often persist into adulthood, but may undergo remission spontaneously.

---

## 👁 Migraine at a glance

**Epidemiology**
<5% school-age children/ adolescents

**Aetiology**
Constriction followed by vasodilatation of intracranial arteries

**History**
Episodic pain (**a**)
Aura
Visual disturbance (**b**)
Older children: throbbing unilateral headache; nausea and vomiting in 90% (**c**)
Younger children: generalized headache; nausea and vomiting
Relief with sleep (**d**)
Family history of migraine common (**e**)
History of travel sickness*

NB *Signs and symptoms are variable

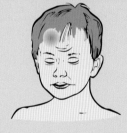

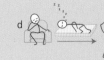

**Physical examination**
Normal

**Confirmatory investigations**
None

**Differential diagnosis**
Tension headaches
(Causes of intracranial pressure)

**Management**
Rest and simple analgesics
Prophylaxis may be needed

**Prognosis/complications**
Spontaneous remission, but may persist into adulthood

## Tension headaches

Tension headaches usually develop towards later childhood. They are thought to be caused by persistent contraction of neck and temporal muscles.

**Clinical features.** Headaches which are constricting or band-like in nature tend to occur towards the end of the day, but do not interfere with sleep. There may or may not be evidence that the child is under stress. Often, other members of the family suffer from similar headaches.

**Management.** The family needs to be reassured that there is no serious underlying pathology. In terms of treatment, rest and sympathy is often all that is required. Simple analgesics such as paracetamol may be given, but dependency should be avoided. Any underlying stress and tensions in the child's life need to be addressed. It is important that school absence is kept to a minimum, and the school may have to be approached directly to develop a strategy for when headaches develop in school hours.

If others at home experience headaches, it helps to advise minimizing attention to them as children can be quite susceptible to the symptoms of others.

**Prognosis.** The headaches often resolve spontaneously or become less frequent.

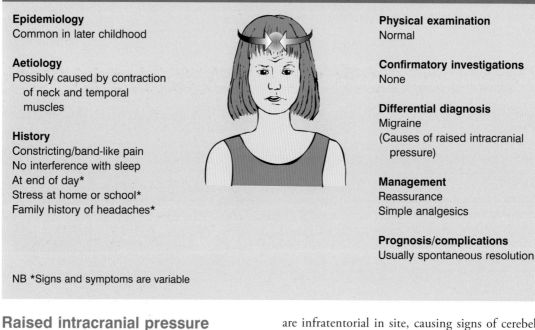

**Tension headaches at a glance**

**Epidemiology**
Common in later childhood

**Aetiology**
Possibly caused by contraction of neck and temporal muscles

**History**
Constricting/band-like pain
No interference with sleep
At end of day*
Stress at home or school*
Family history of headaches*

**Physical examination**
Normal

**Confirmatory investigations**
None

**Differential diagnosis**
Migraine
(Causes of raised intracranial pressure)

**Management**
Reassurance
Simple analgesics

**Prognosis/complications**
Usually spontaneous resolution

NB *Signs and symptoms are variable

## Raised intracranial pressure

Brain tumours, abscesses and chronic subdural haematomas are rare causes of headache in childhood.

**Clinical features.** Headaches which are caused by a rise in intracranial pressure are classically exacerbated by lying down, so it is concerning if a child wakes from sleep with headaches. The headache is often accompanied by vomiting with little associated nausea. Raised intracranial pressure may cause papilloedema, altered neurological function, and, as late signs in severe cases, elevated blood pressure and bradycardia.

The location of the pain is a good localizing sign for the site of the lesion. The commonest tumours are infratentorial in site, causing signs of cerebellar or brainstem dysfunction. Supratentorial tumours may be located in the hypothalamic–pituitary axis, causing endocrine or visual problems, or may be located in the cerebrum, causing epilepsy or spasticity.

**Management.** MRI or CT scans are reliable in detecting intracranial space-occupying lesions. Treatment depends on the pathology of the lesion.

## Hydrocephalus

Hydrocephalus may result from a congenital abnormality of the brain such as aqueductal stenosis, or may be acquired as a result of intracranial haemorrhage, infection or tumour. Premature babies with severe intracranial haemorrhage are particularly at risk. Hydrocephalus is commonly associated with neural tube anomalies and occurs in 80% of babies with spina bifida (see p. 428).

**Clinical features.** The clinical features vary with the age of onset and the rate of rise of intracranial pressure. Irritability, lethargy, poor appetite and vomiting are common. In infants, accelerated head growth is the most prominent sign. The anterior fontanelle is wide open and bulging, the sutures separated and the scalp veins dilated. The forehead is broad and the eyes deviated down, giving the 'setting sun' sign. Spasticity, clonus and brisk deep tendon reflexes are often demonstrable. In the older child the signs are more subtle, with headache and a deterioration in school performance.

**Management.** Cranial ultrasound or MRI scans provide information which determines the appropriate neurosurgical procedure. Most cases of hydrocephalus require extracranial shunts to drain the cerebral fluid away. Most shunts are ventriculoperitoneal, with ventriculoatrial shunts now rarely used. Complications of shunt placement include blockage and infection, and parents must be taught to recognize the features of raised intracranial pressure, which would suggest these problems. They need to seek help urgently if the child becomes lethargic or irritable or there is a change in personality.

**Prognosis.** Children with hydrocephalus are at increased risk for a variety of developmental disabilities and learning difficulties, particularly as related to performance tasks and memory. Visual problems are also common. For these reasons it is important that they receive long-term follow-up.

---

### 👁 Hydrocephalus at a glance

**Epidemiology**
Premature babies with
  intracranial haemorrhage
Common association with
  neural tube anomalies

**Aetiology**
Impaired circulation and
  absorption of CSF leads to
  increased intracranial
  pressure and expansion of
  the head
Causes include:
• Intracranial haemorrhage
• Infection
• Trauma
• Congenital aqueductal
  stenosis

**History**
Irritability
Lethargy
Poor appetite
Vomiting

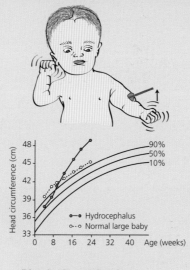

**Physical examination**
Accelerated head growth
Open, bulging fontanelle
Separated sutures
Dilated scalp veins
'Setting sun' eyes
'Cracked pot' sound on skull
  percussion
Transillumination of the skull*
Spasticity, clonus, brisk tendon
  reflexes*

**Confirmatory investigations**
Cranial ultrasound
CT/MRI scan

**Differential diagnosis**
Subdural haematoma
Normal variation large head
Megalencephaly associated with
  some inborn errors of
  metabolism

**Management**
Extracranial, usually
  ventriculoperitoneal, shunt
Long-term follow-up

**Prognosis/complications**
At risk for developmental
  disability
Severe neurological damage if
  pressure is not relieved
Shunt is at risk for blockage
  and infection

NB *Signs and symptoms are variable

# Subdural effusions and haematomas

A subdural haematoma is a collection of bloody fluid under the dura. It results from rupture of the bridging veins that drain the cerebral cortex. Although any form of head trauma may produce subdural bleeding, the physically abused infant who is forcibly shaken is particularly susceptible to this injury (see p. 367). Subdural haematomas may be acute or chronic, in which case they may eventually be replaced by a subdural collection of fluid. Subdural haematomas can lead to blockage of cerebrospinal fluid flow and hydrocephalus.

**Clinical features.** Although an enlarging head is a feature, the infant is more likely to present with fits, irritability, lethargy, vomiting and failure to thrive. Signs of raised intracranial pressure and retinal haemorrhages are common (Figure 20.2). Diagnosis is made by radiological imaging.

**Management.** Management is neurosurgical. All cases of subdural haematoma should be evaluated thoroughly for the possibility of abuse.

**Prognosis.** The prognosis for recovery is variable and depends on the associated cerebral insult.

# Breath-holding spells

Breath-holding spells primarily occur in babies and toddlers. They may be cyanotic or pallid in nature.

## Cyanotic spells

**Clinical features.** The description of an episode is characteristic, as the event is always precipitated by crying because of pain or temper. The child takes a deep breath, stops breathing, becomes deeply cyanotic and the limbs extend. Prolonged attacks of breath-holding can produce transient loss of consciousness and occasionally convulsive jerks of the extremities. The child then becomes limp, resumes respirations and after a few seconds returns to full alertness.

The key to the diagnosis is the typical onset with crying and breath-holding and the absence of a postictal phase.

**Management.** Reassurance alone is required. Parents can become quite terrified of these episodes, and as a result may have difficulty in imposing any form of discipline on the child for fear of provoking an attack.

**Prognosis.** These attacks are always benign, and disappear before the child reaches school age, although children with this history have a higher incidence of vasovagal attacks later in life.

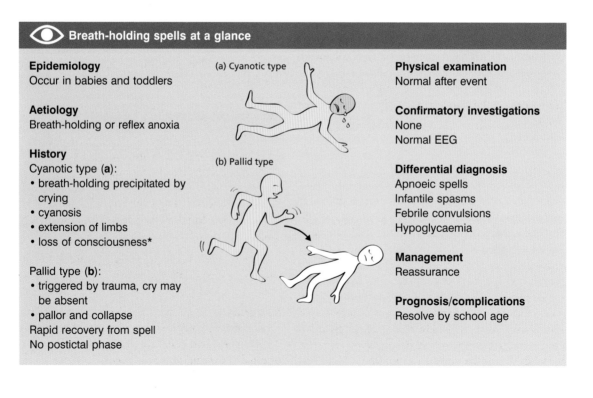

**Breath-holding spells at a glance**

**Epidemiology**
Occur in babies and toddlers

**Aetiology**
Breath-holding or reflex anoxia

**History**
Cyanotic type (**a**):
• breath-holding precipitated by crying
• cyanosis
• extension of limbs
• loss of consciousness*

Pallid type (**b**):
• triggered by trauma, cry may be absent
• pallor and collapse
Rapid recovery from spell
No postictal phase

(a) Cyanotic type

(b) Pallid type

**Physical examination**
Normal after event

**Confirmatory investigations**
None
Normal EEG

**Differential diagnosis**
Apnoeic spells
Infantile spasms
Febrile convulsions
Hypoglycaemia

**Management**
Reassurance

**Prognosis/complications**
Resolve by school age

## Pallid spells (reflex anoxic seizures)

Another form of spell is the pallid spell, or reflex anoxic seizure. The spell classically follows a bump on the head or other minor injury, which triggers vagal reflex overactivity, causing transient bradycardia and circulatory impairment.

**Clinical features.** The child may or may not start to cry, but then turns pale and collapses. There is transient apnoea and limpness, followed by rapid recovery. The typical history, and absence of postictal drowsiness, can help to distinguish these attacks from epilepsy.

**Management.** The electroencephalogram (EEG) is normal, and this can help to establish the diagnosis. Reassurance is all that is required.

**Prognosis.** The attacks disappear spontaneously prior to school age.

## Night terrors

Night terrors usually have their onset in the preschool years.

**Clinical features.** The child wakes from sleep, confused and disorientated, does not recognize his or her parents and appears very frightened. Signs of autonomic activity in terms of dilated pupils, sweating, tachypnoea and tachycardia may be observed. Some minutes may pass before the child becomes orientated again and he or she does not usually recall the event. Night terrors are sometimes mistaken for epilepsy.

**Management and prognosis.** Night terrors require simple reassurance. They are benign and usually self-limited.

## Benign paroxysmal vertigo

These episodes are characterized by acute attacks of vertigo in young children aged 1–4 years old, and are thought to be caused by a disturbance of vestibular function. During a typical attack, the child suddenly becomes unsteady on the feet, appears frightened and may clutch at the parent. There is no alteration of consciousness and the child reverts to normal within a few minutes. The condition is often mistaken for epilepsy, the distinguishing feature being the preservation of normal alertness during an attack. The episodes usually resolve within 1–2 years.

## Syncope

Syncope, or fainting, occurs when there is hypotension and decreased cerebral perfusion. Syncope is quite common, particularly in teenage girls reacting to painful or emotional stimuli. It also occurs in the teenage years in individuals with poor vasomotor reflexes who faint on standing up rapidly or during prolonged standing.

**Clinical features.** Blurring of vision, light-headedness, sweating and nausea precede the loss of consciousness, which is rapidly regained on lying flat. There may be a history of an unpleasant stimulus or prolonged standing. If a person who has fainted is held upright or seated, rather than lain flat, a secondary brief hypoxic seizure can sometimes occur, but a careful history will demonstrate syncope as the primary cause.

**Management and prognosis.** Syncope is rarely a symptom of cardiac arrhythmias or poor cardiac output in childhood. The evaluation should therefore include a clinical cardiac examination, standing and lying blood pressure and an ECG if there is any doubt as to the cause of the faint. Simple syncope usually becomes less of a problem in adulthood.

## Hysterical seizures

Hysterical, psychogenic or pseudoseizures are problems which may mimic epilepsy and not infrequently occur in children with a genuine epileptic condition.

**Clinical features.** Features suggestive of these seizures are:

- episodes provoked by emotional stimuli;
- gradual rather than abrupt onset;
- unusual aura;
- asynchronous flailing movements;
- an abrupt change of the episode in response to a stimulus.

Incontinence, bodily injury and postictal drowsiness are conspicuously absent.

**Management.** A normal EEG recording, particularly if taken during an episode, can be helpful in making the diagnosis, and a full psychological assessment is required if the diagnosis is suspected.

## Hyperventilation

Excitement in some children, particularly teenage girls, may precipitate hyperventilation to the point of losing consciousness.

**Clinical features.** The diagnosis is usually evident in that breathing is excessive and deep, and tetany may also occur. A history of tingling lips and pins and needles may be reported.

**Management.** Rebreathing into a paper bag restores the child back to normality. If episodes occur frequently, psychological therapy may be required.

## Tics

Tics are rapid, repetitive, brief, involuntary movements such as blinking, jerking or facial grimacing. They are common, particularly in school-age children, and are intensified by anxiety, fatigue or excitement. They may resemble simple or complex partial seizures, but can be differentiated by the fact that they can be controlled voluntarily and are not associated with an alteration in consciousness.

## Refractive errors and disorders of vision

As part of child health surveillance children's eyes are tested periodically to identify the common refractive errors – myopia, hypermetropia and astigmatism (Figure 11.3). Refractive errors, if uncorrected, can cause an indifference to schoolwork and have a deleterious effect on educational progress.

### Myopia
Myopia is infrequent in infants and preschool children, other than preterm infants and children of myopic parents. There is increased refractive power of the eye, so that light focuses short of the retina. The result is blurred vision for distant objects.

The incidence of myopia increases during the school years, especially during the preteen and teen years. Concave lenses of appropriate strength are required, with changes in prescription required periodically, particularly during adolescence.

### Hypermetropia
In hypermetropia refractive power is less than normal, resulting in normal vision over distance but greater accommodative effort required for close work. This may result in eyestrain, headaches and fatigue. Convex lenses are required to allow for comfort in focusing on near objects.

### Astigmatism
Astigmatism is a distortion of vision that results from irregularities in the curvature of the cornea or irregularity of the lens. Cylindrical or spherocylindrical lenses are used to provide optical correction.

## Strabismus (squints)

Squints may be convergent, divergent or alternating. If they are untreated, the visual pathways from the squinting eye become irreversibly suppressed and amblyopia develops. Evaluation involves the corneal light reflex and cover tests (see pp. 81–2).

### Paralytic strabismus
Paralytic strabismus is caused by weakness or paralysis of the extraocular muscles. The squint is fixed and characteristically worsens on gazing in the direction of the affected muscle. Paralytic strabismus may be congenital or acquired and, if the latter, is an ominous sign of serious pathology.

### Non-paralytic strabismus
Non-paralytic strabismus is the more common type (see Figure 11.4). The problem is one of malalignment

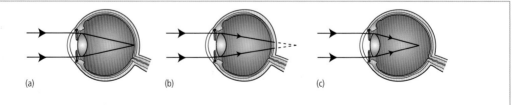

(a)              (b)              (c)

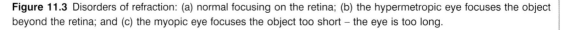

**Figure 11.3** Disorders of refraction: (a) normal focusing on the retina; (b) the hypermetropic eye focuses the object beyond the retina; and (c) the myopic eye focuses the object too short – the eye is too long.

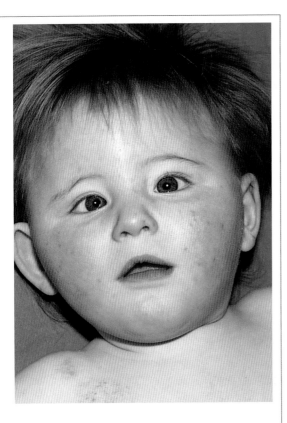

**Figure 11.4** A 6-month-old baby with a convergent squint. Note the asymmetrical corneal light reflex which confirms that the visual axes are not parallel and that this child has a squint rather than simply a wide bridge to the nose.

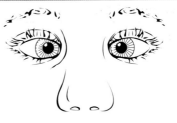

**Figure 11.5** Pseudosquint or false strabismus. A wide nasal bridge and epicanthic folds give the appearance of a squint, but the corneal light reflex test is normal.

mological evaluation. There are two goals of treatment:

**1** To achieve the best possible vision in each eye. This is accomplished by correcting any underlying defect by surgery for a cataract, prescribing glasses for refractive errors and treating amblyopia by occlusion therapy.

**2** To achieve the best possible ocular alignment. In many cases surgery is required; it is particularly important in congenital strabismus. Surgery needs to be carried out at the earliest possible age to give the child the best opportunity of developing normal visual pathways.

## Amblyopia

Amblyopia can be defined as subnormal visual acuity in one or both eyes despite the correction of any refractive error, and is familiarly known as 'lazy eye'.

Under normal conditions the development of visual acuity proceeds rapidly in infancy. However, if interference in the formation of a clear retinal image occurs during this critical period, irreversible suppression of the visual pathway on that side develops. Examples of interference include cataracts and strabismus, where the child tunes out the image of the deviating eye to avoid diplopia (see above).

Treatment of amblyopia includes:

• Providing the clearest possible retinal image, for example by removing the cataract or by prescribing glasses.
• Stimulation or forced use of the amblyopic eye. This is achieved by occlusion therapy or 'patching'. Covering glasses is not very satisfactory and the best results are obtained by adhesive eye patches. Treatment can be trying and must be closely supervised or amblyopia can develop in the patched eye.

of the eyes and no defect is present in the extraocular muscles themselves. The squint may be apparent (manifest) or latent, in which case it is only detected when the child is fatigued or on clinical examination. The underlying causes of non-paralytic strabismus include failure to develop binocular vision at the normal time and, more rarely, underlying ocular defects such as cataracts or high refractive errors.

### 'False' strabismus

Some children, particularly if they have prominent epicanthal folds and broad, flat nasal bridges, give the appearance of being cross-eyed (Figure 11.5). The corneal light reflex and cover test are, however, normal.

### Management

All fixed squints, and any squint persisting beyond 5 or 6 months of age, need to be referred for ophthal-

## Amblyopia at a glance

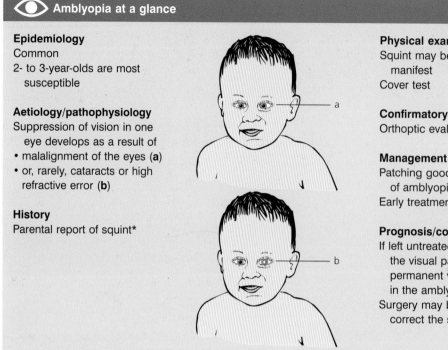

**Epidemiology**
Common
2- to 3-year-olds are most susceptible

**Aetiology/pathophysiology**
Suppression of vision in one eye develops as a result of
• malalignment of the eyes (**a**)
• or, rarely, cataracts or high refractive error (**b**)

**History**
Parental report of squint*

**Physical examination**
Squint may be latent or manifest
Cover test

**Confirmatory investigations**
Orthoptic evaluation

**Management**
Patching good eye to force use of amblyopic eye
Early treatment essential

**Prognosis/complications**
If left untreated, suppression of the visual pathways causes permanent visual impairment in the amblyopic eye
Surgery may be needed to correct the squint

NB *Signs and symptoms are variable

*To test your knowledge on this part of the book, please see Chapter 25.*

# CHAPTER 12

# Development and neurodisability

*There are some who hear a different drummer*
*And who march a different pace.*

*Henry David Thoreau*

## COMPETENCES

### You must . . .

| Know | Be able to | Appreciate |
| --- | --- | --- |
| • The major developmental milestones<br>• Developmental warning signs<br>• How to evaluate developmental delay when it is global or affects talking or walking<br>• How the major disabilities present | • Carry out a developmental assessment on babies and toddlers<br>• Conduct a competent neurological examination on a baby and child<br>• Recognize when development is following a delayed or unusual pattern | • The parental distress of having a child who has delayed or abnormal development<br>• The frustration that even young children experience when development is delayed or abnormal<br>• The difficulties and stress of bringing up a child who has disabilities |

# Developmental concerns

## Finding your way around . . .

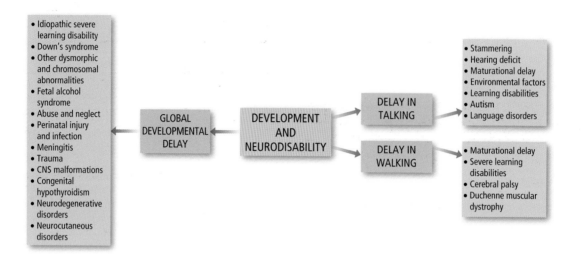

Psychomotor development and growth are issues unique to paediatrics. As in growth, children progress developmentally at different rates and, as in growth, a slower rate of development may be a variation of normal or may be an indicator of serious concern. This chapter discusses the problems of children presenting with delayed or abnormal development and how to manage them.

In order to approach the child with either possible or proven developmental problems, a good understanding of normal development must be acquired along with skill in evaluating a child's developmental progress (Table 12.1).

Given the wide range of normality that occurs in acquiring developmental milestones, it is important to decide when delays should arouse concern. In general, if the skills attained are of good quality and the child continues to progress, somewhat delayed or advanced acquisition is unimportant. For guidelines as to when one should become concerned that a child's development is significantly delayed, see the Red Flag box.

---

### Developmental warning signs

*At any age*
Maternal concern
Regression in previously acquired skills

*At 10 weeks*
Not smiling

*At 6 months*
Persistent primitive reflexes
Persistent squint
Hand preference
Little interest in people, toys, noises

*At 10–12 months*
No sitting
No double-syllable babble
No pincer grasp

*At 18 months*
Not walking independently
Fewer than six words
Persistent mouthing and drooling

*At 2½ years*
No two- to three-word sentences

*At 4 years*
Unintelligible speech

**Table 12.1** Skills required in developmental paediatrics

A grasp of normal development (Chapter 5)

Ability to conduct a developmental evaluation (p. 84)

Recognition of delay

Recognition of abnormal patterns of development

**Table 12.2** Aetiological factors underlying developmental problems

| Factor | Example |
| --- | --- |
| Genetic | Chromosomal anomalies |
| | Inborn errors of metabolism |
| Environmental | Deprivation/neglect |
| | Lead poisoning |
| Injury | |
| Prenatal | Intrauterine infections |
| | Toxins: alcohol, anticonvulsants, etc. |
| At birth | Birth trauma/asphyxia |
| Postnatal | Meningitis |
| | Head trauma |
| Idiopathic | Autism |

It is not always possible to identify the factors underlying a child's delayed or abnormal development. However, it is important to attempt to do so. Important factors underlying some developmental problems are shown in Table 12.2 with examples.

Delayed or abnormal development may affect individual areas of development or the child's overall development, in which case it is known as global delay. Unusual development is commonly identified by the parents, or is detected during child health surveillance, when routine examinations are carried out by the health visitor. In certain circumstances, when a child is known to be at high risk of developmental difficulties, such as after neonatal problems, head injury or meningitis, routine medical follow-up is arranged in order to identify problems early.

The clinical evaluation of a child's development requires time and skill. It is highly dependent on the child's cooperation and often requires evaluation over a period of time. The developmental area in question has to be accurately assessed, and all other developmental areas evaluated too, so that a complete picture of the child's development is obtained. In addition, it is important to look for an aetiology for the difficulties so that when possible a diagnosis can be made.

### History – must ask!

The history is of paramount importance. Children are quite likely to be uncooperative when relating to an unfamiliar person and in unfamiliar surroundings, and a reliable parent's report can provide much information.

The history should include an assessment of the following:

- current developmental skills;
- history of developmental milestones;
- birth history;
- past medical history;
- family history;
- parental anxieties.

Allowances for prematurity must be made during the first 2 years, but beyond that period catch-up in development rarely occurs. Parents often find it difficult to recall their child's developmental milestones, but in the event of delay they are likely to be more accurate. Of particular importance in taking a history is the identification of any developmental skills that the child had previously gained but has subsequently lost (regression).

### Physical examination – must check!

- *Developmental skills.* You should attempt to evaluate development before carrying out any other part of the physical examination, as undressing the child is likely to arouse some antagonism. Assess each developmental area – gross motor, fine motor/adaptive, language and social skills – in turn, and attempt to evaluate the child's vision and hearing.

Checklists of developmental skills can be helpful. In addition, you must assess factors such as alertness, responsiveness, interest in surroundings, determination and concentration, which all can positively influence a child's attainments.

The child may well not cooperate with particular tasks, particularly if they are tired, shy or at the stage of stranger anxiety. You can gain a great deal of information from simply observing the child at play while taking the history.

- *General examination.* You need to carry out a complete physical examination in order to identify medical problems. Particularly relevant are dysmorphic signs, microcephaly, poor growth and signs of neglect.
- *Neurological examination.* This needs to be thorough, looking for abnormalities in tone, strength and coordination, deep tendon reflexes, clonus, cranial nerves and primitive reflexes.

## Investigations

Investigations may be required, depending on the nature of the problem.

## Management

You must address the parents' concerns, whether a particular problem has been identified or not, as ongoing parental anxiety in itself can be damaging to the child. Reassurance may be all that is required, but follow-up is important to ensure that developmental

---

### 👁 General issues for the child with delayed/abnormal development at a glance

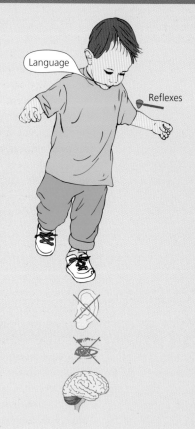

**Causes**
Often no cause is found, but cerebral insults and genetic and environmental factors should be considered

**How the child presents**
Delay may be global or affect individual areas of development
Identified by parents, during child health surveillance, or in medical follow-up of high risk problems

**Clinical evaluation**
Time, skill and cooperation are required
Assess all developmental areas – gross motor, fine motor/ adaptive, language and social skills
Correction for prematurity should be made until 2 years of age

**History**
Current developmental skills
History of developmental milestones
Birth, medical and family history
Parental concerns
Regression in skills

**Physical examination**
**Development**
Observation of the child in free play, assessment of specific skills, vision and hearing, and identification of positive features such as alertness, determination and concentration

**General examination**
Dysmorphic signs, microcephaly, poor growth, signs of neglect

**Neurological examination**
Abnormalities in tone, strength and coordination, deep tendon reflexes, clonus, cranial nerves and primitive reflexes

**Investigations**
Sometimes required

**Management**
Follow-up and reassurance for simple delay
If a developmental problem is identified:
- full discussion with the parents
- consider referral to a therapist
- referral to a child development team if the problems are complex
Caution is needed in predicting outcome

progress is maintained. You may need to refer to an appropriate therapist, either to carry out a more detailed assessment or to provide the child and family with guidance in how to encourage the development of skills. You should always be cautious about developmental predictions, and repeat examinations over time are often needed to predict outcome with any confidence.

When developmental difficulties are complex, the paediatrician alone is unlikely to be able to make a sufficiently detailed assessment of the child's abilities and to advise on appropriate management. In this circumstance the child should be referred to a child development team (see p. 45).

---

### (⚷) Key points: Abnormal or delayed development

- Accurately assess the developmental area which is delayed
- Assess all other developmental areas
- Attempt to make a diagnosis or identify the aetiology for the difficulties
- Remember to correct for prematurity in the first 2 years
- Make sure that the child's developmental skills are not regressing

---

## Delay or difficulty in talking

---

### Causes of speech and language difficulties*

*Speech (or articulation) difficulties*
Stammer
Cleft lip and palate

*Deafness*
*Developmental*
Maturational delay (often familial)
Environmental deprivation and neglect
Learning disabilities (mental retardation)

*Communication difficulties*
Autism

*Language disorder*

*Speech is not delayed by tongue-tiedness, laziness, or 'everything being done for him'.

---

Language is the most highly developed of all human skills. Not only does it allow us to communicate with others, but it is also a vehicle for thought. Disorders of speech and language are extremely common. In many children the problem is one of unclear speech, or a simple delay so that the child's language resembles that of a younger child. However, in some, delay or difficulty in talking is the presenting feature of more serious disorders such as severe learning disabilities, autism and hearing loss.

It is important to appreciate the terminology used in developmental paediatrics. The term *language* refers to the whole process whereby we communicate with others, involving both understanding and expressive processes. *Speech* is the component of language which is articulated.

In order to learn to talk, the child needs normal hearing, intact language pathways in the brain, normal oral structures and, in addition, a certain intellectual ability and the ability to relate to others. Problems in any of these areas will cause a delay or difficulties in the development of speech or language.

Words normally first appear at around the first birthday, and are strung together into two-word phrases by the age of 2 years. Language then develops rapidly, although it is not always initially intelligible to strangers. Parents are often the first to express concern about their child's language development.

As a guide, children need to be evaluated if they have fewer than six words at the age of 18 months, no two- or three-word sentences by 2½ years, or still unintelligible speech at 4 years. Earlier indicators of possible difficulties are the absence of double-syllable babble at a year and persistent mouthing and drooling at 18 months. Evaluation of children for speech and language problems is a complex process and beyond toddlerhood often needs the expertise of a speech and language therapist. However, doctors should be able to identify language difficulties and know when referral is needed.

Children living in socially disadvantaged homes often have language delay, and this is particularly true for neglected and emotionally deprived children. *Maturational delay* refers to an isolated delay in learning to talk. It is frequently familial, and late talkers are more likely to have difficulty in learning to read (dyslexia). This needs to be distinguished from language delay associated with *global learning disabilities,* when delay in fine motor skills and social skills such as toilet training are also usually present.

*Stammering* (or stuttering) is very common. It usually occurs at about the age of 3 years, when the child's thought processes outstrip their ability to express themselves. Language development is normal, the stammer is purely a difficulty in articulation. It is referred to as 'normal non-fluency' and is usually outgrown if not too much attention is paid to the problem. If it proves to be persistent, the school-age child can be helped by speech therapy.

If a child cannot hear clearly, obviously speech cannot develop well. *Conductive hearing loss* resulting from secretory otitis media (glue ear) is the commonest cause of hearing deficit (see p. 120). Once hearing improves, catch-up in language skills occurs. However, if correction does not take place during the critical early years, irreversible difficulties in quality of speech and language may occur. *Neurosensory deafness* is a less common problem, and should be detected by neonatal audiological surveillance before language is affected.

The term *language disorder* refers to the condition when language development follows an abnormal pattern rather than being simply delayed. Receptive or expressive language may be affected. These children are at risk for specific learning difficulties such as dyslexia, and may even require special education. Speech therapy is important.

It is common for a combination of difficulties to occur. For example, the child with a cleft lip is also quite likely to have a conductive hearing loss, and the child with global developmental delay may have autistic tendencies.

### History – must ask!

Even children with normal language skills are shy about talking to strangers, and attempting to assess a child with a language difficulty directly is very likely to be unproductive, so a good history from the parents is essential.

• *Is this a speech or a language problem?* In a speech disorder words are unintelligible, but the child's comprehension of language is normal. If both comprehension and speech is delayed it is likely that there is a language difficulty of some sort.
• *Is there a global delay?* Language strongly reflects a child's ability to learn in a more global sense. Children with severe learning disabilities have poor language skills, but are delayed in their fine motor and social skills too.
• *Is there a hearing deficit?* Language cannot develop if a child cannot hear. You must check whether the parents feel the child has difficulty hearing.

• *Are there non-verbal communication difficulties?* In order to acquire language children need to have well-developed communication skills. Autistic children are likely to have been poor at relating with others from a very young age.

In addition to focusing on language skills, your history should include the following:

• a complete developmental history;
• past medical history including perinatal events;
• a family history of deafness and language delay.

### Physical examination – must check!

• Observation. You can glean valuable information by watching the child at play. You may hear him talk, and you can observe the relationship with the parents. Imaginative play with toys such as dolls, cars and tea-sets gives valuable clues about the child's intelligence.
• Developmental examination. When you assess language, you must try to assess both comprehension and expressive language. Asking questions about pictures and directing the child in play are useful techniques. You should also assess motor and social skills.
• Mouth and ears. The focus of your physical examination should be on the ears and mouth. Look for secretory otitis media, and try to evaluate hearing. Anatomical anomalies are usually obvious on inspection of the mouth.

### Investigations

It is mandatory to carry out a good hearing evaluation on any child with suspected language difficulties. This should be performed by a trained audiologist.

If you confirm language difficulties on your clinical evaluation, a formal assessment by a speech and language therapist is required.

---

**Key points: Speech and language difficulty**

• Assess hearing
• Decide if this is a speech (articulation) or language difficulty
• Decide if the delay is restricted to language or whether there is a global delay
• Look for evidence of a communication disorder (autism)

## Clues to the diagnosis of children with language delay and difficulties

|  | Language development | Other developmental areas | Ability to form interpersonal relationships |
|---|---|---|---|
| **Stammer** | Comprehension and expressive language is normal, but speech is immature, stuttered or unintelligible | Normal | Normal |
| **Hearing deficit** | Comprehension and expressive language delayed | Normal | Normal |
| **Maturational delay** | Comprehension and expressive language delayed | Normal | Normal |
| **Learning disabilities** | Comprehension and expressive language delayed | Delayed | Often normal |
| **Autism** | Comprehension and expressive language delayed | Usually delayed | Abnormal |
| **Language disorders** | Language delayed but also disordered | Usually delayed | Normal |

## Delay in learning to walk

### Commoner causes of delayed walking*

*Delay in motor maturation*
Delayed motor maturation (often familial)
Severe learning disabilities (mental retardation)

*Abnormalities of muscle tone or power*
Cerebral palsy
Hypotonia of any cause
Muscular dystrophy
Other neuromuscular disorders

*Obesity and congenital dislocation of the hip are not causes of delayed walking.

Independent walking is acquired on average at the age of 13 months, although many children walk some months before this. Black babies tend to walk earlier than white. Walking is considered to be delayed if it has not been achieved by the age of 18 months. Delay in walking can result either from delay in maturation of the neuromuscular system or as a result of pathology affecting muscle tone or strength.

You need to determine if the delay is isolated to gross motor skills, or whether there is a more global developmental problem. The quality of motor development to date and a neurological examination should indicate if the problem is simple delay, or if neurological or neuromuscular pathology are present. Look for aetiological factors that might account for the delay.

*Environmental factors* can delay the onset of walking, but emotional deprivation tends to affect gross motor skills less than other developmental skills. In the past, when institutionalized children were restricted to their cots, delay in gross motor skills was common. A similar process is seen in children who have been ill and confined to bed for an extended period. Provided they are given the opportunity to be active, catch-up is seen.

*Delayed motor maturation* is simply a descriptive term for the child who starts to walk late, but is normal in other respects. There is often a family history of late walking, and on examination motor skills are delayed but normal in terms of quality. Mild hypotonia may be present. The diagnosis is made on clinical grounds, and by exclusion of pathology. Parents should be reassured that the child will eventually walk and the prognosis is good, although clumsiness may become apparent and later skills such as running and cycling may be delayed. If there is delay in other developmental areas, more general learning disability should be suspected.

Delayed walking may be the presenting feature of the milder forms of *cerebral palsy*: hemiplegia and spastic diplegia. In more severe cerebral palsy, concerns about developmental progress are likely to have been aroused long before the child is expected to walk. The prognosis depends on the degree of spasticity, but most children with hemiplegia or diplegia eventually learn to walk, although the gait is not normal.

### History – must ask!

Your history should follow the pattern outlined for the presentation of any developmental problem (see p. 226). Make a clear assessment of all four developmental areas. A careful history of motor skills should include the baby's ability to sit supported or unsupported, roll over from both front and back, get to the sitting position independently, crawl, pull to stand and cruise.

A family history of late walking is important as this provides support for the benign diagnosis of maturational delay. It is also important to identify environmental factors such as deprivation or lack of opportunity to exercise gross motor skills.

### Physical examination – must check!

Your physical examination should confirm the developmental history, and identify any abnormal neuromuscular signs. Attempt to assess the child's developmental skills well to clarify whether the delay is generalized or isolated to gross motor skills. A great deal of information can be obtained by placing the child on the floor with some toys in easy reach, while you take the history. You can then observe the child in natural activity, before doing a more formal evaluation.

Your neurological examination should be thorough. Look for abnormalities in tone, deep tendon reflexes, strength, asymmetry of movements and the presence of primitive reflexes.

### Investigations

If the delay in walking is isolated and the child in other respects has normal development, the only investigation required is a creatinine phosphokinase level (CPK or CK) as late walking may be the earliest manifestation of muscular dystrophy (see later).

If you find signs of cerebral palsy or hypotonia, investigations may be required.

---

**⚷ Key points: Delayed walking**

- Determine whether the delay is isolated to gross motor skills or whether there is a more global developmental problem
- Identify any abnormal neurological findings
- Identify any responsible aetiological factors

---

**🔍 Clues to the diagnosis of the child with delayed walking**

| | History | Other developmental milestones | General physical examination | Neurological signs |
|---|---|---|---|---|
| Delayed motor maturation | Family history of delayed walking | Normal | Normal | Normal (or mildly decreased tone) |
| Severe learning disabilities (mental retardation) | | Delayed, usually to a greater degree than gross motor | Dysmorphic features, microcephaly etc. may be found | Normal (or decreased tone) |
| Environmental factors | Lack of opportunity | May be delayed | Normal | Normal |
| Hypertonia– cerebral palsy | | Often delayed | | Increased tone and tendon reflexes in affected limb |
| Muscular dystrophy | Other family members affected | Normal | Later on, large but weak calf muscles | Later on, weakness of the hip girdle muscles |

# Global developmental delay

**Causes of global developmental delay**

| Cause | Example |
|---|---|
| Chromosomal abnormalities | Down's syndrome |
| | Fragile X |
| | |
| Dysmorphic syndromes | |
| Injury | Fetal alcohol syndrome |
| Prenatal | TORCH infection (see p. 407) |
| Perinatal | Hypoxic–ischaemic insult |
| Postnatal | Meningitis |
| | Non-accidental injury |
| | Neglect |
| Central nervous malformations | Neural tube defects |
| | Hydrocephalus |
| Endocrine and metabolic defects | Hypothyroidism |
| Neurodegenerative disorders | |
| Neurocutaneous syndromes | |
| Idiopathic | |

The term *global developmental delay* refers to a delay in acquiring all developmental milestones, but particularly language, fine motor and social skills. It is extremely worrying when this occurs as it usually indicates learning disabilities (mental retardation). Gross motor skills may also be delayed, though they do not reflect intellectual capacity in the same way as the other skills, and are sometimes spared.

The purpose of the clinical evaluation is first of all to ascertain whether the child truly has global developmental delay, and to what extent each area is affected. The next stage is to attempt to seek an underlying cause and consider whether investigations are likely to be helpful.

In about one third of children with global developmental delay, no specific cause is identified, although advances in genetics mean this is changing. *Down's syndrome* (not usually a diagnostic challenge) and *fetal alcohol syndrome* are important causes. Some *inborn errors of metabolism* present with developmental delay, as can *neurodegenerative conditions* – the latter characterized by relentless neurological deterioration. Congenital *hypothyroidism*, once a serious cause, is no longer seen since the introduction of neonatal screening. *Intrauterine infections* such as rubella, cytomegalovirus (CMV) and toxoplasmosis infection cause severe fetal damage and can present with global developmental delay.

*Emotional abuse and neglect* can have serious consequences for a child's developmental progress. The developmental delay is often associated with failure to thrive (see pp. 257, 266) and the child may be apathetic, with evidence of physical neglect or injury.

## History – must ask!

The guidelines given in the previous section (p. 226) are particularly relevant to the child with overall developmental delay. The history needs to cover the following structure.

- *What are the child's current skills?* Obtain a detailed history of the child's current abilities in all four areas. Ask the parents if they have any concerns about the child's hearing or vision.
- *When did the child achieve earlier milestones?* It is important to identify whether development was initially appropriate or whether there were concerns early on. Developmental difficulties may have followed trauma or an illness.

- *Has there been regression in skills?* Children with learning disabilities tend to have a slow but steady acquisition of skills. Regression of skills suggests a neurodegenerative disorder.
- *Past medical history.* A detailed perinatal history is particularly important. Ask about alcohol consumption, medications, prematurity and neonatal complications. The links between developmental difficulties and postnatal events such as meningitis or head trauma are usually obvious.
- *Family history.* A family history of learning disabilities or consanguinity is important as it suggests a possible genetic cause for the problem.

### Physical examination – must check!

Your physical assessment must include a detailed developmental evaluation, followed by a complete physical examination focusing on neurological findings. Assess all four developmental areas. This is described in detail on pp. 84–9. In addition, focus on the following:

- *Growth.* Many children with developmental problems are short. If actual fall-off in growth has occurred, you should consider hypothyroidism and non-organic failure to thrive.
- *Microcephaly.* Microcephaly is a common, often non-specific finding, but if present at birth it suggests intrauterine infections, fetal alcohol syndrome or a genetic disorder. If it develops in the first year of life in association with developmental delay, a neurodegenerative disorder or perinatal cause should be suspected.
- *Dysmorphic signs.* Not uncommonly global developmental delay is associated with congenital anomalies and dysmorphic features. If present they suggestive a genetic defect, chromosomal anomaly or teratogenic effect.
- *General appearance.* Signs of neglect such as an undernourished appearance, skin and hair in poor condition, uncleanliness and irritative rashes in the skinfolds may indicate psychosocial factors responsible for the delay.
- *Skin.* Examine the skin for signs such as café-au-lait spots, depigmented patches and port-wine stains, which are indicative of neurocutaneous syndromes.
- *Hepatosplenomegaly.* The finding of an enlarged liver or spleen suggests a metabolic disorder.

### Neurological examination

Features of particular importance are the following.

- *Hypotonia.* This is often a non-specific finding. It occurs in Down's syndrome.
- *Signs of cerebral palsy* (see p. 237). Cerebral palsy affects motor skills but learning disabilities also commonly occur.
- *Hearing and vision.*
- *Ocular abnormalities.* The finding of ocular abnormalities such as cataracts suggests the presence of a metabolic disorder.

### Investigations

Chromosomal analysis and thyroid function tests should be performed in every child with global developmental delay. More sophisticated investigation of metabolic function or brain imaging may be indicated in some.

### Management

Every attempt should be made to identify an underlying cause for the delay. Although there is rarely specific treatment, parents are helped by being given a diagnosis, and there may be genetic implications for subsequent pregnancies.

The term 'developmental delay' is sometimes used euphemistically as a diagnosis in itself. This is inappropriate. A child should be described as being delayed only up to the point when the diagnosis of learning disabilities becomes clear (usually well before the age of 3 years). The management of the child with global developmental delay is covered in detail in the section on learning disabilities (see p. 242).

---

**Key points: Global developmental delay**

- Correct for prematurity if the child is less than 2 years old
- Confirm that the delay is global
- Assess the extent of the delay in each area
- Determine if there is regression of skills
- Attempt to identify a cause for the delay by examination and investigations
- Refer for a child development team assessment

## Clues to the diagnosis of a child with global developmental delay

| Condition | History | Physical examination | Other features |
|---|---|---|---|
| Down's syndrome | Older maternal age is common | Characteristic facial features, single palmar crease, Brushfield spots, hypotonia | Congenital heart disease, anal/duodenal atresia, growth should be followed on Down's charts |
| Fragile X | Other boys in the family affected | Long face, prominent ears, large jaw, large testes at puberty | Fits, behaviour problems |
| Fetal alcohol syndrome | Possible history of alcohol in pregnancy, intrauterine growth retardation (IUGR) | Short palpebral fissures, maxillary hypoplasia, thin upper lip, microcephaly | Cardiac defects, minor joint and limb abnormalities |
| Dysmorphic syndromes | | Dysmorphic features, +/− congenital anomalies | Poor growth common |
| Abuse and neglect | Family possibly known to social services | Possible signs of neglect or old injuries | Failure to thrive common |
| Inborn errors of metabolism | Consanguinity, neonatal seizures, hypoglycaemia, vomiting, coma | Sometimes coarse features, hepatosplenomegaly, microcephaly, failure to thrive | Developmental regression may occur |
| Congenital hypothyroidism | | May have features of cretinism Plateauing of growth | |
| Neurodegenerative disorders* | Developmental regression | May have coarse features, microcephaly develops | Fits, visual and intellectual deterioration |
| Idiopathic learning difficulties | | Mild dysmorphic features common | |
| Intrauterine infections* | Possible history of contact in pregnancy, IUGR | Visual or hearing deficits common, microcephaly | |
| Neurocutaneous syndromes | Often familial | Characteristic skin lesions | |

*Features vary according to the type of disorder.

# Developmental conditions and disabilities

## Autism

Autism is a condition where there is an inability to relate to others. The symptoms relate to impairment in social interaction, impairment in communication, and restricted interests and repetitive behaviour. Other aspects, such as atypical eating, are also common. There is a spectrum of difficulty, ranging from severe learning disability, where language development is very delayed, to children with normal intelligence (which is also called Asperger's syndrome). Autism has a strong genetic basis, although the genetics of autism are complex

**Clinical features.** Characteristically the child fails to develop social relationships. This may be noticed at a very young age when the baby is not as 'cuddly' as expected, although in others it appears to develop as toddlers. There is very little communication, both verbal and non-verbal, and eye contact is avoided. Ritualistic, repetitive and obsessional behaviour is also characteristic.

**Management.** Autism is one of the hardest conditions for a family to cope with. Children at the severe end of the spectrum have very difficult behaviour and can only attend special school. Others who are of normal intelligence cope educationally in mainstream school but have problems making friends and joining in socially. Input is usually provided by both a speech therapist and psychologist.

**Prognosis.** Children at the severe end of the spectrum need lifelong support and can never achieve independence. Children with autistic spectrum tendencies are less likely to marry and be full members of society.

## Attention deficit disorder

Attention deficit disorder (ADD or ADHD) refers to a difficulty in generally focusing on tasks or activities. Inattention, hyperactivity and impulsivity are the key behaviours, although the diagnosis is also made if hyperactivity (see p. 359) is not a feature. The condition is far commoner in boys than girls.

**Clinical features.** The child is fidgety, has a difficult time remaining in his or her seat at school, is easily distracted and impulsive, has difficulty following instructions, talks excessively and flits from one activity to another. Daydreaming is more obvious if hyperactivity is not a feature. There is often a history of being colicky, temperamentally difficult babies.

**Management.** The child benefits from a regular daily routine with simple clear rules, and firm limits enforced fairly and sympathetically. Overstimulation and overfatigue should be avoided. In school a structured programme is required, with good home communication to ensure consistency.

Attention deficit problems, particularly if associated with hyperactivity, can be very stressful to the family and counselling may be needed. Central nervous system stimulants such as methylphenidate, prescribed during school hours, have been shown to be helpful in selected cases. Therapies such as megavitamins and low-sugar diets have not been proved to be effective. Diets with no artificial colourings or flavourings remain controversial, but in general do not help the majority of these children.

**Prognosis.** Both the hyperactivity and attention difficulties tend to improve through adolescence, but the educational deficit may persist as a handicap later in life.

## Cerebral palsy

Cerebral palsy is a disorder of movement and posture caused by an early permanent and non-progressive cerebral lesion. Fifty per cent of children with cerebral palsy also have a combination of epilepsy, hearing and vision problems, learning or feeding difficulties. Cerebral palsy affects two to three per 1000 children and is the commonest cause of physical disability in childhood.

### Aetiology/pathology (Table 12.3)

Although the brain lesion itself in cerebral palsy is non-progressive, the clinical picture changes as the child grows and develops. The underlying brain lesion may result from different insults occurring at various

| **Table 12.3** Causes of cerebral palsy |
| --- |
| *Prenatal* |
| Cerebral malformations |
| Congenital infection (p. 233) |
| Metabolic defects |
| *Perinatal* |
| Complications of prematurity |
| Intrapartum trauma |
| Hypoxic–ischaemic insult* (p. 403) |
| *Postnatal* (if incurred before 18 months of age) |
| Non-accidental injury |
| Head trauma |
| Meningitis/encephalitis |
| Cardiopulmonary arrest |

\* In term babies this is an uncommon cause. Cerebral palsy should not be attributed to these insults unless they were severe and followed by neurological problems in the neonatal period.

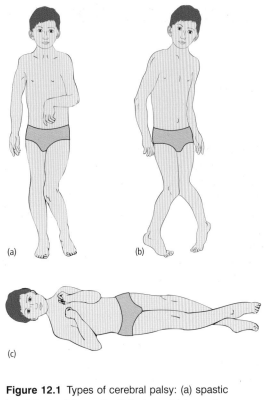

**Figure 12.1** Types of cerebral palsy: (a) spastic hemiplegia, (b) spastic diplegia and (c) spastic quadriplegia.

times in the developing brain. The clinical picture resulting from these insults varies depending on the area of the brain involved.

*Spastic cerebral palsy* is the commonest form and results from damage to the cerebral motor cortex or its connections. *Dystonic (athetoid) cerebral palsy* results from damage to the basal ganglia and is characterized by irregular and involuntary movements which may be continuous or occur on voluntary movement. *Ataxic cerebral palsy* is rare and results from damage to the cerebellum. It is characterized by hypotonia, incoordination and intention tremor.

### Clinical features of spastic cerebral palsy

Spastic cerebral palsy is classified according to the extremities affected (Figure 12.1). Clasp-knife hypertonia, brisk deep tendon reflexes, ankle clonus, and a Babinski response (extensor plantar) are found in the affected limbs.

### Spastic hemiplegia

In spastic hemiplegia (Figures 12.1a, 12.2), only one side of the body is affected, and the arm is often more involved than the leg. During infancy there are decreased spontaneous movements on the affected side. Walking is usually delayed until 18–24 months, and when it develops there is a characteristic gait. The child often walks on tiptoes because of the increased tone, and the affected arm is held in a dystonic posture when running.

### Spastic diplegia

Spastic diplegia (Figure 12.1b) is the commonest type of cerebral palsy seen in survivors of severe prematurity. Both legs are involved, and the arms are less affected, if at all. The first indication of a problem often occurs when the baby starts to crawl and the legs tend to drag behind. There is excessive adduction of the hips and the parents may find difficulty in putting on a nappy. When the baby is suspended under the arms, the legs take up a scissoring posture. Walking is delayed, and the gait is characteristic. The feet are held in the equinovarus position and the child walks on tiptoes.

### Spastic quadriplegia

Spastic quadriplegia (Figure 12.1c) is the most severe form of cerebral palsy because of marked motor

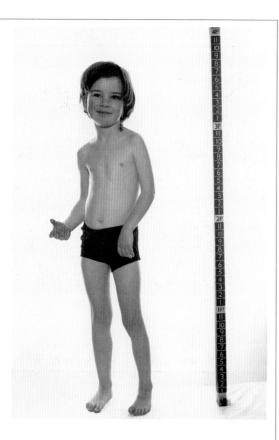

**Figure 12.2** A child with left hemiplegia. Note the flexed posture of the arm and circumduction of the leg.

impairment of all extremities and the high association with severe learning disabilities and fits. Swallowing difficulties and gastro-oesophageal reflux are also common and often lead to aspiration pneumonia. Microcephaly is common, and flexion contractures of the knees and elbows are often present by late childhood. Associated disabilities, especially speech and visual problems, are particularly prevalent.

### Associated problems

Children with cerebral palsy commonly have additional problems, especially if they have the quadriplegic or severe hemiplegic form of the condition. These problems include the following:

- learning difficulties;
- epilepsy;
- visual impairment;
- squint;
- hearing loss;

- speech disorders;
- behaviour disorders;
- feeding difficulties;
- undernutrition and poor growth;
- respiratory problems.

### How cerebral palsy presents and the diagnosis is made

Follow-up of babies who have suffered a cerebral insult perinatally is the commonest way in which cerebral palsy is diagnosed; others may be detected through child health surveillance. In the neonatal period the diagnosis may be suspected if a baby has difficulty sucking, irritability, convulsions or an abnormal neurological examination. However, many of these infants subsequently develop normally, so it is important that cerebral palsy is not mistakenly diagnosed too early.

The diagnosis is usually made late in the first year of life when the following features emerge:

- *Abnormalities of tone.* Initially the tone may be quite reduced, but eventually spasticity develops.
- *Delays in motor development.* Marked head lag and delays in sitting and rolling over are usually found.
- *Abnormal patterns of development.* Movements are not only delayed but also abnormal in quality.
- *Persistence of primitive reflexes.* Primitive reflexes such as the Moro, grasp and asymmetric tonic neck reflex (see p. 78) persist beyond the age at which they normally disappear.

The diagnosis is made on clinical grounds. As the clinical picture takes time to evolve, repeated examinations are often required to establish the diagnosis. Once made, a multidisciplinary assessment is needed to define the extent of the difficulties.

### Investigations

The aetiology of the cerebral palsy is often evident from the history. Rarely, further investigation is required to rule out progressive disorders. Computed tomography (CT) or magnetic resonance imaging (MRI) scans may be useful in demonstrating cerebral malformations, delineating the extent of structural lesions and ruling out very rare progressive or treatable causes such as tumours.

### *Management of cerebral palsy (see Box 12.1)*

The goals of managing cerebral palsy fall into two categories: those specific to cerebral palsy, and those

> **Box 12.1 Managing the child with cerebral palsy**
>
> • Aim to minimize the effects of spasticity and development of contractures
> • Identify and manage any associated problems
> • Ensure the child is provided with appropriate support for their special educational needs
> • Ensure the family has adequate support: financial, practical and emotional
> • Try to maximize the child's integration into society

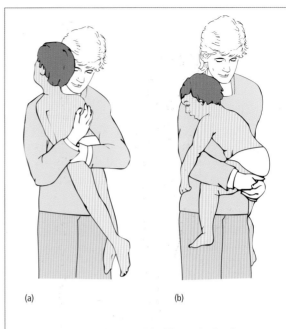

(a)                    (b)

**Figure 12.3** Holding a child with cerebral palsy. (a) Incorrect technique. (b) Correct technique.

related to any child with a disability. As regards cerebral palsy itself, the effects of spasticity and the development of contractures must be minimized by regular physiotherapy. Providing the child with aids may help them to be independently mobile. The associated problems that commonly occur in cerebral palsy must be actively sought and management provided.

As for any child with a disability, appropriate schooling and educational resources must be provided to meet any special educational needs. One must ensure that the family are provided with adequate financial, practical and emotional support, and the child must be helped to integrate as much as possible into society.

## Practical aspects of management

Most children with cerebral palsy have multiple difficulties and require a multidisciplinary input. This is best provided by a child development team, in order to ensure good liaison between professionals and parents, and to structure a coordinated programme of treatment to meet all the child's needs.

### Physiotherapy

The role of the physiotherapist is crucial in the management of the child with cerebral palsy. It is the physiotherapist who advises on handling and mobilization (Figure 12.3). The family must be taught how to handle the child in daily activities such as feeding, carrying, dressing and bathing in ways that will limit the effects of abnormal muscle tone. They are also taught a series of exercises designed to prevent the development of deforming contractures. The physiotherapist may also provide a variety of aids, such as firm boots, lightweight splints and walking frames for the child who is beginning to walk.

### Occupational therapy

The occupational therapist's role overlaps with the physiotherapist. The occupational therapist is trained to advise on special equipment such as wheelchairs and seating, and also on play materials and activities that best encourage the child's hand function.

### Speech therapy

The speech and language therapist is involved in advising on feeding and language. In the early months advice may be required for feeding and swallowing difficulties. Later, a thorough assessment of the child's developing speech and language is often required and help given on all aspects of communication, including non-verbal systems when necessary.

### Medication

Drugs, other than anticonvulsants for epilepsy, have a limited role in cerebral palsy. If spasticity is severe and causing pain, a drug to reduce muscle spasm (baclofen) is sometimes prescribed.

### Orthopaedic surgery

Even with adequate physiotherapy, orthopaedic deformities may develop as a result of long-standing muscle weakness or spasticity. Dislocation of the hips

## Cerebral palsy at a glance

### Definition
Cerebral palsy is a disorder of movement caused by a permanent, non-progressive lesion in the developing brain

### Epidemiology
2–3 per 1000 children

### Aetiology/pathophysiology
Cerebral palsy is caused by pre-, peri- or postnatal insults to the brain. Types include spastic (commonest), dystonic and ataxic cerebral palsy

### Clinical features of spastic cerebral palsy
Hemiplegic, diplegic and quadriplegic forms occur
Neurological signs in affected limbs
- clasp-knife hypertonia (**a**)
- brisk deep tendon reflexes (**b**)
- ankle clonus (**c**)
- Babinski response (extensor plantar) (**d**)

### How the diagnosis is made
The diagnosis is clinical, based on findings of abnormalities of tone, delays in motor development, abnormal movement patterns and persistent primitive reflexes. Diagnosis may be suspected in neonates, but can only be made months later

### Common associated problems
Gastro-oesophageal reflux
Learning disability (mild or severe)
Epilepsy
Visual impairment
Hearing impairment

### Management
- Multidisciplinary assessment and management
- Phsyiotherapy is essential
- Occupational and speech therapy
- Special equipment needs must be met
- Drugs and surgery have a limited place
- Support for the family involving voluntary agencies and social services
- Special educational needs – in mainstream school, if physical access and resources for learning difficulties are adequate. Otherwise, special school for the physically or learning disabled

### Points for routine follow-up
Monitor:
- developmental progress
- medical problems
- development of contractures or dislocation
- behavioural difficulties
- nutritional status
Each child needs a structured programme addressing all needs
Liaison between professionals is important

### Prognosis
Depends on degree and type of cerebral palsy, level of learning disability and presence of other associated problems
Degree of independent living achieved relates to:
- type and extent of cerebral palsy
- degree of learning disability
- presence of associated problems, e.g. visual impairment, epilepsy

may occur as a result of spasticity in the thigh adductors, and fixed equinus deformity of the ankle as a result of calf muscle spasticity. Both of these may require orthopaedic surgery.

### Nutrition

Undernutrition commonly occurs in children with cerebral palsy, and can reduce the chances of achieving physical and intellectual potential. Food must be given in a form appropriate to the child's ability to chew and swallow. Energy-rich supplements and medical treatment for reflux, if present, may be needed. If the child is unable to eat adequate amounts, a gastrostomy may need to be placed.

## Issues for the family

The family has to cope with all the difficulties facing any family with a child with disabilities (p. 45). However, cerebral palsy, if severe, places particularly heavy demands on the family in terms of time and input. Everyday tasks such as dressing and bathing take time, and feeding, in particular, may take hours each day. The child also needs regular physiotherapy at home, and needs to attend for appointments, both for medical follow-up and therapy. In view of this, the family is in need of support, which often goes beyond what family and friends can supply. It is important that they are aware of the support offered by voluntary and social service agencies in terms of babysitting, respite care and benefits.

Very rarely cerebral palsy has a genetic basis. In most cases parents need reassurance that the chance of recurrence is not substantially greater than that for the general population.

## Issues for the school

An important aspect of the child's multidisciplinary assessment is advice about schooling. Children with milder forms of cerebral palsy can cope at mainstream school, provided minor learning difficulties and physical access are addressed. Children with more severe cerebral palsy will need special schooling either in a school for children with physical disabilities, or one for children with severe learning disabilities, depending on the degree of their difficulties.

# Duchenne muscular dystrophy

Duchenne muscular dystrophy is the commonest hereditary neuromuscular disease. It is a progressive

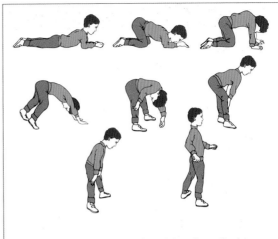

**Figure 12.4** Gower's sign: from lying down the boy uses his hands to 'climb up' his legs.

disorder resulting in death in the early twenties. It is inherited as an X-linked recessive trait.

**Clinical features.** Baby boys are normal at birth, and delayed walking is usually only identified retrospectively. Symptoms appear between the ages of 4 and 6 years and are progressive. They consist of frequent falls, a lordotic waddling gait and difficulty climbing stairs. On examination the child has enlarged but weak calf muscles. The Gower sign is characteristic (Figure 12.4); on rising from a lying position the boy uses his hands to 'climb up' his legs to get to an upright posture. On investigation the creatine kinase level is elevated by at least 10 times the normal level.

**Management.** The child needs physiotherapy, support and help through school. Genetic counselling is extremely important for the family as 50% of sons will be affected. Early detection by finding an elevated CPK level in boys late in starting to walk allows the family to plan future pregnancies, as prenatal diagnosis is now possible.

**Prognosis.** Most of these boys are unable to walk by the age of 8–11 years and become confined to a wheelchair. Chest muscles are also affected. Respiratory insufficiency can be improved by oral steroids or overnight non-invasive breathing support. Life expectancy is improving, but remains poor, with death precipitated by respiratory infections by the mid twenties and early thirties.

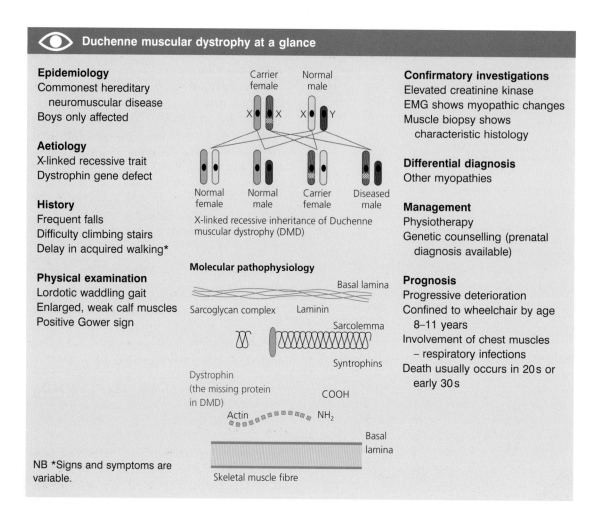

**Duchenne muscular dystrophy at a glance**

**Epidemiology**
Commonest hereditary
   neuromuscular disease
Boys only affected

**Aetiology**
X-linked recessive trait
Dystrophin gene defect

**History**
Frequent falls
Difficulty climbing stairs
Delay in acquired walking*

**Physical examination**
Lordotic waddling gait
Enlarged, weak calf muscles
Positive Gower sign

Carrier female    Normal male

X-linked recessive inheritance of Duchenne muscular dystrophy (DMD)

Normal female    Normal male    Carrier female    Diseased male

**Molecular pathophysiology**

Basal lamina
Sarcoglycan complex    Laminin
Sarcolemma
Syntrophins
Dystrophin
(the missing protein
in DMD)                COOH
Actin           NH₂
Basal lamina
Skeletal muscle fibre

**Confirmatory investigations**
Elevated creatinine kinase
EMG shows myopathic changes
Muscle biopsy shows
   characteristic histology

**Differential diagnosis**
Other myopathies

**Management**
Physiotherapy
Genetic counselling (prenatal
   diagnosis available)

**Prognosis**
Progressive deterioration
Confined to wheelchair by age
   8–11 years
Involvement of chest muscles
   – respiratory infections
Death usually occurs in 20s or
   early 30s

NB *Signs and symptoms are variable.

# Learning disability

The term 'learning disabilities' (or 'difficulties') has replaced the terms 'mental retardation' and 'mental handicap'. Various degrees of learning difficulties occur and are classified into mild, moderate and severe according to intellectual limitations and the degree of independence anticipated or achieved. Individuals with *severe learning difficulties* can learn minimal self care and simple conversation skills, and need much supervision throughout their lives. Those with *profound learning disability* require total supervision, few become toilet trained and language development is generally minimal.

The prevalence of severe learning disability is about four children per 1000. Children with severe learning disabilities are spread throughout the social classes, and usually have an organic basis for their problem. This contrasts with children with milder learning disabilities, where mostly no organic cause is

found and where there is a predominance of children from lower socioeconomic classes.

## Aetiology/pathophysiology

In about one quarter of children with significant learning disability, no specific cause is identified. However, this picture is changing as a result of advances in the field of genetics. Diagnoses are now being made in children who in the past were thought to have idiopathic learning disabilities. Where significant congenital anomalies and dysmorphic features are found, the diagnostic process has been helped by the development of computerized databases.

Chromosome disorders (predominantly Down's syndrome and fragile X) are the commonest cause of severe learning disabilities. (see Table 12.4). *Fragile X* is important as a genetic cause in boys. The chromosomal anomaly consists of a 'fragile site' at the end of one of the long arms of the X-chromosome. The diag-

**Table 12.4** Causes of severe learning disability

| | |
|---|---|
| Chromosome disorders | 30% |
| Other identifiable syndromes | 20% |
| Cerebral palsy, infantile spasms, post-meningitis | 20% |
| Metabolic or degenerative diseases | <1% |
| Idiopathic | 25% |

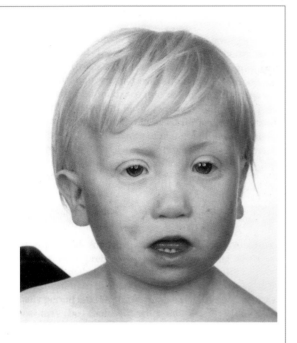

**Figure 12.5** A 3-year-old boy with fetal alcohol syndrome. Note the absent philtrum and short thin upper lip, saddle-shaped nose and maxillary hypoplasia.

tion with these agents occurs for the first time during pregnancy, severe fetal damage can result, leading to multiple disability.

Other causes include the *inborn errors of metabolism,* a group of disorders caused by single gene mutations, inherited in an autosomal recessive manner. They may present in a variety of ways, of which developmental delay is one. As individual conditions they are very rare. Phenylketonuria is the commonest and is routinely screened for in all neonates (p. 22).

*Neurodegenerative diseases* lead to progressive deterioration of neurological function. The causes are heterogeneous and include biochemical defects, chronic viral infections and toxic substances, although many remain of unknown aetiology. The course for all of these conditions is one of relentless and inevitable neurological deterioration.

*Emotional abuse and neglect* have serious consequences for a child's developmental progress. Developmental delay is often associated with failure to thrive (see pp. 254, 266), apathy and evidence of physical neglect. Learning disability can be a consequence even if the child is removed form the home,

### Clinical features

The term 'learning disability' implies reduced intellectual functioning. In early childhood this is seen as a delay in reaching developmental milestones, particularly those relating to language and social tasks. The progress achieved by any child is highly variable and depends on the underlying condition, any associated disabilities, as well as, to some extent, the educational and therapeutic input received. Other factors which affect progress are physical health, a healthy parent–child attachment and a cohesive family unit within a supportive social network.

Severe learning difficulties are often accompanied by problems that further limit the child's abilities. These include epilepsy, impairment of vision and hearing, communication deficits and attention deficit hyperactivity disorder. Feeding problems and failure to thrive may also be an issue.

### How severe learning disability presents

Babies with recognizable syndromes, such as Down's, are usually diagnosed at birth and the degree of their learning difficulties predicted with some confidence. However, the overwhelming majority of children with learning disabilities are identified later when they fail to meet their developmental milestones. Children with severe learning disabilities show marked delays

nosis should be sought in any boy who has unexplained moderate or severe learning disability. Some girls carrying the chromosome have mild learning disabilities.

*Fetal alcohol syndrome* (Figure 12.5) is another relatively common cause. It is caused by a moderate to high intake of alcohol during pregnancy, with the severity of the features related to the quantity of alcohol consumed. The clinical features are characterized by poor growth and microcephaly, a characteristic facial appearance and cardiac defects.

*Intrauterine infections* such as rubella, cytomegalovirus (CMV) and toxoplasmosis still occur. If infec-

---

**Box 12.2 Managing the child with severe learning disability**

- Diagnose the underlying condition where possible, and assess and manage associated problems
- Follow the child's developmental progress
- Provide good general paediatric care
- Ensure appropriate input is provided in the preschool years and that appropriate school placement is found
- Provide a supportive framework for the child and parents

---

in the first year, but children with less severe difficulties typically have normal motor development and present with delayed speech and language in the toddler years.

### Management of a child with severe learning disability (see Box 12.2)

Perhaps the major goal in the management of children with learning disabilities is to support and help the family in coming to terms with the diagnosis and their child's limitations. This is often easier when a specific diagnosis can be made, although that is not always possible. Associated problems need to be identified and the developmental progress of the child followed. Other aspects of management involve providing appropriate educational and therapeutic input throughout the paediatric years, and (it should go without saying) the child with learning disabilities is entitled to the same degree of general paediatric care as any other child.

Once the diagnosis of severe learning difficulties has been made, the most successful approach involves an interdisciplinary effort directed towards education, social activities, behaviour problems and any associated deficits.

#### Diagnosis of an underlying cause

Diagnosing an underlying cause is unlikely to affect the child's prognosis. However, it is of great importance to the family, allows for more accurate genetic counseling, and alerts one to the possibility of associated problems. The process of diagnosing severe learning disabilities is discussed in the section on the child presenting with global developmental delay (p. 233).

#### General paediatric care

The child with learning disabilities requires the same general paediatric care as any other child. This includes immunizations, following their growth and developmental parameters, maintaining dental hygiene and treating intercurrent illnesses.

#### Early intervention and educational programmes

It is important to begin an educational programme early to stimulate cognitive, language and motor development. In the preschool years this may take a number of directions. Therapists from the child development team provide advice to the family on play activities and suitable toys, give guidance in the development of simple skills such as feeding, washing and dressing, and instruct parents on the principles of language development, introducing alternative communication systems where appropriate. Planned programmes such as the Portage system, where a trained worker comes to the home on a regular basis, may also be available. Attendance at special nurseries, such as Mencap, can be stimulating for the child while providing contacts with other families in similar circumstances.

#### School

At the nursery and primary school level many children with learning disabilities can cope and benefit from placement in a mainstream school, with appropriate help provided. Other children, particularly if they have additional disabilities, may be better placed in a special educational setting. Children with learning disabilities require a Statement of Special Educational Needs (see p. 46) to ensure that their needs are met.

#### Behaviour management

Behaviour problems occur with greater frequency in children with developmental disabilities. In milder learning disabilities this may include attention difficulties or hyperactivity (see pp. 236, 359), and in children with severe disabilities, stereotypic or self-injurious behaviour. Psychological help in these circumstances is needed, and occasionally medication, too.

#### Routine review of a child with severe learning disability

The child with severe learning disabilities should have a routine paediatric review, even if perceived to be healthy. Developmental progress should be followed, particularly in the child without a specific diagnosis, as developmental regression suggests an unrecognized degenerative process. Some conditions such as Down's syndrome or congenital CMV infection require routine investigations or hearing tests, as these children are at higher risk for certain problems. Behavioural problems may need special attention. Liaison with other professionals is of great importance, and the family is likely to need on-going support.

## Issues for the family

The diagnosis of severe learning disabilities is devastating, and families require particularly sensitive support (see p. 47) at diagnosis and beyond. Each stage of the child's development brings its own issues. Adolescence is usually a particularly difficult time when issues related to sexuality, vocational training and community living must be addressed.

Genetic counselling is important, whether there is a clearly inherited disorder or not, as the family will want to know the chances of having another affected child. In children with no identified cause, the risks of another sibling being affected is approximately 1 in 25. However, if multiple congenital anomalies are also present the risk falls to 1 in 40.

---

### 👁 Learning disability at a glance

**Definition**
Learning disabilities are considered severe if minimal self-care and simple conversation at most are achievable, and supervision is needed in adult life

**Prevalence**
4 children per 1000

**Aetiology/pathophysiology**
Chromosome disorders: 30% (**a**)
Identifiable disorders or syndromes: 20% (**b**)
Associated with cerebral palsy, microcephaly, infantile spasms (**c**)
Postnatal cerebral insults: 20% (**d**)
Idiopathic: 25%

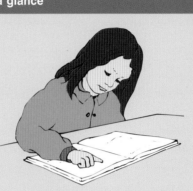

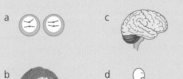

**Presentation and how the diagnosis is made**
Malformations at birth, or later when developmental delay is evident

**Clinical features**
• Reduced intellectual functioning
• Delay in reaching developmental milestones in early childhood, particularly language and social skills
• Dysmorphic features may be evident*

*Symptoms and signs are variable

**Associated problems**
Epilepsy
Vision and hearing deficits
Communication problems
Attention deficit/hyperactivity
Feeding problems and failure to thrive
Specific diagnoses may have own
Complications

**Management**
• Needs to be multidisciplinary
• Diagnosis of underlying cause (see Table 12.4) (parts)
• General paediatric care must not be neglected
• Early intervention and educational programmes to stimulate cognitive, language and motor development.
This may be by individual therapists, planned home programmes or nursery
• School – statementing required and placement in mainstream or special school
• Behaviour difficulties must be addressed
• Support and benefits (see p. 47)

**Points for routine follow-up**
Developmental progress and physical growth need review
Some conditions require screening for specific associated problems
Liaison with other professionals is important
The family needs support

**Prognosis**
Depends on underlying cause and degree of learning disability
Degree of independent living achieved relates to:
• level of learning disability
• underlying aetiology

## Issues for the school

Education for the child with severe learning disability must be realistic, and should include teaching skills such as personal care, hygiene and safety, development of acceptable social behaviour, and maximizing independence. On leaving school, various facilities should be available for the young adult with learning disabilities, including an adult training centre, special hostels, communities and vocational training schemes.

## Down's syndrome

Down's syndrome is the commonest congenital anomaly associated with global developmental delay. The underlying chromosomal abnormality is trisomy

of chromosome 21. The extra chromosome is usually of maternal origin, and the incidence of Down's syndrome increases with maternal age (2% at age 38 years).

**Clinical features.** The features of Down's syndrome are easily recognized – upward sloping palpable fissures, epicanthal folds, Brushfield spots (speckled iris), a protruding tongue, flat occiput, single palmar creases and mild to moderate developmental delay where social skills often exceed the other milestones (Figure 12.6). One third of babies with Down's syndrome are born with gastrointestinal problems, most commonly duodenal atresia, and one third have cardiac anomalies (most commonly atrioventricular

---

### 👁 Down's syndrome at a glance

**Epidemiology**
Commonest congenital anomaly associated with learning disability
Incidence (1 per 650 births) increases with maternal age

**Aetiology**
Trisomy of chromosome 21

**Antenatal diagnosis**
Triple test early in pregnancy, followed by nuchal skin fold thickness, then amniocentesis for those at high risk

**Clinical features**
Mild to moderate developmental delay
Upward sloping palpebral fissures
Epicanthal folds
Brushfield spots
Protruding tongue
Flat occiput
Single palmar creases
Hypotonia
Small stature

**Confirmatory investigations**
Chromosome analysis shows trisomy
21 with non-dysjunction, translocation or mosaicism

| Maternal age | Incidence |
| --- | --- |
| 20 | 1 in 1700 births |
| 40 | 1 in 100 births |
| 44 | 1 in 40 births |

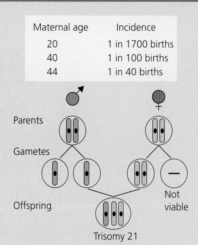

Trisomy 21

Genetics: extra chromosome 21
(Translocation between chromosome 14 and 21 is rarer)

**Differential diagnosis**
Facial features are usually clinically evident from birth

**Management**
Cardiac evaluation at birth
Referral to ophthalmology if squint is present
Routine audiological and thyroid tests
Genetic counselling for family
Arranging for special educational needs

**Complications**
Cardiac anomalies
Duodenal atresia
Secretory otitis media
Strabismus
Hypothyroidism
Atlantoaxial instability
Leukaemia

**Prognosis**
Individuals have varying degrees of learning disability
Children can usually be integrated into mainstream primary school
At risk from Alzheimer's disease in adult life

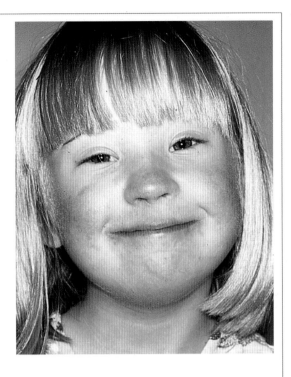

**Figure 12.6** A 5-year-old girl with Down's syndrome.

| Table 12.5 Children at risk for hearing impairment |
| --- |
| Severe prematurity |
| History of meningitis |
| History of recurrent otitis media |
| Significantly delayed or unclear speech |
| Family history of deafness |
| Parental suspicion of deafness |
| Children with cerebral palsy |
| Children with cleft palate |
| Children with absent or deformed ears |

function and skin lesions. In some individuals there may be severe learning disabilities and in others intelligence is normal. Examples of neurocutaneous syndromes include Sturge–Weber syndrome, neurofibromatosis and tuberous sclerosis. The aetiology of these problems is not known, but most are familial.

## Hearing impairment

About 4% of school children have a hearing loss. Most of these are mild, usually resulting from secretory otitis media (p. 120). Two per 1000 children have moderate deafness and require a hearing aid, and a further one per 1000 is severely deaf requiring special education. Some children are at a higher risk for hearing impairment, as shown in Table 12.5.

### Aetiology/pathophysiology (Table 12.6)

Conductive deafness is an extremely common problem in childhood. It results from persistent effusions in the middle ear (a complication of otitis media (see p. 120), and is known as chronic secretory otitis media or glue ear. Sensorineural deafness occurs as a result of damage to the cochlear or auditory nerve. It is rarer, but a cause of more significant disability.

### Presentation and diagnosis

Babies with neurosensory deafness are now being identified in many areas through the introduction of newborn hearing screening. Children may also present when parents become concerned that their child is not responding to sound, or if the child's speech and language development is delayed. If the hearing loss

canal defects). Secretory otitis media, strabismus, hypothyroidism, atlantoaxial instability and leukaemia occur more commonly than in normal children.

**Management.** The medical management of Down's syndrome demands a routine cardiac evaluation at birth. In view of the incidence of hypothyroidism and hearing difficulties, routine audiological and thyroid tests are needed throughout childhood and ophthalmological assessment if there is any evidence of a squint. The child's growth needs to be followed on special Down's growth charts. The family requires genetic counselling.

**Prognosis.** Children with Down's syndrome have varying degrees of learning disability. They can usually be integrated into a mainstream primary school with extra provision made for their educational needs. Individuals with Down's syndrome are at risk for early-onset Alzheimer's disease.

## Neurocutaneous syndromes

The neurocutaneous syndromes are a heterogeneous group of disorders characterized by neurological dys-

**Table 12.6** Causes of deafness in school children

| |
|---|
| *Conductive deafness* |
| Almost all cases due to glue ear following otitis media |
| *Sensorineural deafness* |
| Damage to the cochlear or auditory nerve |
| *Genetic* |
| Various types 50% |
| *Intrauterine* |
| Congenital infection, e.g. rubella, cytomegalovirus (CMV) |
| *Perinatal* (12%) |
| Birth asphyxia |
| Severe hyperbilirubinaemia |
| *Postnatal* (30%) |
| Meningitis |
| Encephalitis |
| Head Injury |

**Box 12.3 Managing the child with hearing loss**

*Conductive hearing loss*
• Correct by placing grommets

*Sensorineural hearing loss*
• Ensure the child has a means of communication
• This may involve sign language
• Maximize hearing by use of a hearing aid
• Ensure schooling is appropriate and that support is provided

is secondary to secretory otitis media, the tympanic membranes look dull and may be retracted.

The hearing deficit is confirmed by audiological testing (see p. 24). If a child is unable to cooperate, or if an objective test is required, brain stem evoked responses (BSER), an electrophysiological measure, is carried out.

### Clinical features

The clinical features vary with the severity of the hearing deficit and the age at which it presents. If it is congenital, the child is delayed in talking. If the onset is later, the child may present with behavioural difficulties which may not be immediately identified as a result of lack of hearing. Deafness is particularly common in certain medical conditions such as cerebral palsy.

Chronic secretory otitis media may be characterized by fluctuating hearing loss, as the middle ear fluid may resolve only to return with each upper respiratory tract infection (URTI).

Hearing deficits frequently occur in association with learning disabilities, visual deficits and neurological disorders.

### Managing the hearing impaired child (see Box 12.3)

If the hearing deficit is secondary to secretory otitis media, the management is surgical (see below). Neurosensory loss is only rarely correctable surgically, and the most important aspect of management therefore is to promote the child's ability to communicate from an early age. If the hearing deficit is significant this will usually require sign language, which is used in conjunction with oral speech.

Deafness is an enormous social barrier, and an important part of management must be to encourage the child to participate fully in school and society at large.

### Conductive hearing loss

Medical treatment in the form of decongestants and antihistamines are ineffectual in the management of middle ear effusion. If the effusion is causing persistent hearing loss, surgical intervention is required. Tiny plastic tubes (grommets) are inserted into the tympanic membrane to aerate the middle ear and drain the fluid. Adenoidectomy may be performed at the same time. When grommets are in place, the child must take care not to allow water to enter the ear canal at bath time or when swimming. The grommets usually eventually fall out spontaneously. They may not need to be replaced as the condition resolves as the child grows.

### Sensorineural deafness
#### Hearing aids

A hearing aid is a device which amplifies sound. It may be worn behind the ear (Figure 12.7) or in a pocket or harness. Some aids have special features such as amplification of low or high frequencies and

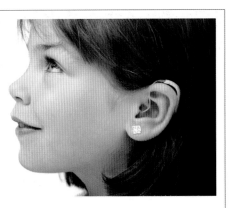

**Figure 12.7** A 10-year-old girl with neurosensory deafness wearing bilateral hearing aids.

circuits to reduce intense peaks of noise. Most aids can be used with the 'loop' wiring system which transmits the teacher's voice, bypassing background noise. Selection of the most suitable aid is made by a paediatric audiologist, who also teaches the family about its management and maintenance.

## Communication

In the past there has been some controversy over teaching sign language on the basis that children must learn to live in a hearing world. However, it is now generally accepted that providing an alternative non-verbal means of communication increases a child's ability to relate to others, reduces the isolation and frustration of being unable to hear, and even encourages language development. Sign language is taught in conjunction with oral speech. Lip-reading is also valuable, and electronic analysers are a new development which can help the child to speak more clearly by converting voice patterns to visual displays.

## Education

The peripatetic teacher of the deaf, who is employed by the local education authority, is responsible for the child's early education and management, and later in advising on school placement.

### Issues for the family

If the hearing deficit is sensorineural, the parents need to learn how to communicate with their deaf child

## Hearing impairment at a glance

**Prevalence**
4% of children have hearing deficits
3 per 1000 are moderately or severely impaired

**Aetiology/pathophysiology**
Most mild to moderate hearing loss is conductive and a result of secretory otitis media
Sensorineural deafness may be genetic, a result of pre- or perinatal problems, or follow a cerebral insult later in life

**Clinical features**
Lack of response to speech
Delayed speech
Behavioural problems

**Associated problems**
Learning difficulties
Neurological disorders
Visual deficits

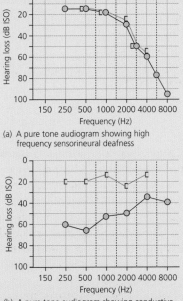

(a) A pure tone audiogram showing high frequency sensorineural deafness

(b) A pure tone audiogram showing conductive deafness. The bone conduction is normal but the air conductive curve is impaired. There is 20–30 dB hearing loss

**Presentation and how the diagnosis is made**
Child health surveillance
Parental concern

**Practical aspects of management**
Grommets for conductive hearing loss
Hearing aids
Communication
Education

**Issues for the family**
Communication with child may involve learning sign language
Genetic counselling

**Issues for the school**
Moderately deaf children can attend a normal school
The severely deaf require specialist education at a school for the deaf or a partially hearing unit attached to a normal school

and promote the child's communication skills. Some causes of deafness are genetic and in these circumstances genetic counselling is required.

### Issues for the school

Many moderately deaf children can attend a normal school. The child is helped by sitting near to the teacher in order to maximize concentration. The 'loop' wiring system is a valuable development. More severely affected children require specialist education either at a school for the deaf or at a partially hearing unit attached to a mainstream school.

## The blind or partially sighted child

Blindness and partial sight are best defined functionally rather than by the degree of visual acuity. A child is defined as blind if he or she requires education by methods which cannot involve sight. If the child is of adequate intelligence this will include Braille. A child is defined as partially sighted if he or she requires special education but can use methods which depend on sight, such as large-print books. In practice, most blind children have some vision even if it is only recognition of light and dark. One in 2500 children is registered blind or partially sighted. Fifty per cent have additional handicaps.

### Aetiology/pathophysiology

The commonest causes of blindness are optic atrophy, congenital cataracts, and choroidoretinal degeneration. In almost half of cases the cause is genetically determined, and in one third it is related to perinatal problems such as retinopathy of prematurity (see p. 432).

### Clinical features

The eyes may be obviously abnormal in appearance, and nystagmus or roving, purposeless eye movements may be present. Babies who have a visual deficit from birth follow an altered pattern of development. Smiling tends to occur at the usual age, but is less consistent and reliable and, as the baby develops, his or her response to sound is unaccompanied by turning towards the source. Motor skills, both gross and fine are likely to be delayed. Hand regard is poor, and reaching for objects and the development of a fine pincer grip is slow. Early language development may be normal, but the acquisition of vocabulary and more complex language may be delayed.

The child with visual deficits frequently develops mannerisms such as eye poking, eye rubbing and rocking. These are known as 'blindisms' and probably occur as they induce pleasurable visual gratification of retinal origin. Neither these mannerisms nor the delayed development should be regarded as evidence in themselves of significant learning difficulties.

Intelligence has an important influence on the child's ability to cope with visual difficulties. However, 50% of children with visual deficits have additional disabilities such as hearing deficits or severe learning difficulties and do less well.

### Presentation and diagnosis

Babies may be identified in the neonatal period if, for example, cataracts are found (p. 404), or nystagmus or roving, purposeless eye movements are present. If, however, the eyes appear normal, it is frequently the mother who first suspects a problem when she fails to elicit eye contact. Children may also be identified in the course of child health surveillance (see p. 25). It must be emphasized that a parent who raises concern about poor vision should be taken seriously.

If a visual defect is suspected, examination by an ophthalmologist is indicated. In the young child, visual evoked response (VER) testing is often required. The VER is an electrophysiological method of evaluating the response to light and special visual stimuli.

### Managing the child with visual impairment (see Box 12.4)

Management is directed towards providing early intervention in order to promote developmental progress, reduce blindisms and to increase parental confidence. The family needs supportive services and the child requires appropriate educational resources.

A peripatetic teacher is provided either by the local authority or the Royal National Institute for the Blind to advise parents in the preschool years.

At school level, improvements in equipment have occurred in recent years so that the child with partial sight may now be able to cope in a mainstream school. These improvements include better optical aids, good

---

**Box 12.4 Managing the visually impaired child**

- Provide early intervention in order to improve developmental progress
- Support the family and increase parental confidence
- Provide appropriate educational resources

**Visual impairment at a glance**

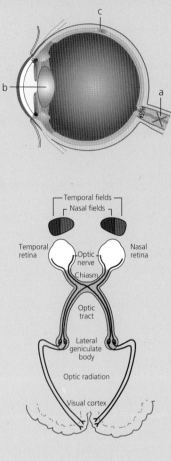

### Definition
A child is defined as blind if education can only be provided by methods not involving sight, e.g. Braille A child is partially sighted if educational methods such as large-print books can be used

### Epidemiology
1 in 2500 children are registered blind or partially sighted 50% have additional handicaps

### Aetiology/pathophysiology
Commonest causes are:
Optic atrophy (**a**)
Congenital cataracts (**b**)
Choroidoretinal degeneration (**c**)

### Clinical features
- The eyes may look abnormal or have unusual movements
- If the deficit is congenital, early smiling is inconsistent and there is no turning towards sound
- Reaching for objects and the pincer grip is delayed
- Early language may be normal, but complex language may be delayed
- 'Blindisms' (eye poking, eye rubbing and rocking) may occur

### Associated problems
Hearing deficit or severe learning difficulties are common

### Presentation and how the diagnosis is made
Malformations at birth, or later when developmental delay is evident

### Practical aspects of management
Early intervention to improve developmental progress, reduce blindisms and increase parental confidence
Preschool: a peripatetic teacher from the Royal National Institute for the Blind
Advice on appropriate schooling
Mobility training
Supportive services

### Issues for the family
Advice on non-visual stimulation and child-rearing
Adaptation of the home

### Issues for the school
Mainstream nursery and nursery school with supportive services are often appropriate
Beyond this, mainstream school, a partially sighted unit, or a school for the blind (depending on learning abilities)

---

illumination, and reading material in very large type. Braille remains the essential method of reading for the child with a severe visual deficit, providing learning disabilities are not present.

Mobility training is an essential part of education. As the child matures, instruction must be given in travel outside of school, initially under supervision and then independently.

## Issues for the family
Parents of a blind child need help at a very early stage. They must be taught to stimulate their infant using non-visual means, such as touch and speech, and must continue to provide stimulation through the early years with appropriate play materials. The home is likely to require adaptation so that the child can explore this environment safely.

## Issues for the school
Mainstream nursery and nursery school are often appropriate for the child with a visual handicap, provided support from the peripatetic teacher is available. Beyond this, factors such as the child's intellect and ability to make use of residual vision, the wishes of the family and the long-term prognosis determine whether placement should be in a mainstream school, partially sighted unit or a school for the blind.

*To test your knowledge on this part of the book, please see Chapter 25.*

# CHAPTER 13

# Growth, endocrine and metabolic disorders

*I knew a little elfman once*
*Down where the lilies blow.*
*I asked him why he was so small,*
*And why he didn't grow*
*He slightly frowned, and with his*
*eyes*
*He looked me through and*
*through:*
*'I'm quite as big for me,' he said,*
*'As you are big for you.'*
*John Kendrick Bangs*
*(1862–1922)*

## COMPETENCES

## You must . . .

| Know | Be able to | Appreciate |
|---|---|---|
| • When a child's growth is of concern<br>• How to diagnose the common and important conditions responsible for poor growth in infants and children, and the principles of managing them<br>• The causes of poor weight gain in young children and babies<br>• How to advise a child who is suffering from obesity<br>• The principles of managing diabetic ketoacidosis | • Plot measures on a growth chart<br>• Weigh and measure a baby and child accurately and correct for prematurity<br>• Calculate BMI<br>• Measure blood glucose using a home monitor | • The stress and anxiety of having a child with weight faltering (FTT), especially if there are eating difficulties<br>• The impact that diabetes has on the child and family<br>• The principles involved in managing diabetes<br>• The importance of good diabetic control to prevent complications |

*Paediatrics and Child Health*, Third Edition. Mary Rudolf, Tim Lee, Malcolm Levene.
© 2011 Mary Rudolf, Tim Lee and Malcolm Levene. Published 2011 by Blackwell Publishing Ltd.

# Symptoms and signs of growth, endocrine and metabolic disorders

## Finding your way around . . .

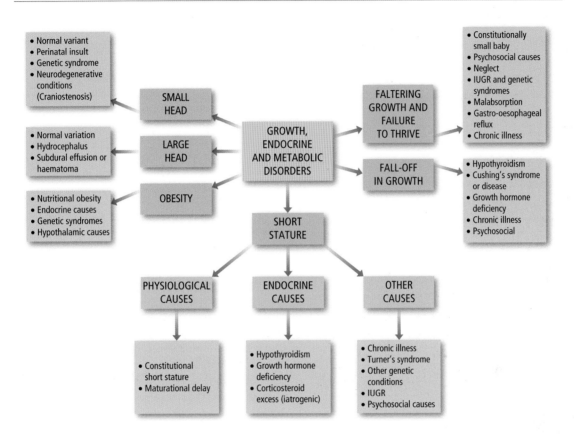

## Short stature

**Causes of short stature**

*Physiological causes*
Normal variant (often familial, also known as 'constitutional short stature')
Maturational delay (often familial)

*Pathological causes*
Endocrine
• Hypothyroidism
• Corticosteroid excess
• Growth hormone deficiency

Chronic illness
• Inflammatory bowel disease, coeliac disease and chronic renal failure may be occult
Genetic
• Turner's syndrome
• Other genetic syndromes
• Skeletal dysplasias
Intrauterine growth retardation
Psychosocial

At birth, a baby's weight and length are influenced mainly by intrauterine factors. This does not correlate well with parental heights, but over the next year or two the baby's growth adjusts, so that by the age of 2 years most children have attained their genetically destined centile. From then until the onset of puberty children usually grow steadily along their centile with little deviation. During puberty it is normal for centiles to be crossed again until final height is achieved, which usually is located midway between the parental centiles. Normal growth reflects a child's well-being, and any deviation may be indicative of adverse physical or psychosocial factors. Guidelines for concern about a child's growth are shown in the Red Flag box.

---

### Guidelines for concern beyond the age of 2 years

- **The short or tall child.** Height or weight beyond the dotted lines on the growth chart (>99.6th or <0.4th centiles, see Figure 4.6) are outside the normal range and pathology is likely to be found. Many children whose height or weight lies in the shaded areas are normal, but an evaluation needs to be considered.
- **Crossing of centiles**. As a rule of thumb, one should be concerned if two centile lines are crossed.
- **Discrepancy between height and weight.** There is a great deal of variation as regards leanness and obesity. The child who is very thin or overweight may have a problem.
- **Discrepancy with parental heights.** A child should be evaluated if there is a large discrepancy between the child's height centile and the midparental centile (an average of the parents' centiles). The child of tall parents who has a growth problem should not wait until he or she falls below the second centile to be evaluated.
- **Parental or professional concern.** A good clinical evaluation should be carried out in any child where the parents or other professionals are concerned about growth.

---

Given the social disadvantage of being short, especially for a man, it is not surprising that short stature commonly causes concern. In most short children height is simply a variant of normal, and delay in physical development (maturational delay) is often a factor. When a short child presents, it is important to exclude organic problems, particularly if a fall-off in growth is observed over time.

Any chronic illness can lead to stunting of growth – however, chronic illnesses rarely present with short stature as the features of the illness are usually all too evident. The exceptions are inflammatory bowel disease (see p. 182), coeliac disease (see p. 180) and chronic renal failure, which can all present with poor growth in advance of other clinical features. Children with genetic syndromes often are short, and Turner's syndrome (gonadal dysgenesis) is important to consider in short girls.

Endocrinological causes of short stature include hypothyroidism, growth hormone deficiency and corticosteroid excess. Hypothyroidism has a profound effect on growth, and the presenting feature is often short stature. Cushing's syndrome and disease are extremely rare in childhood, although iatrogenic growth suppression from exogenous steroids is not uncommon.

Adverse psychosocial factors can severely affect a child's growth. In the young child it is referred to as *failure to thrive* (p. 368). The true incidence of psychosocial short stature is unknown, but it is likely that it is quite common. Children often have a growth spurt on being placed in foster care, even if growth has been apparently normal.

The most important aspect of the evaluation of the child with short stature is the history and physical examination, together with careful measurements of height. The purpose of the evaluation should not only be to discover underlying pathological conditions, but also to understand the impact that short stature has on the child.

### History must ask!

The history needs to focus on symptoms suggestive of underlying conditions such as intracranial pathology, hormone deficiency, chronic illness and gastrointestinal symptoms.

- *Medical history.* You need a careful review of medical symptoms, particularly focusing on headache, diarrhoea and abdominal pain, constipation, cough, wheeze and fatigue. The presence of any chronic condition such as asthma, arthritis or diabetes is obviously relevant, as is any chronic medication.
- *Family history.* A child's growth cannot be interpreted without reference to parental and siblings' heights. A child's height normally falls on the centile between the parents' height centiles, and if there is a disparity a cause should be sought. Enquire into

parental onset of puberty as maturational delay is common and often familial. Most mothers can recall their age at menarche, and maturational delay is likely if it occurred after the age of 14 years. Onset of paternal puberty is harder to identify.

• *Birth history*. Low birthweight is significant. A child born severely preterm or small for gestational age (SGA) may have reduced growth potential, particularly if height as well as weight is affected.

• *Psychosocial history*. Psychosocial factors can severely stunt a child's growth, and you must be alert to the possibility of emotional neglect and abuse. When assessing any short child you should also find out about any social or emotional difficulties *resulting* from their stature.

## Physical examination – must check!

A very thorough examination is required, focusing particularly on the following:

• *Pattern of growth*. Where possible, you should review previous growth measurements as they provide important clues to the aetiology of the condition. Fall-off in growth usually indicates a medical condition requiring treatment.

• *Anthropometric measures*. Take careful measures of length (to age 24 months) or height and weight and plot them on a growth chart (see p. 57).

• *General examination*. Signs of hypothyroidism (see Table 13.4), body disproportion, signs of Turner's syndrome (see below) and dysmorphism are particularly important to identify. Examine each organ system in turn, looking for evidence of occult disease.

## Investigations

Your clinical evaluation should guide any investigations. If you find a decrease in growth velocity, investigations are always required (Table 13.1).

## Managing the short child

The majority of short children will have a physiological cause for their stature: either 'constitutional', or maturational delay. In such cases the family needs reassurance that there is no underlying pathological problem. In addition, it is important to address any psychosocial difficulties the child is having, and occasionally psychological counselling is required. These difficulties are uncommon before adolescence, but become particularly problematic for teenage boys. The use of growth hormone in children with physiological short stature is controversial and probably gives little benefit to final adult height.

---

### Key points: Short stature

• A good history and physical examination will identify most pathological causes of short stature
• The child's height must be related to the parents' heights
• Emotional and social consequences of the short stature should be identified

---

**Table 13.1** Investigations in a child with short stature

| Investigation | Relevance |
| --- | --- |
| Blood count and plasma viscosity or erythrocyte sedimentation rate | Inflammatory bowel disease |
| Urea and electrolytes | Chronic renal failure |
| Coeliac antibodies | Screening test for coeliac disease |
| Thyroxine and thyroid-stimulating hormone | Hypothyroidism |
| Karyotype (in girls) | Turner's syndrome |
| Growth hormone tests | Hypopituitarism, growth hormone deficiency |
| X-ray of the wrist for bone age* (see Figure 1.2) | Delayed bone age suggests maturational delay, hypothyroidism, growth hormone deficiency or corticosteroid excess. A prediction of adult height can be made from it |

## Clues to the diagnosis of short stature

| | Growth pattern | History | Physical examination | Bone age |
|---|---|---|---|---|
| **Constitutional short stature** | Steady growth below the centile lines | Short parents | Normal | Normal |
| **Maturational delay** | Usually short with fall-off of growth in early teens | Family history of delayed puberty/ menarche | Delay in developing secondary sex characteristics | Delayed |
| **Endocrine disorders (hypothyroidism, Cushing's, growth hormone deficiency)** | Fall-off of growth | Symptoms of hypothyroidism, on inhaled or oral steroids, symptoms of brain tumour | Signs of hypothyroidism or Cushing's. Rarely signs of brain tumour | Very delayed |
| **Chronic illness** | Fall-off of growth | Symptoms of inflammatory bowel disease, malabsorption, fatigue | Ill looking. Symptoms of underlying illness, although inflammatory bowel disease and chronic renal failure may be occult | Delayed +/– |
| **Genetic syndromes** | Slow growth below centiles | | Signs of Turner's or other dysmorphism | Variable |
| **Intrauterine growth retardation** | Short from birth | Small for gestational age | Normal but small | Normal |
| **Psychosocial** | Variable depending on social circumstances | Adverse circumstances | Unhappy, signs of neglect or abuse | Usually normal |

## Plateauing in growth

### Causes of fall-off in growth

*Endocrine*
Hypothyroidism (see p. 269)
Corticosteroid excess (see p. 272)
Growth hormone deficiency (see p. 271)

*Chronic illness* (see p. 36)
Inflammatory bowel and coeliac disease, and chronic renal failure may be occult

*Psychosocial causes* (see Chapter 20)

A less common problem than short stature is fall-off in growth. This cannot be identified on one measurement but is a pattern observed over time. If the child is from a tall family, he or she may not be short in relation to peers. Fall-off in growth is always worrying and merits investigation.

The clinical approach and management are the same as those described in the previous section, but the chance of finding pathology is higher.

# Weight and growth faltering

## Causes of weight and growth faltering

*Organic*
Gastro-oesophageal reflux
Malabsorption
Chronic illness
Endocrine dysfunction

*Genetic*
Genetic constitution
Intrauterine growth retardation
Genetic syndromes

*Environmental/psychosocial (non-organic)*
Maternal depression/psychiatric disorder
Disturbed maternal–infant attachment
Eating difficulties
Neglect

'Failure to thrive' implies both a failure to grow and a failure of emotional and developmental progress. The term is sometimes considered pejorative and has been replaced by growth or weight 'faltering'. These terms are usually used in reference to poor weight gain in a toddler or baby, although they may also be used in connection with an older child, and may also refer to height. Because infants commonly cross centiles during the first 2 years of life, expertise is required to differentiate the normal infant from the one with worrying weight faltering.

The following can act as guidelines as to when a clinical evaluation is advisable:

- weight below the 2nd centile;
- height below the 2nd centile;
- crossing down two centile channels for height or weight.

Small parents tend to have small children, and the small healthy normal child of short parents should not arouse concern. Usually in this case growth is steady along the lower centiles, but the large baby born to small parents may cross down centile lines before settling on the destined line. Growth retardation may occur if a fetus experiences adverse uterine conditions. When this occurs early in gestation, length and head circumference in addition to weight can be affected. In this circumstance the potential for postnatal growth may be jeopardized

A child may falter in weight for either organic or psychosocial reasons. In the past children were classified as having organic (OFTT) or non-organic failure to thrive (NOFTT). Children more often than not do not fall simply into one category or the other, and it is important to identify all the factors involved rather than to simplistically seek one cause.

Children and babies with any chronic illness can fail to thrive. They rarely present as a diagnostic dilemma as the manifestations of the disease are usually evident. However, organic failure to thrive may be compounded by psychosocial difficulties, and these need to be addressed. Very rarely, chronic disease can be occult and present as failure to thrive.

Vomiting and possetting are common complaints in a baby, and usually do not deleteriously affect growth. However, reflux in association with oesophagitis can cause poor weight gain. Malabsorption is another important cause, and symptoms of diarrhoea and colic provide diagnostic clues. The commonest childhood causes of malabsorption include coeliac disease (see p. 180) and cystic fibrosis (see pp. 149–51). In the former, the weight characteristically falls off coincident with the introduction of gluten to the diet.

It is very distressing for the family when a young child fails to thrive, and your evaluation needs to be carried out sensitively. The purpose of the evaluation is first to differentiate the child demonstrating normal growth faltering from the child with a problem, and then to identify the contributing factors, whether organic or non-organic.

### History – must ask!

- Nutritional history. Obtain a good dietary history. You should include questions about any feeding difficulties, which may have been present from birth but often develop at weaning and in the toddler years. Eating difficulties may be the cause of the failure to thrive. However, eating difficulties may also be generated from anxiety that naturally occurs when a baby grows poorly because of other causes. It is helpful to ask the mother to keep a food diary for a few days, recording all that the baby has eaten.
- Review of symptoms. Most organic conditions are identifiable by history. Diarrhoea, colic, vomiting, irritability, fatigue and chronic cough are the most features to elicit.
- Past medical history. The birth history is important. A low birthweight may indicate adverse prenatal conditions which affect growth potential. Recurrent illness of any nature may affect growth.

• Developmental history. This is needed for two reasons. First, failure to thrive can affect a baby's developmental progress and, secondly, the child who has neurodevelopmental problems often has associated eating difficulties which may limit nutritional intake.
• Family history. Relate the child's growth to that of other family members. Medical problems affecting other children in the family may suggest a diagnosis. A good social history should identify psychosocial problems that may be causing or at least contributing to the problem.

### Physical examination – must check!

• General observations. The baby's appearance is important. The healthy small baby will look very different from the neglected or ill child. The child who is malnourished for whatever reason will appear thin, with wasted buttocks, a protuberant abdomen and sparse hair. A neglected child may look unclean and uncared for. Observations must also extend to the mother and how she relates to the baby, which can provide valuable clues to maternal–infant attachment difficulties.
• Growth. Plot growth on a growth chart and compare them with previous measurements. The pattern of growth can be very helpful in the diagnostic process (Figure 13.1).
• Physical examination. You need to carry out a full physical examination to complement the history. Occasionally, clinical signs alone can indicate a cause for the poor growth.

### Investigations

There is good evidence that 'fishing' for a diagnosis by carrying out multiple investigations is a futile exercise. Investigations should only be carried out if clues to a problem are obtained on history and physical examination. The only exception is a blood count and ferritin level, as iron deficiency is extremely common in this group of children, and can affect both development and appetite. Other investigations which may be helpful, if clinically justified, are shown in Table 13.2.

### Managing weight faltering

The ability to nurture a baby is perhaps the most basic attribute of parenting. When a child fails to thrive it usually causes extreme distress, anxiety and feelings of inadequacy. It is important therefore that a normal, healthy but small baby is not wrongly labelled as having a problem. On the other hand it is important that both organic and psychosocial problems are identified and addressed, as failure to thrive has important consequences on the child's developmental progress as well as growth. A thorough clinical evaluation, together with information from the health visitor, can usually sort out the problem. Occasionally it may be helpful to admit the baby to hospital for observation.

---

### Key points: Weight faltering and failure to thrive

• Differentiate the normal baby who is crossing centiles from the baby who is failing to thrive
• Identify any symptoms and signs that suggest an organic condition
• Only perform laboratory investigations if there are clinical leads in the history and physical examination
• Identify psychosocial problems that might be affecting the baby's growth

---

### Clues to the differential diagnosis of weight and growth faltering

| | Growth pattern* | History | Physical examination |
|---|---|---|---|
| **Constitutional** | Steady growth below centiles, or 'catch-down' for larger baby | Short parent(s) | Normal |
| **Psychosocial** | Crossing down of centiles at any age | Eating difficulties common Maternal depression may be present | Usually normal Poor or disturbed maternal–infant attachment may be evident |

## Clues to the differential diagnosis of weight and growth faltering (*Continued*)

| | Growth pattern* | History | Physical examination |
|---|---|---|---|
| **Coeliac disease** | Crossing down of centiles classically occurring at introduction of wheat solids | Frequent stools or diarrhoea<br>Irritability | Distended abdomen<br>Wasted buttocks (late sign) |
| **Cystic fibrosis** | Crossing down of centiles | Appetite often fine<br>Chest infections<br>Frequent loose fatty stools | Protuberant abdomen<br>Decreased muscle mass<br>Chest signs possible<br>Poorly child |
| **Gastro-oesophageal reflux** | Crossing down centiles early in life | Vomiting, irritability, occasionally apnoea | Normal |
| **Intrauterine growth retardation** | Low birthweight with subsequent poor weight gain. Length and head circumference may be reduced | Possible placental insufficiency, difficult pregnancy, smoking, alcohol | Small normal. Look for signs of intrauterine infection (TORCH ) |
| **Neglect** | Crossing down of centiles, catch up if removed from home | Difficult or troubled family circumstances | Poorly cared for, nappy rash, developmental delay common |

*Usually refers to weight in the first instance.

# Obesity

## Causes of obesity in childhood

*Common*
Nutritional

*Rare*
Hypothyroidism
Cushing's syndrome or disease
Various genetic syndromes

Obesity is increasing as a problem in childhood. The vast majority of overweight children have nutritional obesity, and this diagnosis can be simply made on the basis of the clinical evaluation. The importance of identifying the obese child is principally in order to provide support and advice and to attempt to prevent the complications of obesity later in life. Although there is a folk belief that obesity is caused by a child's 'glands', this is very rarely the case.

Weight alone is not a measure of obesity in childhood, but must be related to the child's height. Your clinical evaluation should firstly focus on excluding the rare endocrine and genetic causes of obesity. As all of these are accompanied by poor growth, they can be excluded on clinical grounds fairly easily. You then need to assess those aspects of the child's lifestyle that predispose to obesity and any emotional and behavioural difficulties the child is having.

### History – must ask!

- *Diet.* Ask what the child and family eat on a normal day, bearing in mind that this may be a sensitive issue. Nonetheless. it can form a basis for advice.
- *Lifestyle.* Ask about physical activity during the day and also about sedentary activities.
- *Sleep problems.* Sleep apnoea is a common complication of obesity so ask about snoring, and lethargy or tiredness during the day.
- *Complications.* Musculoskeletal symptoms are common due to the increased load on the joints. It is rare for diabetes or cardiovascular disease to develop in childhood, although there may be biochemical indicators present.
- *Emotional and behavioural problems.* Social and school problems are very common. Children may be bullied or be bullies, or may suffer from significant depression.

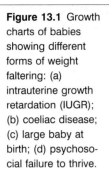

**Figure 13.1** Growth charts of babies showing different forms of weight faltering: (a) intrauterine growth retardation (IUGR); (b) coeliac disease; (c) large baby at birth; (d) psychosocial failure to thrive.

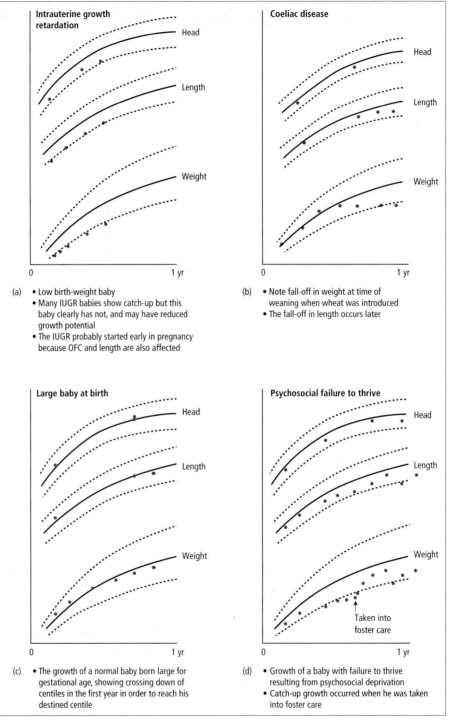

(a) • Low birth-weight baby
• Many IUGR babies show catch-up but this baby clearly has not, and may have reduced growth potential
• The IUGR probably started early in pregnancy because OFC and length are also affected

(b) • Note fall-off in weight at time of weaning when wheat was introduced
• The fall-off in length occurs later

(c) • The growth of a normal baby born large for gestational age, showing crossing down of centiles in the first year in order to reach his destined centile

(d) • Growth of a baby with failure to thrive resulting from psychosocial deprivation
• Catch-up growth occurred when he was taken into foster care

• *Learning difficulties.* Children with a genetic syndrome associated with obesity are likely to have special educational needs.
• *Physical symptoms.* Ask about any physical symptoms that might suggest hypothyrodism (Table 13.4) or Cushing's disease (p. 272) as a cause.

• *Family history.* As obesity is a familial condition (genetically and environmentally), a family history is important. It is important to ask about any family members who have developed or died from diabetes or early heart disease.

**Table 13.2** Investigations to consider in the evaluation of weight faltering

| Investigation | What you are looking for |
|---|---|
| Full blood count, ferritin | Iron deficiency is common in failure to thrive and can cause anorexia |
| Urea and electrolytes | Unsuspected renal failure |
| Stool for elastase | Low faecal elastase and the presence of fat globules suggest malabsorption |
| Coeliac antibodies and jejunal biopsy Sweat test | Coeliac disease and cystic fibrosis are causes of malabsorption |
| Thyroid hormone and thyroid-stimulating hormone | Congenital hypothyroidism causes poor growth and developmental delay |
| Karyotype | Chromosomal abnormalities are often associated with short stature and dysmorphism |
| Hospitalization | Hospitalization can be a form of investigation Observation of baby and mother over time can provide clues to the aetiology |

### Physical examination – must check!

- *Growth.* This is the most important indicator of a non-nutritional cause. In nutritional obesity the child is relatively tall. With pathological causes, the child is either short or demonstrates a fall-off in height as the weight increases. You should also calculate the body mass index (BMI) and plot this on a BMI chart (see Figure 4.8). Figure 13.2 illustrates the growth patterns seen with different causes of obesity.
- *Signs of an endocrinological cause.* In the child with poor growth, look for signs of hypothyroidism (goitre – see Figures 13.5 and 13.6 and Table 13.4; developmental delay; slow return of deep tendon reflexes; bradycardia) and steroid excess (moon face, buffalo hump, striae, hypertension, bruising).
- *Signs of dysmorphic syndromes.* Certain dysmorphic syndromes are characterized by obesity. These children are invariably short. Look in particular for microcephaly, hypogonadism, hypotonia and congenital anomalies.
- *Signs of complications.* Check the blood pressure and look for acanthosis nigricans (a dark velvety appearance at the neck and axillae) as this is a sign of insulin resistance.

### Investigations

Investigations are required if you are concerned that there is a non-nutritional cause for the obesity, par-

ticularly if the child is short, dysmorphic, is demonstrating a fall-off in height or has learning difficulties. In this case thyroid function tests, diurnal cortisol levels and genetic studies are indicated. If the child is very obese, investigation for heart disease, diabetes and steatohepatitis may be needed. Possible investigations are shown in Table 13.3.

### Managing obesity

Lifestyle management is the mainstay of treating obesity (see p. 267) (see Figure 13.4). At present there are no medications licensed for use in children.

---

**Key points: Obesity**

- Exclude rare causes of obesity, remembering that most children with an organic cause will be growing poorly
- Calculate the BMI and plot on BMI growth charts
- Assess the child for early complications resulting from obesity
- Obtain a clear picture of the child's lifestyle, focusing on physical activity and diet
- Find out about emotional and behavioural problems

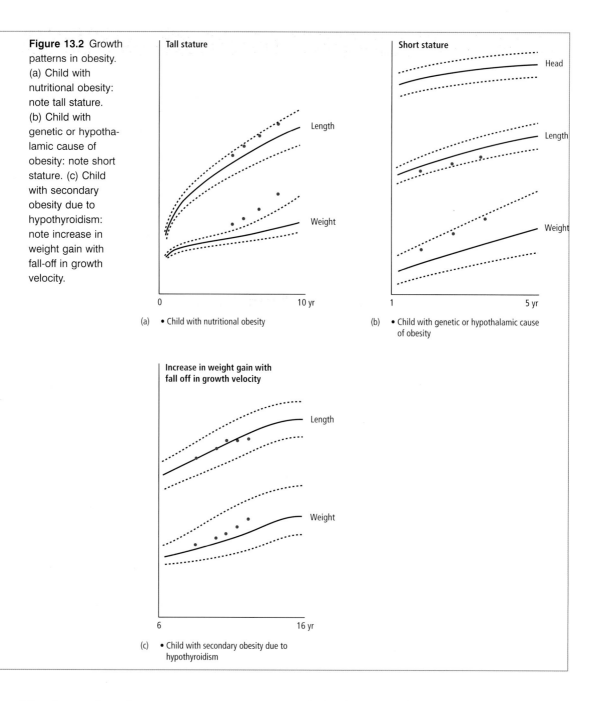

**Figure 13.2** Growth patterns in obesity. (a) Child with nutritional obesity: note tall stature. (b) Child with genetic or hypothalamic cause of obesity: note short stature. (c) Child with secondary obesity due to hypothyroidism: note increase in weight gain with fall-off in growth velocity.

(a) • Child with nutritional obesity

(b) • Child with genetic or hypothalamic cause of obesity

(c) • Child with secondary obesity due to hypothyroidism

## The large head

### Causes of a large or enlarging head

Normal variation (often familial)
Hydrocephalus
Subdural effusion or haematomas
Feature of certain dysmorphic syndromes

The head grows rapidly in the first 2 years of life and then slows down, but continues to grow throughout childhood. In the early years the sutures are open, and then fuse around the age of 6 years. Prior to fusion they can separate in response to raised intracranial pressure. The posterior fontanelle usually closes by 8 weeks of age, and the anterior by 12–18 months.

Head size is not directly proportional to body size, but large children are more likely to have large heads, and vice versa. As in body growth, it is not unusual

**Table 13.3** Investigations that may be indicated in the obese child

| | Investigation | Relevance |
|---|---|---|
| Looking for a cause | T4, TSH | Low T4 and high TSH are found in hypothyroidism |
| | Urinary free cortisol | High in Cushing's disease |
| | Karyotype and DNA analysis | Genetic syndrome |
| | MRI of the brain | Hypothalamic cause |
| Looking for consequences of obesity | Urinary glucose, fasting glucose and insulin or an oral glucose tolerance test | Diabetes |
| | Fasting lipid screen | Hyperlipidaemia |
| | Liver function tests | Fatty liver |

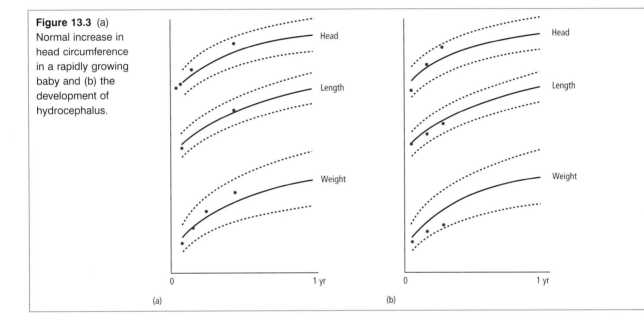

**Figure 13.3** (a) Normal increase in head circumference in a rapidly growing baby and (b) the development of hydrocephalus.

for head circumference measurements to cross centiles in the first year. However, when this occurs clinical assessment is needed to exclude pathological causes.

A large head is usually a normal variant, and often is a familial feature. An unusually large head may indicate hydrocephalus, in which case evidence of raised intracranial pressure may be present. Large heads may also be a feature of certain genetic syndromes.

### History – must ask!

- *Is the baby developing normally?* Abnormal developmental progress in a child with a large head is strongly indicative of pathology.

- *Are there symptoms of raised intracranial pressure?* The baby with hydrocephalus or subdural effusion is likely to be irritable and lethargic, have a poor appetite and vomit.

### Physical examination – must check!

- *Growth measures.* The pattern of head growth is important. Crossing of centile lines is more concerning than steady growth of a large head. Length and weight indicate whether the head is disproportionately large (Figure 13.3).
- *Signs of hydrocephalus.* The child with hydrocephalus has characteristic features (see p. 219).

• *Development.* A developmental examination should accompany the developmental history.

### Investigations –

If raised intracranial pressure is suspected, immediate investigation is required. If the anterior fontanelle is still open, a cranial ultrasound can be performed to detect hydrocephalus, effusions or haemorrhage. If the fontanelles are closed, a magnetic resonance imaging (MRI) scan is required to delineate underlying pathology.

### Management –

Frequent measurements of head circumference can generate anxiety, and should not be performed if the head size is considered to be a variant of normal. If pathology is suspected, investigations should be carried out and the baby referred for neurosurgery.

---

### Key points: The large head

• An enlarging head is more concerning than a steadily growing large head
• Parental head size is helpful in deciding if this is a normal variant
• Assess the baby's developmental skills
• Evidence of raised intracranial pressure indicates hydrocephalus or subdural collection of fluid

---

## The small head (microcephaly)

---

### Causes of microcephaly or poor head growth

*Normal variant (often familial)*

*Limited brain growth*
Perinatal insult to the brain, e.g. hypoxic–ischaemic insult
Genetic syndromes usually associated with learning disability
Neurodegenerative conditions

*Craniosynostosis (very rare)*

---

A small head can be familial and of no concern, but as the head grows in response to brain growth, a small head often indicates limited brain growth. For this reason microcephaly is a feature of many dysmorphic syndromes, the commonest being Down's syndrome. The sort of insults to the developing brain that can be responsible for poor growth of the head include:

• hypoxic–ischaemic encephalopathy (see p. 403);
• congenital infections (see p. 407);
• genetic disorder or syndrome;
• antenatal toxins, such as alcohol;
• malnutrition;
• meningitis.

Very rarely, poor head growth occurs as a result of premature fusion of cranial sutures (craniosynostosis). If all the sutures are involved, skull growth is restricted, resulting in raised intracranial pressure.

### History – must ask!

• *Is the baby developing normally?* If a baby is developing normally, it is unlikely that the head size is a cause for concern. If developmental delay is present, the baby needs to be evaluated for perinatal insults or genetic syndromes.
• *Past medical history.* The perinatal history may throw light on factors such as infection, alcohol or hypoxic–ischaemic events which may have affected brain growth.

### Physical examination – must check!

• *Growth measures.* The length and weight of the baby indicate whether the head size is disproportionately small. The pattern of head growth is important. Crossing of centile lines is more concerning than steady growth of a small head.
• *Parental head size.* Microcephaly in normal individuals is often familial.
• *Developmental skills.* Confirm the developmental history by carrying out a good developmental assessment.
• *Dysmorphic features.* Dysmorphic features suggest the diagnosis of a genetic syndrome.

### Investigations

A skull X-ray shows premature fusion of the sutures if craniosynostosis is present. A karyotype and neurometabolic screen is indicated if you suspect a neurodegenerative or dysmorphic syndrome.

**Key points: The small head**

- Determine whether the child is developing normally
- Check parental head size

## Management

If craniosynostosis is demonstrated, the child should be referred for urgent neurosurgical intervention. If you suspect developmental disability, close follow-up is required (see p. 228).

# Growth, metabolic and endocrine disorders

## Constitutional short stature

As stature is largely genetically determined, short parents tend to have short children. 'Constitutional' or 'familial' short stature is the term used of children who are short because of their genetic constitution.

**Clinical features.** The history and physical examination is normal, and the bone age is appropriate for age. Social difficulties are common in the adolescent years, particularly for boys.

**Management and prognosis.** Reassurance is often all that is required. Occasionally children need psychological support in the adolescent years. There are social disadvantages to being short.

## Maturational delay

Children with maturational delay are often called 'late developers' or 'late bloomers'. The biological clock operates more slowly than usual. It may be associated with constitutional short stature, in which circumstance the child may have particular difficulty coping with their height. It is not uncommonly a cause of bullying, especially for boys.

**Clinical features.** Children are short and reach puberty late, their final height depending on their genetic constitution, which may be normal. A family history of delayed puberty and menarche is often obtained. The bone age is delayed.

**Management and prognosis.** Most families simply require reassurance that final height will not be affected. Occasionally teenage boys find the social pressures to be so great that it is helpful to artificially trigger puberty early, thus causing an early growth spurt. Treatment does not have an effect on final height.

## Non-organic failure to thrive

The commonest causes for failure to thrive are psychosocial. The problems include difficulties in the home, limitations in the parents, disturbed attachment between the mother and child, maternal depression/psychiatric disorder and eating difficulties. Neglect is the underlying factor in only a few children.

**Clinical features.** Weight gain is usually affected first, but eventually a reduction in linear growth and head circumference follows and the child's developmental progress may be delayed.

Children with failure to thrive range across a spectrum of backgrounds. At one end of the spectrum is the child from a caring home who appears well looked after. The parents are anxious and concerned and interact well with the child. The problems are often eating difficulties, where the child has a minimal appetite or refuses to eat, meals are very stressful and the parents have been drawn into excessive measures (sometimes force feeding) to persuade the child to eat. At the other end of the spectrum is the neglected child who shows physical signs of poor care and emotional attachment. In this case the problem is often denied and compliance with intervention is poor.

**Management.** Management of failure to thrive must fit the problem. Most families can be helped by appropriate intervention, usually consisting of dietary advice and psychological support. Practical support can ease the stress, and nursery placement can be very helpful in this regard as well as helping to resolve eating difficulties. In those cases where neglect is the cause and the family are not amenable to help, social services must be involved (see pp. 31, 366).

**Prognosis.** With appropriate intervention, the problem usually resolves or at least stabilizes. A few children need to be removed from their homes.

## Non-organic failure to thrive at a glance

**Epidemiology**
2% hospital admissions

**Definition**
Diagnosis is considered when height or weight below 2nd centile *or* cross down two centiles *and* organic causes have been excluded

**Aetiology/pathophysiology**
Psychosocial problems such as
• disturbed maternal–child attachment
• maternal depression/psychiatric disorder
• eating difficulties
• neglect

**History**
• Poor weight gain (a)
• Eating difficulties* (b)
• Inadequate diet* (c)
• Maternal anxiety/depression*

NB *Signs and symptoms are variable.

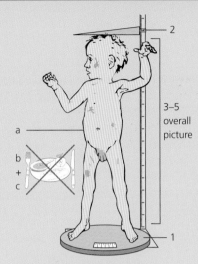

3–5 overall picture

**Physical examination**
• Fall-off in weight velocity (1)
• Fall-off in linear growth and head circumference* (2)
• Developmental delay* (3)
• Signs of malnutrition: thin child, wasted buttocks, thin hair* (4)
• Signs of neglect: dirty, unkempt, nappy rash, unusual reaction to strangers* (5)

**Confirmatory investigations**
Exclusion of organic causes of failure to thrive (see Causes box, p. 257)
Iron status (iron deficiency is common)
Good weight gain in hospital with standard diet

**Differential diagnosis**
Organic causes of failure to thrive (see Causes box, p. 257)

**Management**
Dietary advice
Psychological support
Social support (nursery placement particularly effective)
Referral to social services in some cases

**Prognosis**
With good early intervention, the process is likely to reverse
Without intervention the child is at severe risk for emotional and intellectual deficits and poor growth

## Intrauterine growth retardation

Intrauterine growth retardation can result from a variety of causes (see p. 410). The impact on postnatal growth depends on at which stage of the pregnancy the growth retardation occurred. If the insult occurred early in gestation, the baby is born not only underweight but also short and often with a small head. Many short newborns have a reduced growth potential and remain short throughout life. If catch-up growth occurs, it does so in the first 2 or 3 years.

## Nutritional obesity

The metabolic factors that predispose some individuals to becoming obese have yet to be determined. Certainly the correlation between nutrient intake and development of obesity is not simple.

**Clinical features.** The nutritionally obese child tends to be tall for his or her age, and tends to develop puberty early, so that final height is not excessively tall. Boys' genitalia may appear deceptively small if buried in fat. Knock-knees are common. Obese children have a high incidence of emotional and behavioural difficulties.

**Management.** Rapid decreases in weight should not be attempted, and during the growing years maintenance of weight, while the child increases in height, is a reasonable goal (Figure 13.4). The family needs encouragement to take a whole-family approach towards a healthier lifestyle, rather than targeting the child with the weight problem.

Lifestyle management programmes, if available in the community, can be a helpful way to tackle diet and eating behaviour and encourage an increase in physical activity. If the child is reluctant to participate

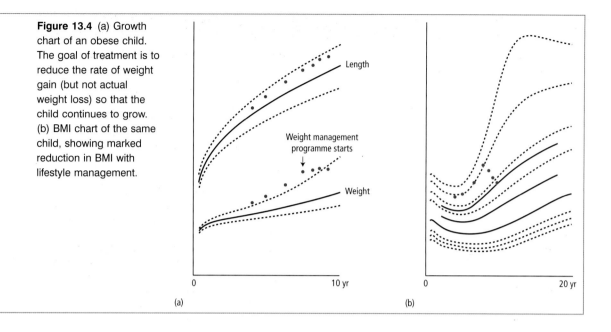

**Figure 13.4** (a) Growth chart of an obese child. The goal of treatment is to reduce the rate of weight gain (but not actual weight loss) so that the child continues to grow. (b) BMI chart of the same child, showing marked reduction in BMI with lifestyle management.

in organized sports, everyday exercise such as walking to school may be more acceptable. Obese children are often the victims of teasing by peers, and psychological disturbance is common. Even if weight control is not successful, continuous support is necessary to help these children cope with their condition.

**Prognosis.** Despite medical intervention, reduction of obesity once it is well established is difficult. Psychological difficulties may well persist into the adult years. Society deals harshly with the obese, and studies show that obesity is a handicap later in life.

In childhood, overt medical complications are few, although metabolic markers for cardiovascular disease, diabetes and fatty liver are common. Obese children are more susceptible to musculoskeletal strain and slipped capital femoral epiphyses (see p. 291). Rarely, insulin-resistant diabetes mellitus develops in child-

hood. If these children become obese adults, the morbidity is significant, with diabetes and hypertension common, leading to early mortality from ischaemic heart disease and strokes. Gallstones and certain cancers are also more prevalent.

**Prevention.** As in most conditions, prevention is better than cure. There is some evidence that breastfeeding in infancy is protective, and promotion of good nutrition in the early years, when food habits are developing, is important. Physical activity needs to be encouraged in all children, not simply the obese. There is a need for these health issues to be addressed in school, particularly during adolescence, when a high intake of high-fat foods and decrease in exercise is common. If intervention is provided early in the course of obesity, weight control is likely to be more successful.

## Nutritional obesity at a glance

**Epidemiology**
14% of school-aged children

**Definition**
BMI >98th centile

**Aetiology**
- Excessive nutritional intake (**b**)
- Inadequate physical activity (c)
- Familial factors (**a**)

**History**
Dietary intake in excess of requirements*
Emotional/behavioural difficulties*

**Physical examination**
Excessive weight
Tall stature
Boys' genitalia apparently small
Genu valgus*

**Confirmatory investigations**
Endocrine tests if child is short or a fall-off in growth is observed
Fasting oral glucose tolerance test
Lipid screen liver fuction test to ascertain co-morbidity

**Differential diagnosis**
Hypothyroidism, Cushing's *only* if obesity is associated with poor growth
Certain genetic or hypothalamic syndromes if the child is short

**Management**
Dietary advice
Increased physical activity
Support

**Prognosis/complications**
Obese children/adolescents at high risk for adult obesity
High risk of psychological problems
Susceptible to slipped capital femoral epiphysis and musculoskeletal strain

NB *Signs and symptoms are variable.

## Congenital hypothyroidism

Lack of thyroid hormone in the first years of life has a devastating effect on both growth and development. However, since neonatal screening has been introduced (see p. 22), congenital hypothyroidism is a rare cause of developmental delay. The underlying pathological defect is either abnormal development of the thyroid gland or inborn errors of thyroxine metabolism.

**Clinical features.** Babies usually appear normal at birth, and rarely have the characteristic features of cretinism. These include coarse facies, hypotonia, a large tongue, an umbilical hernia, constipation, prolonged jaundice and a hoarse cry (Figure 13.5). In the older baby or child, delayed development, lethargy and short stature are found. Thyroid function tests reveal low T4 and high thyroid-stimulating hormone levels.

**Management.** Congenital hypothyroidism is one of the few treatable causes of learning disabilities. Thyroid replacement is required throughout life and must be monitored carefully as the child grows.

**Prognosis.** If therapy is started in the first few weeks of life, and if compliance is good, the prognosis for normal growth and development is excellent.

## Thyroiditis (Figure 13.6)

Thyroiditis is more common in girls than boys.

**Clinical features.** In thyroiditis, the gland is diffusely enlarged, smooth and non-tender, although nodules may occur. The onset is usually insidious, with the goitre noticed as an incidental finding or observation (see Figures 13.6 and 13.7). The child may be clinically euthyroid or hypothyroid (see Table 13.4),

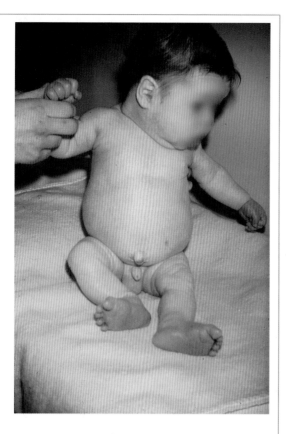

Figure 13.5 A baby with congenital hypothyroidism: note coarse facies and the umbilical hernia.

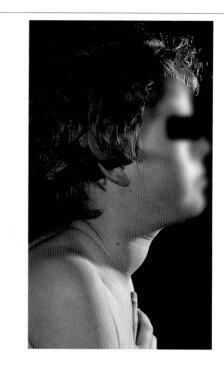

Figure 13.6 A 12-year-old girl who presented with a swelling in the neck, which proved to be due to thyroiditis.

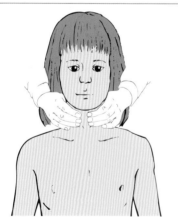

Figure 13.7 Palpation of the thyroid gland. Stand behind the child and ask the child to swallow.

| Table 13.4 Signs of hypo- and hyperthyroidism |
| --- |
| *Hypothyroidism* |
| Sluggishness |
| Constipation |
| Dry skin |
| Poor growth |
| Developmental delay |
| Underachievement at school |
| Bradycardia, hypotension |
| Delayed tendon reflexes |
| *Hyperthyroidism* |
| Nervousness |
| Hyperactivity |
| Increased appetite |
| Tremor |
| Increased sweating |
| Tachycardia and hypertension |
| Lid lag and retraction |

although thyroid overactivity (tremor, palpitations, diarrhoea, sweating) is sometimes seen at the onset. Hypothyroidism is manifested by deceleration of growth with a marked delay in bone age, lethargy, constipation, dry skin and sluggish deep tendon reflexes. Surprisingly, school work does not appear to suffer, although following treatment the child is often transformed from a quiet personality into a spirited child.

**Investigations.** Laboratory investigations show either normal thyroid function tests, or evidence of

primary hypothyroidism with a normal or low T4 and elevated thyroid-stimulating hormone (TSH). Antithyroid antibodies (antimicrosomal and antithyroglobulin) may be present.

**Management.** If there is evidence of hypothyroidism, replacement treatment with thyroxine is indicated. The goitre usually shows some decrease in size. Even if untreated, all children require follow-up of their thyroid status. If nodules persist despite treatment, biopsy should be performed as thyroid cancer can develop.

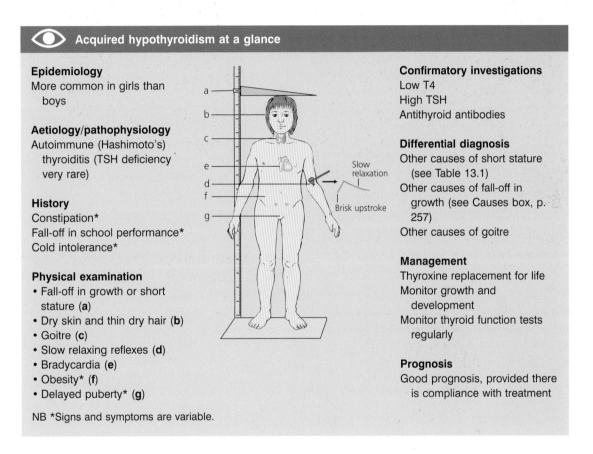

### Acquired hypothyroidism at a glance

**Epidemiology**
More common in girls than boys

**Aetiology/pathophysiology**
Autoimmune (Hashimoto's) thyroiditis (TSH deficiency very rare)

**History**
Constipation*
Fall-off in school performance*
Cold intolerance*

**Physical examination**
• Fall-off in growth or short stature (a)
• Dry skin and thin dry hair (b)
• Goitre (c)
• Slow relaxing reflexes (d)
• Bradycardia (e)
• Obesity* (f)
• Delayed puberty* (g)

NB *Signs and symptoms are variable.

Slow relaxation

Brisk upstroke

**Confirmatory investigations**
Low T4
High TSH
Antithyroid antibodies

**Differential diagnosis**
Other causes of short stature (see Table 13.1)
Other causes of fall-off in growth (see Causes box, p. 257)
Other causes of goitre

**Management**
Thyroxine replacement for life
Monitor growth and development
Monitor thyroid function tests regularly

**Prognosis**
Good prognosis, provided there is compliance with treatment

## Growth hormone deficiency

Growth hormone deficiency is a rare cause of short stature. It may occur secondary to lesions of the pituitary such as tumours or cranial irradiation. Growth hormone deficiency can be isolated or accompanied by deficiency of other pituitary hormones.

**Clinical features.** Growth hormone deficiency causes poor growth, with a delay in bone age. This deficiency can be confirmed by growth hormone testing. Brain

imaging is needed to identify any underlying pathology.

**Management.** Growth hormone deficiency is treated with daily subcutaneous injections of synthetic growth hormone until the child stops growing. Underlying lesions, if any, need to be treated.

**Prognosis.** As regards growth, the prognosis is dependent on the age at which growth hormone therapy was initiated; the younger the child, the greater the chances that final height will be in the normal range. In secondary growth hormone deficiency, the prognosis is related to the underlying lesion.

## Cushing's syndrome and cortico-steroid excess

Cushing's syndrome and disease, resulting in excessive levels of cortisol in the blood, are extremely rare in childhood, growth suppression from exogenous steroids being much more common. In children requiring long-term high steroid therapy, the deleterious effects on growth can often be minimized by giving the steroids on alternate days.

## Turner's syndrome

Turner's syndrome (gonadal dysgenesis) is an important cause of short stature and delayed puberty in girls. It is a genetic disorder caused by the absence of one X-chromosome. The resulting phenotype is female, with gonads which are merely streaks of fibrous tissue. Mosaicism is common. Intelligence is usually normal.

**Clinical features (Figure 13.8).** As neonates, babies with Turner's syndrome often have marked webbing of the neck and lymphoedematous hands and feet. In childhood, short stature is marked and the classic features of webbing of the neck, shield-shaped chest, wide-spaced nipples and a wide carrying angle, may or may not be evident. Some girls are only diagnosed in adolescence when puberty fails to occur.

**Management.** During childhood, growth can be promoted by small doses of growth hormone and oestrogen. Puberty must be initiated and maintained by oestrogen therapy.

**Prognosis.** Women with Turner's syndrome, despite treatment, are generally short. Recent advances in infertility treatment have resulted in a few women becoming pregnant through *in vitro* fertilization with donated ova.

---

### 👁 Turner's syndrome at a glance

**Epidemiology**
One in 2500 female births

**Aetiology/pathophysiology**
45 XO karyotype leads to streak gonads (gonadal dysgenesis) and failure of oestrogen production
Mosaicism is common

**Clinical features**
• Short stature (a)
• Delayed puberty (b)
• Webbing of the neck (c)
• Shield-shaped chest, widely spaced nipples (d)
• Wide carrying angle (e)
  Classic features are often absent*

**Confirmatory investigations**
Chromosome analysis
May be diagnosed at amniocentesis

NB *Signs and symptoms are variable.

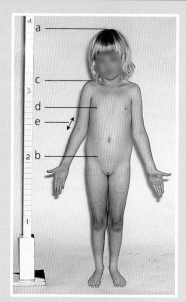

**Differential diagnosis**
Other causes of short stature (see Table 13.1)
Other causes of delayed puberty (see Table 23.6)

**Management**
Promotion of growth in childhood by low-dose growth hormone and oestrogen therapy
Induction of puberty and maintenance with oestrogen replacement therapy

**Associated problems**
Coarctation of the aorta
Renal malformations

**Prognosis**
Generally remain short despite treatment
New advances provide some chance of fertility

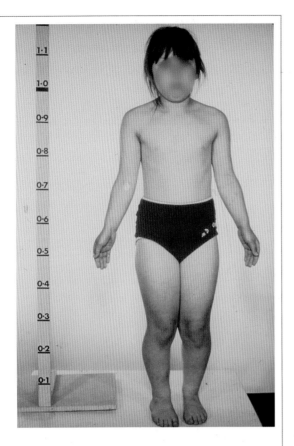

**Figure 13.8** A 10-year-old girl with Turner's syndrome. Note the short stature, webbing of the neck, shield shaped chest and wide carrying angle.

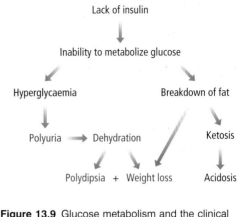

**Figure 13.9** Glucose metabolism and the clinical features of diabetes (shown in blue).

# Diabetes mellitus

Diabetes occurs in one in 500 children. It is an important condition as it has such a major impact on the child and family in terms of daily life, the possibility of unpredictable emergencies and the severity of the medical problems that occur later in life.

## Aetiology of diabetes

Diabetes mellitus is the medical condition that results from insulin deficiency. In childhood this almost always occurs as a consequence of failure of the beta cells in the islets of the pancreas. This aetiology contrasts with that of adult-onset diabetes, which usually results from a peripheral resistance to the action of insulin and high rather than low insulin levels occur.

The process by which the beta cells in the pancreatic islets of Langerhans are destroyed is yet to be elucidated. It is likely that the process is generated by environmental factors, possibly viral, which affect genetically susceptible individuals. An autoimmune process has also been implicated.

## Pathophysiology of diabetes

In order to appreciate the management of diabetes it is necessary to review normal glucose metabolism. Insulin in the normal individual is secreted in response to a rise in blood glucose. Its release is finely modulated by the fluctuation in glucose levels which occur on eating and exercise, and are also under hormonal and neural influence. Insulin facilitates the utilization of glucose as energy for immediate use and its storage as fat for later use. In the fasting state, the fall in blood glucose cuts off insulin secretion, so allowing for mobilization of fat with resultant ketone production. The result is regular swings between the high-insulin anabolic rate and the low-insulin catabolic state.

In the diabetic individual the lack of insulin results in an inability to utilize glucose, causing hyperglycaemia and breakdown of fat. This is responsible for the clinical features of the untreated diabetic state (Figure 13.9).

High levels of blood sugar place the individual in a hyperosmolar state. The resultant osmotic diuresis causes polyuria and dehydration, precipitating thirst and polydipsia. Despite the high glucose levels, the calories cannot be utilized and their loss in the urine causes weight loss. As insulin levels are low, fat is broken down to ketones and ketoacidosis ensues.

Management of the condition requires replacement of insulin. It is impossible to mimic the normal physiological state exactly; however, regular injections of insulin should maintain blood sugar levels near the normal range. This is important not only to avoid the immediate symptoms and dangers of hyperglycaemia, but also the long-term complications of diabetes.

## Diabetic complications

There are four major long-term complications which occur in diabetes and which account for the major morbidity of the condition:

- retinopathy (the commonest cause of blindness in developed countries);
- nephropathy (affects 25–40% of diabetic individuals);
- neuropathy;
- heart disease.

Complications tend to occur some years after onset and therefore are uncommon in the childhood years. These complications have been shown to be directly related to the degree of long-term glycaemic control, and it is for this reason that every effort must be made to maintain the child in as close to a euglycaemic state as possible.

In addition to these complications, hypothyroidism, other autoimmune diseases and coeliac disease occur more commonly in the child with diabetes.

## Initial presentation of diabetes

In childhood diabetes, symptoms are usually present for only a number of weeks before the diagnosis is made. This contrasts with adult-onset diabetes, where symptoms may occur for months or even years before diagnosis. Most children are diagnosed following recognition of the symptoms of polyuria, polydipsia, thirst and weight loss, although rarely they present in diabetic ketoacidotic coma. In young children polyuria may present as secondary nocturnal enuresis. Accompanying symptoms may include lethargy, anorexia and constipation, and if prolonged also vomiting, abdominal pain and the features of diabetic ketoacidosis (DKA) (see Figure 13.10).

Physical examination is often not helpful but may confirm weight loss, and there may be signs of dehydration and the smell of acetone on the breath. The diagnosis is confirmed by the finding of hyperglycaemia, either on random blood sampling or by testing the urine for the presence of sugar. An elevated blood sugar is confirmation in itself, and no further tests

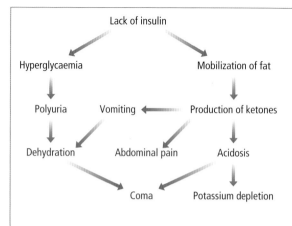

**Figure 13.10** Metabolic cycle leading to the features of diabetic ketoacidosis (shown in blue).

such as fasting blood sugar or glucose tolerance tests are indicated.

Referral to a paediatric specialist team is always required. The child is usually admitted to hospital for a few days even if not in ketoacidosis, as intensive education is essential for both the child and the family.

### Correction of the metabolic state

Most children are admitted with hyperglycaemia and ketonuria, but not in frank ketoacidosis. Normoglycaemia is usually easily achieved by subcutaneous insulin injections and oral rehydration. If marked dehydration and ketoacidosis are present, these demand treatment as described in Table 13.6.

### Education of the child and parents

The diagnosis of diabetes involves a change in lifestyle, probably greater than any other chronic medical condition. The initial education period is crucial in establishing and maintaining these changes. By the end of this period the family should have acquired the following skills:

- insulin administration;
- blood glucose monitoring;
- testing urine for ketones;
- nutritional understanding and a dietary plan;
- an understanding of the relationship of food, insulin, exercise and infection;
- ability to identify and manage hypoglycaemic attacks;
- an understanding of the importance of good control;
- knowledge as to how to obtain advice at any time.

In addition, the school should have been visited to ensure that the staff likewise understand and are trained to cope.

**The diabetic team**

The team of professionals required to manage diabetes successfully in childhood usually consists of:

- a paediatrician with a special interest in diabetes;
- a diabetes nurse specialist;
- a dietitian;
- a social worker.

In some teams a psychologist or psychiatrist, chiropodist and dentist are also involved.

*Management of diabetes*

The goals of management in diabetes, as for any chronic condition of childhood, are to encourage the child to live as normal a life as possible while accepting the limitations that good management of the condition allows (Box 13.1; see also pp. 37–8). This entails maximizing diabetic control, not only to ensure a minimum of hypoglycaemic and hyperglycaemic episodes, but also to minimize the risks of complications in later life. As a lifelong condition the child needs to learn to take responsibility for managing their diabetes in all its aspects (see Box 13.2).

Medication

Insulin preparations have varying durations of action (see Table 13.5). The goal of therapy is to approximate insulin levels to physiological insulin secretion. This is achieved by mixing short- and long-acting insulins.

---

**Box 13.2 Medical management of diabetes**

*Insulin*
- Insulin is given subcutaneously by syringe or pre-mixed insulin 'pen'
- A mixture of short- and medium-acting insulin is given to approximate to the fluxes in insulin that occur physiologically
- At least two injections a day are needed to ensure good control
- The insulin dose should be adjusted on the basis of blood glucose monitoring and $HbA_{1c}$ levels

*Hypoglycaemia*
- Treat with carbohydrate snack or dextrose tablets if the child is able to eat
- Apply glucose gel to buccal mucosa if level of consciousness does not permit oral intake
- If unconscious, give glucagon intramuscularly if available
- Intravenous glucose can be given in hospital (10–25% only)

*Diabetic ketoacidosis*
- Rehydrate with normal saline and replace electrolytes, especially potassium
- Give continuous low-dose intravenous insulin until glucose levels fall to 12 mmol/L and then continue with the addition of dextrose to clear ketones
- When clear and able to drink fluids, change to short-acting insulin using a sliding scale, or child's regular regimen
- Treat any precipitating infection

---

**Box 13.1 Goals in managing diabetes**

- Good metabolic control – maintaining blood glucose levels as normal as possible, without episodes of DKA and a minimum of hypoglycaemic events
- A good understanding of the condition by the family such that they can competently manage the child's diabetes and adjust insulin requirements to diet, exercise, stress and infection
- Minimize complications
- Normal growth and development with full participation in school and social activities
- Work towards the child taking maximal responsibility for his or her diabetes as appropriate for age and intelligence

---

**Table 13.5** Types of insulin preparation and their action

| Type of insulin | Onset | Peak | Duration |
| --- | --- | --- | --- |
| Short-acting | 30 minutes | 2–4 hours | Up to 8 hours |
| Medium- to long-acting | 1–2 hours | 4–12 hours | 16–35 hours |

The commonest insulin regimen is called 'basal-bolus', and consists of a once-a-day long-acting insulin to give a basal background of insulin, with boluses of fast-acting insulin given with each meal. The dose of the boluses is often determined by the parent assessing the approximate carbohydrate content of each meal, a process termed 'carbohydrate counting'. In young children who have low insulin requirements, a twice-daily regimen consisting of a pre-mix of fast- and medium-acting insulin is sometimes used.

Children usually require 0.5–1.0 units of insulin/kg per day, giving approximately half of the dose as fast-acting boluses and half as the once-a-day basal dose. These proportions form a very rough guide and the dose needs to be adjusted on a regular basis according to blood glucose measurements, which should be monitored regularly. Insulin is usually given before meals to match the rise in insulin with the rise in postprandial glucose. Figure 13.11 shows the relationship of blood glucose and insulin levels to meals and insulin injections.

**Mode of delivery.** Insulin is given subcutaneously by syringe or by using preloaded insulin 'pens' (Figure 13.12). The site of injection is unimportant, but children are encouraged to rotate the site between upper arms, thighs, abdomen and buttocks, in order to avoid lipoatrophy and lipohypertrophy, which are unsightly and can affect absorption rates. Some children are managed using insulin pumps that give a continuous infusion via a permanently sited subcutaneous needle (Figure 13.13).

## Dietary management

The other mainstay of treatment is diet. This is often seen to be a major restriction for the family, but in fact the requirements are simply a normal 'healthy' diet which is high in fibre in amounts sufficient to promote normal growth. High-sugar foods must be kept to a minimum as they cause excessive swings in glucose levels.

In children as opposed to adults it is important not to adjust food intake to counteract rises in blood sugar, as this may jeopardize growth. Unless obesity is an issue, the child's requirements should be guided by appetite and hunger, and the dietary recommendations and insulin dose adjusted accordingly.

Families require the guidance of a dietitian, particularly in the early stages. In order to allow for

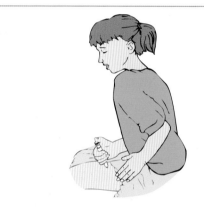

**Figure 13.12** A girl with diabetes injecting insulin with a pen.

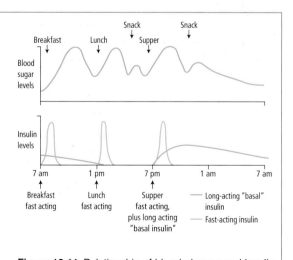

**Figure 13.11** Relationship of blood glucose and insulin levels to meals and insulin injections.

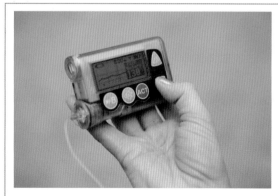

**Figure 13.13** An insulin infusion pump.

flexibility and consistency, the family is taught to recognize foods as easily identifiable 10-g portions which allow for ready and sensible adjustments.

## Monitoring the condition

### Blood glucose monitoring and diary

Confirmation of symptoms and adjustments in insulin dose are guided by regular blood glucose monitoring (Figure 13.14) using glucose testing strips and a monitor. The goal is to keep glucose levels as close to the normal range of 4–6 mmol/L as possible. Most children adjust to the demands of testing, and it is usually recommended that it is carried out at least 3–4 times per day, 2 days per week, and whenever the child has symptoms of hypo- or hyperglycaemia. Results are recorded in a diary (Figure 13.15) and allow for sensible adjustments in insulin dose to be made on a regular basis. If measurements are running high for a period, especially if the child is unwell, the family is taught to test for ketosis by measuring the level of ketones in the urine or blood using reagent strips.

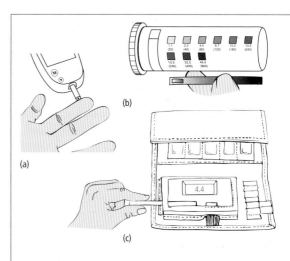

**Figure 13.14** Blood glucose monitoring. (a) A drop of blood is obtained and dropped on to a blood monitoring strip. (b) The colour, after flushing, is compared with a chart or (c) inserted into a meter for reading.

| Date | Insulin injection | | Blood | | | | | | | | Urine | | | | Comments |
|---|---|---|---|---|---|---|---|---|---|---|---|---|---|---|---|
| Time | Human Mixtard 30 Pen 7.30 a.m. | Human Mixtard 30 Pen 6.00 p.m. | Before breakfast | 2 hours after breakfast | Before midday meal | 2 hours after midday meal | Before evening meal | 2 hours after evening meal | Before bed | During night | Before breakfast | Before midday meal | Before evening meal | Before bed | |
| 1st | 28u | 20u | 5.1 | 8.4 | | | 5.8 | | 7.1 | | | | | | |
| 4th | | | 5.2 | | 6.3 | | 5.5 | 6.4 | | 1.5 | | | | | Hypo during night - 3 a.m. - Forgot evening snack |
| 7th | | | 6.0 | 8.5 | | | 4.7 | | 6.5 | | | | | | |
| 9th | | | 5.1 | 8.3 | | | 5.2 | | 7.6 | | | | | | |
| 11th | | | | | 5.1 | 7.3 | | | 8.2 | | | | | | |

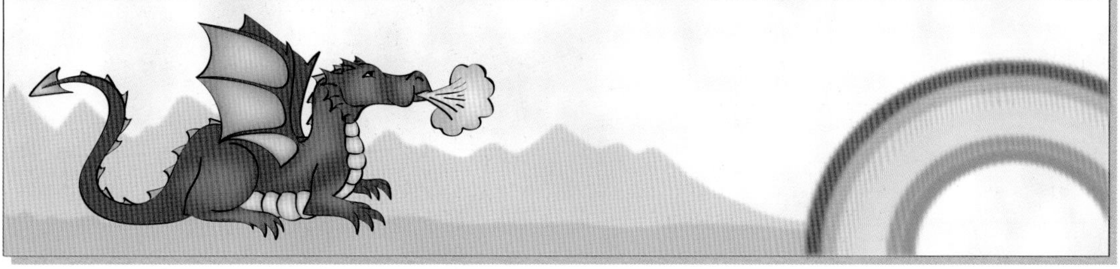

**Figure 13.15** Diabetic diary showing good control. Note hypoglycaemia during one night.

### Glycosylated haemoglobin (HbA₁c)

Blood glucose monitoring is very dependent on the compliance of the individual. Glycosylated haemoglobin ($HbA_{1c}$) levels have the advantage of providing an objective measure of the child's control, and are the benchmark for changes in management and give motivation to both the family and the physician.

$HbA_{1c}$ reflects the prevailing blood glucose levels over the previous couple of months. In simplistic terms the $A_{1c}$ fraction of haemoglobin becomes irreversibly 'sticky' (or glycosylated) in proportion to the degree of hyperglycaemia. In normal individuals 4–6% of the $HbA_{1c}$ fraction is glycosylated. For diabetic individuals in good control, $HbA_{1c}$ levels are almost normal, but levels above 10% reflect poor control which has been running over a number of months at least.

## Management of acute problems

### Diabetic ketoacidosis

Diabetic ketoacidosis is precipitated when insulin levels fall below the child's requirements. This may occur as a result of non-compliance or because of increased requirements, as occurs with infection. Some individuals, particularly adolescents, have brittle diabetes and develop ketoacidosis very easily. The cycle of events is shown in Figure 13.10 (see also p. 95).

Diabetic ketoacidosis is a medical emergency and must be treated immediately. Treatment requires skill, the particular dangers being hypokalaemia or cerebral oedema, which may cause death. Management consists of careful rehydration, provision of insulin, replacement of electrolytes and treatment of any precipitating infection (Table 13.6).

### Hypoglycaemia

Virtually all diabetic children experience some hypoglycaemic attacks at some time. They are an almost inevitable accompaniment to management, which emphasizes the importance of good control. The symptoms and signs include pallor, hunger, sweating, trembling and tachycardia, and may proceed to drowsiness, mental confusion, seizures and coma. Hypoglycaemia is easily differentiated from ketoacidosis as it occurs over a span of minutes as opposed to hours or days.

Hypoglycaemia indicates that there is too much insulin relative to food intake and energy expenditure. Common causes include errors in insulin dose, inadequate caloric intake, and physical activity in the absence of food intake.

**Table 13.6** Management of diabetic ketoacidosis

| |
|---|
| General resuscitation if in shock (see p. 378) |
| Clinical assessment including weight and signs of infection |
| Cardiac monitor |
| Intravenous line and investigations (glucose, blood gases, electrolytes, full blood count, cultures) |
| *Rehydration* (see p. 388) |
| Normal saline should be used initially |
| Care must be taken, as overzealous fluid replacement can precipitate lethal cerebral oedema |
| *Insulin* |
| Low-dose intravenous insulin is given continuously by pump |
| Blood glucose monitoring must be carried out frequently to titrate the insulin dose. Once the blood glucose level has fallen, dextrose is added to the solution and insulin continued as it is still required to clear the ketones |
| *Electrolytes* |
| Acidosis drives the potassium out of the cells and depletion occurs as a result of diuresis. Potassium must be replaced and is added to the intravenous solution once the child has passed urine (so ensuring functional kidneys) |
| *Identification of infection* |
| Clinical and laboratory search for infection is required |
| When the diabetic ketoacidosis is under control, subcutaneous insulin can be introduced, initially using regular doses of short-acting insulin on a sliding scale, followed by the child's normal dose. Oral fluids followed by a regular diet can be introduced |

Hypoglycaemia is treated, if the child is conscious, by giving dextrose tablets or a carbohydrate-containing snack or drink. If the child is unable to drink or eat, a glucose gel can be squeezed on to the buccal mucosa. The family should also be taught how to inject glucagon (which releases hepatic glucose stores) intramuscularly if the child is unconscious. Intravenous 10% glucose solution is administered if medical personnel are available. It is important that the family has an understanding of the precipitating factors of the attack, and that adjustments in snacks or insulin dose are considered.

### Routine follow-up of the child with diabetes (see Checklist)

In most areas special diabetes clinics are established, which often incorporate education sessions and opportunities for families to meet as well as routinely reviewing the child's diabetic condition. In addition to these clinic visits, families must have access to appropriate medical advice at all times to help them cope competently with acute problems as they occur.

There are particular periods when families are likely to need extra advice and input:

- *At diagnosis.* Obviously at the onset of the condition the family will require a great deal of input in order for them to grasp the principles and practicalities of management. Initially glucose control is usually smooth as the child often has some reserves of insulin which buffer glucose swings. This period after diagnosis is called the honeymoon period and may last for several months.
- *In toddlerhood.* These years are characterized by the child asserting him- or herself in a typically unreasonable manner. Two particular difficulties may occur as a result. The first is picky eating and food refusal, which can result in hypoglycaemia. If food refusal is a consistent problem, insulin may have to be given after the meal and adjusted to the quantity of food eaten. The second problem is recognition of hypoglycaemia. Normal temper tantrums may be impossible to distinguish from hypoglycaemia, and it is hardly advisable to treat them with sweet rewards. Blood glucose tests differentiate the two.
- *In the adolescent years.* Adolescence is a difficult period for the family with a diabetic. The stresses of adolescence, hormonal changes, often erratic lifestyle and compliance all contribute to disrupting diabetic control. The adolescent also requires extra advice about avoiding smoking, alcohol excesses and contraception.
- *During illness.* Illness places an extra stress on the child and demands extra insulin. It is often the trigger for diabetic ketoacidosis. Interestingly, the first sign of an infection can be a rise in glucose levels.
- *During stress.* Stress, whether physical such as in accidents, or psychological, increases insulin demands. This may be mediated by secretion of the stress hormones cortisol and adrenaline.

**Clinical assessment**

**History.** A well-kept diary will provide all the details required to review the child's condition. However, in

---

### ✓ Checklist for review of a child with diabetes

**If the child is new to you or the clinic, check:**
- ☐ Family's understanding of diabetes and their ability to make adjustments in insulin dose
- ☐ Who gives the insulin and whether by pen or syringe
- ☐ Blood glucose monitoring is being performed
- ☐ School is well informed
- ☐ Family is aware of the British Diabetes Association

**At routine follow-up, review:**
*History*
Review diary and ask about:
- ☐ Blood glucose levels
- ☐ Symptoms of hypo- and hyperglycaemia
- ☐ Dietary difficulties
- ☐ Problems at school, related or unrelated to diabetes
- ☐ If in poor control, assess compliance with injections and diet, and any new stresses

*Physical examination*
- ☐ Height and weight
- ☐ Injection sites for lipoatrophy or hypertrophy
- ☐ Fundi and blood pressure

*Investigations*
- ☐ HbA$_{1c}$
- ☐ Thyroid function tests if thyromegaly or fall-off in growth
- ☐ Ophthalmological exam yearly from 8 years after onset

*Action*
- ☐ Advise on adjustments in insulin and diet
- ☐ Encourage child to take more responsibility as he or she grows
- ☐ Counsel about particular issues such as:
  - food refusal in toddlers
  - compliance, smoking, alcohol and contraception in adolescence

its absence the family should be asked about symptoms of hypo- and hyperglycaemia, dietary difficulties, blood glucose levels and any problems at school related or unrelated to diabetes. If the child is in poor control, any new stresses should be sought and compliance with injections and diet should be gently ascertained.

**Physical examination.** A full physical examination is not required at every review. However, monitoring of growth is important, both as a measure of control and also as an indication of hypothyroidism or coeliac disease. Injection sites should be inspected for lipoatrophy or lipohypertrophy, as this can both be unsightly and affect the absorption of insulin. Fundi should be inspected and blood pressure measured annually.

**Investigations.** Glycosylated haemoglobin levels are an objective measure of blood glucose control. It is most helpful if a recent level is available at the time of the review, as encouragement or advice can be given accordingly. Assessment of thyroid function and coeliac disease is required if a fall-off in growth is observed. Every child needs an eye examination by an ophthalmologist if the diabetes is of more than 8–10 years' duration.

### Advice

The visit should not only focus on advice about adjustments in insulin and diet, although this of course is important. The issues discussed in the introductory section on chronic illness (p. 36) are particularly relevant to the diabetic child as the condition has implications in every facet of his or her life. The family will need advice as the child grows and passes through stages, each of which brings its own problems. Over the years the child has to be encouraged to take on more responsibility for him- or herself. It is important that the transition from the paediatric to the adult clinic should be smooth so that the individual can face the problems of diabetes in adult life with good support.

## Prognosis

The survival of young people with diabetes is excellent. The prognosis no longer depends on overcoming the potentially life-threatening problems of hypoglycaemia and ketoacidosis, but depends on the long-term complications which develop years if not decades after onset. As the development of these problems is related to preceding metabolic control, how the individual is managed in childhood will have repercussions on the long-term quality of life.

## Issues for the family
### Education

The education given at the onset of diabetes is critical in providing the family with a good approach as well as giving them the practical skills required to manage the condition. Apart from having to adjust to a life-long medical condition, they have to cope with learning the technicalities of insulin injections, blood glucose monitoring, managing potentially life-threatening hypoglycaemia and ketoacidosis, and dietary changes.

### Coping with crises

Experienced families can cope with episodes of hyperglycaemia and even mild diabetic ketoacidosis at home with support by giving frequent injections of short-acting insulin. They should always have a snack and glucose gel at hand to cope with hypoglycaemia, and should also have glucagon available for a severe reaction. The other life crises of toddlerhood and adolescence may be more problematic.

### Reactions of others

Diabetes is a condition that, although not obviously visible, is very evident to others, and often provokes negative reactions and even fear.

### Genetic

Although diabetes is not a genetic disease, there is an increased risk of about one in 20 for first-degree relatives. Special care is required during pregnancy, as there are risks for the fetus if control is not exemplary. Teenage girls therefore need advice about contraception and planning pregnancies.

### Support

Families with diabetes need plenty of support. On the medical front, arguably the most important person is the diabetic nurse specialist. Diabetes UK gives families the opportunity to be mutually supportive, and children often find it helpful to attend their camps.

## Issues at school

The school has to be aware of the child with diabetes and understand the implications of the condition. The

## The child with diabetes at a glance

### Epidemiology
1 in 500 children

### Aetiology/pathophysiology
Destruction of the beta cells in the islets of Langerhans, resulting in insulin deficiency

### How the diagnosis is made
Children usually present with polyuria, polydipsia, and weight loss. Diagnosis is confirmed by finding raised blood sugar levels. A glucose tolerance test is not required in children

### Clinical features
*Poor control (hyperglycaemia)*
*History*
- Polydipsia
- Polyuria and enuresis
- Hypoglycaemic episodes*

*Physical examination*
- Poor growth
- Lipoatrophy/dystrophy

*Investigations*
- High blood sugar
- High HbA$_{1c}$

### Ketoacidosis
*History*
- Thirst and polyuria
- Vomiting
- Abdominal pain

*Physical examination*
- Acetone smell on breath
- Dehydration
- Kussmaul breathing
- Hypovolaemic shock*
- Drowsiness/coma*

*Investigations*
- Very high blood sugar, ketonuria
- Blood gases – metabolic acidosis
- Urea and electrolytes deranged

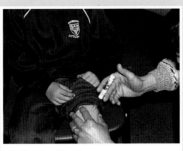
Injecting insulin using a pen

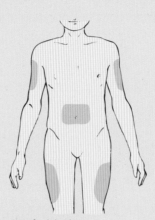
Sites for injections

### Clinical features (cont.)
*Hypoglycaemia*
*History*
- Hunger
- Shakiness

*Physical examination*
- Pallor
- Sweating
- Tachycardia
- Tremor
- Drowsiness
- Seizures
- Coma

*Investigations*
- Low blood sugar often followed by rebound high blood sugar

### General management
A specialist team should be involved

### Initial management: correction of metabolic state and education of the family
*Medication:*
Insulin (see Table 13.5 and Box 13.2)
Nutritional control
*Monitoring:*
Blood glucose by finger prick at home
HbAlc levels
*Education:*
Self-management of diabetic control
Injection technique
Diet
Coping with hypo/hyperglycaemia
Liaison with school

### Management of acute problems
Hypoglycaemia (see Box 13.2)
Diabetic ketoacidosis (see Table 13.6 and Box 13.2)

### Points for routine follow-up

*Monitor*
- diary of symptoms of hypo- and hyperglycaemia
- dietary difficulties
- intercurrent illness and stress
- growth
- injection sites
- blood pressure
- fundi

*Investigations*
HbA$_{1c}$, thyroid function tests, ophthalmological exam

### Prognosis
Lifelong condition. Complications of retinopathy, nephropathy, neuropathy and atherosclerosis are not usually seen until beyond childhood and are related to the degree of diabetic control attained

diabetes nurse specialist makes a point of going to the school at the outset to prepare school staff for the newly diabetic child's return, but it must be remembered that re-education is needed over time and when there is a change of school. The school must be able to recognize and manage hypoglycaemia, and cope with the dietary requirements of snacks at odd times. Staff can also be very helpful in reporting untoward symptoms and non-compliance.

*To test your knowledge on this part of the book, please see Chapter 25.*

# CHAPTER 14

# Musculo-skeletal disorders

*A general pain of all the joints . . . The disease lies concealed for a long time, when the pain and the disease are kindled up by any slight cause . . . It is incredible how far the mischief spreads.*
*Aretaeus, 1st century AD*

## COMPETENCES

### You must . . .

| Know | Be able to | Appreciate |
|---|---|---|
| • How to diagnose and manage common condition presenting with leg pain, limp or swollen joints<br>• The common presentations of juvenile chronic arthritis | • Examine the knee and hip joints competently<br>• Recognize the common conditions that can alter gait<br>• Recognize associated features of rare but significant causes of limp such as leukaemia | • The importance of rapidly diagnosing septic arthritis before destruction of the joint occurs<br>• The impact that juvenile chronic arthritis has on the child and family |

# Musculoskeletal symptoms and signs

## Finding your way around . . .

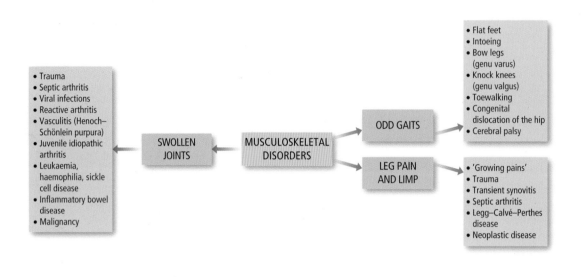

## Leg pain and limp

**Causes of leg pain and limp**

| | |
|---|---|
| *Organic* | Osteomyelitis |
| Transient synovitis | Neoplastic disease |
| Septic arthritis | Systemic disease |
| Legg–Calvé–Perthes disease | |
| Slipped capital femoral epiphysis | *Non-organic* |
| Trauma | Growing pains |

The complaint of leg pain alone, unaccompanied by physical signs, is usually non-organic in nature. Limp, however, is likely to have an underlying organic explanation. *Transient synovitis* is the commonest cause of limp and must be distinguished from *septic arthritis*, which if missed can lead to destruction of the joint.

*Trauma* when acute is an obvious cause of pain; however, chronic pain can result from stress fractures or prolonged healing of muscle haematoma. The pain of *osteomyelitis* is usually accompanied by swelling, erythema and tenderness, but it may present subclinically. Leg pain caused by sickling crisis is a cardinal sign in *sickle cell anaemia*, and children with *haemophilia* may have leg pain as a result of bleeding into the tissues. *Juvenile idiopathic arthritis* and the *collagen vascular diseases* tend to present with swelling of the joints (see p. 286) rather than arthralgia. Both *Legg–Calvé–Perthes disease* (avascular necrosis of the femoral head) and *slipped capital femoral epiphyses* are paediatric causes of leg pain. *Neoplastic disease*, such as leukaemia or osteosarcoma, is the most potentially serious cause. Leg pain without an organic cause is commonly called *growing pains*.

In a child presenting with acute or recurrent leg pain, a good history and physical examination should differentiate non-organic from organic causes. Investigations may be required to identify the aetiology where organic disease is suspected.

## History – must ask!

Focus on the characteristics of the pain and any systemic symptoms that the child might have.

- *What is the pain like?* Pain from organic causes tends to be persistent, occurring day and night, and interrupts play as well as schooling. Particularly significant is a limp or refusal to walk. Organic pain is often unilateral or located to a joint. By contrast, non-organic pain usually occurs at night and primarily on school days. It does not interfere with normal activities, and the parents report a normal gait. It is often bilateral and located between joints.
- *Are there systemic symptoms?* Systemic symptoms such as weight loss, fever, night sweats, rash and diarrhoea point to organic causes.

## Physical examination – must check!

Examine the child lying down and then walking. Remember that pain in the hip may be referred to the knee, so that a child presenting with knee pain requires a full examination of the leg and groin.

- *The limb.* Look for signs of point tenderness, redness, swelling and muscle weakness or atrophy. Examine the joints for limitation of movement. In non-organic pain the examination is normal, although you may see minor changes such as coolness or mottling of the leg.
- *General examination.* Look for evidence of fever, rash, pallor, lymphadenopathy or organomegaly, which suggest infectious or systemic causes.

## Investigations

If the leg pain is thought to be pathological, the investigations listed in Table 14.1 may be indicated.

**Table 14.1** Laboratory tests helpful in diagnosing leg pain

| Investigation | What you are looking for |
| --- | --- |
| Blood count | Leukaemia |
| | Infections |
| | Collagen vascular disease |
| Plasma viscosity | Infections |
| Erythrocyte sedimentation rate | Collagen vascular disease |
| C-reactive protein | Inflammatory bowel disease |
| | Tumours |
| X-ray | Bone tumours |
| | Infection |
| | Trauma |
| | Avascular necrosis |
| | Leukaemia |
| | Slipped capital femoral epiphysis |
| Bone scan | Osteomyelitis |
| | Stress fractures |
| | Malignant tumours |
| Muscle enzymes | Damage to muscle cells |

## Managing leg pain

In the child where no organic cause is suspected, the approach described in Box 9.1, p. 168, may be helpful.

> ### Key points: Leg pain or a limp
>
> - Organic and non-organic causes can be differentiated on clinical grounds
> - Important features suggesting organic disease are limp or refusal to walk, and any physical signs
> - Pain in the hip is referred to the knee, so children with knee pain require a full examination of the leg and groin

| Q | Clues to the differential diagnosis of leg pain |
|---|---|

|  | **Organic** | **Non-organic** |
|---|---|---|
| **Characteristics** | Day and night | Only at night |
|  | Interrupts play | Primarily school days |
|  | Unilateral | No interference with normal activities |
|  | Located in joint | Located between joints |
|  | Limp or refusal to walk | Bilateral |
|  |  | Normal gait |
| **History** | Weight loss | Otherwise healthy child |
|  | Fever |  |
|  | Night sweats |  |
|  | Rash |  |
|  | Diarrhoea |  |
| **Physical examination** | Point tenderness | Normal examination or minor changes such as coolness or mottling of leg |
|  | Redness |  |
|  | Swelling |  |
|  | Limitation of movement |  |
|  | Muscle weakness or atrophy |  |
|  | Fever, rash, pallor, lymphadenopathy, organomegaly |  |

## Swollen joints

| **Causes of swollen joints** | |
|---|---|
| Trauma | |
| Infection | Septic arthritis, viral |
| Reactive arthritis | Post-streptococcal or gastrointestinal infections |
| Vasculitis | Henoch–Schönlein purpura |
| Collagen vascular disease | Juvenile chronic arthritis, systemic lupus erythematosus |
| Haematological disease | Leukaemia, haemophilia, sickle cell disease |
| Gastrointestinal disease | Ulcerative colitis, Crohn's disease |
| Malignancy | Leukaemia |

Swollen joints from causes other than trauma are not very common in childhood. They include viral or reactive causes, but more serious pathology must be excluded, the most critical being *septic arthritis*, which demands urgent diagnosis and treatment.

A number of conditions can lead to persistent or recurrent joint swelling. *Juvenile chronic arthritis* (JCA), a chronic condition of childhood, is the most important and has three different patterns of presentation. Children with *ulcerative colitis* or *Crohn's disease* can also experience arthritis, which tends to coincide with periods of active bowel disease. *Leukaemia* and other malignancies occasionally present with swelling of one or more joints and pain, which is often severe. These need to be considered particularly if anaemia, thrombocytopenia or white blood cell abnormalities are present.

Haemarthrosis affecting elbows, knees and ankles is a hallmark of *haemophilia*. The bleeding often seems to be spontaneous, but does not form a diagnostic problem as children present earlier in life with obvious bleeding. Children with *sickle cell disease* may have symmetrical, painful swelling of the hands and feet as a result of vaso-occlusive crises. *Henoch–Schönlein purpura*, a diffuse allergic vasculitis characterized by a distinctive rash (see Figure 17.14), is often accompanied by pain in the joints with or without swelling.

Viral infections, notably rubella, can resemble chronic rheumatic disease. *Reactive arthritis* is a sterile arthritis affecting one or more joints which may follow any streptococcal infection or bacterial gastro-enteritis. The arthritis is generally transient and the outcome good.

As ever, a thorough clinical evaluation is essential, as the history and distribution of the joints involved provide clues to the underlying problem.

### History – must ask!

• *Joint symptoms.* Stiffness is an important complaint which may be localized or generalized. In most inflammatory arthropathies, the stiffness that occurs in the morning or after periods of inactivity is alleviated by activity, whereas mechanical problems are exacerbated by activity. A history of pain or swelling of other joints is obviously relevant.
• *Systemic symptoms.* Once you have discounted trauma, you must establish whether the child's symptoms are specific to the joint(s) or whether there are clues present, such as fever, anorexia, weight loss, rash, weakness and fatigue, that suggest a systemic cause.
• *Past medical and family history.* Important information in the past medical and family history includes inflammatory bowel disease, autoimmune conditions, blood dyscrasias and psoriasis: these are all associated with arthritis.

### Physical examination – must check!

• *Musculoskeletal system.* Your examination should include all four limbs and the spine. Carefully examine the affected joints by inspection and palpation, looking for skin colour changes, heat, tenderness, range of motion and asymmetry. In the young child it is very helpful to observe normal active motion, especially gait, to pinpoint the joints involved.
• *General examination.* Unless there is a clear history of trauma to the joint, the child needs a full physical examination looking for signs such as anaemia, hepatosplenomegaly, cardiac murmurs and rash, which might be associated with systemic disease.

### Investigations

Most children presenting with arthritis or joint swelling require investigations. These are described in Table 14.2.

**Table 14.2** Useful investigations in the child with swollen joints and their relevance

| Investigation | Relevance |
| --- | --- |
| Full blood count | Elevated white count and shift to the left with bacterial infection<br>Anaemia in collagen vascular diseases, inflammatory bowel disease, malignancy<br>Characteristic features of the haemoglobinopathies |
| ESR and plasma viscosity | Elevated in bacterial infection, very high in collagen vascular disease and inflammatory bowel disease |
| Blood culture | Positive in septic arthritis |
| ASO titre | Indicative of recent streptococcal infection – reactive arthritis or, very rarely, rheumatic fever |
| Viral titres | Viral arthritis |
| Rheumatoid factor and antinuclear antibodies | Negative in most forms of juvenile chronic arthritis |
| X-ray of the joint | Characteristic depending on the underlying aetiology |
| Joint aspiration | Microscopy and culture to exclude/confirm septic arthritis. May be helpful in other conditions |

ESR, erythrocyte sedimentation rate.

### Key points: Swollen joints

• Trauma is the commonest cause of an isolated swollen joint
• If the joint is acutely swollen, rule out septic arthritis as the cause
• Elicit any systemic symptoms
• Clues to the underlying diagnosis are provided by the history and distribution of the joints involved
• An isolated swollen joint that does not settle within a few days should be X-rayed to rule out a bone tumour

# Unusual gait

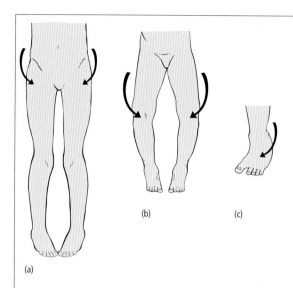

**Figure 14.1** Types of intoeing: (a) femoral anteversion, (b) tibial torsion, and (c) metatarsus adductus.

Parents not uncommonly have concerns about the shape of their child's legs or their gait. They are rarely of significance, and reassurance is usually all that is required. The child should be observed walking independently and without a nappy, trousers, socks or shoes, and then on standing still, from in front and from behind. All the joints should be examined lying down (see p. 78).

**Flat feet.** Most babies have flat feet, the arch gradually developing through childhood. Flat feet in childhood are painless and need no therapy.

**Intoeing.** Intoeing (see Figure 14.1) may occur as a result of rotation of the leg at the hip (femoral anteversion), at the tibia (medial tibial torsion) or in the foot (metatarsus adductus). The diagnosis is made clinically. The only condition which requires orthopaedic intervention is metatarsus adductus, as buying shoes is problematic if the feet are curved. Otherwise intoeing usually resolves by 4 or 5 years of age.

**Bow legs and knock-knees.** During the first 2 years the legs are naturally bowed in shape. During the third and fourth year a physiological knock-knee pattern emerges, which straightens by the age of 10 years, although may persist in the obese. Only rarely nowadays are bow legs indicative of rickets or other pathology.

**Toewalking.** Some children start to walk on their toes. This is usually a normal variant, but is occasionally a sign of cerebral palsy, which can be determined by neurological examination of the legs.

**Congenital dislocation of the hip.** This is usually detected through screening before the child starts to walk, but should be considered if there is a limp (see p. 284).

**Cerebral palsy.** Occasionally mild forms of cerebral palsy present with an abnormal hemiplegic or diplegic gait (see pp. 72, 237). The diagnosis is made clinically by the finding of spasticity, increased deep tendon reflexes and an extensor plantar response in affected legs.

# Musculoskeletal disorders

## Growing pains

'Growing pains' is a term used for the common complaint of leg pain in children where organic disease has been excluded. The complaint tends to occur in the 3- to 6-year-old age group. The term is a misnomer as the pain does not appear to be related to growth, but may be caused by oedema in the fascial sheaths.

**Clinical features.** Limp is not a feature. The pain classically occurs at night, often after a day of vigorous activity. These children also not infrequently experience headaches and abdominal pain.

**Management.** Symptoms usually respond to heat and massage and may need simple analgesia. As in all cases of functional pain, psychosomatic factors should be considered. The approach described in Box 9.1, p. 168, may be helpful.

## Trauma

Trauma is a common cause of joint pain and swelling in childhood, and in this case the cause of the swelling is obvious. Two paediatric forms of joint trauma are worthy of particular mention.

*Pulled elbow* or *'nursemaid's' elbow* is a common mishap which occurs in the toddler age group. The child may not complain of pain but refuses to use the arm and holds it in a flexed position. The precipitating cause is sudden forceful traction on the arm, causing dislocation at the elbow. This usually happens when a reluctant child is dragged by the arm, or trips while being held by the hand (Figure 14.2). The condition is treated by simply supinating the arm fully causing the head of the ulnar to click back into place. No post-reduction fixation is necessary. The parents need to be alerted to the cause in order to avoid recurrence.

The other traumatic joint problem peculiar to childhood is *fracture of the growth plate*. When a child traumatizes a joint, the most vulnerable structure is the growth plate, rather than the ligaments. Children presenting with swelling of a joint following trauma may well have a fracture through the growth plate rather than a ligamentous sprain. The fracture is not easily seen on X-ray. Treatment consists of immobilizing the joint for some weeks.

## Osteomyelitis

Osteomyelitis affects the metaphyses of long bones and is usually haematogenous in origin. The commonest organisms are *Staphylococcus aureus*, *Haemophilus influenzae* and *Streptococcus pyogenes*.

**Clinical features.** Children may present with pain or PUO, and the infected limb is obviously tender and held immobile. Swelling and redness eventually appear. The adjacent joint may contain a sterile 'sympathetic' effusion. The erythrocyte sedimentation rate (ESR) is high and the white cell count elevated.

**Management.** Repeated blood culture determines the causative organism. X-rays are not of any diagnostic help in the first 10 days as it takes time for the radiological changes of the subperiosteum to develop.

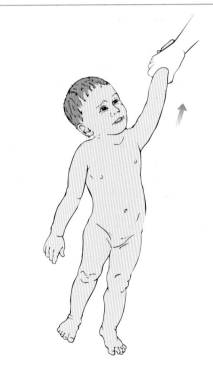

**Figure 14.2** Nursemaid's elbow. Sudden forceful traction dislocates the elbow joint.

Bone scans, however, are useful early in the course of the disease. High-dose intravenous antibiotics are required initially. Once blood inflammatory markers and temperatures settle, the child can be changed to high-dose oral antibiotics, which should be continued for a total of at least 4 weeks. If there is no immediate response, surgical exploration and drainage is required. If the infection is inadequately treated, irreversible bone necrosis, draining sinuses and limb deformity can occur.

## 👁 Osteomyelitis at a glance

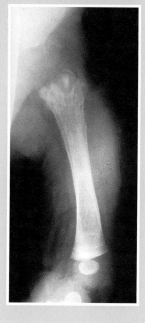

**Aetiology**
Infection of the metaphysis
  (usually blood-borne)
Organisms: *Staphylococcus
  aureus*
*Haemophilus influenzae*
*Streptococcus pyogenes*

**History**
Fever
Painful limb

**Physical examination**
Swelling and redness at site
Sympathetic effusion of
  adjacent joint*

**Confirmatory investigations**
High white cell count and
  erythrocyte sedimentation rate
Blood culture (repeat samples
  needed)

Bone scan to detect early
  changes
Subperiosteal changes on X-ray
  seen only after 10 days

**Differential diagnosis**
Soft tissue infection
Trauma
Malignancy
Septic arthritis

**Management**
High-dose antibiotics for 4
  weeks
Surgical exploration and
  drainage

**Prognosis/complications**
If inadequately treated may lead
  to bone necrosis, draining
  sinuses, limb deformity

NB *Signs and symptoms are variable.

## Transient synovitis

Transient synovitis is the commonest cause of limp in young children, usually affecting boys aged 2–8 years. It is a benign condition, the major significance being the possibility of overlooking septic arthritis of the hip.

**Clinical features.** There is a sudden onset of limp with hip and/or knee pain. A mild UTI may precede the symptoms. On examination there is limited abduction, extension and internal rotation of the hip. Transient synovitis can be differentiated from septic arthritis by the lack of systemic symptoms and signs, a normal white cell count, normal or only mildly elevated erythrocyte sedimentation rate, and a normal hip X-ray.

**Management and prognosis.** Transient synovitis lasts for a few days or weeks and treatment consists of rest and simple analgesia.

## Septic arthritis

Septic arthritis is a serious cause of joint swelling which, if untreated, rapidly leads to destruction of the joint. Infection usually affects the larger weight-bearing joints such as hip, knee and ankle. The commonest organism is a staphylococcus, but *Haemophilus influenzae* may also be responsible. These organisms are blood-borne.

**Clinical features.** Children present with fever and a hot, tender, swollen joint. Occasionally more than one joint may be involved. Movement of the joint is limited and extremely painful. When the hip is involved, the leg is held in a flexed and abducted posture and may not appear swollen or hot to the touch. In neonatal septic arthritis, the baby usually looks very ill and holds the limb immobile ('pseudo-paralysis').

**Investigations.** Supportive evidence of bacterial infection may be found in the white cell count and elevated erythrocyte sedimentation rate and C-reactive protein. Ultrasound or X-ray of the joint may show widening of the joint space caused by fluid accumulation, and in some cases signs of an adjacent osteomyelitis. Aspiration of the joint should be carried out urgently for microscopy and culture. The joint fluid is purulent with organisms found on Gram's stain.

**Management.** Treatment involves intravenous antibiotics, and local instillation of antibiotic into the affected joint may be beneficial. Intravenous flucloxacillin plus a penicillin or cephalosporin is the treatment of choice. The joint needs to be splinted in the acute stage. Once temperatures and inflammatory markers settle, antibiotics are switched to the oral route and 2–4 weeks of therapy are necessary. As soon as pain has subsided, a full range of joint mobility needs to be encouraged, with physiotherapy to prevent joint flexion deformities.

**Prognosis.** With early and effective treatment the prognosis is very good. If the diagnosis is delayed, destruction of the joint may occur. This is most likely in the neonate.

## Legg–Calvé–Perthes disease

Legg–Calvé–Perthes disease (avascular necrosis of the femoral head) is a relatively common condition affect-

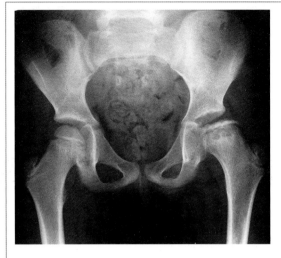

**Figure 14.3** X-ray of the hips of a 5-year-old child with Legg–Calvé–Perthes disease. Note the increased density, flattening and fragmentation of the left capital femoral epiphysis.

ing children, principally boys, between the ages of 4 and 10 years. It may follow on from an episode of transient synovitis. The aetiology of the avascular necrosis is unknown.

**Clinical features.** The condition is initially painless, but once a crush fracture develops, pain in the hip or knee and limp are major features. Diagnosis is made by X-ray (Figure 14.3) or bone scan.

**Management and prognosis.** Treatment involves bracing or traction and recovery may take 2–3 years.

## Slipped capital femoral epiphysis

Slipped capital femoral epiphysis is a condition classically occurring in overweight sedentary teenage boys.

**Clinical features.** Pain is experienced in the groin or medial side of the knee, often gradual in onset. On examination the hip is held in abduction and external rotation with limitation of internal rotation. X-ray confirms the diagnosis (Figure 14.4).

**Management.** Treatment is surgical.

## Neoplastic disease

Neoplastic disease is the most potentially serious of all causes of limb pain, and should always be considered if limb pain or limp persists for more than a few days. Malignant tumours usually initially present with pain, and in some cases are palpable as a tender mass, which is seen as a destructive bony lesion on X-ray. Benign tumours also occur and may also present as a mass or pain. Leukaemic bone disease is harder to diagnose.

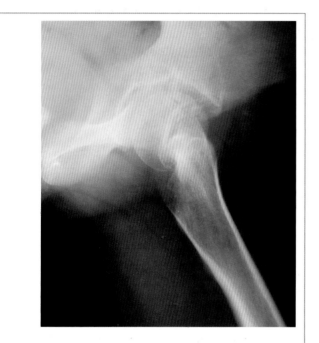

**Figure 14.4** X-ray of an obese boy with slipped capital femoral epiphysis.

The pain is described as deep and throbbing and often wakes the child at night. Diagnosis is often made on the blood count, but X-rays are only sometimes helpful.

## Juvenile idiopathic arthritis

Juvenile idiopathic arthritis (JIA) is one of the most common rheumatic disease of children and is a major cause of chronic disability. It is characterized by synovitis of the peripheral joints, with soft tissue swelling and effusion. There are three main patterns of presentation – systemic, poly- and pauci-articular arthritis. Each form has distinctive clinical features and the prognoses differ. The various features are summarized in Table 14.3.

### Systemic juvenile idiopathic arthritis (Still's' disease)

This is the rarest form of JIA. It often presents as a diagnostic puzzle as the child may not have any joint symptoms at the outset. He or she looks ill with a remitting fever, variable rash, hepatosplenomegaly, anaemia, weight loss or abdominal pain. Joint symptoms may be overlooked in view of the other systemic features. Sepsis and malignancy are often considered in the diagnosis. There are no characteristic laboratory findings, and rheumatoid factor is negative, making the diagnosis at times difficult to confirm.

### Polyarticular juvenile idiopathic arthritis

Children with polyarticular JIA present with painful swelling and restricted movement of both large and

**Table 14.3** Features of juvenile idiopathic arthritis

| Type | Characteristics | Sex ratio | Rhesus factor/ ANA* | Iridocyclitis | Severe arthritis |
|------|-----------------|-----------|---------------------|---------------|------------------|
| Systemic | Large and small joints affected | M>F | Negative | No | 25% |
| Polyarticular | Large and small joints affected | F>M | RhF negative, ANA may be positive | No | 12% |
| Pauciarticular | <5 joints, usually large | F>M | RhF negative, ANA may be positive | High risk | No usually |

*ANA, antinuclear antibody.

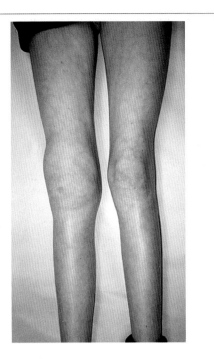

**Figure 14.5** A 10-year-old girl with pauciarticular juvenile idiopathic arthritis affecting the right knee.

small joints. This is commonly symmetrically distributed. Systemic features are not prominent, although poor weight gain and mild anaemia may occur. Morning stiffness is common and young children may be quite irritable. Rheumatoid factor is usually negative, although antinuclear antibodies may be positive. The prognosis for this type of JIA is generally good.

### Pauciarticular juvenile idiopathic arthritis (Figure 14.5)

Pauciarticular JIA commonly affects girls under the age of 4 years. By definition it involves few (fewer than five) joints, commonly knees, ankles and elbows. Systemic symptoms are minimal and the appearance of the joints is identical to those in the polyarticular

form. Rheumatoid factor is again negative, although antinuclear antibodies may be positive.

The important distinction between the two latter forms, apart from the number of joints involved, is the risk of chronic iridocyclitis. In pauciarticular arthritis, inflammation of the inner structures of the eye may lead to loss of vision and even permanent blindness. The changes are only detectable by slit lamp examination, and for this reason regular ophthalmological examinations are necessary.

### Management of the child with juvenile idiopathic arthritis

The aims of management are twofold:

- to preserve joint function;
- to help the child to achieve optimal psychosocial adjustment.

The goals of medical treatment are to reduce joint inflammation, maintain function and prevent deformity. Non-steroidal anti-inflammatory drugs are used to suppress the inflammation. Corticosteroids are indicated for severe systemic disease unresponsive to other therapies. Steroid injection into selected joints may be helpful, but should not be used repeatedly. Hydroxychloroquine, penicillamine, gold injections, methotrexate and immune regulatory drugs are used in severe disease.

Physical and occupational therapy are important to improve movement and physical strength in affected joints and to maintain the function of the child as a whole. Treatment consists of daily exercises, hydrotherapy, and day and night splints.

The family needs support, and children should be encouraged to lead as normal and self-sufficient lives as possible. Unpredictable exacerbations are disheartening, and families need encouragement to work at maintaining joint mobility. The prognosis in the various subgroups differs, but overall most children have a good prognosis with no or only minor disability in adulthood. Children with residual handicaps need help in vocational planning.

*To test your knowledge on this part of the book, please see Chapter 25.*

## Juvenile idiopathic arthritis at a glance

### Epidemiology
Three patterns occur: systemic (Still's disease) and pauciarticular in young children; polyarticular in older children

### Aetiology
Immune disorder

### Clinical features
*A. Systemic JIA:*

*History*
- fever and shaking chills
- malaise
- weight loss
- arthralgia*

*Physical examination*
- ill child
- high, spiking fever
- hepatosplenomegaly

*Lymphadenopathy*
- salmon pink rash*
- arthritis at onset*

*B. Pauciarticular JIA:*
*History*
- painful swollen joints

*Physical examination*
- <5 swollen joints (knees, ankles or elbows)

*C. Polyarticular JIA:*
*History*
- painful swollen joints
- poor weight gain

*Physical examination*
- swollen, tender large and small joints

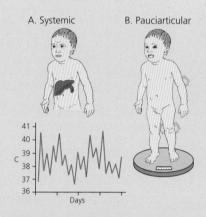

A. Systemic          B. Pauciarticular

C

Days

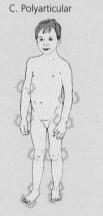

C. Polyarticular

NB Rule out sepsis

### Confirmatory investigations
High erythrocyte sedimentation rate
Anaemia with high white cell count
Rheumatoid factor – negative
ANA (antinuclear antibody) may be positive in pauci- and polyarticular types
X-ray: soft tissue swelling, periostitis, early loss of cartilage, bone destruction and fusion

### Differential diagnosis
Sepsis and malignancy in systemic type
Other causes of swollen joints in pauci- and polyarticular types (see Causes box, p. 286)

### Management
Reduction of inflammation using non-steroidal anti-inflammatory drugs
Steroids for severe disease
Physio- and occupational therapy
Psychosocial support

### Prognosis/complications
- Generally good, with eventual resolution of arthritis in most
- 25% of systemic type develop chronic disabling arthritis
- Pauciarticular form at high risk for chronic iridocyclitis

NB *Signs and symptoms are variable.

# CHAPTER 15

# Renal and urinary tract disorders

*And this little piggy went Wee, Wee, Wee all the way home.*
*English nursery rhyme*

## COMPETENCES

### You must . . .

| Know | Be able to | Appreciate |
| --- | --- | --- |
| • How to diagnose and manage the important and common conditions that cause urinary symptoms<br>• The criteria for diagnosing UTI on urine culture<br>• Advice for a child with dysuria due to perineal irritation<br>• How to manage nocturnal enuresis<br>• How to differentiate psychogenic from organic causes of enuresis | • Dipstick a urine specimen<br>• Interpret urinalysis findings | • How common the problem of nocturnal enuresis is in children and teenagers |

*Paediatrics and Child Health*, Third Edition. Mary Rudolf, Tim Lee, Malcolm Levene.
© 2011 Mary Rudolf, Tim Lee and Malcolm Levene. Published 2011 by Blackwell Publishing Ltd.

# Renal and urinary symptoms and signs

## Finding your way around . . .

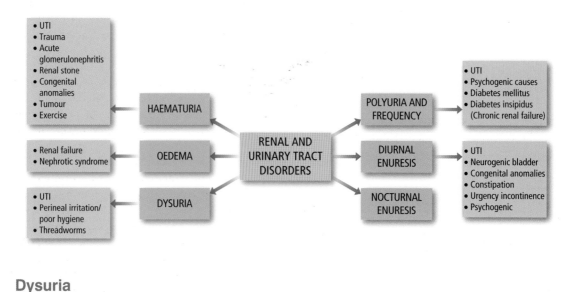

## Dysuria

**Causes of dysuria**

Urinary tract infections (see p. 303)
Irritation secondary to poor hygiene
Sensitivity to bubble baths or washing powder

Irritation secondary to threadworm infestation
(p. 190)

Dysuria, or pain on micturition, is commonly experienced by little girls secondary to vulval irritation and inflammation. Poor hygiene, bubble bath sensitivity and threadworms all irritate the delicate skin and mucous membranes and cause soreness. Poor hygiene may be a particular problem in young girls who have just achieved independent toileting but may not wipe themselves well or wash carefully. Paradoxically, bubble baths and soaps also cause dysuria by irritating the sensitive skin in this area.

Other causes include urinary tract infection (UTI), which is less frequently a cause but needs to be considered, particularly if fever is also present. Itching and soreness can be a problem for girls infested with threadworms, when the worms emerge from the anus and enter the perineal area. Candida infection is often overdiagnosed as a cause of dysuria in children who are out of nappies.

### History – must ask!

A history of UTIs or symptoms such as frequency, fever and abdominal pain suggest urine infection. Anal itching indicates irritation from threadworms.

### Physical examination – must check

The perineal area should be inspected for signs of inflammation and poor hygiene, and evidence of a discharge may be found in underwear.

### Investigations (see also p. 96)

Urine dipstick and urinalysis may be helpful, although it may well show protein, red and white cells from irritation even if there is no urine infection. If it tests positive for nitrites, infection is more likely. A urine culture is needed to assess if a UTI is present. If

- Take daily baths or wash with simple, non-perfumed soap or, if not too dirty, water alone
- Avoid bubble baths and talcum powder
- Only wear pure cotton knickers and preferably wear skirts. Constricting clothing such as nylon tights or tight trousers trap moisture and exacerbate irritation
- A barrier cream or nappy cream may help
- An empirical trial of mebendazole against threadworms can be given

itching is a problem, the child needs to be investigated for threadworms (see Figure 9.10) or empirically treated with mebendazole.

### Management

The management, if there is no urinary infection, lies in improving hygiene and reducing factors which lead to inflammation of the area (see Box 15.1). Treatment of urine infections is covered on p. 303.

## Diurnal enuresis

**Causes of diurnal enuresis**

*Organic*
Urinary tract infection
Neurogenic bladder
Congenital anomalies
Constipation (or, rarely, other pelvic masses)

*Physiological*
Urgency incontinence

*Psychogenic*

Diurnal enuresis can be defined as a lack of bladder control during the day in a child old enough to maintain bladder continence. Most children experiencing daytime enuresis also have nocturnal enuresis. In our culture bladder control usually occurs by the age of 2½ years, but it can be delayed beyond this without being abnormal.

The commonest cause of daytime wetting is *psychological*. When stressed, young children are likely to wet themselves. Common triggers are the birth of a sibling and school entry, when children may be too shy or embarrassed to ask permission to go to the

toilet. These children are helped by sympathy and support both at home and at school. However, enuresis may be part of a wider behavioural problem, when children become resistant and negative about using the toilet. Bowel continence may also be affected. Usually the toilet training has been highly pressurized, either in terms of endless lecturing or physical punishment. Management needs to be directed towards reducing pressure on the child and giving positive encouragement.

In contrast to nocturnal enuresis alone, which is nearly always non-organic in nature, diurnal enuresis requires exclusion of organic disease. This can usually be done on clinical grounds. *Urinary tract infections* are a consideration, although they usually present with symptoms of dysuria, frequency, abdominal pain and/or fever rather than enuresis alone.

Enuresis can result from *neurological dysfunction* of the bladder. It is usually evident that the child already has a neurological problem such as cerebral palsy or spina bifida, and gait disturbance or inadequate bowel control generally accompany the complaint. Neurological dysfunction can range from a spastic small bladder which empties suddenly without warning, to a large hypotonic bladder which fills to capacity and overflows. A neurogenic bladder may result from either an upper or lower motor neurone lesion, and features which suggest this are a distended bladder, abnormal perianal sensation and anal tone, and abnormal neurological findings in the legs. The finding of hairy patches or lipoma overlying the lower spine suggests a spinal anomaly responsible for the problem. Neurogenic bladder dysfunction is serious, not only because of the difficulties of incontinence, but also because such children are at risk for damage to the kidneys.

The commonest *congenital urinary tract anomalies* causing enuresis are ectopic ureters in girls and posterior urethral valves in boys. The ectopic ureter commonly ends in the vagina, causing continuous dampness and dribbling. Posterior urethral valves cause lower urinary tract obstruction and bladder distension with overflow incontinence. Both conditions are treated surgically.

*Pelvic masses*, the commonest being faecal impaction, may lead to stress incontinence which is particularly troublesome when running, coughing or lifting.

*Urgency incontinence* is more common in girls when bladder spasms lead to abrupt voiding. There is usually a lifelong history of urgency, but it is sometimes triggered by a UTI. Children may become very distressed by the problem and are usually well motivated to tackle it; treatment involves voiding at frequent intervals and training the child to increase control by practicing stream interruption exercises, such as those recommended in antenatal classes.

## History – must ask!

- *Is the enuresis primary or secondary?* Find out how old the child was when he or she was toilet trained. Enuresis is primary if bladder control has not yet been attained and secondary if a relapse in control has occurred.
- *Is the child ever dry?* Most enuresis is intermittent through the day, but if there is continuous dampness or leakage of urine, you must suspect an organic problem such as an ectopic ureter.
- *Are there other symptoms?* Symptoms of dysuria, frequency and haematuria or a prior UTI suggest a UTI. Suspect a neurogenic bladder if the child has coexisting bowel and gait difficulties.

## Physical examination – must check!

Examine the genitalia, abdomen, anus and legs, and if possible observe the urinary stream (in girls it is easier to listen than observe).

- *The abdomen.* A distended bladder suggests bladder outlet obstruction. This can be caused by abdominal masses – hard faeces or another mass.
- *The genitalia.* If the history suggests continuous wetting, inspect the vulval area for seepage of urine.

- *The back and legs.* Examine the back for a midline lipoma, hairy patch or spinal deformity, and the legs for neurological signs which would suggest spina bifida occulta (see p. 429) and a neurogenic bladder.
- *The anus.* Rectal examination is now only rarely carried out in children, but abnormal perianal sensation and anal tone suggest a neurogenic bladder, and a pelvic mass obstructing the urinary outlet may be felt.

## Laboratory investigations

The only baseline tests required are a urinalysis and urine culture, and even the latter is probably unnecessary in boys. If organic causes are suspected, imaging of the urinary tract by ultrasound, renal scan, intravenous pyelogram and uroscopy may be indicated, along with spinal X-rays.

---

**🔑 Key points: Diurnal enuresis**

- Establish if the enuresis is primary or secondary
- The commonest organic cause is urinary tract infection
- Continuous leakage of urine indicates an anatomic cause
- Features of a neurogenic bladder include a distended bladder, abnormal perianal sensation and anal tone, and abnormal neurological findings in the legs

---

**🔍 Clues to the diagnosis of diurnal enuresis**

| Condition | Type of enuresis | Other features |
|---|---|---|
| Urinary tract infection (UTI) | Secondary | Frequency, dysuria |
| Neurogenic bladder | Primary or secondary, depending on problem | Distended bladder, abnormal perianal sensation and anal tone, abnormal neurological findings in the legs, spinal deformity, lipoma and hairy patch |
| Congenital anomalies | Primary (or secondary if triggered by UTI) | Continuous leakage of urine<br>Distended bladder<br>Urinary tract infection in the preschool years |
| Constipation | Secondary | Infrequent stools<br>Faecal mass palpable in abdomen and per rectum |
| Physiological | Primary or secondary | Lifelong history of urgency |
| Psychogenic | Primary or secondary | Stress such as sibling birth or starting school<br>Behaviour problems |

# Nocturnal enuresis

## Causes of nocturnal enuresis

*Common*
Delayed maturation (often familial)
Emotional difficulties

*Rare*
Urinary tract infection
Causes of polyuria (see p. 299)

Nocturnal enuresis or bedwetting can be defined as being a problem when it occurs during more than one night a month. Enuresis may be primary (dryness never achieved) or secondary (a relapse of bladder control). Unlike diurnal enuresis, an organic problem is rarely implicated, although it is usual to exclude infection by urinalysis and culture, particularly if the problem is secondary rather than primary.

Enquiry may reveal stresses which have triggered the enuresis, common triggers being the birth of a sibling, moving to a new house or family dissension. As enuresis frequently runs in families, particularly among the males, it is important to enquire into a family history too. The physical examination usually contributes little to the diagnosis. Relevant signs are as described for diurnal enuresis.

# Polyuria and frequency

## Causes of frequent and excessive urination

Urinary tract infection
Psychogenic causes
Diabetes mellitus
Diabetes insipidus
(Chronic renal failure)

Polyuria and frequency may be difficult to differentiate on clinical grounds unless urine volume measurements are made, so these two problems are considered together. Both may result from organic disease but may also, and more commonly, arise from psychogenic causes. In your clinical evaluation you must differentiate the psychogenic causes from organic disease, which you need to go on and identify.

Urine infections are an important cause of *frequency*. However, more commonly frequency is a behavioural symptom. Young children around the time of acquiring bladder control often test and try their parents by frequent demands for the potty or toilet. This may be irritating for parents, but is rarely a major diagnostic problem. At a later age children often experience frequency and sometimes urgency when excited or frightened, and this too can usually be handled sensibly. More rarely, urinary frequency can be an indicator of more serious emotional problems and stress.

The commonest cause of *polyuria* is polydipsia. Obviously a child who drinks excessively will pass very large quantities of dilute urine. Usually the problem is simply one of habit, particularly in the toddler who is attached to a bottle.

Very rarely, polydipsia can be a sign of significant psychopathology. Children with diabetes mellitus commonly present with symptoms of polyuria and weight loss and are usually diagnosed within a few weeks of the onset, often before diabetic acidosis has developed. Unlike adults, they rarely present with chronic polyuria.

Diabetes insipidus is a rare condition in which there is an inability to concentrate urine. Polyuria also occurs in chronic renal failure and is caused by the loss of the kidney's ability to concentrate urine. It is unlikely to be the presenting symptom.

### History – must ask!

- *Pattern of urination.* You may be able to differentiate frequency and polyuria by taking a good history. In general, parents are more aware of the child who frequently urinates than the child who passes large quantities of urine at normal intervals. In any child who has only recently attained bladder control, any condition causing polyuria or frequency is likely to cause enuresis. If symptoms are absent through the night, a psychogenic cause is likely, although the reverse cannot be stated. UTIs may be associated with dysuria, abdominal pain and fever, although they may also be asymptomatic.
- *Thirst and pattern of drinking.* The key question by which to decide if polyuria rather than frequency alone is present, is to ask if the child is experiencing thirst. Thirst and polydipsia always accompany polyuria, whether it comes from an organic or psychogenic cause. Organic causes precipitate thirst secondary to decreased hydration and, conversely, excessive drinking for any reason results in increased urine output. However, thirst does not accompany frequency if there is no polyuria.

- *Behaviour.* Ask about behavioural and emotional issues, as the commonest causes of both frequency and polyuria are psychogenic.
- *Past medical history.* A history of poor growth, weight loss and head injury are significant in identifying the child with a chronic illness.

### Physical examination – must check!

The physical examination rarely contributes to the diagnosis of urinary symptoms. Height and weight measurements are important if only to provide a baseline for the future. Any signs of dehydration and weight loss are clearly concerning. It is good practice to examine the abdomen for bladder distension, kidney size and abdominal masses.

### Investigations

The most important bedside action is to obtain a sample of urine and carry out urinalysis prior to culture. Sugar in the urine indicates diabetes mellitus, blood and protein a UTI, and a low-specific-gravity polyuria, whether caused by diabetes insipidus or psychogenic polydipsia.

Psychogenic polydipsia can usually be differentiated from true diabetes insipidus by withdrawing fluids. In psychogenic polydipsia, urinary output should be reduced and urine concentration (specific gravity) increased. However, in long-standing cases the kidneys may become 'washed out' and may take a period to recover normal concentrating capacity. If there is serious concern that diabetes insipidus is present, the trial of fluid withdrawal must be carried out in hospital as the child in this case can become seriously dehydrated.

## Haematuria

**Causes of haematuria**

Urinary tract infection
Trauma
Acute glomerulonephritis
Stones and hypercalciuria
Congenital anomalies
Tumour
Bleeding disorder
Exercise
Drugs

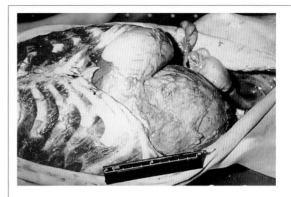

**Figure 15.1** Post-mortem photograph of an infant with Wilms' tumour.

Haematuria may be gross and evident to the eye, or microscopic and identified on dipstick or microscopy of the urinary sediment. It may occur as an isolated symptom or accompanied by signs of a systemic disorder. The commonest cause is UTI, whether bacterial or viral. Another important cause in childhood is acute glomerulonephritis, in which glomerular damage is inflicted by the formation of immune complexes, most commonly following a streptococcal infection. Gross or microscopic haematuria may also follow vigorous exercise. The source of bleeding is probably in the lower urinary tract. It resolves within 48 hours of cessation of exercise.

Blunt or penetrating injury to the abdomen may injure the kidney and cause haematuria, and if there is a urinary tract malformation, even minor trauma to the flank can result in bleeding. Renal stones are rare and can result from chronic infection or excessive secretion of calcium and other metabolites. The commonest tumour is Wilms' tumour (Figure 15.1), which may present with haematuria, but more commonly presents with a loin mass.

### History – must ask!

- *What colour is the urine?* The colour of the urine indicates the site of damage. Haematuria originating from the kidney is brown or cola-coloured, and that originating from the bladder or urethra has a red to pink colour and may contain clots. Not all red urine is caused by blood – urine may turn red on eating certain foods, notably beetroot and blackberries.
- *Are there other urinary symptoms?* Frequency and dysuria suggest a UTI.
- *Is there pain?* Abdominal pain or renal colic suggest a clot, calculus or obstructive malformation.

- *Was there a precipitating factor?* Trauma to the loin or abdomen can cause kidney damage. Upper respiratory tract or skin infections often precede acute glomerulonephritis. Intense exercise may precipitate haematuria.
- *Family history.* A family history of a bleeding disorder, hypertension or kidney disease may be relevant.

### Physical examination – must check!

- *Blood pressure.* It is mandatory to measure blood pressure in any child presenting with haematuria. Hypertension suggests renal malfunction and you should admit the child to hospital.
- *Oedema.* Look for oedema periorbitally and at the ankles. It can be a feature of glomerulonephritis.
- *Renal mass.* Palpate the abdomen carefully for tenderness, and for renal masses. If you find a mass, the most likely diagnoses are hydronephrosis, polycystic kidneys or tumour.

### Investigations (Table 15.1)

A dipstick test of urine is not a precise diagnostic test. If haematuria is suspected or identified, urinalysis is required on the sediment of a centrifuged sample of urine. The presence of red cell casts and proteinuria indicate the glomeruli to be the source of the damage.

Urinalysis and culture is required in any child with haematuria, but beyond this investigations are guided by clinical evaluation. If acute glomerulonephritis is suspected, confirmation of streptococcal infection is required by throat culture, antistreptolysin (ASO) titre and complement (C3) levels, and serum creatinine concentration to assess renal function. Further investigations are only required in this condition if renal failure ensues or the course is atypical for post-streptococcal disease.

---

### 🔑 Key points: Haematuria

- Identify the site of the urinary tract damage by the colour of the urine and microscopy of the sediment
- Measure blood pressure
- Palpate carefully for renal masses

---

**Table 15.1** Investigations and their relevance in haematuria

| Investigation | Relevance |
|---|---|
| Urinalysis | Red cell casts and proteinuria indicate a glomerular lesion. Pyuria and bacteriuria point to infection |
| Urine culture | Urinary tract infection |
| Full blood count | Anaemia |
| ASO titre and throat culture | Recent streptococcal infection often precedes acute glomerulonephritis |
| Serum creatinine, urea and electrolytes | Elevated creatinine and urea indicate impaired renal function |
| 24-hour urine for creatinine, protein and calcium | Creatinine clearance quantifies the degree of renal impairment |
| Serum C3 level | Low C3 is specific for certain types of glomerulonephritis |
| ANF/autoantibodies | Positive in systemic lupus erythematosus |
| Abdominal/pelvic ultrasound and intravenous pyelogram (IVP) | Structural abnormalities of the kidney |
| Renal biopsy | Required if haematuria is persistent with proteinuria, hypertension or impaired renal function |

## Clues to the diagnosis of haematuria

| Condition | Urine | Symptoms | Possible signs |
|---|---|---|---|
| Urinary tract infection | Bloody | Dysuria, frequency, urgency | |
| Glomerulonephritis | Smoky, Coca-cola coloured, granular and red cell casts | Malaise, oliguria | Hypertension, oedema |
| Renal stone | Bloody | Renal colic | |
| Tumour | Bloody | Abdominal pain | Renal mass |
| Congenital anomalies | Bloody | Painless | Renal mass |

## Oedema

Generalized oedema is an uncommon problem and invariably results from some form of the nephrotic syndrome. It is important to remember that peripheral oedema is not a feature of congestive heart failure in childhood, which is manifested by liver enlargement rather than oedema.

# Renal and urinary conditions

## Urinary tract infection

Acute urinary tract infection is the commonest bacterial infection in childhood and occurs in 3% of girls and 1% of boys. *Escherichia coli* is the causative organism in 90% of cases. A clear diagnosis of UTI is important as it may be the first sign of a congenital anomaly of the urinary tract or vesicoureteric reflux (VUR) which, if untreated, may lead to renal failure.

**Clinical features.** Symptoms are often non-specific and include fever, irritability, vomiting and diarrhoea. In the neonate, prolonged jaundice, apnoea, weight loss and collapse may be the presenting signs. Older children are more likely to present with more specific symptoms including dysuria, frequency, bed-wetting and loin pain. Dysuria and frequency as isolated symptoms are very common and are often not caused by UTI, but this must always be excluded. Clinically it may be impossible to differentiate between cystitis and pyelonephritis in young children as both may present with fever.

**Diagnosis.** UTI can only be reliably diagnosed by identifying a pure growth of bacteria in a urine specimen. Unfortunately, the collection of uncontaminated urine may be difficult. In older, cooperative and continent children a mid-stream urine sample is the most reliable method. An alternative in younger children is a 'clean catch' specimen. Stimulation by tickling or gently pressing on the suprapubic region may encourage the passage of urine. Sterile cotton wool placed in the nappy, or a bag specimen of urine is often taken in babies, but even with careful cleansing of the genital region, bacterial contamination often occurs. If there is a doubt as to whether organisms in the urine are the result of contamination, a suprapubic aspirate is necessary. The growth of $>10^5$ colony-forming units together with $>50$ white cell count in a fresh urine specimen indicates UTI. Any organisms present in a suprapubic specimen indicate UTI (see also p. 96).

**Management (see Box 15.2).** The principles of management can be summarized as antibiotics, copious fluid intake and analgesia appropriate to the degree of pain. In all cases a urine sample should be obtained

> **Box 15.2 Managing the child with a urinary tract infection**
>
> - Always obtain a urine sample for culture before starting antibiotics
> - Prescribe the appropriate antibiotic for the organism found on culture
> - In an infant <3 months of age, or in older children with signs of systemic illness, give intravenous antibiotics
> - Investigate children with atypical or recurrent UTIs
> - Consider prophylactic antibiotics at low dose in children with recurrent UTIs
> - Treat any constipation and give advice on hygiene, maintaining a good fluid intake, and not delaying voiding

for culture prior to commencing antibiotics. Trimethoprim is the first-line antibiotic and should be given for 3 days for uncomplicated lower urinary tract infection, or 7–10 days if there are concerns that the upper urinary tract is involved. In an infant below 3 months of age, or an older child who is acutely ill, intravenous antibiotics are necessary. Advice should be given to the parents to reduce the risk of further UTIs. If symptoms resolve there is no need for a follow-up urine culture after completion of the course of antibiotics. Antibiotic prophylaxis is now only recommended following recurrent UTIs. Advice should be given to the parents to reduce the risk of further UTIs.

**Investigations (see Table 15.2).** Infants less than 6 months of age with a single confirmed UTI require an ultrasound of their urinary tract, even if they respond rapidly to antibiotics. Children with atypical or recurrent UTIs need further investigation (see Table 15.2). The first-line investigation is an ultrasound scan, which can identify renal tract anomalies such as megaureters and bladder abnormalities. DMSA radioisotope scans are performed to detect renal scarring. A micturating cystourethrogram (MCUG) (Figure 15.2) is indicated in infants less than 6 months of age, or older children when there are specific concerns, to look for bladder neck outflow and vesicoureteric reflux. MCUG is an

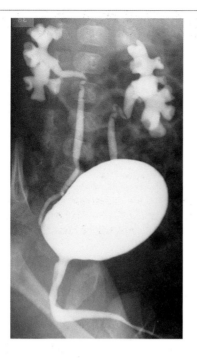

**Figure 15.2** Micturating cystourethrogram (MCUG) in a child with recurrent urinary tract infection. Gross bilateral vesicoureteric reflux (VUR) is seen as the child micturates.

unpleasant procedure as it requires catheterization, and should be covered with a short course of oral trimethoprim. It must not be performed immediately after a UTI as the acute infection can cause transient ureteric reflux.

Persistent proteinuria in the presence of sterile urine suggests renal compromise, possibly as the result of the UTI. If present, biochemical assessment of renal function (creatinine clearance) should be monitored.

**Prognosis.** Recurrence of UTI occurs in 50% of girls within 5 years. If it becomes a recurring problem, and vesicoureteric reflux has been excluded, long-term prophylactic antibiotics may be required. Permanent renal damage as a result of UTI is rare in children, but in infants, infection, particularly in the presence of vesicoureteric reflux, may cause permanent renal scarring with loss of function. Renal scarring is associated with hypertension in adult life and, rarely, chronic renal failure. Chronic pyelonephritis is usually a result of untreated reflux.

## 👁 Urinary tract infection at a glance

**Epidemiology**
3% of girls, 1% boys

**Aetiology**
*Escherichia coli* causative
  organism in 90%

**History**
Non-specific symptoms in
  infants
Fever*
Dysuria
Frequency
Enuresis
Abdominal/loin pain

**Physical examination**
Often normal

NB *Signs and symptoms are variable

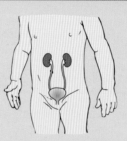

**Confirmatory investigations**
• Clean urine for culture (bag
  urine in babies; though
  suprapubic aspiration
  sometimes necessary)
• >10$^5$ colony-forming units on
  culture (any number if
  suprapubic specimen)
  *and* >50 white cell count
• Dipstick may show haematuria and proteinuria

**Differential diagnosis**
Any febrile illness in babies
Poor perineal hygiene in older
  girls

**Management**
Rapid sterilization of urine with
  antibiotics (IV in neonate or ill
  child)
Encourage fluid intake
Investigation of renal structure
  and vesicoureteric reflux (see
  Box 15.2)

**Prognosis/complications**
10–20% develop hypertension if
  scarring of the kidney occurs
Chronic renal failure very rare

**Table 15.2** Investigations required according to urinary tract infection characteristics

| UTI type | UTI age <6 months | Atypical UTI | Recurrent UTI |
|---|---|---|---|
| **Features** | • Single confirmed UTI<br>• Respond rapidly to treatment | • Seriously ill<br>• Septicaemia<br>• Poor urine flow<br>• Abdominal or bladder mass<br>• Raised serum creatinine<br>• Failure to respond to antibiotics within 48 hours<br>• Non *E. coli* organisms | • 3 or more episodes of cystitis/lower urinary tract infection<br>• 2 or more episodes of urinary tract infection if any episode involved upper urinary tract |
| **Investigations required** | • Ultrasound urinary tract | • Ultrasound urinary tract<br>• DMSA scan 4–6 months later<br>• MCUG if age <6 months | • Ultrasound urinary tract<br>• DMSA scan 4–6 months later<br>• MCUG if age <6 months |

## Vesicoureteric reflux

Vesicoureteric reflux (VUR) refers to reflux of urine from the bladder up the ureter on micturition. It can be found in children who present with atypical or recurrent UTI, and its importance lies in the risk of renal scarring (reflux nephropathy).

**Clinical features and diagnosis.** There are no specific clinical features of VUR. It is identified by investigation following atypical or recurrent UTI, or may be suspected in a fetus found to have dilated renal pelvices or scarring on antenatal ultrasound screening. It is diagnosed by a MCUG (Figure 15.2) and graded as shown in Figure 15.3.

**Management.** The majority of children with VUR tend to have less severe reflux as they get older. Long-term prophylactic trimethoprim or nitrofurantoin is the recommended treatment, with careful surveillance for normal renal growth. Mild degrees of VUR tend to resolve, but children with grade 3 reflux require very close surveillance and may require surgical reimplantation of the ureter into the bladder, particularly if repeated UTI occurs on prophylactic treatment.

**Prognosis.** More than half of children with severe VUR have renal scars. Renal scarring carries a 10–20% risk of hypertension in adult life, and, less commonly, chronic renal failure.

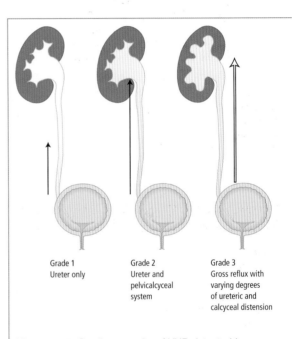

Grade 1
Ureter only

Grade 2
Ureter and pelvicalyceal system

Grade 3
Gross reflux with varying degrees of ureteric and calyceal distension

**Figure 15.3** Grading severity of VUR detected by MCUG. For clarity only one side is shown.

## Vesicoureteric reflux at a glance

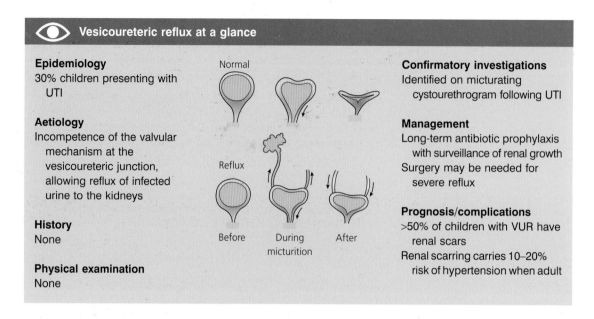

**Epidemiology**
30% children presenting with UTI

**Aetiology**
Incompetence of the valvular mechanism at the vesicoureteric junction, allowing reflux of infected urine to the kidneys

**History**
None

**Physical examination**
None

Normal

Reflux

Before        During        After
              micturition

**Confirmatory investigations**
Identified on micturating cystourethrogram following UTI

**Management**
Long-term antibiotic prophylaxis with surveillance of renal growth
Surgery may be needed for severe reflux

**Prognosis/complications**
>50% of children with VUR have renal scars
Renal scarring carries 10–20% risk of hypertension when adult

## Nocturnal enuresis

Nocturnal enuresis is very common, occurring in 30% of children at 4 years old, 10% at 6 years old, 3% at 12 years old and 1% at 18 years old. Enuresis may be primary (dryness never achieved) or secondary (a relapse of bladder control). Various mechanisms have been implicated in nocturnal enuresis, such as immaturity of the pathways for voluntary bladder control, inadequate nocturnal antidiuretic hormone secretion, small bladder capacity and deep sleeping.

**Clinical features.** There may be stresses that have triggered the enuresis, such as the birth of a sibling, moving to a new house or family dissension. Boys are affected more than girls, and the problem frequently runs in families, particularly among the males – it is interesting how often fathers seem to conceal this information from their suffering sons. There are no signs on physical examination.

**Investigations.** Urinalysis and culture are negative.

### Management of nocturnal enuresis
Intervention is usually delayed until a child is 7 years old and at a stage of maturity when he or she can take some responsibility for tackling the problem. Needless to say, even before this age wet beds can cause a lot of tension within the family and embarrassment for the child.

**Preliminary tactics.** Parents usually try tactics such as fluid restriction in the evening and lifting a child from bed to urinate at night, with varying degrees of success. Understanding how prevalent bedwetting is in childhood, and how counterproductive it can be to address the problem at too early an age, can help relieve the frustration and exasperation of some parents.

**Behavioural management.** Many children respond to good behavioural management in the form of star charts (see p. 355) and rewards for dry nights, provided they are mature enough to understand and motivated enough to try.

A more intensive behavioural approach is the use of the enuresis alarm, which is triggered by urine touching a sensor attached to the pyjama bottoms or sheet (Figure 15.4). The child is woken in time to

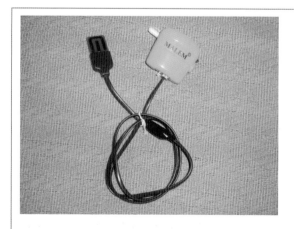

**Figure 15.4** An enuresis alarm.

complete voiding in the toilet. This alarm is very successful in training the motivated child and is often not required beyond a period of 2–3 weeks. It is best to reserve this method until the child is responsible enough to connect the alarm system him- or herself, and to change clothes and bedding too, if necessary.

**Medication.** Medication is an alternative to the alarm system. Vasopressin is available as a nasal spray or orally. Some children respond to a course of treatment by remaining dry, but others relapse on withdrawal of the medication. Vasopressin can also be effectively used to ensure a dry night on an occasional basis, such as at cub camp or staying with a friend. In the past the antidepressant imipramine was used, and was generally effective for the duration of administration, but children frequently relapsed when it was discontinued.

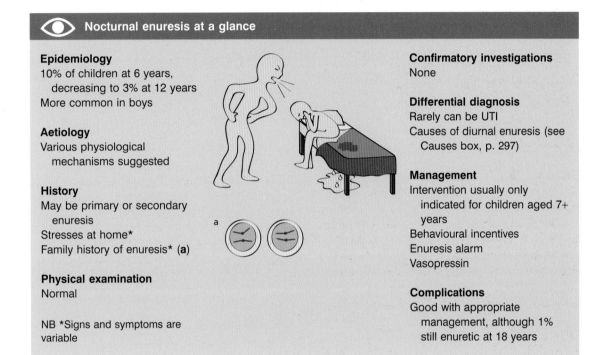

### Nocturnal enuresis at a glance

**Epidemiology**
10% of children at 6 years, decreasing to 3% at 12 years
More common in boys

**Aetiology**
Various physiological mechanisms suggested

**History**
May be primary or secondary enuresis
Stresses at home*
Family history of enuresis* (a)

**Physical examination**
Normal

NB *Signs and symptoms are variable

**Confirmatory investigations**
None

**Differential diagnosis**
Rarely can be UTI
Causes of diurnal enuresis (see Causes box, p. 297)

**Management**
Intervention usually only indicated for children aged 7+ years
Behavioural incentives
Enuresis alarm
Vasopressin

**Complications**
Good with appropriate management, although 1% still enuretic at 18 years

## Acute glomerulonephritis

Acute glomerulonephritis results from immunological damage to the glomerulus. The commonest form in childhood occurs as a result of the formation of immune complexes following infection by a nephritogenic form of streptococcus. Haematuria characteristically occurs 1–2 weeks after a throat or skin infection. Other forms of glomerulonephritis are much rarer and need only be considered if the course of the illness is atypical.

**Clinical features.** The presenting complaint is the appearance of smoky or cola-coloured urine. The child may otherwise be asymptomatic, although malaise, headache and vague loin discomfort may occur. Oedema may be seen around the eyes, and the backs of the hands and feet. Urine microscopy shows gross haematuria with granular and red cell casts. Proteinuria is also evident. In most children mild oliguria only occurs, but the course may be complicated by renal failure, hypertension, seizures and heart failure.

**Management.** Evidence that the condition is the post-streptococcal form is sought by taking a throat swab and ASO titre. Low complement (C3) levels provide further evidence. There is no specific therapy for glomerulonephritis, and the management is similar to that of acute renal failure. Creatinine clearance and fluid balance need to be monitored, and if oliguria develops, salt and water restriction is imposed. Diuretics and hypotensive drugs are needed if there is hypertension, and rarely peritoneal dialysis is required.

Eradication of streptococcal infection with penicillin is recommended to limit the spread of nephritogenic organisms, but there is no evidence that it affects the course of the disease. Members of the family should also be cultured and, if the organism is found, treated with penicillin.

**Prognosis.** The long-term prognosis for post-streptococcal glomerulonephritis is excellent. Other forms have a poorer prognosis. The illness usually resolves in 10–14 days, but if renal impairment persists, a renal biopsy is justified to define the nature of the glomerular pathology.

---

### 👁 Acute glomerulonephritis at a glance

**Prevalence**
Age 3+ years

**Aetiology**
Immunological damage to the glomerulus, usually caused by immune complexes resulting from streptococcal infection

**History**
Smoky/cola-coloured urine (a)
Malaise/headache* (b)
Loin discomfort* (c)
Throat or skin infection 1–2 weeks previously* (d)

**Physical examination**
Oedema*: periorbital and backs of hands/feet (1)
Hypertension* (2)

**Confirmatory investigations**
Gross haematuria
Urinalysis: haematuria, proteinuria
Urine microscopy: granular and red cell casts
Throat swab/ASO titre for streptococcal infection
Low C3 (as opposed to normal in nephrotic syndrome)

NB *Signs and symptoms are variable

**Differential diagnosis**
UTI
Other causes of haematuria (see Causes box, p. 300)

**Management**
Monitor fluid balance and creatinine clearance

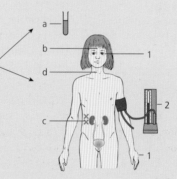

Salt and water restriction if oliguric
Diuretics and hypotensive agents for hypertension
Rarely dialysis
Penicillin to eradicate streptococcus in child and family
Renal biopsy if course is atypical

**Prognosis/complications**
Good prognosis for post-streptococcal glomerulonephritis
Usually resolved by 10–14 days
Complications include:
• renal failure
• hypertension
• seizures
• heart failure

**Pathophysiology**

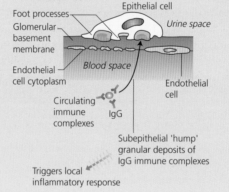

---

## Nephrotic syndrome

The nephrotic syndrome is characterized by proteinuria, hypoproteinaemia, oedema and hyperlipidaemia. The underlying pathology is an increase in glomerular capillary wall permeability, which leads to urinary protein loss, and as a result of hypoalbuminaemia

oedema develops. Three histological patterns are seen in nephrotic syndrome, the commonest being 'minimal change', which is seen in 85% of cases.

**Clinical features (Figure 15.5).** Nephrotic episodes may follow a viral URTI. Periorbital or pitting oedema of the legs is usually noticed first. With time it

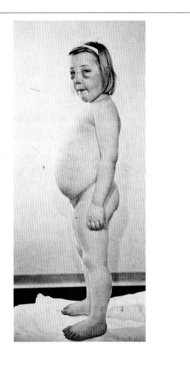

**Figure 15.5** A girl with severe nephrotic syndrome.

**Table 15.3** Typical investigations in nephrotic syndrome

| Urinalysis | 3+ or 4+ or protein/ microscopic haematuria |
|---|---|
| Serum albumin | Low |
| Serum cholesterol and triglycerides | High |
| C3 levels | Normal |

Excessive fluid intake is discouraged and sodium intake is limited to 'no added salt'. Steroid treatment (prednisone) is given to induce remission, which may take 2 weeks to occur. Recovery is monitored by daily weights and proteinuria. Low-dose steroids are continued for 4–6 weeks. During steroid treatment children are at risk if exposed to chicken pox or live vaccines. Prophylactic penicillin is given because of the risk of infection when hypoproteinaemic (antibodies are lost in the urine).

Approximately 75% of children who initially respond to steroids experience a subsequent relapse with proteinuria. Children who frequently relapse or who show signs of steroid toxicity should be treated with cyclophosphamide. A renal biopsy is not necessary unless the child is resistant to steroid treatment.

**Prognosis.** Most children experience relapses over the subsequent 10 years or so, which must be treated in the same way as the initial episode. The long-term prognosis for minimal change nephrotic syndrome is good and residual renal impairment is rare. The prognosis for other forms of nephrotic syndrome is more guarded.

*To test your knowledge on this part of the book, please see Chapter 25.*

becomes more generalized and is associated with weight gain, ascites, pleural effusion and declining urinary output. Symptoms of anorexia, abdominal pain and diarrhoea are common, but hypertension is rare. An increased susceptibility to infection occurs.

**Investigations.** Typical results of investigations are shown in Table 15.3. Renal biopsy is only necessary if the clinical picture does not appear to be typical of minimal change nephrotic syndrome, or if the child does not respond to steroids within a month.

**Management.** It is usual to hospitalize the child for diagnostic, therapeutic and educational purposes.

## 👁 Nephrotic syndrome at a glance

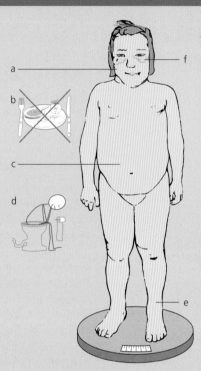

### Epidemiology
'Minimal change' form most
   common

### Aetiology
Idiopathic
Increase in glomerular
   permeability leads to
   proteinuria,
   hypoalbuminaemia and
   oedema

### History
Puffiness (**a**)
Anorexia (**b**)
Abdominal pain* (**c**)
Diarrhoea* (**d**)
Preceding URTI*

### Physical examination
Pitting oedema of the legs (**e**)
Periorbital oedema (**f**)
Weight gain
Ascites and pleural effusion*
Reduced urine output

NB *Signs and symptoms are variable.

### Confirmatory investigations
Proteinuria +/– haematuria
Low serum albumin
High cholesterol
High triglycerides
Normal C3
Renal biopsy if presentation
   atypical or poor response to
   steroids

### Differential diagnosis
Other causes of oedema are
   extremely rare

### Management
Hospitalize, monitor weight and
   urinary protein loss
Moderate fluid and salt intake
Steroids to induce remission
Low-dose steroids for 3–6
   months (NB child at risk for
   severe chicken pox)
Prophylactic penicillin
Cyclophosphamide if steroids
   ineffective

### Prognosis/complications
Relapses are common
Long-term prognosis good for
   minimal change
Other forms can lead to renal
   impairment

# CHAPTER 16

# Genitalia

There was a young infant named Paul
Who seemed to have only one ball
But kind doctor Hynd
Was able to find
That there really were two after all.

*Anon.*

## COMPETENCES

### You must ...

| Be able to | Appreciate |
|---|---|
| • Competently examine for retractile or undescended testes<br>• Distinguish a hydrocoele from an inguinal hernia<br>• Carry out a developmental assessment on babies and toddlers | • That it is important to operate on undescended testes before the age of 2 years<br>• The importance of sensitivity in examining the genitalia beyond infancy |

*Paediatrics and Child Health*, Third Edition. Mary Rudolf, Tim Lee, Malcolm Levene.
© 2011 Mary Rudolf, Tim Lee and Malcolm Levene. Published 2011 by Blackwell Publishing Ltd.

# Symptoms and signs relating to the genitalia

## Finding your way around . . .

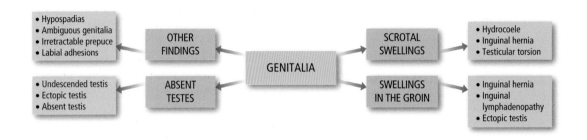

## Scrotal swellings

A swelling in the scrotum may present for attention because of parental concern, or may be an incidental finding identified during child health surveillance.

### History – must ask!

*   *Characteristics*. An inguinal hernia characteristically causes intermittent swelling, particularly when intra-abdominal pressure is increased, as in crying or straining. Hernias (unless incarcerated) and hydrocoeles are painless, although parents may think a hernial swelling is painful as it tends to occur when the baby cries. Testicular torsion, in contrast, is acutely painful.

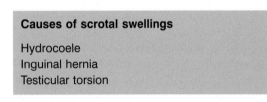

**Causes of scrotal swellings**

Hydrocoele
Inguinal hernia
Testicular torsion

Hydrocoeles are often present at birth and show little variation in size over time.

### Physical examination – must check!

*   *Observation*. The boy with testicular torsion is obviously in acute pain. The swelling caused by an inguinal hernia extends up into the groin, whereas the hydrocoele usually does not.
*   *Palpation*. On palpation the inguinal hernia can be felt to reach up to the inguinal region, and can usually be reduced through the inguinal ring. The testis is palpable separate from the hernial swelling. A hydrocoele, in contrast, does not usually extend up into the groin and the testis cannot be palpated through the fluid. Neither is usually tender, although the hernia becomes so if incarcerated. A testicular torsion is so tender that palpation is not possible. Reduction of an inguinal or inguinoscrotal mass, whether spontaneously or by manipulation, is diagnostic of a hernia.
*   *Transillumination*. When a torch is held to the scrotum, a hydrocoele transilluminates, whereas a hernia does not.

### Investigations

The differentiation between these conditions is clinical. No investigations are indicated.

## Clues to diagnosing scrotal swellings

|  | Hernia | Hydrocoele | Torsion |
|---|---|---|---|
| **Usual age** | Infants, particularly premature | Babies | Boys under 6 years |
| **Pain** | No (unless incarcerated) | No | Intense |
| **Extends to groin** | Yes | Usually not | No |
| **Transilluminates** | No | Yes | No |

## Swellings in the groin

### Causes of swelling in the groin

Inguinal hernia
Inguinal lymphadenopathy
Ectopic testis

Like scrotal swellings, lumps in the groin are distinguishable clinically. The features of *inguinal hernias* are described in the previous section. In contrast, the *inguinal lymph node* has a firm consistency with clear borders. It may be tender, and a responsible infected lesion may be found on the legs. If an enlarged lymph gland is found, the child must be fully examined for more generalized lymphadenopathy and hepatosplenomegaly, which if found may be suggestive of a serious cause such as lymphoma.

Rarely, the lump may be an *ectopic testis*, and the scrotum should be examined for the presence of both testes. Small 'shotty' inguinal nodes are very common in young children, and are related to the degree of minor trauma that the legs incur at this age. They are of no significance.

## Impalpable testes

### Causes of impalpable testes

Undescended or ectopic testes
Retractile testes
True testicular absence

The commonest reason for a testis or testes to be impalpable is an exaggerated cremasteric reflex which retracts the testes high into the scrotum. Retractile testes can be brought down by careful palpation when the child is relaxed in a warm room, and scrotal examination is made easier if the child is in a squatting or cross-legged position. Often more than one examination is required to establish whether the testis is truly absent from the scrotum.

Cryptorchidism (undescended testes) is an important condition to identify in babies and is screened for during child health surveillance, as there is a risk of infertility and malignancy if it is left uncorrected. Undescended testes may descend into the scrotum spontaneously before the age of 1 year. Beyond that age, if the testes cannot be palpated and brought down into the scrotum, referral to a paediatric surgeon is required. Surgery should be carried out before the age of 2 years to minimize the risk of complications.

Approximately 20% of non-palpable testes are absent. In most cases this is presumed to be a result of a vascular accident. If absent bilaterally, intersex must be considered and the chromosomal sex confirmed.

### Key points: Impalpable testes

• Examine the child in a warm room with warm hands
• Scrotal examination is facilitated if the child is in a squatting or cross-legged position

# Conditions affecting the genitalia

## Hydrocoele

A hydrocoele is an accumulation of fluid in the tunica vaginalis. Hydrocoeles do not fluctuate in size, unless they communicate with the peritoneal cavity. Most hydrocoeles resolve by the age of 1 year, but occasionally large ones persist and require surgical treatment. Rarely, the development of a hydrocoele in an older boy is indicative of malignancy.

## Inguinal hernia

Inguinal hernias in childhood are indirect. They are far more common in boys and result from persistent patency of the processus vaginalis, which normally closes at birth (Figure 16.1). They are particularly common in premature infants.

**Clinical features.** A swelling is evident in the groin which may extend down into the scrotum (Figure 16.2). It tends to be most obvious when intra-abdominal pressure is raised as a result of crying, straining or coughing, and often disappears when the baby or child is relaxed and lying down. A hernia is usually not painful unless incarcerated, in which case signs of intestinal obstruction may occur. The observation of an inguinal or inguinoscrotal mass that reduces spontaneously or on manipulation is diagnostic of a hernia.

**Management.** Management of a hernia is surgical. Rarely, if a hernia is incarcerated and irreducible, this must be carried out as an emergency. More commonly the hernia can be gently reduced by the doctor or parent (relaxing the child in a warm bath or with a drink can help). Surgery can then be carried out as an elective procedure.

---

### 👁 Inguinal hernia at a glance

**Epidemiology**
Boys more than girls, particularly premature infants

**Aetiology**
Herniation of bowel through a defect caused by a persistently patent processus vaginalis

**History**
Swelling in groin particularly prominent on crying/straining
Painful only if incarcerated

**Physical examination**
Swelling in groin extending to scrotum
No transillumination
Reducible by manipulation unless incarcerated

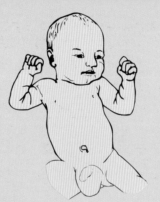

**Confirmatory investigations**
The diagnosis is clinical

**Differential diagnosis**
Hydrocoele

**Management**
Reduce by manipulation, and plan elective surgery
Instruct parents about signs of incarceration
Urgent surgery if hernia becomes strangulated

**Prognosis/complications**
Risk of strangulation of bowel and testis is low
Excellent prognosis following surgery

**Anatomy**

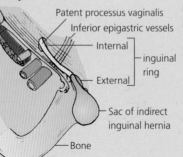

Patent processus vaginalis
Inferior epigastric vessels
Internal ⎤
　　　　⎥ inguinal
　　　　⎥ ring
External ⎦
Sac of indirect inguinal hernia
Bone

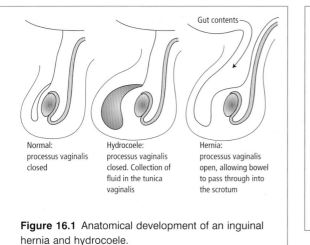

Figure 16.1 Anatomical development of an inguinal hernia and hydrocoele.

Normal:
processus vaginalis closed

Hydrocoele:
processus vaginalis closed. Collection of fluid in the tunica vaginalis

Hernia:
processus vaginalis open, allowing bowel to pass through into the scrotum

Gut contents

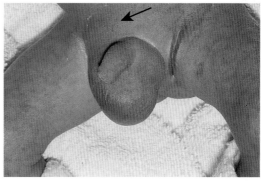

**Figure 16.2** Right inguinal hernia.

## Undescended and ectopic testes

Undescended and ectopic testes can only be differentiated from each other at operation, and both conditions are referred to as cryptorchidism. Testes usually descend from their fetal intra-abdominal position through the processus vaginalis and into the scrotum during the seventh month of gestation (see Figure 16.1). The undescended testicle is found along the normal path of descent and the processus vaginalis is usually patent. If bilateral, the diagnosis of hypopituitarism should be considered. The ectopic testis is one that has completed its descent through the inguinal canal, but lands up at the wrong destination, usually in the groin.

**Clinical features.** The distinction between retractile testes and cryptorchidism is discussed above. One or both testes may be affected. Undescended testes are more common in premature babies than in term babies, and are often accompanied by an inguinal hernia.

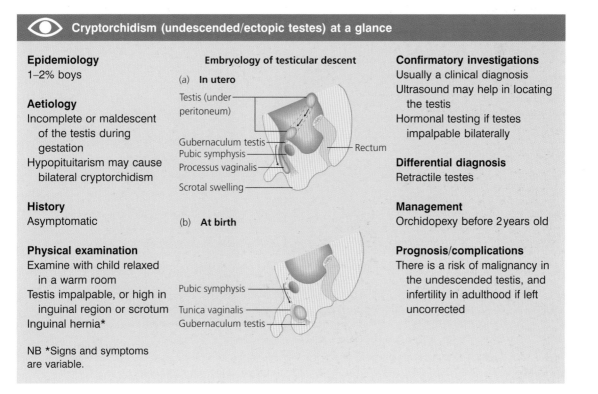

### Cryptorchidism (undescended/ectopic testes) at a glance

**Epidemiology**
1–2% boys

**Aetiology**
Incomplete or maldescent of the testis during gestation
Hypopituitarism may cause bilateral cryptorchidism

**History**
Asymptomatic

**Physical examination**
Examine with child relaxed in a warm room
Testis impalpable, or high in inguinal region or scrotum
Inguinal hernia*

NB *Signs and symptoms are variable.

**Embryology of testicular descent**

(a) **In utero**
Testis (under peritoneum)
Gubernaculum testis
Pubic symphysis
Processus vaginalis
Scrotal swelling
Rectum

(b) **At birth**
Pubic symphysis
Tunica vaginalis
Gubernaculum testis

**Confirmatory investigations**
Usually a clinical diagnosis
Ultrasound may help in locating the testis
Hormonal testing if testes impalpable bilaterally

**Differential diagnosis**
Retractile testes

**Management**
Orchidopexy before 2 years old

**Prognosis/complications**
There is a risk of malignancy in the undescended testis, and infertility in adulthood if left uncorrected

**Management and prognosis.** Surgery should be performed before the age of 2 years, as by this age the number of germ cells in undescended testes is already reduced and the risk of infertility is increased whether the cryptorchidism is unilateral or bilateral. There is also an increased risk of testicular tumour occurring in the third and fourth decade if surgery is delayed.

## Testicular torsion

Testicular torsion usually occurs below the age of 6 years. The testes in young boys are unusually mobile and torsion results when the testis rotates on the spermatic cord. Prompt diagnosis and treatment is required for the testis to survive.

**Clinical features.** The boy presents with acute pain and swelling of the scrotum. On examination the scrotum looks tender and swollen and examination is resisted.

**Management and prognosis.** Prompt surgical exploration is required to untwist and fix the testis to the scrotum. If this takes place within 6 hours, the majority of gonads survive. The contralateral testis must also be fixed as it is also prone to torsion.

## Hypospadias (Figures 16.3, 16.4)

Hypospadias is a condition where the urethra is abnormally sited. It occurs in approximately one in 500 boys. The meatus may be sited anywhere from the ventral aspect of the glans penis (the commonest type) to the penoscrotal junction or even the perineum. With increasing degrees of severity the penis is curved ventrally (chordee).

Severe cases require repair to allow the boy to void standing, to allow future sexual function and to avoid the psychological consequences of malformed genitalia. Management is surgical reconstruction before the age of 2 years. Severe cases require reconstruction using the foreskin and the parents must be given strict instructions not to have the child circumcised.

## Ambiguous genitalia

Rarely, babies are born with ambiguous genitalia and indeterminate sex. This should be considered to be a medical emergency as it may be associated with major electrolyte imbalance. The indeterminate nature of the child's gender should be discussed with the parents and a decision regarding gender only made when investigations are complete. This depends as much on the surgical possibility of producing a functional penis as the genetic sex. Delay in naming the child is advised until gender determination is made. The diagnostic approach to the baby with ambiguous genitalia is beyond the scope of this book.

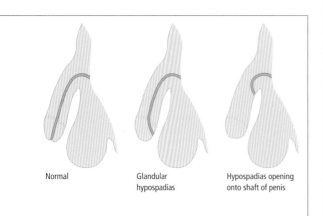

Normal     Glandular hypospadias     Hypospadias opening onto shaft of penis

**Figure 16.3** Hypospadias showing sites of opening of the meatus.

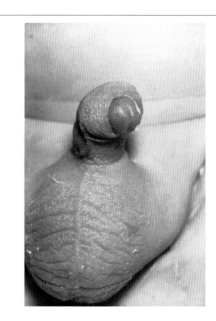

**Figure 16.4** Hypospadias. The meatus is at the junction of the glans and shaft.

## Irretractable prepuce

In the majority of boys the prepuce becomes retractable by the age of 3 years. Inability to retract before this age is not pathological.

True phimosis (the inability to retract the prepuce) can be congenital or a sequel of inflammation, and requires surgery.

## Labial adhesions

The labia majora are sometimes found to be adherent in young girls who are still in nappies. The adhesions probably develop as a result of irritation secondary to nappy rash. There is no need for the labia to be forcibly separated as the adhesions resolve in later childhood.

*To test your knowledge on this part of the book, please see Chapter 25.*

# CHAPTER 17
# Dermatology and rashes

*If there is a white spot on the skin, . . . . . . then the priest shall quarantine the affected person for 7 days*
*Leviticus 13:4*
*If the skin is covered with dull white spots, it is a simple rash . . . . . .*
*Leviticus 13:39*

## COMPETENCES
### You must . . .

| Know | Be able to | Appreciate |
|---|---|---|
| • How to recognize acute and chronic skin rashes in childhood<br>• How to recognize other systemic conditions presenting with rash<br>• How to manage eczema | • Differentiate and describe lesions of the skin<br>• Identify the common childhood exanthems clinically<br>• Recognize common birth marks<br>• Advise a parent about caring for a baby's nappy rash | • The social consequences of having a chronic skin condition<br>• The danger of excessive use of topical steroid creams<br>• The significance of finding purpuric and petechial rashes |

*Paediatrics and Child Health*, Third Edition. Mary Rudolf, Tim Lee, Malcolm Levene.
© 2011 Mary Rudolf, Tim Lee and Malcolm Levene. Published 2011 by Blackwell Publishing Ltd.

# Dermatological symptoms and signs

## Finding your way around . . .

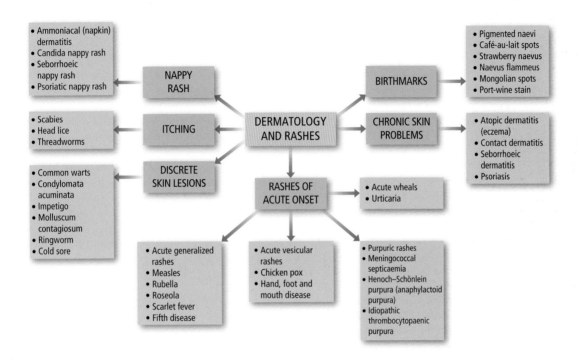

Parents commonly bring their child to the doctor for diagnosis of rashes and skin lesions. In most situations a diagnosis can be made clinically, and treatment, if required, can be given without further investigation. Experience is required to identify these skin manifestations, and the process of identification is rather like identifying wild flowers or bird-spotting – if you have encountered it before, you are likely to recognize it again. It is important, however, to learn to describe the features, just as in bird-spotting; this increases one's powers of observation and enhances the learning process.

The various types of skin lesion are described and illustrated in Table 17.1.

Unlike with almost any other condition in medicine, it is reasonable to examine the child presenting with a rash or skin lesion *before* embarking on a detailed history.

### Description of the rash or lesion

If you are unsure of the correct dermatological term for lesions, you should carefully describe them. The following features are important to include:

* raised or flat;
* crusty or scaly;
* colour;
* blanching on pressure;
* size of the lesions;
* distribution (discrete, generalized or limited to certain sites in the body).

### Other features

The child's age, changes in the rash over time, current health and any accompanying features contribute to the diagnosis.

**Table 17.1** Types of skin lesion

| Type of lesion | Description | Example |
|---|---|---|
| Macules | Discrete flat lesions of any size or shape that are pink or red in colour. Characteristically they fade on pressure | Rubella<br>Roseola |
| Papules | Solid palpable projections above the surface of the skin | Insect bite |
| Maculopapular | Mixture of macules and papules which tend to be confluent | Measles<br>Drug rash |
| Purpura and petechiae | Purple lesions caused by small haemorrhages in the superficial layers of the skin. In general, they indicate a serious condition. Characteristically they *do not fade on pressure*. Petechiae are tiny purpuric lesions | Meningococcal septicaemia<br>Idiopathic thrombocytopenic purpura<br>Henoch–Schönlein purpura<br>Leukaemia |
| Vesicles | Raised fluid filled lesions <0.5 cm in diameter. If large, they are called bullae | Chicken pox |
| Wheals | Raised lesions with a flat top and pale centre of variable size | Urticaria |
| Desquamation | A loss of epidermal cells producing a 'scaly' eruption | Post-scarlet fever |

On the basis of this brief evaluation, the problem can be classified according to the following criteria:

- acute onset of rash;
- chronic rashes;
- nappy rash;
- individual skin lesions;
- birthmarks;
- itchy conditions.

Each of these is discussed in the following sections.

## Acute rashes (Figure 17.1, 17.2)

Most children presenting with acute onset of a rash have one of the common infectious diseases of childhood and are unwell with a temperature. These conditions are covered in Chapter 7. Purpuric conditions always need attention as they may be a sign of a life-threatening condition and must be identified promptly.

### History – must ask!

- *Is the child ill or febrile?* Most of the exanthematous diseases are accompanied by fever and malaise (see Chapter 7). In Henoch–Schönlein purpura (HSP)

**Causes of acute rash**

| Type of rash | Causes |
|---|---|
| Macular and maculopapular | Exanthems of childhood infections (see p. 321)<br>Allergy |
| Vesicular | Chicken pox<br>Hand, foot and mouth disease |
| Purpuric | Meningococcal septicaemia<br>Henoch–Schönlein purpura (see p. 334)<br>Idiopathic thrombocytopenic purpura (see p. 349) |
| Wheals | Urticaria |

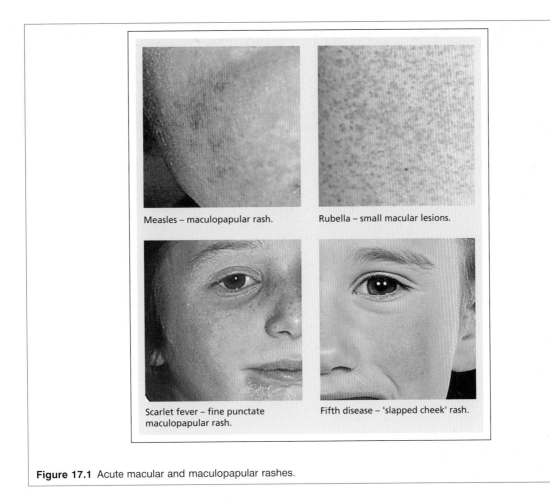

Measles – maculopapular rash.

Rubella – small macular lesions.

Scarlet fever – fine punctate maculopapular rash.

Fifth disease – 'slapped cheek' rash.

**Figure 17.1** Acute macular and maculopapular rashes.

and idiopathic thrombocytopenic purpura (ITP) fever is usually absent.

• *Is the rash itchy?* Itchiness suggests an allergic response, or chicken pox if the rash is vesicular. If you suspect allergy, ask about possible allergens such as food, washing powder, soaps and lotions. However, it is rare to identify the allergen.

• *Are there associated symptoms?* These are particularly important in the purpuric conditions. In ITP there may be bruising, and bleeding from the gums and nose. In HSP, arthritis and abdominal pain, melaena and haematuria commonly occur. In hives, wheezing or stridor may rarely be present.

• *Past medical history.* A history of a previous attack of an infectious disease makes a further attack unlikely, but there is a high incidence of inaccurate diagnoses, particularly with maculopapular rashes. It is obviously relevant to ask about the child's immunization history. An atypical rash commonly follows some 10 days after measles, mumps and rubella (MMR) vaccination.

• *Contact with anyone ill.* Enquire whether anyone else in the family, or at school or nursery has been diagnosed as having an infectious disease.

### Physical examination – must check!

You need to describe the rash carefully, focusing on the following:

• *Characteristics.* Is the rash macular, papular, maculopapular, purpuric or petechial, vesicular or wheals? An important part of the examination is to test the rash for blanching, as purpuric and petechial rashes do not blanch on pressure whereas maculopapular rashes do.

• *Distribution.* Measles and rubella both start on the face and work their way down the body. Roseola and chicken pox are mostly on the trunk. Both HSP and fifth disease have characteristic distributions.

• *The presence of an enanthem.* Look in the mouth for an enanthem (see p. 111).

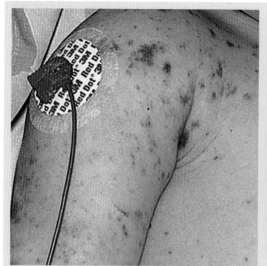

Meningococcaemia. Note the typical purpuric rash.

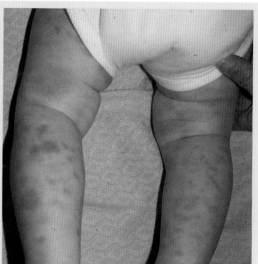

Henoch–Schönlein purpura. Note the typical distribution.

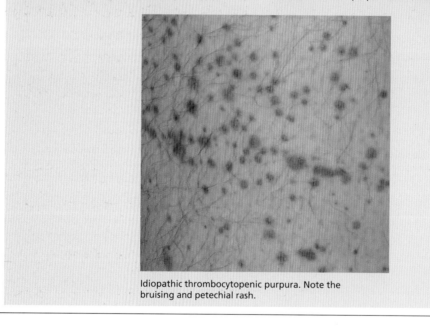

Idiopathic thrombocytopenic purpura. Note the bruising and petechial rash.

**Figure 17.2** Acute purpuric and petechial rashes.

### Investigations

In general, the viral exanthems do not need a serological confirmation of the diagnosis, unless for public health reasons. The exception, of course, is if rubella is suspected in a pregnant girl. If meningococcal septicaemia is suspected, blood cultures, meningococcal PCR, clotting screen, full blood count, and calcium profile are performed urgently. If the rash is petechial, a platelet count is required to make the diagnosis of thrombocytopenia.

### Management

Prior to the advent of immunization, there was little difficulty in recognizing the childhood exanthems as they were so common. It is important to recognize them so that appropriate advice about incubation periods and isolation can be made (Table 7.2). Maculopapular rashes are often overdiagnosed clinically as being caused by measles or rubella. As these diagnoses are difficult to make unless in the midst of an epidemic, it is preferable to make the diagnosis of viral exanthem rather than a wrong diagnosis. If accurate diagnosis is required, confirmation by serological testing is necessary.

If meningococcal septicaemia is suspected (see p. 128), the child should immediately be given intramuscular penicillin as rapid deterioration can occur, and urgent admission to hospital arranged. The child with suspected ITP also requires urgent hospital evaluation and admission if the platelet count is dangerously low.

> **Key points: Acute rashes**
>
> • Decide if the rash is macular, maculopapular, vesicular, purpuric or wheals
> • Determine if the child is febrile or ill
> • If the rash is petechial or purpuric and the child is unwell, treat with penicillin IM and admit for investigation
> • Beware of making a specific diagnosis of measles or rubella clinically. Without serological confirmation, 'viral exanthem' should be diagnosed

## Clues to diagnosing acute generalized rashes in childhood

| | Type of rash | Characteristics of the rash | Other features |
|---|---|---|---|
| **Measles** | Maculopapular | Begins on the face and spreads downwards | Koplik spots, coryza, cough and conjunctivitis, ill child |
| **Rubella** | Macular | Tiny pink macules on the face and trunk, works downwards | Well child, lymphadenopathy sometimes |
| **Roseola** | Macular | Faint pink rash on the trunk | Rash occurs after fever defervesces |
| **Scarlet fever** | Maculopapular | Fine punctate red rash with sandpapery feel, followed by peeling | Strawberry tongue, perioral pallor, tonsillitis |
| **Fifth disease** | Maculopapular | 'Slapped cheek' appearance. Lace-like rash on the arms, trunk and thighs | Well child, lasts up to weeks |
| **Allergic reaction** | Papular | Itchy rash, often generalized | The allergen is usually not identified |
| **Chicken pox** | Vesicular | Occurs in crops on face and trunk. Papules, vesicles and crusts are present | Shallow ulcers of the mucous membranes |
| **Meningococcal septicaemia** | Purpuric | Morbilliform, petechial or purpuric | May progress rapidly to shock and coma |
| **Henoch–Schönlein purpura** | Purpuric | Typical rash characteristically distributed over the buttocks, thighs and legs | Abdominal pain, arthralgia, melaena, haematuria. Child usually appears well |
| **Idiopathic thrombocytopenic purpura** | Petechial | Petechial rash over body, with bruising | Bleeding from other sites, e.g. venepuncture, gums, nose. Child usually appears well |
| **Urticaria** | Wheals | Well circumscribed, itchy wheals of different sizes | Rarely accompanied by wheezing or anaphylactic shock |

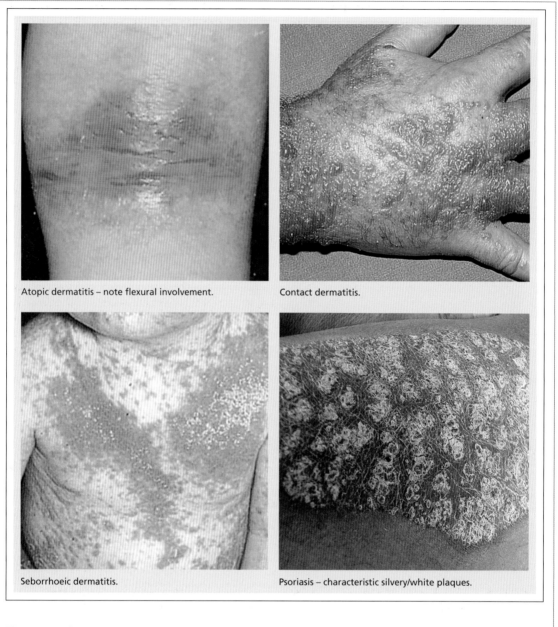

Atopic dermatitis – note flexural involvement.

Contact dermatitis.

Seborrhoeic dermatitis.

Psoriasis – characteristic silvery/white plaques.

**Figure 17.3** Common chronic skin conditions.

## Chronic skin rashes (see Figure 17.3)

**Common chronic skin rashes**

Eczema (atopic dermatitis)
Contact dermatitis
Seborrhoeic dermatitis
Psoriasis

Most chronic skin conditions in childhood are eczematous. Acute eczema (the generic term used to designate a particular type of skin reaction) is characterized by erythema, weeping and microvesicle formation within the epidermis. Chronic eczema is characterized by thickened, dry, scaly, coarse skin (lichenification). The commonest type of eczema in children is atopic dermatitis, although contact dermatitis and seborrhoeic dermatitis are also relatively common.

Most children presenting with a chronic skin rash have atopic dermatitis, but it is important to learn to distinguish other rashes.

### History – must ask!

• *Is the rash itchy?* Itchiness is characteristic of atopic and contact dermatitis. It may also be present in seborrhoeic dermatitis.
• *Are there precipitating factors?* Certain foods such as cow's milk, wheat and eggs may precipitate or exacerbate atopic dermatitis. Saliva, citrus juices, bubble bath, detergents, occlusive synthetic shoes and topical medication are common irritants that cause contact dermatitis.
• *Is there a family history?* Children with eczema often have a family history of atopy. The presence of psoriasis in a parent may support a diagnosis of psoriatic rash in a child. A recent history of scabies in the family or at school would suggest a diagnosis of scabies rather than atopic dermatitis.

### Physical examination – must check!

• *Characteristics of the rash.* Examine the child completely so that you can assess the rash and its distribution adequately. Note that the pattern of involvement of atopic dermatitis changes during childhood.
• *Other helpful features.* The presence of cradle cap or a rash behind the ears and skin folds suggests seborrhoeic dermatitis. Nail pitting or joint involvement point towards psoriasis.

### Management of chronic skin complaints

The skin is visible, so skin disease poses an additional problem not usually found in diseases of other systems. This means that the child and family are subject to the stares and curiosity of others, and possibly stigmatization. It is important to remember that management should involve not only the skin condition but the whole child too.

Topical corticosteroids form an important part of the management of a variety of chronic skin conditions. They must be used with care as long-term use, particularly of the fluorinated variety, leads to atrophy of the skin and an increase in hair growth in some patients. Small amounts of cream applied frequently is more effective than large amounts applied infrequently. The more potent topical steroids should not be applied to the face. If they are applied over the body using occlusive dressings, systemic absorption with adrenal suppression can occur.

---

**🔍 Clues to diagnosing chronic skin conditions**

| | Atopic dermatitis | Contact dermatitis | Seborrhoeic dermatitis | Psoriasis |
|---|---|---|---|---|
| **Lesions** | Erythema, weepiness and crusting leading to dry, thickened scaling skin | Erythema and weeping | Dry scaly and erythematous; red plaques may be present | Plaques of thick silvery or white scales with sharp borders |
| **Distribution** | See At a glance box p. 330 | At sites of contact with the irritant | Face neck, axillae and nappy area | Scalp, knees, elbows and genitalia |
| **Itchiness** | +++ | +++ | +/– | – |
| **Other features** | Starts in infancy; family history of atopy | | Cradle cap | Nail pitting |

## Nappy rash (see Figure 17.4)

---

**Causes of nappy rash**

| | |
|---|---|
| Ammoniacal dermatitis | Seborrhoeic dermatitis |
| Candidiasis | Psoriasis |

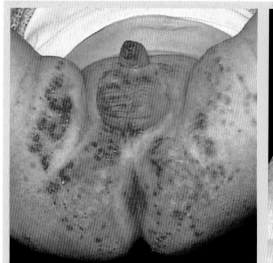

Ammoniacal nappy rash.

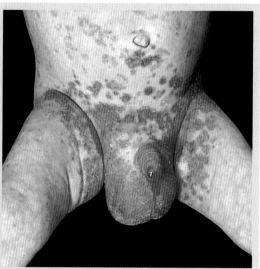

Candida nappy rash – note rash involving the inguinal folds with satellite lesions.

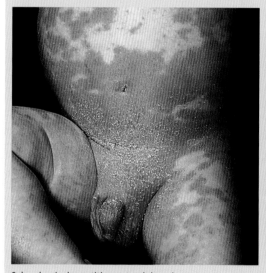

Seborrhoeic dermatitis – note pink and greasy looking lesions.

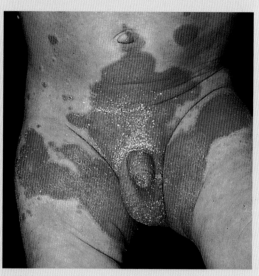

Psoriatic nappy rash.

**Figure 17.4** Nappy rashes.

The nappy area is very prone to rash as it is an area that is warm and moist, usually tightly enclosed in an occlusive waterproof covering, and is in contact with urine, which is an irritant. Mostly the rash is a simple irritative rash, commonly with candidiasis superim-posed, but in a prolonged, resistant rash, conditions such as seborrhoeic dermatitis and psoriasis should be considered. The baby needs to be examined, paying particular attention to the intertriginous areas, scalp and mouth.

## Clues to distinguishing nappy rashes

| | |
|---|---|
| **Ammoniacal dermatitis** | Erythematous +/− papulovesicular or bullous lesions, fissures and erosions |
| | Patchy or confluent |
| | Skin folds characteristically spared |
| **Candida** | Bright red, with sharply demarcated edge and satellite lesions |
| | Inguinal folds involved |
| | Oral thrush may be found |
| **Seborrhoeic dermatitis** | Pink, greasy lesions with yellow scale |
| | Often in the skin folds |
| | Cradle cap may be found |
| **Psoriatic nappy rash** | Like seborrhoeic dermatitis |
| | Positive family history for psoriasis |

## Itching

### Conditions causing itching

Atopic dermatitis
Contact dermatitis
Urticaria
Scabies
Chicken pox
(Seborrhoeic dermatitis)
Head lice
Threadworms

Itching is an unpleasant symptom which, if generalized, is usually associated with a rash. Certain measures can help reduce the discomfort of itching, whatever the cause. Cool baths are soothing, and tight synthetic or woollen clothing should be avoided. It is important to discourage scratching, and fingernails should be kept short and clean to minimize secondary infection. Antihistamines prescribed at night can increase the chances of a more restful night.

## Infectious skin lesions

### Common infectious skin lesions

Warts
Impetigo
Molluscum contagiosum
Tinea
Herpes simplex (cold sores)
Birthmarks

Diagnosis of these common lesions requires visual recognition (Figure 17.5). You should learn to distinguish them by studying the photographs, and looking for characteristic distinguishing features.

## Clues to diagnosing infectious skin lesions

| | |
|---|---|
| **Common warts** | Roughened keratotic lesions with an irregular surface |
| **Impetigo** | Sticky, heaped-up, honey-coloured crusts |
| **Molluscum contagiosum** | Pearly, dome-shaped papules, with central umbilicus |
| **Tinea corporis** | Dry, scaly papule which spreads centrifugally with central clearing |
| **Cold sore** | Single or grouped vesicles/pustules sited periorally |

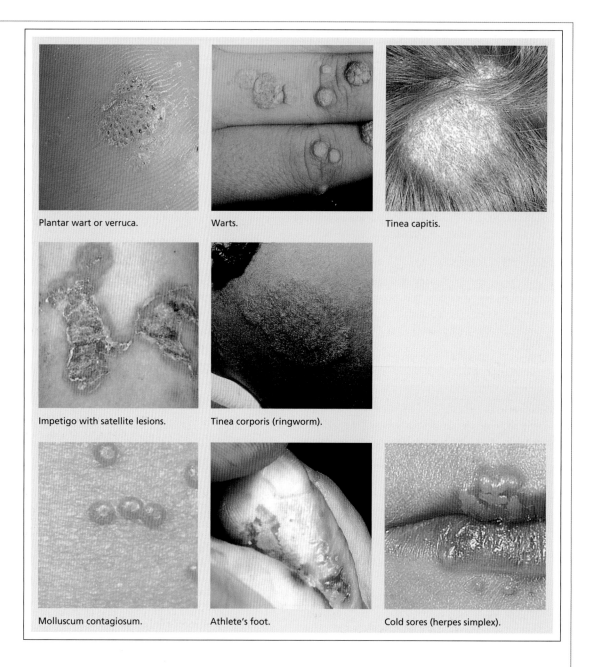

Plantar wart or verruca.

Warts.

Tinea capitis.

Impetigo with satellite lesions.

Tinea corporis (ringworm).

Molluscum contagiosum.

Athlete's foot.

Cold sores (herpes simplex).

**Figure 17.5** Infectious skin lesions.

# Dermatological conditions and other rashes

## Atopic dermatitis (eczema) (Figure 17.6)

Atopic dermatitis is an inflammatory skin condition characterized by erythema, oedema, intense itching, exudation, crusting and scaling. There appears to be a genetically determined predisposition, and infants with atopic dermatitis tend to subsequently develop allergic rhinitis and asthma. It most often begins in the first 2–3 months of life, and the onset frequently coincides with the introduction of certain foods such as cow's milk, wheat and eggs into the diet. There is some evidence that genetically susceptible infants have a reduced risk of developing eczema if they are exclusively breast-fed. There is often a family history of atopy.

**Clinical features.** The clinical features vary according to the stage of childhood. In infancy the lesions are erythematous, weepy patches on the cheeks which subsequently extend to the rest of the face, neck, wrists, hands and extensor surfaces of the extremities. Pruritus is marked, and the infant makes efforts to scratch by face-rubbing on the sheets. This leads to weeping and crusting, and commonly secondary infection.

By preschool age (3–5 years) there is a tendency towards remission, although some children have per-sistent mild to moderate dermatitis in the popliteal and antecubital fossae, on the wrists, behind the ears and on the face and neck.

During school years recurrence tends to occur, with antecubital and popliteal involvement and extension to the neck, forehead, eyelids, wrists and dorsa of the hands and feet. The skin becomes dry and thickened and the face can take on a whitish hue. Hyperpigmentation, scaling and lichenification become prominent.

**Investigations.** The diagnosis is a clinical one. Serum IgE levels are often raised and eosinophilia may be present. Although skin testing is frequently positive, it is rarely helpful clinically.

**Management (see Box 17.1).** Scratching has a major role in the production of skin lesions, and treatment is directed at trying to interrupt the itch–scratch–itch cycle. Dietary restriction is controversial and generally of limited value. Arbitrary exclusion of a number of foods can lead to malnutrition.

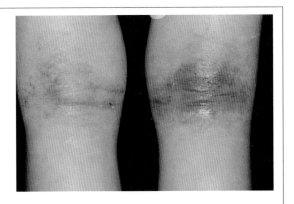

**Figure 17.6** Atopic dermatitis. The legs of a child with atopic dermatitis, showing flexural involvement.

> **Box 17.1 Advice for children with atopic eczema**
>
> • Avoid food and environmental factors known to trigger itching (but arbitrary exclusion of numerous foods from infants' diets is irrational and can lead to malnutrition)
> • Avoid extremes of temperature and humidity
> • Keep fingernails short to help control scratching
> • Clothes should be of smooth cotton and avoid wearing wool
> • Avoid medicated soap, though a superfatted, simple soap is acceptable
> • Bath oils and creams are intended to seal moisture into the skin. Apply them after the child has soaked in the bath for 15 minutes or so
> • A pet-free household is advisable, given the common development of asthma in atopic children
> • Breast-feeding with avoidance of cow's milk protein for the first several months is advisable in subsequent siblings

During an acute flare-up wet dressings are helpful as they have an anti-inflammatory and antipruritic effect. Topical steroids are then applied between dressing changes. Antihistamines can be useful for their sedative and antipruritic effect. Scratching often causes infection even if this is not obviously apparent, and so topical or oral antibiotics are often required.

After the acute phase, while the dermatitis is still active, topical steroids are applied in the form of creams or ointments. The more potent steroid creams must be kept to a minimum to control the disease and should not be applied to the face. Systemic corticosteroids are only rarely used.

Lubricants are used after application of steroid creams and continued on a prophylactic basis to keep the skin moist. Bath oils can be added to the bath water after the child has soaked well, so that moisture is sealed into the well-hydrated skin.

**Prognosis.** The course of atopic dermatitis is fluctuating; fortunately the condition resolves entirely in some 50% of infants by the age of 2 years. A few cases continue to be problematic beyond childhood. Reasonable control of this chronic condition can usually be achieved in most children.

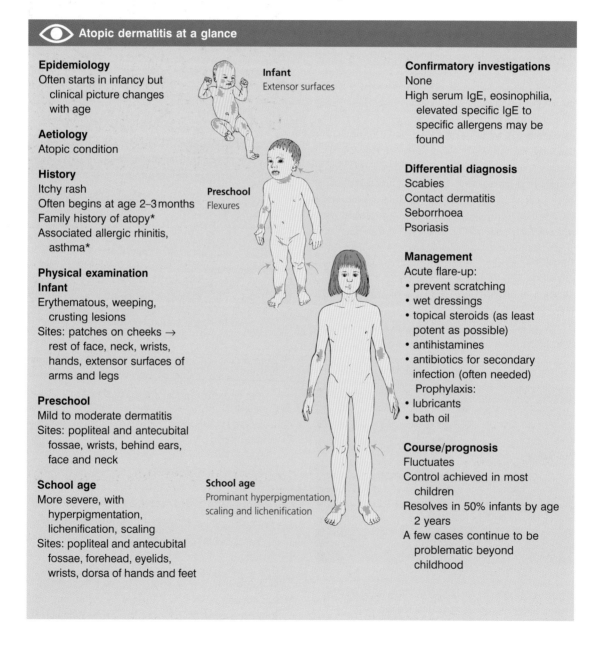

## Atopic dermatitis at a glance

**Epidemiology**
Often starts in infancy but clinical picture changes with age

**Aetiology**
Atopic condition

**History**
Itchy rash
Often begins at age 2–3 months
Family history of atopy*
Associated allergic rhinitis, asthma*

**Physical examination**
**Infant**
Erythematous, weeping, crusting lesions
Sites: patches on cheeks →
   rest of face, neck, wrists, hands, extensor surfaces of arms and legs

**Preschool**
Mild to moderate dermatitis
Sites: popliteal and antecubital fossae, wrists, behind ears, face and neck

**School age**
More severe, with hyperpigmentation, lichenification, scaling
Sites: popliteal and antecubital fossae, forehead, eyelids, wrists, dorsa of hands and feet

**Infant**
Extensor surfaces

**Preschool**
Flexures

**School age**
Prominant hyperpigmentation, scaling and lichenification

**Confirmatory investigations**
None
High serum IgE, eosinophilia, elevated specific IgE to specific allergens may be found

**Differential diagnosis**
Scabies
Contact dermatitis
Seborrhoea
Psoriasis

**Management**
Acute flare-up:
• prevent scratching
• wet dressings
• topical steroids (as least potent as possible)
• antihistamines
• antibiotics for secondary infection (often needed)
   Prophylaxis:
• lubricants
• bath oil

**Course/prognosis**
Fluctuates
Control achieved in most children
Resolves in 50% infants by age 2 years
A few cases continue to be problematic beyond childhood

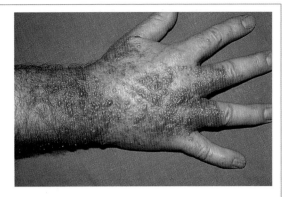

**Figure 17.7** Contact dermatitis. A severe rash that erupted on contact with holly.

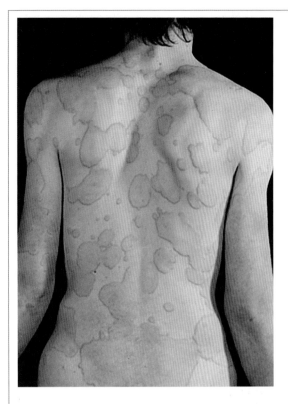

**Figure 17.8** Urticaria (hives). Note the characteristic, well-circumscribed wheals.

## Contact dermatitis (Figure 17.7)

Clinically, contact dermatitis may be indistinguishable from atopic dermatitis, although a detailed history, the sites involved and the age of the child often provide clues. It can either be caused by irritants or, in susceptible individuals, by allergens. It results from prolonged or repetitive contact with a variety of substances that include saliva, citrus juices, bubble bath, detergents and occlusive synthetic shoes. Topical medications, jewellery and chemicals used in the manufacture of clothing are all potential allergens.

**Clinical features.** Saliva may cause dermatitis on the face and neckfolds of a drooling child. It also occurs in older children who habitually lick their lips. 'Trainer' or 'sneaker' dermatitis can result from the leaching out of chemicals in the shoe rubber by excessive sweating. Bubble baths can be a cause of severe pruritus.

**Management.** In general, contact dermatitis clears on removal of the irritant or allergen and temporary treatment with a topical corticosteroid preparation.

## Urticaria (hives)

Urticaria is an allergic reaction characterized by well-circumscribed but sometimes coalescent wheals of various sizes (Figure 17.8). It is usually difficult to identify the allergen. Certain individuals may develop urticaria when exposed to insect bites (papular urticaria), cold, exercise, hot showers and anxiety.

**Clinical features.** The lesions may be intensely pruritic. Each wheal resolves within 2 days, but new ones continue to occur and urticaria may become chronic, persisting for many weeks. In angioneurotic oedema deeper tissues are also involved, including the upper respiratory and gastrointestinal tract. Urticaria may also be seen in the child presenting in anaphylactic shock.

**Management.** In most instances urticaria is a self-limited condition requiring no treatment, other than that aimed at reducing itching. Antihistamines are the drug of first choice. The allergen is usually not identified, although it is worth taking a good food and drug history.

## Seborrhoeic dermatitis (Figure 17.9)

Seborrhoeic dermatitis is a chronic inflammatory condition which is commonest during infancy and adolescence. It is often most troublesome in the first year of life.

**Clinical features.** Cradle cap is the commonest manifestation and is seen as diffuse or focal scaling and yellow crusting of the scalp. A dry scaly erythematous

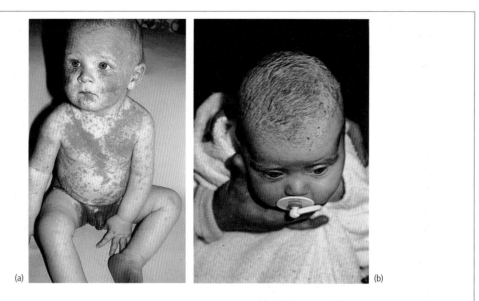

**Figure 17.9** Seborrhoeic dermatitis. (a) Note the baby's erythematous rash involving the face, neck, chest and nappy area. (b) Severe cradle cap in a baby, with widespread scaling and crusting of the scalp.

dermatitis may also involve the face, neck, axillae and nappy area and behind the ears. If the scaling is prominent it may look like psoriasis, and red scaly plaques may appear. Itching may or may not be present. Seborrhoeic nappy rash is characterized by pink, greasy lesions with a yellow scale. It is most commonly seen in the intertriginous areas.

**Management.** Scalp lesions are usually controlled with antiseborrhoeic shampoo. Inflamed lesions respond to topical corticosteroid therapy. Secondary bacterial infections and superimposed candidiasis are not uncommon. Seborrhoeic nappy rash usually responds to mild topical corticosteroid cream.

## Psoriasis (Figure 17.10 and 17.11)

Psoriasis is a common chronic skin disorder among adults, one third of whom become affected during childhood. Girls are more affected than boys and there is usually a family history.

**Clinical features.** The lesions consist of erythematous papules which coalesce to form plaques of thick silvery or white scales and sharply demarcated borders. They tend to occur on the scalp, knees, elbows, umbilicus and genitalia. Nail involvement, a valuable diagnostic sign, is characterized by pitting of the nail plate. Guttate psoriasis is a variant affecting children where multiple small oval or round lesions appear over the body, often following a recent streptococcal infec-

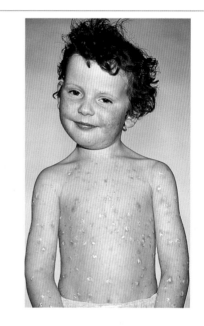

**Figure 17.10** Psoriasis. Note the characteristic silvery/ white plaques over the upper body.

tion. Psoriasis in the infant can present as a persistent nappy rash, similar to that of seborrhoeic dermatitis.

**Management.** Therapy is mainly palliative and should be kept to a minimum. The application of coal tar preparations after a bath is helpful. Salicylic acid ointment is useful in removing scale, but extensive

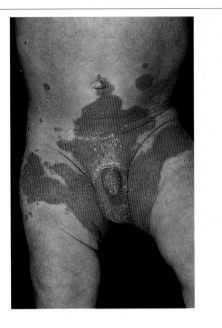

**Figure 17.11** Psoriatic nappy rash.

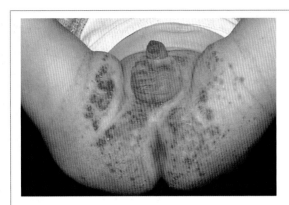

**Figure 17.12** Ammoniacal nappy rash.

application can result in salicylate poisoning, particularly in young children. Topical corticosteroids are effective but must be used with caution.

# Ammoniacal (napkin) dermatitis (Figure 17.12)

Nappy rash can be considered the prototype of irritant contact dermatitis. The rash results as a reaction to overhydration of the skin, friction, maceration, and prolonged contact with urine, faeces, nappy detergents and chemicals. There is some controversy as to whether disposable or cloth nappies are less likely to cause rash.

**Clinical features.** The rash is erythematous, often with papulovesicular or bullous lesions, fissures and erosions. The eruption can be patchy or confluent, but the skin folds are characteristically spared as they are in less contact with urine than the exposed areas are. Secondary infection with bacteria and yeasts is common.

## Nappy rash at a glance

**Epidemiology**
Universal

**Aetiology**
Prolonged contact with urine, faeces, detergents, chemicals
Candidal superinfection common

**Physical examination**
Erythema
Patchy or confluent
Sparing of skin folds (unless candida present too)
Papules, vesicles, bullae, fissures, erosions*
Oral thrush*

NB *Signs and symptoms are variable.

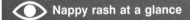

**Confirmatory investigations**
None

**Differential diagnosis**
Candida
Seborrhoeic nappy rash
Psoriatic nappy rash

**Management**
Regular changing and washing area
Exposure to air
Protective creams
Consider use of mild hydrocortisone cream, anticandida creams

**Management.** The rash often responds to simple measures, including regular changing and washing of the genitalia with warm water and mild soap, exposure of the area to air as much as possible, and the application of protective creams such as zinc and castor oil ointment. When these measures do not suffice, limited application of mild hydrocortisone cream can be used. As superimposed candida infection is so common, use of anticandidal agents is also justified.

## Candida nappy rash (Figure 17.13a)

Candida superinfection of other rashes is common. It also commonly follows a course of oral antibiotics as the gut flora is changed, so allowing the candida to flourish opportunistically.

**Clinical features.** Candidal dermatitis classically appears as a bright red rash with a sharply demarcated edge and satellite lesions beyond the border. Unlike in ammoniacal dermatitis, the inguinal folds are usually involved as the warm moist area promotes growth of the yeast.

Thrush (oral candidiasis) may be found on inspection of the mouth. It appears as white 'curds' coating the tongue, gums and buccal mucosa (Figure 17.13b).

**Management.** The diagnosis is usually made on clinical grounds, but confirmation can be made on potassium hydroxide (KOH) preparation. Treatment consists of application of an anticandidal agent such as nystatin, at each nappy change, until the rash has resolved.

If oral thrush is present oral nystatin suspension should be prescribed.

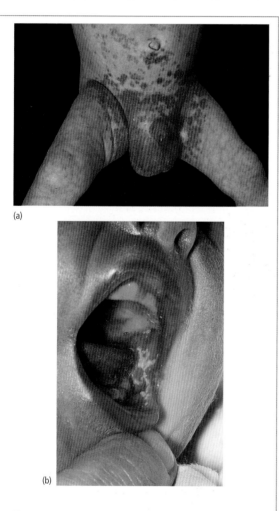

(a)

(b)

**Figure 17.13** Candidal nappy rash. (a) Note the bright red rash involving the inguinal folds and the satellite lesions. (b) Oral thrush appearing like white curds on the buccal mucosa.

## Henoch–Schönlein purpura (anaphylactoid purpura)

Henoch–Schönlein purpura is a form of systemic vasculitis which is presumed to be caused by immune-complex-mediated disease.

**Clinical features.** The child presents with a purpuric rash in a typical distribution over the buttocks, thighs and legs (Figure 17.14). The lesions are purple, raised and a few millimetres in diameter. Arthritis or arthralgia and abdominal pain are commonly experienced, and occasionally melaena occurs. Seventy per cent of the children develop haematuria and/or proteinuria, but the glomerulonephritis is usually asymptomatic and non-progressive.

**Management.** The diagnosis is usually made by the clinical constellation of the typical rash, and abdominal and joint complaints, with a normal platelet count. Treatment is simply supportive. The rash resolves over a week or two, although microscopic haematuria can persist for over a year. Children with renal manifestations should continue to have urinary examinations and blood pressure measurements at periodic intervals to detect late development of hypertension and renal impairment.

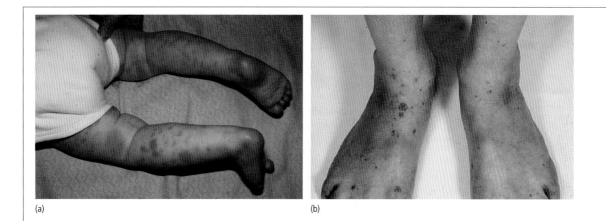

(a)              (b)

**Figure 17.14** Henoch–Schönlein purpura. (a) Note the distribution; (b) close-up of the rash over the feet.

## 👁 Henoch–Schönlein purpura at a glance

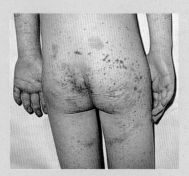

**Epidemiology**
Any age

**Aetiology**
Systemic vasculitis presumed to
   be mediated by immune
   complexes

**History**
Arthralgia*
Abdominal pain*
Melaena*

**Physical examination**
Purple raised lesions
Typical distribution over
   buttocks, thighs and legs*
Arthritis*

NB *Signs and symptoms are variable.

**Confirmatory investigations**
Clinical diagnosis
Haematuria/proteinuria in 70%
Normal platelet count

**Differential diagnosis**
Usually unequivocal
(Septicaemia)
(Bleeding diathesis)

**Management**
Supportive
Urinalysis and blood pressure
   periodically if renal
   manifestations are present

**Prognosis/complications**
Rash lasts 1–2 weeks
Haematuria may persist for
   many months
Hypertension and renal
   impairment may occur

## Impetigo (Figure 17.15)

Impetigo is a skin infection occurring most commonly in children, particularly in the hot humid summer months. The organisms responsible are group A haemolytic streptococci or staphylococci (which commonly also causes a bullous lesion). Infection may be spread to other parts of the body by the fingers, clothing and towels. Insect bites, dermatitis and scabies serve as portals of entry for the organism, which does not penetrate intact skin.

**Clinical features.** The skin lesions pass rapidly through a vesiculopustular phase, and following rupture sticky, heaped-up, honey-coloured crusts are formed. The sites involved are usually exposed areas.

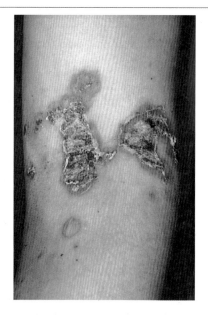

**Figure 17.15** Impetigo. Note the honey-crusted lesions. Spread has occurred with satellite lesions.

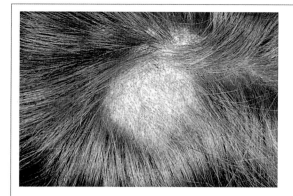

**Figure 17.16** Tinea capitis. Note the circumscribed patch of hair loss with patchy scaling of the scalp.

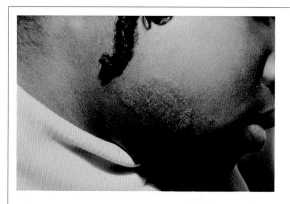

**Figure 17.17** Tinea corporis (ring worm) contracted from a pet dog. Note the typical ring-like patches with central clearing.

**Management.** Impetigo can be contagious, and in all cases simple rules of hygiene must be followed to prevent spread. Antibiotic cream is prescribed if the number of lesions is small (fewer than five), and is applied after the crusts have been soaked off with warm water and soap. In more extensive impetigo, oral antibiotics are required, erythromycin being the drug of choice as it covers both streptococcal and staphylococcal infections

## Ringworm (tinea)

Children can be affected by ringworm, which is either anthropophilic (exclusive to humans) or zoophilic (primarily parasites of other animals). Differing organisms cause lesions at different sites.

### Tinea capitis
In tinea capitis the child presents with a circumscribed patch of hair loss and patchy scaling of the scalp (Figure 17.16). Close examination shows the hair to be broken off close to the follicle, giving a 'black dot' appearance. It may present as a kerion – a boggy inflammatory mass with local lymphadenopathy. The common form of tinea capitis infection fluoresces brilliant green on Wood's light examination, and can be seen microscopically in a wet-mount KOH prepa-ration. Topical therapy alone is ineffective: griseoful-vin needs to be taken orally for at least 4 weeks.

### Tinea corporis
Tinea corporis can be acquired from infected persons or pets or simply by contact with shed scales or hairs. The typical lesion (Figure 17.17) begins as a dry scaly papule which spreads centrifugally, clearing centrally as it does so. The diagnosis can be confirmed by microscopical examination of the scrapings in a KOH wet mount. Lesions usually respond to topical anti-fungal agents applied for 2–4 weeks, but griseofulvin may be required in extensive cases.

### Tinea pedis
Tinea pedis (or athlete's foot) (Figure 17.18) is uncom-mon and is overdiagnosed in young children, where

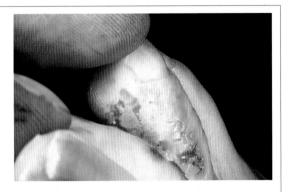

**Figure 17.18** Athlete's foot in a teenage boy. Maceration and peeling are seen in the interdigital space.

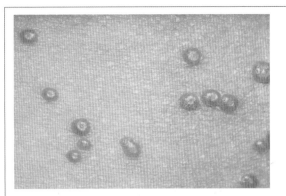

**Figure 17.20** Lesions of molluscum contagiosum. Note the characteristic pearly dome-shaped papules.

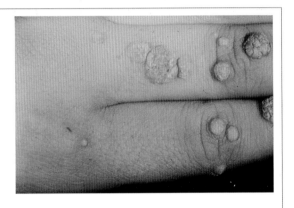

**Figure 17.19** Warts. Note the roughened, irregular, keratotic appearance.

contact dermatitis is a more likely diagnosis. It does occur with some frequency during adolescence. The interdigital spaces between the toes become macerated, with peeling of the surrounding skin. An odour and severe itching are characteristic. Simple measures such as avoidance of occlusive footwear, drying between the toes and the use of antifungal powder usually suffices for most infections.

## Common warts (Figure 17.19)

Common warts are harmless and self-limiting. They are transferred by direct contact, but once acquired are spread by autoinoculation.

**Clinical features.** Warts occur most frequently on the hands, face, knees and elbows, and are well-circumscribed papules with a roughened keratotic, irregular surface. If they are situated on the soles of the feet, they are called verrucas or plantar warts, and are usually flush with the surface of the sole because of the pressure of weight bearing. Plantar warts may be painful.

**Management.** Warts tend to disappear spontaneously within 2 years. No special precautions are indicated for school activities other than swimming, when plantar warts should be covered by a latex sock. If painful, warts can be treated either by the application of a salicylic-acid-based wart paint, or frozen using liquid nitrogen.

## Condylomata acuminata

Condylomata acuminata (venereal warts) are moist, fleshy, papillomatous lesions that occur on the perianal mucosa and genitalia. When untreated they proliferate, forming large cauliflower-like masses. They can be transmitted with or without sexual contact, and in prepubertal children they suggest sexual abuse. Cervical infections may become latent and are associated with cervical cancer. Condylomata are treated by repeated application of podophyllin in tincture of iodine.

## Molluscum contagiosum (Figure 17.20)

Molluscum contagiosum is a common skin infection caused by a DNA virus. The disease is acquired by direct contact and spread by autoinoculation.

**Clinical features.** The lesions are discrete, pearly, dome-shaped papules which typically have a central umbilication from which a plug of cheesy material can be expressed. The papules may occur anywhere on the body, but particularly on the face, axillae, neck and thighs.

**Management.** Molluscum contagiosum is a self-limited disease, but can persist for months if not years. Treatment, for example with phenol or liquid nitrogen, is generally not required, although should be considered in children who also have atopic dermatitis as the infection may spread rapidly.

## Cold sore (Figure 17.21)

Recurrent herpes simplex infections are common as cold sores around the mouth. The virus persists in a latent form after primary infection and appears as single or grouped vesicles perorally. They tend to recur during respiratory tract infections, menstruation and stress. There is minimal therapeutic benefit from the use of topical aciclovir. Children do not need to be excluded from day care or school.

## Scabies (Figure 17.22)

Scabies infection is caused by a mite which is transmitted by direct contact.

**Clinical features.** The eruption is intensely pruritic, particularly at night, and consists of wheals, papules, vesicles and a superimposed eczematous dermatitis. A characteristic lesion occurs which, if seen, is pathognomonic for scabies – the mite burrow appears as a thread-like line, commonly seen in the interdigital spaces, but this is often obliterated by scratching. In older children and adults the head, neck, palms and soles are usually spared, but these areas are often affected in babies.

**Management.** The diagnosis is made by microscopic examination of the mites obtained from scrapings. Treatment requires application of scabicides (malathion or permethrin), but these must be used with extreme caution in babies because of their toxic effects. The eczematous reaction and pruritus may persist for some time because of ongoing hypersensitivity to dead mites. All the household should be treated and bedding and clothes laundered in hot water.

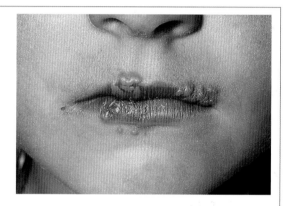

**Figure 17.21** Cold sores caused by herpes simplex infection. The lesions are at the pustular stage prior to crusting.

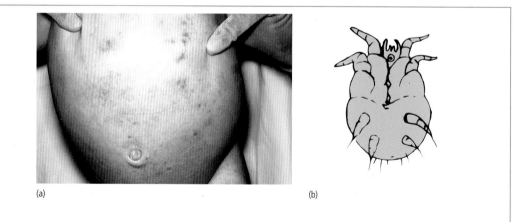

(a)  (b)

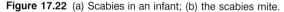

**Figure 17.22** (a) Scabies in an infant; (b) the scabies mite.

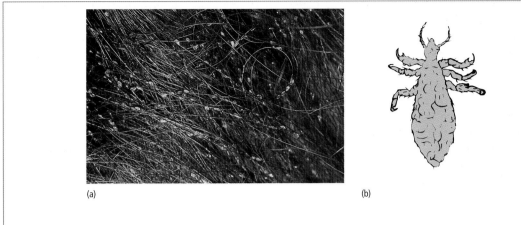

(a)                                                    (b)

**Figure 17.23** (a) Nits; (b) a head louse.

## Head lice (pediculosis capitis) (Figure 17.23)

Head lice are the only common lice infestation in children. They cause intense itching of the scalp. The lice can be transmitted on infested clothing, combs, brushes or direct human contact. The lice themselves are not always visible, but their eggs (or nits) can be readily identified as white specks adherent to the hair shaft, close to the scalp (Figure 17.23a). The adult louse can be extracted by combing the hair with a fine-tooth comb, particularly if this is carried out after washing with conditioner. Combing in this way provides a good preventive measure. Treatment involves the use of a variety of anti-pediculosis shampoos (e.g. carbaryl). After treatment, removal of nits is not necessary to prevent spread.

## Threadworms (enterobiasis)

Threadworm infection causes intense itching of the anus and occasionally the vulval area. It is a common infestation particularly affecting preschool children. The threadworms reside in the gut, and the gravid females migrate by night to the perianal region to deposit their eggs. Scratching transmits the eggs to the fingers and the eggs become disseminated and ingested.

**Clinical features.** The infestation may be asymptomatic or may be recognized if a child is seen to be scratching or complains of itching or anal pain.

**Management.** The diagnosis can sometimes be made by examining the anal area during itching, when a tiny (5 mm) white worm may be seen. Alternately, the sticky-tape test can be applied (see Figure 9.10). Sticky tape is applied around the end of a tongue depressor, with the sticky side outermost. This is placed against the child's anus on rising in the morning, and then applied to a glass slide. The threadworm eggs can then be visualized microscopically. Examination of stool specimens does not identify threadworms. Treatment consists of a single dose of mebendazole. The whole family may need to be treated. Reinfection is very common.

## Birthmarks (Figure 17.24)

### Pigmented naevi

These naevi are rarely present at birth and start to appear at the age of 2 years. In childhood they are usually flat or only slightly elevated. The risk of malignancy is extremely rare unless they are large congenital naevi.

### Café-au-lait spots

Café-au-lait spots are uniformly pigmented, sharply demarcated, macular lesions, which can vary greatly in size. They may be present at birth or develop during childhood. Extensive café au lait spots are a feature of neurofibromatosis (see p. 340).

### Strawberry naevus (superficial haemangioma)

These are bright red, protuberant, compressible, sharply demarcated lesions. Almost all of these lesions, even if large, resolve spontaneously. They may increase in size in the first year of life before fading. Temptation to treat should therefore be resisted unless the lesion's location interferes with a vital function such as vision.

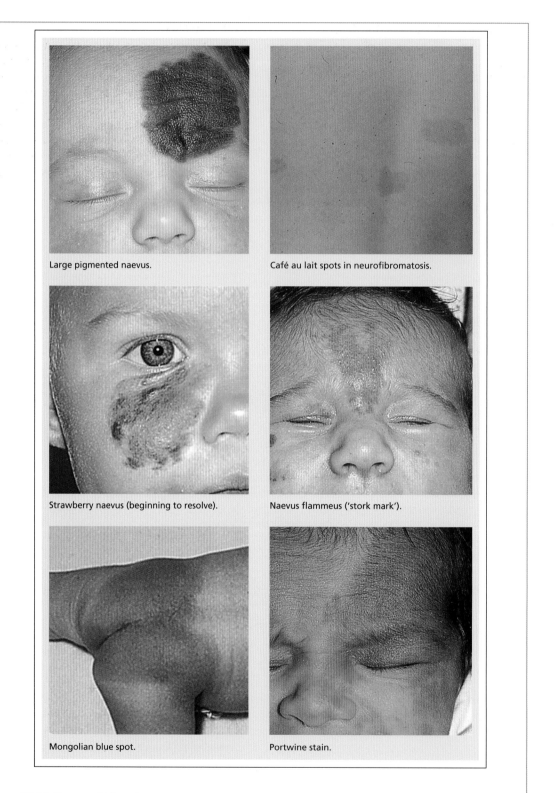

Large pigmented naevus.

Café au lait spots in neurofibromatosis.

Strawberry naevus (beginning to resolve).

Naevus flammeus ('stork mark').

Mongolian blue spot.

Portwine stain.

**Figure 17.24** Common birthmarks.

### Naevus flammeus (salmon patch)

These are small pink flat lesions that occur most commonly on the eyelids, neck and forehead. The lesions on the face usually fade and disappear entirely. They are popularly called stork marks – signs left by the beak of the stork at delivery!

### Mongolian spots

These are blue or slate-grey lesions which occur most commonly in the sacral area. More than 80% of black and Asian babies are born with them. They usually fade during the first few years of life.

### Port-wine stain

Port-wine stains are present at birth. They consist of mature, dilated, dermal capillaries. The lesions are macular, sharply circumscribed, pink to purple in colour and vary in size. If localized to the trigeminal area of the face, the diagnosis of Sturge–Weber syndrome must be considered. In this syndrome there is an underlying meningeal haemangioma and intracranial calcification which can be associated with fits.

*To test your knowledge on this part of the book, please see Chapter 25.*

# CHAPTER 18

# Haematological disorders

And as pale sickness
does invade
Your frailer part, the
breaches made
In that fair lodging,
still more clear
Make the bright
guest, your soul,
appear.

*Edmund Waller*
*(1606–1687)*

## COMPETENCES

### You must . . .

| Know | Be able to | Appreciate |
| --- | --- | --- |
| • How to investigate and manage a child with anaemia<br>• When to suspect leukaemia and therefore request a blood film<br>• The outcomes for leukaemia in childhood | • Diagnose children presenting with a hypochromic microcytic blood film | • That iron deficiency is very common in young children<br>• The impact that chronic haematological conditions have on the child and family<br>• The doctor's role in supporting the family of a child with a chronic haematological condition |

*Paediatrics and Child Health*, Third Edition. Mary Rudolf, Tim Lee, Malcolm Levene.
© 2011 Mary Rudolf, Tim Lee and Malcolm Levene. Published 2011 by Blackwell Publishing Ltd.

# Haematological symptoms and signs

## Finding your way around . . .

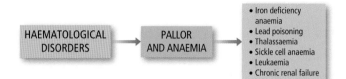

## Anaemia and pallor

**Causes of anaemia/pallor in childhood**

*Common causes* (all hypochromic microcytic)
Iron deficiency anaemia
Thalassaemia trait

*Less common causes*
Lead poisoning
Haemolysis, e.g. thalassaemia major, sickle cell anaemia
Chronic infection
Chronic renal failure
Malignancy, e.g. leukaemia

Anaemia is usually detected when a blood count is performed routinely or on investigating another problem. It may also be suspected if a child is noted to look pale.

Iron deficiency anaemia is very common in childhood, as it is difficult to sustain iron stores when growing rapidly and eating inadequate amounts of iron-rich foods, as is common in toddlers. If a child is ill, serious causes of anaemia must be considered. Chronic infection and chronic renal failure give a normochromic normocytic picture. The haemoglobinopathies have characteristic clinical features. The commonest malignancy is leukaemia, which can usually be suspected on the peripheral blood count.

Haemoglobin levels vary during childhood (Table 6.1, p. 91) and blood counts need to be interpreted accordingly. The neonate starts life with a polycythaemic picture, and a physiological fall occurs in the first years.

In adulthood, anaemia is always investigated before treatment is started. In childhood, nutritional iron deficiency is so common that it is usual to give a therapeutic trial of iron first, and to investigate only if the response is inadequate.

If a child fails to respond to iron, and the picture is microcytic and hypochromic, thalassaemia trait and lead toxicity should be considered, and haemoglobin electrophoresis and testing for lead should be carried out (Figure 18.1). If the child is ill, investigations should not be delayed (see Table 18.1).

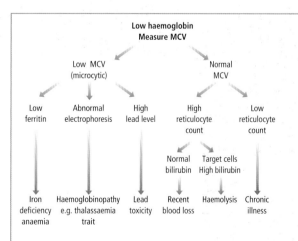

**Figure 18.1** Flow diagram to show the investigation of anaemia.

**Table 18.1** Possible investigations in the child with anaemia who is ill or unresponsive to iron treatment

| Investigation | Relevance |
|---|---|
| Full blood count | Degree of anaemia |
| | Type of anaemia (microcytic, hypochromic, etc.) |
| Blood film | Presence of bizarre cells |
| | Presence of blast cells (suggest leukaemia) |
| Ferritin | Low in iron deficiency |
| Lead level | High in lead toxicity |
| Haemoglobin electrophoresis | Abnormal in haemoglobinopathies (e.g. thalassaemia) |
| Urea and electrolytes | Abnormal in renal failure |
| Blood and urine culture | Chronic infection |
| Bone marrow aspiration | Presence of leukaemic cells |

# Haematological disorders

## Iron deficiency anaemia

In the early childhood years, the demand for iron is high to keep up with the rapid growth that occurs at this time. Babies and children commonly have a poor intake of iron-rich foods, and the combination of these two factors results in a high prevalence of iron deficiency. Blood loss may exacerbate the problem if babies are given whole cow's milk too early, as it can induce chronic microscopic bleeding. The incidence of iron deficiency anaemia can be as high as 50% in some populations, depending on dietary and social habits.

**Clinical features.** Pallor is the most important clue to iron deficiency. If the haemoglobin level falls significantly, irritability and anorexia occur. Iron deficiency may also have a detrimental effect on neurological and intellectual functioning. A number of reports suggest that iron deficiency, even in the absence of anaemia, affects attention span, alertness and learning.

**Investigations.** The initial finding in iron deficiency is a low ferritin level, reflecting inadequate iron stores. As the deficiency progresses, the red blood cells become smaller and the haemoglobin content decreases. With increasing severity, the red blood cells become deformed and misshapen and present characteristic microcytosis, hypochromia and poikilocytosis (see Figure 6.2, p. 92).

**Management.** The treatment is iron salts given orally over 2–3 months so that iron stores are adequately built up. Parents should be advised to limit the consumption of milk to 1 pint daily and to encourage the consumption of more iron-rich foods. The haemoglobin level starts to increase within 1 week of starting treatment. If it does not, this suggests non-compliance or an incorrect diagnosis.

**Prevention.** Breast milk is somewhat protective against the development of iron deficiency. Although it has a relatively low iron content, the iron is absorbed more efficiently because of the iron-binding protein lactoferrin. Since unmodified cow's milk can cause subtle chronic intestinal blood loss, it should not be given during the first year of life. Tea is also inadvisable as it reduces the absorption of iron. In many countries, screening for anaemia is carried out routinely in the first year of life.

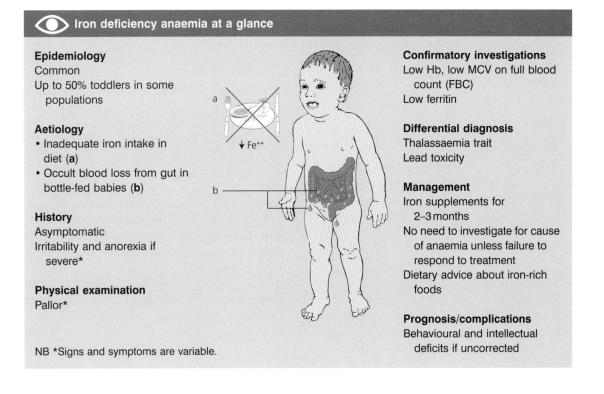

**Iron deficiency anaemia at a glance**

**Epidemiology**
Common
Up to 50% toddlers in some populations

**Aetiology**
- Inadequate iron intake in diet (a)
- Occult blood loss from gut in bottle-fed babies (b)

**History**
Asymptomatic
Irritability and anorexia if severe*

**Physical examination**
Pallor*

**Confirmatory investigations**
Low Hb, low MCV on full blood count (FBC)
Low ferritin

**Differential diagnosis**
Thalassaemia trait
Lead toxicity

**Management**
Iron supplements for 2–3 months
No need to investigate for cause of anaemia unless failure to respond to treatment
Dietary advice about iron-rich foods

**Prognosis/complications**
Behavioural and intellectual deficits if uncorrected

NB *Signs and symptoms are variable.

## Lead poisoning

Lead affects many enzyme systems, but particularly those involved in haem synthesis. The main sources of lead poisoning used to be lead paint and water from lead pipes. More recently, there has been concern regarding inhalation of atmospheric lead from car exhaust fumes.

**Clinical features.** Symptoms are usually subtle and non-specific, consisting of irritability, anorexia and decreased play activity. Colic may be present and pica (the chronic ingestion of non-nutrient substances) is a feature of lead poisoning. Acute encephalopathy with vomiting, ataxia and seizures is now rare.

**Investigations.** The blood picture is one of hypochromic microcytic anaemia. High lead levels confirm the diagnosis. X-ray of the abdomen may demonstrate radiopaque flecks if foreign matter containing lead was recently ingested. X-ray of the long bones may show bands of increased density at the growing ends of the bone (leadlines).

**Management.** Treatment is directed at removing lead from the body. This is achieved by using lead chelating agents which increase lead excretion. The source of lead must be identified and removed.

**Prognosis.** Chronic lead exposure has a detrimental effect on intellectual development. Severe lead poisoning carries a high mortality and survivors are often neurologically handicapped.

## Thalassaemia

The thalassaemias are a heterogeneous group of heritable hypochromic anaemias of varying degrees of severity. The underlying genetic defect results in a suppression of haemoglobin polypeptide chain synthesis. Beta thalassaemia is the commonest form, and affects individuals from Asian and Mediterranean backgrounds.

**Clinical features.** Heterozygous beta thalassaemia produces a mild anaemia, known as thalassaemia trait. Homozygous thalassaemia results in a severe haemolytic anaemia, where compensatory bone marrow hyperplasia produces a characteristic overgrowth of the facial and skull bones (see Figure 18.2).

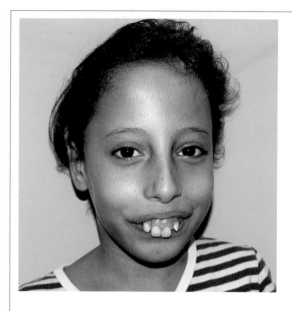

**Figure 18.2** A child with thalassaemia. Note the characteristic facial features with frontal bossing and maxillary overgrowth, and skin pigmentation due to haemosiderosis.

Haemosiderosis with cardiomyopathy, diabetes and skin pigmentation occur as a result of repeated blood transfusions, although these complications have become reduced since the introduction of desferrioxamine.

**Investigations.** A hypochromic, microcytic anaemia is found in thalassaemia trait, which may be confused with iron deficiency. In the homozygous state there is severe anaemia, with hypochromia and microcytosis, bizarre fragmented poikilocytes and target cells. Precise diagnosis of the type of thalassaemia can be made by haemoglobin electrophoresis. In beta thalassaemia major $HbA_1$ is absent and $HbA_2$ and HbF greatly increased.

**Management.** Thalassaemia trait requires no treatment. The main importance of diagnosing the condition is to prevent the child from undergoing unnecessary investigation and treatment. In thalassemia major, blood transfusions are given on a regular basis to maintain haemoglobin levels. Haemosiderosis (overload with iron) is an inevitable consequence, but can be minimized by the use of subcutaneous or intravenous infusions of the chelating agent desferrioxamine. Oral iron chelating agents have been developed and are also used.

## Thalassaemia major at a glance

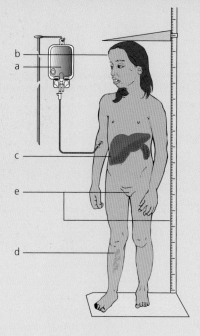

### Epidemiology
Beta thalassaemia is the commonest form
In the UK, it is seen predominantly in children of Greek Cypriot or Bangladeshi origin

### Aetiology/pathophysiology
A genetic defect of globin chain synthesis causing ineffective erythropoiesis in the bone marrow and premature destruction of circulating red blood cells by the spleen
Clinical features are related to haemosiderosis caused by treatment

### History
Anaemia and jaundice from babyhood
Family history of thalassaemia

### Physical examination
- Anaemia (**a**)
- Maxillary overgrowth, frontal bossing (**b**)
- Hepatosplenomegaly (**c**)
- Skin pigmentation due to haemosiderosis (**d**)
- Short stature and delayed puberty (**e**)

### Confirmatory investigations
Hypochromic microcytic anaemia
High HbF and HbA$_2$ on haemoglobin electrophoresis
Antenatal diagnosis is available

### Differential diagnosis
Thalassaemia major: other causes of severe haemolytic anaemia
Thalassaemia minor: iron deficiency, lead toxicity

### Management
Regular blood transfusions to maintain haemoglobin levels
Subcutaneous intravenous or oral iron chelate to excrete iron overload
Genetic counselling for family

### Prognosis/complications
Without treatment, life expectancy is only a few years
Haemosiderosis caused by frequent blood transfusions leads to cardiomyopathy, cirrhosis, diabetes and endocrinopathies
Thalassaemia minor (the heterozygous carrier state) is asymptomatic, and detected by a hypochromic microcytic blood film, and high HbF and HbA$_2$ on electrophoresis

## Sickle cell anaemia

Sickle cell anaemia is the commonest of the haemoglobinopathies, and principally occurs in black populations. The homozygous condition is referred to as sickle cell anaemia and the heterozygous condition as sickle cell trait. The underlying genetic defect is a substitution of one of the amino-acid sequences in the globin chain, causing an unstable haemoglobin (HbS). When HbS is deoxygenated, it forms highly structured polymers which cause brittle, spiny red cells. The clinical manifestations of the disease are caused by ischaemic changes, which result from occlusion of blood vessels by masses of sickled cells.

**Clinical features.** Sickle cell anaemia is a serious disease characterized by chronic haemolytic anaemia. Children experience recurrent, acute, painful crises which can be precipitated by dehydration, hypoxia or acidosis. Painful swelling of the hands and feet is a common early presentation. Repeated splenic infarctions tend to occur in the early years, eventually leaving the child asplenic and susceptible to serious infections. Renal damage leads to a reduced ability to concentrate urine, making dehydration a severe problem. Sickle cell trait is asymptomatic other than in conditions of low oxygen tensions such as occur at high altitude or under general anaesthesia.

**Investigations.** The peripheral blood smear in the homozygote state typically contains target cells, poikilocytes and irreversibly sickled cells (Figure 18.3). Diagnosis is made by haemoglobin electrophoresis, which may also be used for screening in susceptible populations.

**Management.** Treatment of crises is largely symptomatic with analgesics, antibiotics, warmth, adequate fluids, and oxygen if required to maintain normal oxygen saturations. In severe cases with a high proportion of HbS, exchange transfusion is considered. It is important to maintain immunization status, and daily lifelong prophylactic penicillin must be given to reduce the risk of pneumococcal disease.

**Prognosis.** Antenatal screening with specialist counselling of prospective parents is important. Neonatal screening programmes can ensure early identification of affected children and reduce morbidity and mortality by enabling early recognition and treatment of crises.

## 👁 Sickle cell anaemia at a glance

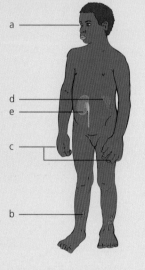

### Epidemiology
Commonest haemoglobinopathy
Predominantly seen in black Americans, Africans, Afro-Caribbeans

### Pathogenesis
Genetic mutation of the Hb chain results in unstable haemoglobin (HbS)
When deoxygenated, HbS causes sickling of red cells which occlude the microcirculation
Crises are precipitated by dehydration, hypoxia, acidosis

### History
Recurrent acute painful crises affecting any organ

### Physical examination
Chronic anaemia
Flow murmur
• Jaundice* (a)
• Chronic leg ulcers* (b)
• Dactylitis (c)
• Splenomegaly in young child only (d)
• Haematuria* (e)

### Confirmatory investigations
Low haemoglobin, sickle cells on smear
HbS and absent HbA on haemoglobin electrophoresis
Abnormal liver function tests

NB *Signs and symptoms are variable.

### Differential diagnosis
Leukaemia
Arthritis

### Complications
Chronic haemolysis
Recurrent painful crises due to ischaemic occlusions
Aplastic crises
Sequestration crises causing circulatory collapse
Pneumococcal infection due to asplenism
Osteomyelitis
Renal damage with reduced ability to concentrate urine
Gallstones
Heart failure from chronic anaemia

### Management
Analgesics, antibiotics, warmth, fluids during crises
Blood transfusion if Hb falls markedly during an aplastic, sequestration or haemolytic crisis
Maintenance of immunizations
Penicillin prophylaxis to prevent pneumococcal infection
Genetic counselling for family

### Prognosis
High mortality from sepsis under age 3 years 85% survive to age 20 years
Heterozygous state is asymptomatic (unless in very low oxygen tensions as with GA or high altitude)

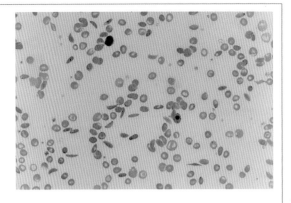

**Figure 18.3** Sickle cell anaemia. Peripheral blood smear with target cells, poikilocytes and irreversibly sickled cells.

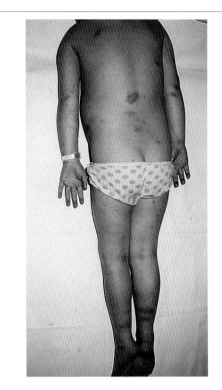

**Figure 18.4** Idiopathic thrombocytopenic purpura.

## Splenectomy and hyposplenism

Children who lack an effective spleen are at increased risk of sepsis. Hyposplenism may occur as a result of sickle cell disease, splenectomy for trauma and some metabolic and haematological conditions.

**Clinical features.** The major risk of hyposplenism is infection, including an increased risk of overwhelming sepsis or meningitis. This is especially high in children under 5 years old. As the spleen is responsible for filtering the blood and early antibody responses, sepsis can progress rapidly, leading to death within 24 hours.

**Treatment and prevention.** Penicillin reduces the risk of infection in hyposplenic children. Other measures include prompt evaluation and treatment of fevers. Pneumococcal vaccination should be given to at-risk children.

## Idiopathic thrombocytopenic purpura

As its name suggests, the features of ITP are caused by thrombocytopenia due to platelet destruction. It presents with petechiae and superficial bruising (Figure 18.4), but mucosal bleeding from the gums and nose may also occur. It often follows 1 or 2 weeks after a viral infection and is thought to have an immunological basis underlying the destruction of circulating platelets.

**Clinical features.** The onset is frequently acute, and apart from the signs of bleeding the child appears clinically well. The most serious complication is intracranial haemorrhage, which occurs in less than 1% of cases.

**Investigations.** Diagnosis is made on the finding of a platelet count which is reduced to below $40 \times 10^9$/L and may be below $5 \times 10^9$/L. The white cell count is normal and there is no anaemia unless significant blood loss has occurred. As the differential diagnosis includes an aplastic or neoplastic process of the bone marrow, bone marrow aspiration may be indicated. In ITP a normal or increased number of megakaryocytes is seen, reflecting the increased turnover which occurs as a result of the destruction of platelets peripherally.

**Management.** In those who have only mild symptoms no treatment is necessary, but where there is a risk of severe bleeding a short course of steroids or immunoglobulin infusion may produce a rise in the platelet count. Platelet transfusion is of little benefit as the transfused platelets survive only briefly. They should be administered, however, if life-threatening haemorrhage occurs.

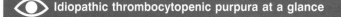

## Idiopathic thrombocytopenic purpura at a glance

**Aetiology**
Destruction of circulating
platelets by immune
mechanism

**History**
Generally well
Bleeding from nose and gums*
Preceding viral infection
1–2 weeks before*

**Physical examination**
Petechial rash (**a**)
Superficial bruising (**b**)

**Confirmatory investigations**
Low platelet count (<20 × 10⁹/L)
Normal white cell count, normal
haemoglobin
Bone marrow aspirate shows
normal or increased number
of megakaryocytes

NB *Signs and symptoms are variable.

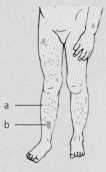

**Differential diagnosis**
Leukaemia
Aplastic anaemia

**Management**
Monitor platelet count
Short course of steroids or IV
gamma globulin for frank
bleeding
Platelet transfusion for life-
threatening haemorrhage

**Prognosis/complications**
85% of patients have simple
limited course
Spontaneous haemorrhage or
intracranial bleeding are the
worrying complications
A few patients develop chronic
ITP and need splenectomy and
immunosuppressive therapy

**Pathogenesis**

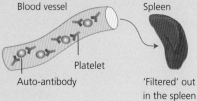

Blood vessel
Spleen
Platelet
Auto-antibody
'Filtered' out
in the spleen

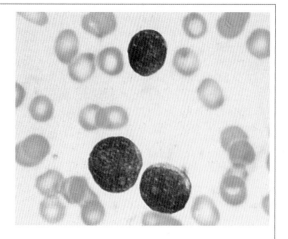

**Figure 18.5** Acute lymphoblastic leukaemia (ALL).
Peripheral blood smear. Note blast cells.

**Prognosis.** Idiopathic thrombocytopenic purpura has an excellent prognosis, with 85% having a self-limited course. Severe spontaneous haemorrhage and intracranial bleeding are usually confined to the initial phase of the disease, and the majority of children recover spontaneously within 6 months. In a few children ITP becomes chronic. Splenectomy and immunosuppressive therapy may be required in these cases.

## Leukaemia

Leukaemia is characterized by a malignant proliferation of white cell precursors which occupy the bone marrow. These blast cells may also circulate in the blood and deposit in various tissues. The commonest leukaemia in childhood is acute lymphoblastic leukaemia (ALL), in which the blast cells resemble primitive precursors of lymphoid origin. It can occur at any age, but the peak incidence is 5 years.

**Clinical features.** The onset is usually insidious with anorexia, irritability and lethargy. As the bone marrow fails, pallor, bleeding and fever occur. Bone pain may be an important presenting complaint. Rarely, signs of increasing intracranial pressure such as headache and vomiting indicate meningeal involvement. On examination, petechiae or mucous membrane bleeding may be present, and lymphadenopathy and splenomegaly may be found.

**Investigations.** Most patients have an markedly elevated white cell count, anaemia and thrombocytopenia on the peripheral blood smear. Blast cells may also be seen (Figure 18.5) The definitive diagnosis is made on examination of the bone marrow, which is replaced by leukaemic lymphoblasts.

**Management.** The basic components of treatment include induction chemotherapy, which is given until the child no longer shows leukaemic cells, prophylactic treatment to the central nervous system and a continuation of systemic treatment for 2–3 years. The child needs to be followed closely for relapse and, if this occurs, intensive retreatment is required.

**Prognosis.** The prognosis varies with the type of ALL. In some forms a cure rate of more than 75% is achieved. The prognosis is less favourable if the child is less than 2 or more than 10 years of age.

*To test your knowledge on this part of the book, please see Chapter 25.*

---

## 👁 Leukaemia at a glance

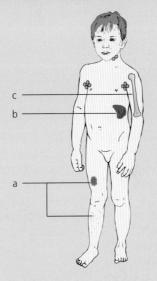

**Epidemiology**
Commonest childhood
  malignancy
80% of childhood leukaemias
  are acute lymphoblastic
  leukaemia (ALL)

**Aetiology**
Malignant proliferation of white
  cell precursors

**History**
Insidious onset
Anorexia, irritability, lethargy
Fever
Bone pain*
Mucous membrane bleeding*

**Physical examination**
Pallor
• Petechiae, bruising* (**a**)
• Lymphadenopathy, spleno-
  megaly* (**b**)
• Bone tenderness* (**c**)

**Confirmatory investigations**
Peripheral blood: high white cell
  count, anaemia,
  thrombocytopenia, blast cells
Bone marrow: replaced by
  leukaemic lymphoblasts

**Differential diagnosis**
Chronic infection
Bleeding diatheses
Other causes of
  lymphadenopathy
Other tumours infiltrating the
  bone marrow

**Management**
Chemotherapy to induce
  remission
Ongoing less intense
  chemotherapy for 2 years
Prophylaxis (chemotherapy/
  radiation) to the CNS
Close monitoring and treatment
  of relapses
Psychosocial support

**Prognosis**
Depends on the leukaemia. In
  favourable presentations of
  ALL, 75% are cured. There is
  a less favourable outcome of
  <2 years or >10 years

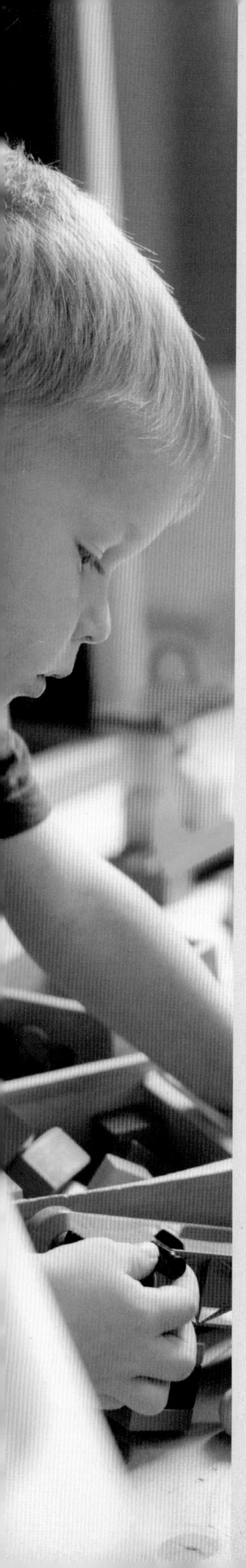

# CHAPTER 19

# Emotional and behavioural problems

She was not really
bad at heart,
But only rather rude
and wild;
She was an aggravat-
ing child.

'Rebecca, Who
Slammed Doors for
Fun', Hilaire Belloc

Common difficulties

## COMPETENCES

## You must . . .

| Know | Be able to | Appreciate |
|---|---|---|
| • Family and school stresses that contribute to the development of behavioural problems<br>• Circumstances that protect against emotional and behavioural difficulties<br>• Types of behaviour indicative of serious disturbance<br>• The sort of advice for common behavioural difficulties that may be helpful for parents | • Obtain a good picture of a child's behavioural and emotional difficulties<br>• Make a good assessment of the family issues | • How common behavioural problems are<br>• How stressful these problems can be for the family<br>• That good parenting is a difficult task<br>• That a good evaluation does not focus on the child alone<br>• That smacking is an inappropriate form of discipline and that praise is more powerful than punishment |

*Paediatrics and Child Health*, Third Edition. Mary Rudolf, Tim Lee, Malcolm Levene.
© 2011 Mary Rudolf, Tim Lee and Malcolm Levene. Published 2011 by Blackwell Publishing Ltd.

# Emotional and behavioural difficulties

## Finding your way around . . .

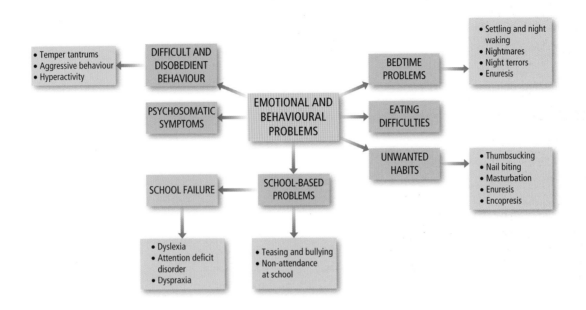

**Common emotional and behavioural problems in childhood**

Sleeping difficulties
Eating problems
Unwanted habits
Difficult and disobedient behaviour
School-based problems
Psychosomatic symptoms
Enuresis

This chapter covers some common problems that are rather different from other conditions presenting to a doctor during childhood, as in the main they do not require a differential diagnosis. On the surface they may seem to lie more in the province of a psychologist, but parents very commonly turn to their doctor for advice about these problems and it is very important that a doctor learns to feel comfortable in addressing them.

Many of these emotional and behavioural problems occur to some degree in all children, but can become exaggerated for a variety of reasons, either related to the child, or as a result of the way they are handled. Other difficulties arise as a result of stresses in the family, such as death or divorce, or are caused by problems at school.

Some childhood behaviours, notably deliberate destructive conduct and self-harm, running away, encopresis and age-inappropriate sexual behaviour are indicative of serious disturbance (see Red Flag box).

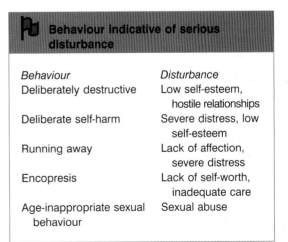

**Behaviour indicative of serious disturbance**

| Behaviour | Disturbance |
|---|---|
| Deliberately destructive | Low self-esteem, hostile relationships |
| Deliberate self-harm | Severe distress, low self-esteem |
| Running away | Lack of affection, severe distress |
| Encopresis | Lack of self-worth, inadequate care |
| Age-inappropriate sexual behaviour | Sexual abuse |

**Table 19.1** Factors contributing to emotional and behavioural problems

| |
|---|
| *In the child* |
| Difficult temperament |
| Developmental delay |
| Poor self-image |
| School failure |
| Abuse |
| *In the family* |
| Marital problems |
| Death of a relative, friend or pet |
| Poor discipline |
| Poverty |
| *In school* |
| Change of school |
| Bullying |
| Poor peer relationships |

**Table 19.2** Factors that protect against emotional/behavioural problems

| |
|---|
| Consistent loving relationships |
| Adequate income |
| Stable family relationships |
| Support outside the family |

Factors that contribute to emotional and behavioural problems, and those that protect against their development, are shown in Tables 19.1 and 19.2.

In addressing emotional and behavioural problems, more than any other problems in childhood, it is essential that the focus does not rest on the child alone. An understanding of the difficulties must be seen in the context of the family and the child's environment. Even if these factors are not directly responsible for the problem (and they often are), it is impossible to address the issue without a good understanding of the broader picture. It is also important to remember that handling these problems well takes both time and empathy.

### History – must ask!

- *The problem.* Obtain a full picture of the problem or difficulty, with the parents' perceptions of the cause, and how the situation is handled. It is worthwhile to include the child in this process if he or she is old enough.
- *The child.* Gain an understanding of the child's temperament and personality, how the child is viewed by the parents, and how he or she relates to friends and family.
- *Recent events.* Childhood disturbances often occur as a reaction to events in the family. Common triggers include the birth of a sibling, the death of a grandparent or a move to a new house or school.
- *The family.* An understanding of family circumstances is essential. Marital friction is a common source of childhood emotional and behavioural problems, and single parents are likely to have more difficulties in disciplining and coping with their children single-handed. Isolation compounds any problem, and it is important to assess the level of support from relatives and friends.
- *School or nursery.* School life brings its own problems and also affects how the child adjusts to difficulties at home. Peer and teacher relationships are as important to assess as the level of academic achievement.

### Management of the child with emotional and behavioural problems

While emotional and behavioural problems differ from one another and from family to family, there is a commonality to approaching their management. Perhaps the most important aspect is to listen well, hearing a full account of the problem. This in itself can be therapeutic, and can lead the family to find solutions themselves. The process of listening cannot be rushed: adequate time must be given.

Many parental concerns relate to normal behaviour, for example, food fads in toddlers or night waking in infants, and it may be adequate simply to provide reassurance. Other concerns relate to difficult behaviour, and guidance regarding effective discipline is required.

The general principles of effective discipline include providing structure and routine in everyday life, setting clear limits of acceptable behaviour, rewarding good behaviour, and being consistent with punishments. Punitive anger is often ineffective and

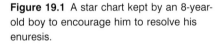

| | 1st Week | 2nd Week | 3rd Week | 4th Week | |
|---|---|---|---|---|---|
| Monday | | ★ | | ★ | |
| Tuesday | | | ★ | ★ | |
| Wednesday | ★ | | ★ | ★ | |
| Thursday | | ★ | ★ | ★ | |
| Friday | | | | ★ | |
| Saturday | | ★ | ★ | ★ | |
| Sunday | ★ | | | ★ | |

**Figure 19.1** A star chart kept by an 8-year-old boy to encourage him to resolve his enuresis.

does not encourage the child to learn to control his or her actions and emotions. It is helpful to remind parents that positive results can be obtained by simply 'catching their child being good', rather than always looking to punish negative behaviour (see Box 19.1).

## Star charts (Figure 19.1)

A useful strategy in overcoming difficult behaviour is using a star chart, which can be adapted to improve and motivate a variety of behaviours, from enuresis to temper tantrums and disruptive behaviour at school. A calendar is drawn up, and each day the child has behaved as required, a star or smiley face is awarded. When a certain number of stars have been earned, the child is rewarded with a prize. This method can be very effective in reinforcing desirable behaviour, while alleviating focus on the negative.

## Time out

Time out is a strategy used during an episode of difficult behaviour. The child is required to stay in a quiet spot for a fixed short period of time. One minute per year of age is a good guide, and a kitchen timer a useful way of enforcing the time. This method allows the child (and the parent) time to cool off, and also gives the parent a clear but limited non-violent means of discipline.

An important aspect of good management is to arrange a follow-up appointment for the parents. Other professionals may also provide support and help for the child. The health visitor is a particular asset for the preschool child, and the teacher for the child at school. More intransigent cases may require referral to a child psychologist or psychiatrist.

**Key points: Emotional and behavioural problems**

• Allow adequate time to make a full assessment
• Ensure that you obtain a full picture of the problem, the child, the family and the environment. If the child is old enough, obtain his or her account too
• Family and school issues must be addressed as well as the child's problems. Where relevant, confer with others involved such as grandparents, teachers, childminders, etc.
• Parents need to be provided with guidelines for effective discipline, to be enforced with love and affection
• Do not wait for a child to grow out of a problem. Even if the problem resolves, the child may remain psychologically damaged
• Medication has a very limited role and should only be prescribed by specialists

# Common behavioural and emotional problems

## Difficulties in settling to sleep and waking through the night

Babies and children differ in their requirements for sleep, and parents vary in their ability to tolerate their child waking in the night. A substantial number of children have struggles around bedtime, and reports indicate that as many as one third of preschool children have disturbed sleep.

In most babies sleeping 'difficulties' are simply habit. They result from a lack of early establishment of routine, and develop so that toddlers readily realize that by playing up at bedtime they can control their parents. Sleep difficulties can also occur as a result of conflict in the family, or anxieties, such as starting school or fear of dying.

**Clinical features.** Sleeping problems include a refusal to settle at night and waking through the night. Difficulties in settling commonly develop if babies are only put to bed once they are already asleep, and may also persist after a child wakes at night as a result of having been unwell. A common mistake is for parents to take the child into their bed or to sleep with the child for comfort. Once this pattern is established, it is difficult to break.

**Management.** Parents may be resigned to sleepless nights and may not be aware that they are capable of controlling the situation. The problem can only be overcome if they are determined to tackle it. This is most easily achieved at an age when the child cannot

> **Box 19.2 Parental guidelines for preventing and managing sleeping problems**
>
> - Set a bedtime
> - Have a relaxing bedtime routine
> - Say goodnight
> - If the child cries, ignore or at least give no positive attention
> - If the child gets out of bed, return him or her promptly and firmly
> - Give positive reinforcement following good nights

climb out of bed. Night sedation is best avoided and should only be used as a last resort.

Successful management involves the following principles (see Box 19.2). A regular routine should be firmly established with parents adopting a calm, understanding but determined attitude, while avoiding angry threats and punishments. Bedtime should be set at a regular time, with time for a quiet, restful pre-bedtime routine, which might include a warm bath, light snack and reading a story. At the set time the child should resolutely be put to bed. If the child cries then, or later through the night, the crying should be ignored, or if that proves to be too stressful for the parent, the child may be checked but no positive attention given. On no account should the child be taken to the parental bed. If the parents are resolute, the sleeping problem resolves within a short period. However, it is usually a stressful undertaking and plenty of support, reassurance and encouragement are required.

## Nightmares and night terrors

In a *nightmare* the child wakes as a result of a bad dream, becomes lucid quickly and usually remembers the dream's content. The child can often simply be reassured and returned to sleep. Nightmares may occur as a result of stresses, and if persistent may need psychological help.

*Night terrors* (see p. 221) are a sleep problem of the preschool years. By contrast with a nightmare, the child wakes confused, disorientated and frightened, and fails to recognize the parent. Minutes pass before orientation occurs, and the dream cannot usually be recalled. Night terrors should not be confused with epilepsy. They are shortlived and reassurance alone is required.

## Eating difficulties

Most children at some stage or another develop food fads. Difficulties frequently result if there is excessive parental insistence on eating and subsequent anxiety when the child refuses to do so. In fact, most of the worry about children's eating is unnecessary, and the majority of children come through this phase thriving and unscathed. Mismanagement by the parent can result in a great deal of conflict and stress at mealtimes, which is particularly distressing as it challenges the parents' basic need to nurture. The problems are compounded if the eating problems are associated with failure to thrive (see p. 257).

Occasionally, severe eating problems are caused by emotional stress and can be associated with problems in the parent–child relationship. Eating disorders in adolescence are discussed in Chapter 23.

**Clinical features.** Eating difficulties may present early in infancy, or more commonly develop during weaning. They may follow a minor illness, where appetite is naturally reduced, and negative reactions to food are set up as a result of parental insistence to eat. The child then develops adversive behaviour such as refusing to eat, spitting out or throwing food, or even vomiting (Figure 19.2). Parents may respond by force-feeding, playing games, preparing alternative meals or persisting with lengthy mealtimes in order to get just another mouthful in.

**Management.** Eating difficulties can be hard to tackle. It is important to reduce the parents' anxiety, and it is often helpful to demonstrate that the child is growing normally according to a growth chart. Battles over food are always best avoided, and relaxed,

social family meals should be encouraged (see Box 19.3). A high chair is invaluable for the toddler at mealtimes, both for comfort and restraint. The child's appetite should be respected and no attempts made to make the child eat by bribery, games or force. With reduction in anxiety and pressure the problem usually resolves. Although the diet often lacks variety, it is usually nutritionally adequate and prescription of vitamins is not necessary.

## Unwanted habits

Children not infrequently indulge in habits that concern their parents. These include thumb-sucking, head-banging, body-rocking, nail-biting, hair-pulling, teeth-grinding and tics. The child may not be able to control these habits, which may be further reinforced by parents attempting to stop the child exhibiting them. As the child grows older he or she often learns to inhibit the habit, particularly in social situations.

### Thumb-sucking

Thumb-sucking is normal in early infancy. However, beyond a certain age it makes the older child appear immature and may interfere with normal alignment of the teeth. It is a difficult habit to influence, and it is best to ignore it as it resolves over time. The child who actively tries to restrain thumb-sucking should be given praise and encouragement.

### Nail-biting

Nail-biting is a difficult habit to break, and it is only possible to influence if the child is resolved to do so. Application of bitter tasting nail varnish can be helpful. In some children nail-biting is a sign of tension.

### Masturbation

Masturbation is common in children, and this sometimes presents as a problem, particularly if it occurs

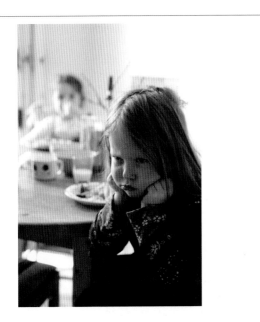

**Figure 19.2** Eating difficulties are very common in young children.

> **Box 19.3 Parental guidelines for preventing and managing eating difficulties**
>
> • Be guided by the child's appetite
> • Mealtimes should be relaxed social events
> • Do not resort to bribery, games or force
> • End the meal at the first sign of adverse behaviour
> • Do not provide alternatives if a meal is refused

publicly. It is more likely to appear when the child is bored, anxious or tired, and the child can often be distracted at these times. Dressing the child in clothes that make access more difficult may help. Parents should be told to ignore the habit in younger children. The older child should not be reprimanded, but does need to be informed that it is not a social activity and should not be carried out publicly.

### Enuresis

Failure to achieve toilet training, or regression to wetting, may be, and often is, a sign of stress. Common precipitating events include the birth of a sibling, death in the family, move to a new home and marital conflict. Enuresis may also result from inadequate or inappropriate toilet training. Enuresis is fully discussed in Chapter 15 (p. 297).

### Encopresis

Encopresis, or the passage of faeces in inappropriate places, usually indicates a serious emotional disturbance. It needs to be distinguished from soiling, which results from leakage of liquid faeces around hard stool when a child is constipated. Encopresis and soiling are covered in Chapter 9 (p. 188).

## Psychosomatic symptoms

Some children manifest emotional problems in the form of psychosomatic symptoms. The commonest of these symptoms are abdominal pain in the younger child and headaches in the older child. Once organic causes for these complaints have been excluded (see Chapters 9 and 11), the possibility of an underlying emotional cause must be explored.

## Difficult and disobedient behaviour

### Temper tantrums (Figure 19.3)

Temper tantrums are a normal aspect of a child's development and peak at around the ages of 18 months to 3 years.

**Clinical features.** Frustration, anger and tantrums are typical for toddlers, and may involve hitting, biting and other potentially harmful behaviour. Some babies and toddlers may resort to breath-holding (see p. 220) as part of the tantrum, and this is often a frightening event to witness.

**Management.** The parental response to tantrums is very important. Caregivers who respond to toddler

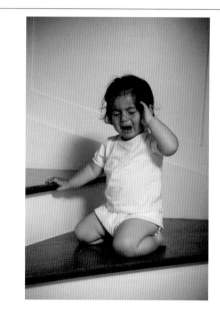

**Figure 19.3** A toddler having a temper tantrum. These are best handled firmly and can often by diverted by giving the child a choice of acceptable activity. Time out is a helpful strategy.

> **Box 19.4 Parental guidelines for preventing and managing temper tantrums**
>
> • Prevent tantrums by avoiding high-risk situations such as hunger and tiredness
> • Attempt to divert the tantrum if possible
> • Teach control by example
> • Reward good behaviour
> • Ignore the behaviour and leave the child until calm
> • Use time out as a strategy

defiance with punitive anger run the risk of reinforcing defiance, and teach the child that out-of-control emotions are a reasonable response to frustration. Temper tantrums need firm handling, without anger and aggression (see Box 19.4). They can often be averted by avoiding high-risk situations like hunger and tiredness, and the episode diverted by providing distraction or allowing the child to have simple choices of activities. Once the tantrum is in full cry, it is best to ignore it until the child has calmed down. Time out is an excellent strategy for managing the tantrum after the event.

### Aggressive behaviour

Young children often have aggressive outbursts, ranging from temper tantrums to hurting others or destroying toys or furniture. This behaviour usually results from frustration and the child's inability to deal with it. Most children learn to control their aggression, but some fail to do so, and it escalates as a problem, leading to bullying in primary school and delinquency beyond. If the behaviour is extreme, the psychiatric term "conduct disorder" is applied.

**Clinical features.** Several factors contribute to aggression. Boys more than girls, large, active children and children from larger families tend to show more aggressive behaviour. Marital discord and aggression within the home contribute to its expression, and exposure to aggression on television may also have an effect. There is a relationship between aggression and emotional disturbance, school failure, brain damage and overactivity.

**Management.** Parents need to be consistent in their management of the child exhibiting aggressive behaviour, and, difficult though it may be, must resist from counteracting aggression with more aggression. Both time out and star charts are positive methods for managing the child. It is important for the doctor to explore whether frustration, disturbance and tensions in the home can be reduced.

For the school-age child, management must involve the staff at school in order to address any academic or social problems, and to gain cooperation in instituting behaviour modification. If aggression and bullying (see below) are general problems for the school, instituting school-based intervention can be effective.

### Hyperactivity (see Attention deficit disorder, pp. 236 and 361)

Hyperactivity is characterized by poor ability to attend to a task, motor overactivity and impulsivity. In the preschool years, children are naturally active and tend to have a short attention span for activities. How this is viewed often depends on parental perceptions, and a child with high spirits in one family may be perceived to be hyperactive in another.

Boys tend to suffer from hyperactivity more than girls, and there is often a family history. Babies who have been temperamentally difficult are more likely to develop into hyperactive children, and it is more common in children with delay of developmental milestones. Hyperactivity is also seen in children who have never been given limits or taught to develop self-control, and it occurs as a reaction to tensions and problems in the home.

**Clinical features.** It is important to be aware that the hyperactive child may not demonstrate the extent of his or her hyperactivity in the visit to the doctor, and the history is therefore more important than observation in the clinical setting. The hyperactive child is restless, impulsive and excitable, and fails to focus on any activity for long. The child tends to have little sense of danger, and requires great vigilance. As such children are unable to concentrate for long on any quiet activity, they often have difficulties on starting school.

**Management.** The hyperactive child benefits from routine and regularity in everyday life. He or she needs to have firm boundaries set for his or her behaviour and consistency in discipline. On starting school, the support of the teacher is essential in helping with adjustment. Medical management is discussed on p. 236.

## School-based problems

### Teasing and bullying

Bullying is a major problem for many children. Overall, about 10% of children report being bullied once per week, and 7% of children are identified as bullies. It is important to remember that victims may be bullies themselves and that most bullying goes undetected by parents and teachers. Bullying tends to be more common in primary schools, and varies from school to school according to the ethos.

**Clinical features.** A child may or may not admit to being a victim of bullying, and it should therefore be considered as a possible cause of distress whenever a schoolchild is disturbed. The child may react to bullying by becoming withdrawn or aggressive or developing psychosomatic symptoms. Bullying is a common cause for school refusal.

**Management.** In schools where bullying is a problem, a whole-school approach is most effective so that the ethos of bullying becomes unacceptable, and both the victims and the bullies are helped. The individual child needs help in handling the situation and increasing self-esteem. Any school refusal must be addressed instantly.

| **Table 19.3** Reasons for school absence |
| --- |
| Illness |
| Kept at home by parent |
| School refusal |
| Truancy |

| **Table 19.4** Causes for failing at school |
| --- |
| *Educational* |
| Limited intellect |
| Attention deficit disorder |
| Hearing or visual deficit |
| Dyslexia |
| Dyspraxia |
| *Social* |
| Problems at home |
| Peer problems |
| Absence from school |

## Non-attendance at school

Most absences from school (Table 19.3) occur as a result of illnesses, which are usually minor. These absences may be prolonged through parental anxiety, particularly if the child has a chronic illness (see p. 36). In some circumstances, parents may keep their child at home to help care for younger siblings or elderly relatives, or even to help out at work. The two situations where the doctor may become involved are school refusal and truancy.

**Clinical features.** The main distinction between school refusal and truancy is that in the former everyone knows where the child is, but in the latter the child's whereabouts are unknown during school hours.

School refusal may result from either separation anxiety or school phobia. Anxiety on separating from parents is common on first starting school, and also may be precipitated by a traumatic event, such as a family death. School phobia is usually triggered by distressing events at school, such as problems with peers or teachers. In both types of school refusal the child is usually well behaved with no academic problems, although there may be associated neurotic behaviour.

Truancy is commonest in secondary school, particularly in the last years, and is probably universal to a degree. Persistent truancy is associated with generally antisocial behaviour, poor academic achievement and unsettled family background.

**Management.** Management of school absenteeism must involve close collaboration between the parents and the teachers. In most cases of school refusal the child should be returned to school as quickly as possible, while addressing underlying problems. Delaying the return only exacerbates the problem. Truancy is harder to tackle and requires a total treatment package. The needs of the child must be met, including any learning problems. The education welfare officer should become involved if the truancy is persistent.

## School failure

Failure at school has profound effects for the individual not only in terms of his or her achievements in adult life and chances of employment, but also in terms of quality of life in the school years. School failure is associated with low self-esteem, behavioural difficulties and psychosomatic disorders. Children may fail at school for a number of reasons, both educational and social, that may compound each other (Table 19.4). From the educational point of view it is particularly important to address causes such as dyslexia, attention deficits and visual or hearing impairments that reduce the child's potential to learn, and can lead to frustration and other negative psychological reactions.

## Dyslexia

Dyslexia is the commonest type of specific learning difficulty. The dyslexic child is unable to process effectively the information required in order to read. The result is a reading ability below that expected for the child's general level of intelligence. Dyslexia must be differentiated from slow reading as a result of limited intellect or inadequate teaching. It is much more common in boys and there is often a family history.

**Clinical features.** The child often has a history of delay in learning to talk. There may be difficulties other than reading, and spelling is affected more than reading. If the difficulty is not recognized, the child is likely to fail at school and commonly responds by withdrawing or exhibiting disruptive behaviour.

**Management.** If suspected, the diagnosis must be confirmed on testing by an educational psychologist. The child needs individual help in overcoming the difficulty, and may need 'statementing' (see p. 46).

### Attention deficit disorder

'Attention deficit disorder' refers to a general difficulty in focusing on tasks or activities. It may or may not occur with hyperactivity (see pp. 236, 359) and is far commoner in boys than girls. These children often have a history of being colicky, temperamentally difficult babies.

**Clinical features.** The child is fidgety, has a difficult time remaining in his or her seat at school, is easily distracted and impulsive, has difficulty following instructions, talks excessively and flits from one activity to another. Daydreaming is more obvious if hyperactivity is not a feature.

**Management.** The child benefits from a regular daily routine with simple clear rules, and firm limits enforced fairly and sympathetically. Overstimulation and overfatigue should be avoided. In school, a structured programme is required with good home communication to ensure consistency.

Attention deficit problems, particularly if associated with hyperactivity, can be very stressful to the family and counselling may be needed. Central nervous system stimulants such as methylphenidate, prescribed during school hours, have been shown to be helpful in selected cases. Therapies such as megavitamins and low-sugar diets have not been proved to be effective. Diets with no artificial colourings or flavourings remain controversial, but in general do not help the majority of these children.

**Prognosis.** Both the hyperactivity and attention difficulties tend to improve through adolescence, but the educational deficit may persist as a handicap later in life.

### Dyspraxia

Clumsiness, or dyspraxia, can cause problems at home and at school. Fine motor incoordination leads to untidy writing, and gross motor incoordination leads to difficulty with sports. The academic and social difficulties that ensue can cause the child considerable unhappiness and lead to behavioural problems if they are not recognized and dealt with helpfully. An occupational therapist can assist the school in devising a programme which will help overcome the difficulties and build self-confidence.

*To test your knowledge on this part of the book, please see Chapter 25.*

# CHAPTER 20

# Social paediatrics

There was an old woman
who lived in a shoe,
She had so many children
she didn't know what
to do!
So she gave them some
broth without any bread,
And she whipped them all
soundly and sent them
to bed!

*English nursery rhyme*

## COMPETENCES

### You must . . .

| Know | Be able to | Appreciate |
|------|-----------|-----------|
| • How to proceed if you suspect that a child has been abused or neglected<br>• Features that are characteristic of non-accidental injury | • Recognize signs of abuse and neglect | • The impact that abuse and neglect have on a child<br>• The assessment of abuse should only be carried out by a skilled paediatrician in an appropriate setting |

# Symptoms and signs of child abuse

## Finding your way around . . .

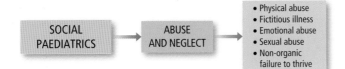

During the course of child health surveillance children may be identified as being the victims of neglect or abuse. This may emerge on finding characteristic physical signs at a routine examination, or witnessing abnormal behaviour on the part of the child. The older child may take the opportunity of a routine contact with a doctor or nurse to disclose abuse.

The clinical evaluation of a child who is the sus-

---

### Types of child abuse

Physical neglect
Emotional abuse
Non-accidental injury
Sexual abuse
Non-organic failure to thrive (see p. 266)

---

pected victim of abuse or neglect requires skill. Enough time must be allowed so the evaluation is not rushed, and the setting must be private to ensure confidentiality. The doctor's attitude is important as it is vital to gain both the child's and, where possible, the family's trust. There is no place for the doctor to be accusatory in any way.

The evaluation must be thorough, including a full history and physical examination, or important clues may be missed. If injuries are present, it is important to decide whether they were incurred accidentally or could have been inflicted.

It is important to contact other professionals such as social workers, the GP and the school, who may throw light on the child's home circumstances.

### History – must ask!

• *How did the injury occur?* The most important part of the history is the explanation given for any injuries, as this helps you decide whether the

lesions were likely to be non-accidental (see Red Flag box). Characteristically, in non-accidental injury the explanation given does not match the appearance of the injury and often sounds unconvincing. Injuries occurring in young, non-mobile infants should arouse particular suspicion. There is often a delay before medical advice is sought, and the child may communicate details which conflict with the parental explanation.

• *Past medical history.* A history of previous injuries is obviously relevant.

• *Developmental history and behaviour.* A child's psychosocial development can be severely affected by neglect and abuse, and an assessment can also be useful to serve as a baseline for the future.

• *Social history and family history.* In order to gain a complete picture you need a full social history. It is important to know who is in the home, and if anyone other than the mother is responsible for caring for the child. Child abuse is more likely to occur in unstable homes where there are changes of partner. Other professionals such as health visitors and nursery nurses can often provide important details about the family.

---

### 🚩 Characteristics of non-accidental injury

• Injuries in very young children
• Explanations which do not match the appearance of the injury and sound unconvincing
• Multiple types and age of injury
• Injuries which are 'classic' in site or character
• Delay in presentation
• Things the child may communicate during the evaluation

## Physical examination – must check!

You must always carry out a thorough physical examination with the child undressed.

- *General appearance.* Note how the child looks. He or she may show signs of neglect, such as an unkempt dirty appearance, sores and untreated nappy rash. The child's reaction to you is important. A child who has experienced prolonged abuse may have a 'frozen watchful' appearance: appear motionless, with an expressionless face and wary eyes. The neglected child may be abnormally affectionate to strangers, as if seeking any human contact.
- *Growth.* Abused and neglected children commonly fail to thrive. Height, length, weight and head circumference need to be measured, plotted and compared with previous measurements.
- *Injuries* (see Box 20.1). Examine the child for signs of injury. Many non-accidental injuries have a characteristic appearance, and multiple injuries at different sites and of different ages are particularly suspect.
    - *Bruises.* Multiple bruises are commonly found on the legs of any toddler, but bruises at other sites may be suspicious. The age of the bruises can be estimated from the colour and may help in refuting an implausible explanation. The pattern of the bruise may indicate how it was acquired (Figure 20.1 a–d).
    - *Burns and scalds.* When a toddler accidentally scalds him- or herself the scald is usually irregular and asymetrical in shape with additional splash marks. Inflicted scalds are classically symmetrical and may cause a doughnut-shaped lesion on the buttocks, which are centrally spared where the bottom of the bath protects the skin from contact with the hot water (Figure 20.1f). Inflicted cigarette burns cause deep circular ulcers (Figure 20.1e) as compared with the superficial lesions seen with accidental burns.
    - *Bites.* Bites have the shape of a dental impression. These can be used forensically to identify the perpetrator (Figure 20.1g).
    - *Hidden head injuries.* Examine the fundi for retinal haemorrhages (Figure 20.2), as they may occur when a baby is shaken and can be associated with the presence of subdural haematomas (see p. 220).
    - *Bone injuries* (Figure 20.3). You may find evidence of fractures.
- *Signs of sexual abuse.* If the child discloses sexual abuse or is suspected of being a victim, the genitalia and anus must be carefully examined. Signs of sexual abuse may be overt, such as bruising and tears, or may be more subtle, but it is important to remember that the absence of physical signs does not in any way mean that a child has not been sexually abused. This examination should only be carried out by an experienced paediatrician in a setting where the child's privacy can be respected.

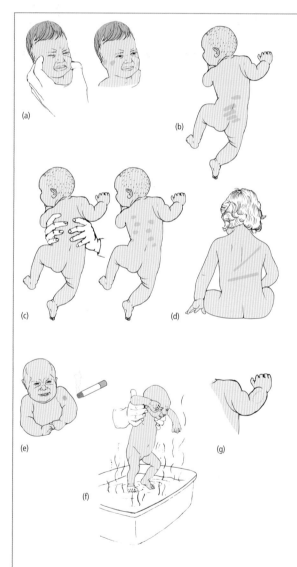

**Figure 20.1** Skin lesions indicative of non-accidental injury: (a) facial squeeze, (b) slap marks, (c) grip marks, (d) stick marks, (e) cigarette burns, (f) scalding, and (g) bite marks.

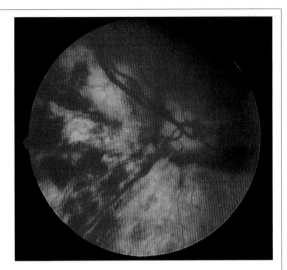

**Figure 20.2** Retinal haemorrhages seen in an infant who was admitted with fits and lethargy following a severe shaking injury.

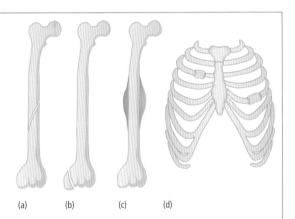

**Figure 20.3** Types of fractures associated with non-accidental injury: (a) spiral fractures, (b) metaphyseal chips, (c) periosteal bleeds, and (d) callus around ribs.

**Box 20.1  Clinical features of physical abuse**

- Physical neglect
- Failure to thrive
- Bruises
- Fractures
- Burns and scalds
- Bites
- Ligature marks

**Table 20.1** Investigations in suspected child abuse

| Investigation | Relevance |
| --- | --- |
| Photographs | Useful for further consultation and evidence in court |
| Full blood count, prothrombin time and partial thromboplastin time | To rule out thrombocytopenia or other haematological disorder as a cause for excessive bruising |
| Skeletal survey (X-rays) | Characteristic fractures and fractures at various stages of healing may be found in non-accidental injury |
| Head CT scan | Particularly important in infants presenting with probable abuse, to detect subdural haemorrhages which may otherwise be easily missed |
| Pregnancy test and cultures for sexually transmitted disease | In children suspected of sexual abuse, the finding of sexually transmitted disease is strong corroborative evidence (and needs treating) |

### Investigations

Table 20.1 shows the investigations which may be helpful in children suspected of being victims of abuse. If suspicious injuries are found, photographs should be taken so that they are available for future consultation and evidence in court.

As the implications of non-accidental injury are so serious, rare medical causes of excessive bruising or fragile bones must be ruled out. A full blood count and clotting screen will exclude a haematological cause for bruising. In the case of fractures, osteogenesis imperfecta (brittle bone disease) may be considered and can usually be ruled out on clinical evaluation.

In any child <2 years old suspected of being a victim of abuse or neglect, a skeletal survey (X-ray of the entire body) should be requested to determine whether there have been previous unreported injuries. Fractures that have been inflicted often have a characteristic appearance and tend to occur through the growth plate, as this is the most vulnerable part of growing bones. Spiral fractures are particularly likely to result from violent inflicted trauma. When multiple fractures are found, they are often seen to be at different stages of healing.

The child who has disclosed sexual abuse needs to be investigated for sexually transmitted diseases, and forensic samples taken. A pregnancy test is needed in the postpubertal girl who has been raped.

### Management of the child suspected of being a victim of abuse (see also Chapter 5)

Where there is any suspicion that a child has suffered abuse or neglect, the child should be referred immediately for the specialist opinion of a paediatrician experienced in child protection work. If the paediatrician concludes that the child has been abused or is at risk of abuse, the social services department is immediately informed.

If the child is deemed to be in danger, or further assessment is required, he or she needs to be admitted to a place of safety, usually a hospital ward or a social services institution, until a fuller inquiry can be made. An emergency care order can be obtained from court if the family resists admission or investigation.

The social work team usually take the lead in planning the strategy for management. Initial policy is worked out at a case conference, attended by all professionals involved and the parents. Many children are allowed home, initially under supervision and with appropriate support. Occasionally it is necessary to take the child away from the parents. This is generally a difficult decision and requires a court order. The child may be placed with another member of the family, in foster care or, in the case of an older child, a group home.

For the child returned to his or her home, support must be provided. This may be in the form of placement in a social services day nursery, or voluntary and self-help groups may be available to help the parents overcome their difficulties. Social Care keep a record of children who have been abused or neglected so that professionals can readily determine if a child or others in the family are known to be at risk.

---

### Key points: When abuse is suspected

- Evaluations should be conducted in privacy and the child's trust gained
- Helpful information can be obtained from other health professionals and social services
- If injuries are present, indications that they have been inflicted must be sought in the history and physical appearance
- A thorough examination, including growth and general appearance, must be made to identify other injuries, failure to thrive and signs of neglect
- Comprehensive clear notes must be made and where necessary photographs taken as they may be required for evidence

# Forms of abuse and neglect

## Physical abuse (non-accidental injury)

Parents who abuse their children come from all ethnic and socioeconomic groups. In most cases the abuser is a related caretaker or male friend of the mother. Most have neither psychotic nor criminal personalities, but tend to be unhappy, lonely, angry adults under stress, who have often themselves experienced physical abuse as children. The event often coincides with the loss of a job or a home, marital strife or physical exhaustion.

**Clinical features.** Injuries may range in severity from minor bruises to fatal subdural haematomas. Characteristic injuries are shown in Figures 20.1 and 20.3.

**Management.** The injuries, if severe, require medical attention. The general management of abused children is discussed above.

---

### 👁 Physical abuse at a glance

**Epidemiology**
Occurs in all ethnic and socioeconomic groups

**Aetiology**
Most perpetrators are close contacts of the child, often abused themselves as children

**History**
Delay in seeking medical advice*
Explanation does not match appearance of injury*
Inconsistent history*
Past injuries*

**Physical examination**
Injuries typical of abuse
Multiple injuries of different ages*
Failure to thrive*
Signs of neglect*

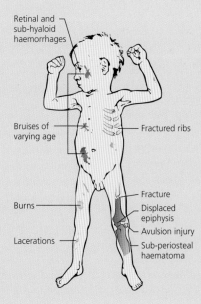

Retinal and sub-hyaloid haemorrhages

Bruises of varying age

Fractured ribs

Burns

Lacerations

Fracture

Displaced epiphysis

Avulsion injury

Sub-periosteal haematoma

**Confirmatory investigations**
It is essentially a clinical diagnosis
Blood dyscrasias need to be ruled out by an FBC and clotting screen
Skeletal survey is needed to assess presence of fractures
Consider head CT

**Differential diagnosis**
Accidental injury
Blood dyscrasias
Osteogenesis imperfecta very rare

**Management**
Medical care for injury
Involve social services
Admit to place of safety if child in ongoing danger
Case conference
Child Protection Register
Removal from home if child remains at risk

**Prognosis/complications**
Without intervention 5% of abused children are killed, 25% are seriously injured
Neurological damage is common from repeated CNS insults
Emotional/behavioural disturbance
Commonly become perpetrators of abuse as adults

NB *Signs and symptoms are variable.

**Prognosis.** About 5% of abused children who are returned to their parents without intervention are killed and 25% seriously injured. Children with repeated injury to the central nervous system may develop brain damage with learning disabilities or epilepsy. Abused children are commonly fearful, aggressive and hyperactive, and many go on to become delinquent, violent and the next generation of abusers.

## Emotional abuse and neglect

Emotional abuse can be defined as the frequent rejection, scapegoating, isolation or terrorizing of a child by caretakers. It is usually very difficult to prove, and has long-term emotional and developmental consequences for the child.

**Clinical features.** Emotional abuse is commonly associated with developmental delay and failure to thrive (see pp. 233, 266). On presentation the child may be apathetic, and show evidence of physical neglect such as dirty clothing, unkempt hair and nappy rash. There may be signs of non-accidental injury, and if there is any suggestion of regression of developmental skills, the diagnosis of chronic subdural haematomas (which can occur as a result of shaking injuries) should be considered.

**Management.** Intensive input and support is required. Day nursery placement can provide good stimulation, nutrition and care. If the child continues to be at risk for ongoing abuse or neglect, he or she must be removed from the home (see pp. 30, 366).

**Prognosis.** The prognosis depends on the degree of the damage incurred and how early the intervention is provided. Children who require removal from the home often have irreversible learning and emotional difficulties.

## Sexual abuse

Sexual abuse may take the form of inappropriate touching, forced exposure to sexual acts, vaginal, oral or rectal intercourse and sexual assault. Secrecy is often enforced by the offender, who is usually male and a family member or acquaintance of the family, but rarely a stranger.

**Clinical features.** Sexual abuse may come to light if disclosure is made as a result of genital infections or trauma, or if a child exhibits inappropriate sexual behaviour. Signs of trauma may be evident in the mouth, anus or genitalia, but absence of signs is common and less than half of the victims have any substantiating physical evidence.

**Management.** Particularly sensitive and skilled management is required and should only be undertaken by those experienced in the work. All victims require psychological support, and the offender too may be amenable to help.

**Prognosis.** With intervention most incest victims can lead normal adult lives. Without intervention they are likely to become seriously disturbed and grow up unable to form close relationships. Victims commonly enter abusive relationships with men later in life and often need psychiatric help.

## Non-organic failure to thrive

A proportion of young children whose weight falters or who fail to thrive (see p. 257) do so as a result of neglect, the principal factor being inadequate nutrition. The mother is commonly deprived and unloved herself and often is clinically depressed.

**Clinical features.** The child looks malnourished and uncared for, and immunizations are often not up to date. Delays in development are common, and signs of physical abuse may be seen. When admitted to hospital these babies often show rapid weight gain.

**Management.** If the problem is clearly one of neglect, child protection procedures must be initiated.

**Prognosis.** Without detection and intervention a small proportion of these children die from starvation. With intervention, catch-up growth may occur, but brain growth may be jeopardized and emotional and educational problems are common.

## Fabricated illness (Munchausen by proxy)

In this bizarre form of abuse the carer fabricates the child's symptoms or signs. The child is likely to become subject to extensive hospitalization and investigations, and may be in actual physical danger (as when apnoea is fabricated by suffocation or drugs administered without prescription). The diagnosis is difficult to make, but must be suspected if the presentation is unusual and incongruous, and if symptoms and signs emerge in the parent's presence alone.

*To test your knowledge on this part of the book, please see Chapter 25.*

# CHAPTER 21

# Emergency paediatrics

Elisha came into the house and behold! – the boy was dead, laid out on his bed. He entered and shut the door behind them both. Then he went up…and placed his mouth upon his mouth…and he warmed the flesh of the boy…the boy sneezed seven times, and the boy opened his eyes.

*2 Kings 4: 32–34*

## COMPETENCES

## You must . . .

### Know

- How severely ill children may present
- How to rapidly assess a child presenting as an emergency
- The basics of cardiopulmonary resuscitation
- How to diagnose key emergency paediatric conditions
- The principles of managing key emergency paediatric conditions
- How to clinically estimate the severity of dehydration and principles of treating it
- Advice given in the Back to Sleep campaign

### Be able to

- Carry out the Heimlich manoeuvre
- Place the comatose child in the recovery position
- Advise a parent about first aid management of a fitting child
- Advise a parent about the use of rectal diazepam or buccal midazolam

### Appreciate

- That in emergencies management precedes history and physical examination

*Paediatrics and Child Health*, Third Edition. Mary Rudolf, Tim Lee, Malcolm Levene.
© 2011 Mary Rudolf, Tim Lee and Malcolm Levene. Published 2011 by Blackwell Publishing Ltd.

# Emergency paediatric presentations

## Finding your way around . . .

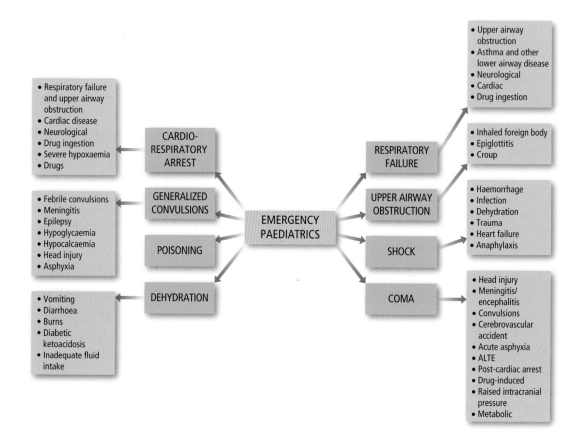

This part of the book discusses the presentation and treatment of children with acute life-threatening disorders and emergency problems. Children may become critically ill very rapidly, and survival depends on rapid recognition of the ill child, appropriate first aid, rapid transfer to hospital and appropriate use of therapies.

The commonest cause of severe illness in children is infection. The immune response may be impaired by prematurity, malnourishment, drugs (steroids in particular), malignant disease and its management and, rarely, an inherited or acquired abnormality in immune function (Table 21.1). AIDS and congenital immune deficiency are very rare cause of immune deficiency in childhood. Newborn babies are particularly prone to infection. This is usually bacterial and

acquired perinatally from the mother or nosocomially from carers.

### How do acutely ill children present?

Presentation to some extent depends on the age of the child. Babies and young children obviously cannot verbalize their distress. The older child is likely to have more specific symptoms and an ability to describe the site of any pain. Physical signs may also vary with age: for example, signs such as Kernig's or neck stiffness are specific in older children, but in very young children they may not occur at all or only very late in the illness. For these reasons, assessing whether a baby of 6 months of age or less is significantly ill may be difficult, and attempts have been made to develop easily applied rating scores to evaluate how ill a baby is.

**Table 21.1** Factors predisposing to the development of severe and acute illness in children

| Factor | Risk group |
|---|---|
| Age | Neonates |
| | Infants <1 year |
| Impaired immune function | Premature infants |
| | Steroid treatment |
| | Malignancy |
| | Immune deficiency (AIDS) |
| | Splenectomy |
| Malnutrition | E.g. malabsorption |
| Chronic disease | E.g. cystic fibrosis |
| Immunization status | |
| Exposure to infectious agents | Children in hospital |
| | Institutionalized children |

**Table 21.2** Features to look for in determining whether a baby in the first 6 months of life is acutely ill. (From Baby Check*)

| Symptom | Particular features to consider |
|---|---|
| Vomiting | Regular vomiting |
| | Bile-stained vomiting |
| Fluid intake | Reduction of one-third on normal 24-hour volume |
| Urine output | Fewer wet nappies than expected |
| Blood in stool | Frank blood in stool |
| Drowsiness | Abnormally drowsy most of time |
| Abnormal cry | High-pitched |
| Floppiness | Persistent and generalized |
| Alertness | Less watchful of mother |
| | Less interested in environment |
| Wheeze | Expiratory |
| Recession | Deep indrawing of intercostal or subcostal area |
| Pallor | |
| Cyanosis of periphery | |
| Skin perfusion | Is there a significant delay in reperfusion of big toe after squeezing? |
| Swelling in groin | Is there an inguinal hernia? |
| Rash on trunk | Generalized? |
| Pyrexia | Temperature >38.0°C (less than 3 months of age) or >39.0°C (more than 3 months of age) |

*C.J. Morley, A.J. Thornton, T.J. Cole, P.H. Hewson and M.A. Fowler. Baby check: a scoring system to grade the severity of acute systemic illness in babies under 6 months old. *Archives of Disease in Childhood* 1991, **66**, 100–6.

Baby Check* is a system designed to be used by parents to guide them in seeking medical help. It consists of a number of symptoms over the previous 24 hours as well as examination findings, which are scored and indicate whether the baby is mildly, moderately or seriously ill (see Table 21.2).

Older children with severe illness are easier to assess. Signs of acute and potentially severe illness in older children are shown in Table 21.3.

Critically ill children must be rushed to hospital for resuscitation and supportive care without delay as they can deteriorate very rapidly. Clearly, children with the following conditions need urgent hospitalization:

- shock (see p. 378 for definition);
- coma;
- acute cyanosis;
- profound apnoea;
- major trauma;
- progressive purpuric rash (see p. 322).

## Assessment and management in an emergency

Although life-threatening disorders often start insidiously, it is important to remember that progression from minor symptoms to moribund state may occur very rapidly. This is particularly likely if the child has an underlying predisposition to severe illness (Table 21.1).

The homeostatic physiological milieu is relatively fragile in children and particularly so in infancy. The

**Table 21.3** Signs of acute and severe illness in older children

| Symptom | Features |
|---|---|
| Toxicity | This includes a high fever with marked facial flushing and confusion |
| | Hallucinations may occur with high fever |
| Severe pain | Associated with pallor, tachycardia, immobility or writhing |
| Change in consciousness level | This is always significant of severe illness |
| Shortness of breath | Causing difficulty in speaking |
| Dehydration | See p. 385 |
| 'Going off their feet' | Any acute difficulty in walking or unsteadiness of gait |

child has an ability to preserve intravascular volume against abnormal fluid losses as occur in diarrhoea or excessive vomiting, but once these physiological mechanisms have been fully deployed, collapse with shock can rapidly occur.

Unlike in any other aspect of paediatrics, management of the emergency must precede history and examination. After very rapid assessment, the critically ill child must be resuscitated, the airway secured and the child's condition stabilized. The initial management of the critically ill child is discussed below, but the difference between life and death may depend on the management in the first hour after the collapse.

Once the initial resuscitation has taken place, the child must be carefully assessed for evidence of disease in other systems that may have caused the initial collapse, although the underlying disease may be obvious as in trauma or asthma.

### History – must ask!

• *Description of the events leading up to the collapse.* A detailed history from a witness of the collapse may be very helpful. This may be a teacher or a playmate if the child collapsed away from home. Establish whether the child was well immediately before the collapse or whether there was a rapidly progressive illness.

• *Previous medical history.* It is very important to establish whether the child has an underlying illness such as diabetes, allergy or asthma predisposing to collapse. Find out if the child has been on prescription drugs or could have been indulging in substance abuse. In infants, a recent minor illness may be significant, and the severity of diarrhoea and vomiting may have been underestimated by the parents.

### Physical examination – must check!

After the initial emergency assessment of the child, a more careful physical examination must be carried out. Important clues as to the cause of the collapse may be obtained from the physical examination; the Red Flag box lists the important features to assess.

---

**⚑ Signs that may help in the diagnosis of a severe illness**

Rashes, particularly petechial or purpuric (see p. 322)
Depth of coma (Figure 21.3)
State of hydration (p. 387)
Vital signs (blood pressure, pulse, respiratory rate, temperature)
Signs of respiratory distress
Stridor
Signs of injury
Surface area of burns

---

### Investigations

Investigations are directed towards:

• *Diagnosis.* The appropriate investigations are discussed below in the relevant sections on causes of collapse.
• *A guide to appropriate management.* If the child requires respiratory support, a chest X-ray and regular blood gases are essential to guide management.

### Management

Emergency treatment should occur where the child presents. In practice, this is in an Accident and Emergency room. A guide to the immediate assessment, resuscitation and management is shown in Box 21.1. As soon as the child is stable, he or she

## Box 21.1 Assessment and management in an emergency

*Assessment*
This must be conducted rapidly
Is the airway clear?
Is the child breathing?
Is there adequate circulation?
Are there obvious injuries?
  • fractures
  • lacerations
  • burns
What is the level of consciousness?

*Resuscitation*
Clear the airway
Give inflation breaths if not breathing
Cardiopulmonary resuscitation if cardiac output is poor
Establish intravenous access
Pressure to stop bleeding
Immobilize fractured limbs, and neck if trauma suspected

*Problem-directed management*
Blood gases
Treat shock with fluids (p. 378)
Investigate cause of illness
Investigate function of other organs
Ensure adequate hydration
Specific drugs once a diagnosis is made

## Key points: The child presenting as an emergency

• Rapidly assess the state of the child
• Stabilize the condition
• Only then take a full history and carry out a physical examination
• Assess the child for evidence of disease in other systems which may have precipitated the emergency

tion. Once the child is stabilized, the most senior member of the team should inform the parents of the situation and answer their questions as honestly as possible.

# Cardiorespiratory arrest

## Commoner causes of cardiorespiratory arrest

*Severe respiratory disease*

*Upper airway obstruction*

*Cardiac disease*
Arrhythmia
Cardiac failure
Myocarditis

*Neurological disorder*
Birth asphyxia
Cerebral oedema
Coning
Head injury

*Drug or toxin*

*Severe hypoxic–ischaemic insult*
Suffocation
Drowning

*Anaphylaxis*

should be moved to an intensive care unit for further monitoring and management.

Management of the pulse-less or moribund child must be prioritized into these four areas in sequence.

| A | Airway | *plus* | D | Don't |
|---|--------|--------|---|-------|
| B | Breathing | | E | Ever |
| C | Circulation | | F | Forget |
| D | Drugs | | G | Glucose |

Management of shock is discussed on p. 378. Management of the traumatized child is beyond this book's scope.

### Support for relatives
During resuscitation, relatives must be kept closely informed. A member of the resuscitation team – usually a nurse – should stay with the relatives and keep them informed of progress and give emotional support. It is best if only one person is involved in talking to the relatives during the process of resuscita-

There must be a well-rehearsed protocol for cardiac arrest that occurs in hospital. All medical staff involved in resuscitation should be appropriately trained. It is beyond the scope of this book to describe the detailed approach to the management of cardiac arrest, but the important principles are shown in Box 21.2.

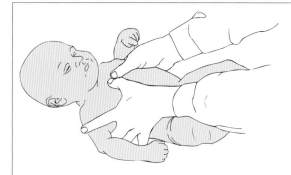

**Figure 21.1** External cardiac massage in an infant. The compression rate should be 100 per minute with 30 compressions to two ventilatory breaths.

---

**Box 21.2 Managing cardiorespiratory arrest**

*Call for help*

*Airway*
Open airway
Clear oropharynx

*Breathing*
Ventilate initially with high-concentration oxygen via a facemask and self-expanding resuscitation bag
Mouth-to-mouth if nothing else available
Intubate once experienced operator available

*Circulation*
Check pulse
External cardiac massage, rate of 100/min
Alternate 30 cardiac compressions with two lung inflations
Display ECG trace and defibrillate if appropriate

*Drugs*
Establish vascular access for drug and fluid administration
Alternatively, some drugs can be given down the endotracheal tube or by direct intracardiac injection
Check blood sugar, give glucose if low

---

*Management*

The process of resuscitation is a team effort and requires an experienced paediatrician and anaesthetist together with nursing support. The most senior doctor on the team should take charge of the resuscitation, and if necessary be the person who decides how long resuscitation should continue if there is no response.

The principles of managing the child with cardiac arrest is the same for any critically ill child. Proceed in the sequence:

• Open the airway (chin lift/jaw thrust).
• Clear the airway by suction under direct vision if necessary.
Secure the airway by means of a tracheal tube if necessary
• Establish ventilation with inflation breaths using high-concentration oxygen.
• Give external cardiac massage (Figure 21.1).
• Give cardiac stimulant drugs.

Once the initial resuscitation has been established, consideration should turn to the cause of the collapse and the child should be monitored very closely in an intensive care environment.

## Respiratory failure

---

**Causes of respiratory failure**

*Upper airway obstruction*
Inhaled foreign body
Epiglottitis
Croup

*Lower airway disease*
Asthma
Bronchiolitis
Pneumonia
Cystic fibrosis
Neonatal lung disease

*Neurological*
Head injury
Meningitis
Raised intracranial pressure
Muscle disorder

*Cardiac*
Severe cardiac failure

*Toxic*
Drug ingestion

*Allergic*
Anaphylaxis

---

Respiratory failure is the end result of a large number of causes, but its definition is usually based on abnormal arterial blood gases with both severe hypoxia and hypercapnia (see p. 95). A careful history and physical examination should elicit the underlying cause of the child's respiratory failure, and a diagnosis is essential for specific management of the condition.

The clinical diagnosis of respiratory failure is obvious if the child is apnoeic or severely cyanosed, but impending respiratory failure may be more difficult to recognize.

### History – must ask!

Asthma is the commonest cause of respiratory failure in children over 1 year of age, and a careful history of previous episodes should be taken. Wheeze and night cough are important features of this condition. Record a list of prescribed medication and find out how much of each drug has been given in this episode.

In infants, infection, particularly bronchiolitis (p. 153), is the commonest cause, and the history should focus on exposure to infectious agents, recent fever and a history of apnoea associated with the present illness.

### Physical examination – must check!

Inability to speak because of breathlessness is a worrying sign that should be carefully assessed. Signs of respiratory distress include dyspnoea, recession, cyanosis and grunting in babies, but these may all be present in children who do not go on to develop respiratory failure.

### Investigations

The relevant investigations and their significance are shown in Table 21.4. Children with impending respiratory failure due to stridor should have their airway secured (e.g. by intubation by an experienced anaesthetist) before investigations are performed.

### Management

Management is directed at the underlying cause of the respiratory failure, and supporting the respiratory physiology. If the child is hypoxic (cyanosed), but the $Pa\text{CO}_2$ is normal, he or she requires oxygen therapy and careful observation. A rising $Pa\text{CO}_2$ indicates the need for respiratory support with mechanical ventila-

tion. This should take place only on an intensive care unit. Oxygen saturation monitoring may be helpful in following the progress of the illness.

Antibiotics are required for infection (p. 151), steroids and bronchodilators for asthma (p. 142) and bronchoscopy for removal of a foreign body.

**Table 21.4** Investigations and their relevance in a child with respiratory failure

| Investigation | Relevance |
|---|---|
| Blood gases | Falling pH and increasing $Pa\text{CO}_2$ indicates respiratory failure with need for ventilation<br>Low $Pa\text{O}_2$ indicates need for additional oxygen |
| Oxygen saturation | Monitor progress of respiratory disease<br><br>Oxygen should be given to maintain saturations >92% |
| Chest X-ray | Lobar or segmental collapse<br><br>Aspiration |

### Key points: Respiratory failure

- Assess arterial blood gases and regularly reassess
- Attach an oxygen saturation monitor and if desaturated give oxygen
- Mechanically ventilate if $Pa\text{CO}_2$ is increasing (but the need for ventilation is based on the whole clinical picture, not just blood gases)
- Investigate cause of respiratory failure
- Treat underlying cause:
  antibiotics for infection (p. 151)
  steroids and bronchodilators for asthma
    (p. 142)
  remove foreign body via bronchoscope

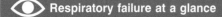

## Respiratory failure at a glance

**Aetiology (see Causes box, p. 374)**
Upper airway obstruction
Lower airway disease
Neurological
Toxic

**Clinical features**
- Dyspnoea
- Tachypnoea
- Cyanosis
- Alar flaring
- Grunting in babies
- Intercostal, subcostal and suprasternal retractions
- Symptoms and signs of underlying disease
- In severe asthma, wheezing may not be heard because of poor air entry
- Restlessness, dizziness
- Impaired consciousness and confusion

**Investigations**
Blood gases
Chest X-ray

**Management**
Oxygen saturation monitor
Consider ventilation
Investigate and treat underlying cause

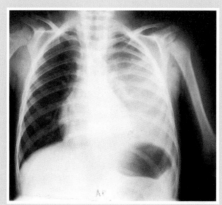

## Upper airway obstruction

Acute upper airway obstruction is an acute medical emergency as death may occur rapidly if it is unrelieved. Obstruction may be intrinsic (e.g. epiglottitis) or extrinsic, caused by a foreign body in the upper airway. The major symptom of upper airway obstruction is inspiratory stridor, which is discussed fully on p. 139.

Acute upper airway obstruction is most likely to occur as the result of aspiration of a foreign body. This is particularly likely in toddlers, who tend to put small objects into their mouths. Peanuts are a particularly common object to inhale. Larger objects are most likely to obstruct above the level of the carina, and the symptoms are immediate and dramatic. The presentation is acute with sudden onset of choking, coughing and cyanosis.

### History – must ask!

Specific questions to be asked include whether there is the possibility of aspiration of foreign body (has the child had access to beads, peanuts, etc.?) or whether there has been a history of progressive stridor and malaise suggestive of acute epiglottitis or croup (p. 155).

### Physical examination – must check!

If obstruction is severe, the child will be cyanosed and collapsed. Stridor may be present if the child is able to move enough air around the obstruction. Marked recession will be present. If epiglottitis is suspected, the doctor must not examine the child's throat.

### Investigations

All investigations must be delayed until a safe airway has been established. Undertaking any painful procedure such as blood tests or moving the child from the mother's arms to examine or take to an X-ray may precipitate complete airway obstruction.

### Management

If an object is blocking the larynx or trachea, it must be removed as rapidly as possible as death may occur within minutes. Every effort must be made to avoid pushing the object further down as this may cause complete airway obstruction.

Tracheostomy may be necessary as a life-saving procedure in hospital.

## The Heimlich manoeuvre (see Figure 21.2)

This is a first-aid measure to relieve acute upper airway obstruction such as occurs as a result of choking on a piece of food or partially aspirating a foreign body. The operator stands behind and embraces the child, with his or her hands grasping each other under the costal margin. The operator then pulls sharply inwards and upwards, increasing intra-abdominal pressure and forcing the air out of the lungs. This should also result in the foreign body being blown out.

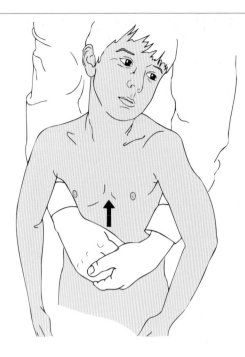

---

### 🔑 Key points: Upper airway obstruction

- If a foreign body is suspected in the trachea, perform the Heimlich manoeuvre
- If cardiorespiratory arrest occurs, first establish the airway by intubation (or tracheostomy if that is impossible)
- If intubation is required, avoid distressing the child until an anaesthetist arrives
- Support the child with cardiopulmonary resuscitation if necessary

**Figure 21.2** The Heimlich manoeuvre. Stand behind with hands grasping each other under the costal margin. Pull sharply inwards and upwards.

---

### 👁 Upper airway obstruction at a glance

**Aetiology**
Intrinsic: epiglottis, croup
Extrinsic: foreign body

**Clinical features**
- Choking, coughing
- Inspiratory stridor
- Decreased air movement
- Marked recession
- Cyanosis
- Collapse if complete obstruction occurs

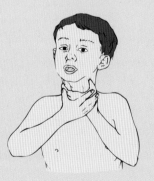

**Investigations**
Delay until airway is established

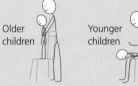

Older children      Younger children

Heimlich manoeuvre

**Management**
Heimlich manoeuvre if foreign body
Consider intubation
CPR if necessary

# Shock

| Causes of shock | | |
|---|---|---|
| **Hypovolaemic** | **Cardiogenic** | **Anaphylactic** |
| Haemorrhage | Myocardial impairment | Allergic reaction |
| Infection (e.g. meningococcal) | Heart failure | |
| Loss of intravascular fluid (p. 386) (e.g. vomiting, diarrhoea) | | |
| Diabetic ketoacidosis | | |
| Trauma | | |
| Burns | | |

'Shock' is the term used to describe a state where the cardiac output is insufficient to perfuse the tissues adequately. The easiest clinical measure of shock is the capillary refill time, which is the time taken for the skin to turn pink again once the pressure from the observer's finger has been removed. A capillary refill time longer than two seconds is prolonged and may suggest shock. Blood pressure is maintained in the normal range by children until the very late stages of shock: once the blood pressure starts to fall, cardiac arrest is imminent unless urgent action is taken. Hypotension will cause perfusion to fall in vital organs, resulting in failure of multiple organs, of which the brain and kidneys are the most vulnerable. The body has a variety of physiological mechanisms to protect vital organs during periods of hypotension; these include redistribution of blood flow from the skin, muscles and bowel to the vital organs, brain, myocardium and kidneys. This is why children in shock are pale with poor skin perfusion.

## History – must ask!

Take a careful history to elucidate the cause of the shock. Enquire into obvious sources of fluid loss (e.g. diarrhoea, vomiting, history of diabetes). Ask whether the child has had a cardiac problem and enquire about allergies (e.g. bee stings, peanuts, etc.). Enquire whether there was a close relationship between ingesting an unusual food and the onset of shock.

## Physical examination – must check!

Two distinct assessments must be made on physical examination: the severity of the shock and its underlying cause.

- *Signs of shock.* It is important to recognize the signs of shock in its relatively early stages before the child collapses. Early symptoms include restlessness, tachycardia with a thready pulse and pallor with cold clammy extremities. At this stage the blood pressure may be normal. Poor skin perfusion can be assessed by blanching the skin by pressing on it with a finger and seeing how long it takes for the capillaries to refill. Oliguria is a common feature of the shocked child. Once hypotension occurs, the child is extremely ill.
- *Signs of the underlying cause of the shock.* Signs include petechial or purpuric skin lesions in meningococcaemia, evidence of trauma, and hepatomegaly in cardiac failure. The focus of a septicaemic illness may be otitis media (examine tympanic membranes), meningitis (assess for neck stiffness), osteomyelitis and septic arthritis (examine joints and limbs for sites of swelling and tenderness).

## Investigations

The relevant investigations and their significance are shown in Table 21.5.

- *Temperature.* The failure of skin perfusion will result in the child having a widening difference between peripheral temperature and core temperature.
- *Blood gases.* Metabolic acidosis occurs as the result of anaerobic tissue metabolism.
- *Electrolytes* and *urea* to assess dehydration.
- *Blood glucose* to exclude hypoglycaemia or diabetic ketoacidosis.
- *ECG* to evaluate cardiac function.
- A *central venous pressure* (CVP) line is helpful to assess the degree of fluid loss and to monitor replacement.

## Management (see Box 21.3)

In shock, the key to management is to give intravenous fluid irrespective of the cause. Isotonic saline should be given rapidly in large volume (20 mL/kg) to restore the blood pressure. Blood is essential if there has been acute blood loss. Drugs to improve cardiac output may also be useful. These include dobutamine, dopamine, adrenaline, and noradrenaline, which have

**Table 21.5** Investigations in shock and their relevance

| Investigation | Relevance |
|---|---|
| Temperature difference between core and periphery | Wide difference (rectal/skin) suggests peripheral shutdown |
| Full blood count (FBC) | Neutrophilia suggests infection |
| Blood cultures | Septicaemia |
| Blood pH | Metabolic acidosis suggests tissue hypoxaemia |
| Serum electrolytes and urea | High urea/creatinine indicates dehydration or renal impairment |
| Blood glucose | Hypoglycaemia |
|  | Hyperglycaemia as a result of diabetic ketoacidosis |
| ECG | Cardiac function |
| Central venous pressure | Low in dehydration |
|  | High in cardiac failure |

the effect of improving cardiac output by increasing heart rate, improving myocardial contractility and causing peripheral vasoconstriction.

Specific treatment must be directed towards the cause of the shock, such as antibiotics for infection and corticosteroids for anaphylaxis.

---

**Box 21.3 Management of shock**

- Give intravenous cefotaxime if meningococcaemia suspected (pp. 128, 322)
- Give rapid intravenous fluid bolus 20 mL/kg irrespective of cause
- Give blood to replace haemorrhagic loss
- Monitor fluid replacement by central venous pressure line
- Give inotropes if cardiac performance is impaired
- Investigate and treat underlying cause(s)
- Continue monitoring in an intensive care environment
- Treat complications: coma, renal failure, etc.

---

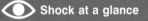 **Shock at a glance**

**Aetiology**
Hypovolaemia, anaphylaxis, cardiogenic (see Causes box, p. 378)

**Clinical features**
- Restlessness
- Tachycardia
- Thready pulse
- Tachypnoea
- Mottled pale cold skin
- Clammy extremities
- Hypotension (late finding)
- Oliguria
- Metabolic acidosis

**Specific signs:**
- Fever in sepsis (core temp > skin temp)
- Purpuric rash in meningococcaemia
- Hepatomegaly in cardiac failure
- Focus of infection

**Investigations**
Full blood count
Infection screen
Blood gases
Urea, electrolytes and glucose
ECG
CVP

**Management**
IV cefotaxime if meningococcaemia suspected
IV fluids or blood
Inotropes
Treat cause and complications

## Prognosis

Approximately 20% of children who present with hypotensive shock will die. A small proportion of the survivors will sustain irreversible brain injury as a result of failure of brain perfusion. The two most important prognostic factors are the duration of shock prior to adequate treatment and the underlying cause of the shock.

> ### 🔑 Key points: Shock
>
> • Recognize the signs of shock before the child collapses
> • Elucidate the cause clinically and carry out investigations
> • Give intravenous fluids

## Coma

> ### Causes of coma
>
> Head injury (accidental or non-accidental)
> Meningitis/encephalitis
> Convulsions, particularly status epilepticus
> Cerebrovascular accident
> Acute asphyxial event
>   birth asphyxia
>   post-cardiac arrest
> Drug-induced
> Raised intracranial pressure
> Metabolic disorders
>   hypoglycaemia
>   diabetic ketoacidosis
>   inborn errors of metabolism

Coma is a poorly understood condition and refers to a markedly reduced state of consciousness caused by a reduction in cerebral metabolic rate. Sometimes the term 'encephalopathy', which refers to altered state of consciousness, is used to describe a precomatose state. Prolonged epileptic seizures are an important cause of coma and are a medical emergency.

In any child presenting with coma, the first task is to stabilize the child (see below) prior to further evaluation.

### History – must ask!

Once the child is stable, take a careful history. Focus particularly on whether there has been a prodromal illness, history of recent contacts with infectious diseases, possibility of drug ingestion (either deliberate or accidental in young children) or a recent head injury. Be aware of the possibility of non-accidental injury. If there has been a convulsion, ascertain its duration and whether there has been a history of previous convulsions. Document the neurodevelopmental state of the child prior to the status. Clarify if there were precipitating factors such as playing computer games or a history of diabetes.

### Physical examination – must check!

Carry out a careful neurological examination to establish the degree of coma.

*   *Vital signs.* Bradycardia suggests raised intracranial pressure, and fever with tachycardia suggests infection. Cardiac arrhythmia occurs in some types of drug overdose. Tachypnoea occurs in respiratory distress and deep sighing (Kussmaul) respirations are a feature of diabetic ketoacidosis.
*   *Focus of infection.* Examine the child for a focus of infection that might have precipitated coma. This includes signs of consolidation in the chest, meningeal irritation and otitis media.
*   *Depth of coma.* This can be determined clinically by assessing the child's best response to commands (Figure 21.3). The lighter the coma, the more appropriate the response, and the deeper the coma, the less the response. In deep coma there is no response at all. The AVPU score is the simplest classification, where the child is classified as either **A**: Alert; **V**: responds to Voice; **P**: responds to Pain; or **U**: Unresponsive.

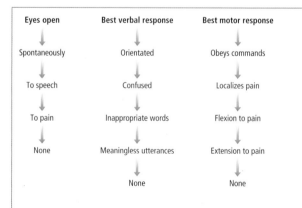

**Figure 21.3** Clinical assessment of depth of coma. The less the response, the deeper the coma.

- *Papilloedema.* Examine the fundi for papilloedema: a sign of raised intracranial pressure that may be accompanied by a slow pulse and raised blood pressure.
- *Pupillary light reflex.* A unilateral dilated pupil with impaired light reflex indicates a third nerve palsy caused by temporal lobe herniation.

## Investigations

Investigations required and their relevance are shown in Table 21.6. The commonest and most treatable metabolic cause of coma is hypoglycaemia, and all

children with an altered level of consciousness should have an urgent fingerprick stick test for blood glucose.

All unconscious children must have a brain scan before lumbar puncture (LP) to assess for any risk of coning (p. 209). Computed tomography (CT) or magnetic resonance imaging (MRI) scans will show focal pathology (tumour, haemorrhage, infarction) and will indicate whether severe oedema is present. If cerebral oedema is not present, lumbar puncture should be performed.

## Management

Specific therapy for cerebral oedema includes the use of osmotic agents (e.g. mannitol). Steroids are only used for focal oedema around a tumour. High-dose barbiturates are commonly used to reduce cerebral metabolic rate once a child is ventilated.

If the child is convulsing on admission, rapid treatment should be given to terminate the episode (see p. 384). If the child is postictal, the level of consciousness should be ascertained (see Figure 21.3). Examination for signs of head injury, pupillary reflex and formal neurological assessment should be carried out.

Drug ingestion may require specific therapy (see p. 391).

## Prognosis

This depends largely on the underlying cause of the coma. The concept of brainstem death is now accepted in most countries, and life support can be withdrawn in such patients despite continued cardiac activity. Brain death should be diagnosed by two consultant doctors who are not responsible for the child's care.

**Table 21.6** The relevance of various investigations in elucidating the cause of coma

| Investigation | Relevance |
|---|---|
| Blood glucose | Hypoglycaemia: rapid coma |
| | Hyperglycaemia: ketoacidosis and slower onset of coma |
| Full blood count | Elevated WCC and shift to left in infection |
| | Decreased PCV and decreased Hb in acute haemorrhage |
| Blood and urine culture | Organisms identified if infection |
| Urea and electrolytes | Elevated urea if dehydrated |
| Blood gases | Indicates metabolic or respiratory acidosis (see p. 95 for interpretation) |
| Chest X-ray | Infection or cardiac failure |
| CT or MRI scan | Focal pathology (tumour, haemorrhage, abscess) |
| | Cerebral oedema |
| Lumbar puncture | Only if no cerebral oedema or features of raised ICP on imaging |
| | Positive in meningitis (see Table 6.8, p. 97, for interpretation) |

WCC, white cell count; PCV, packed cell volume; Hb, haemoglobin; CT, computed tomography; MRI, magnetic resonance imaging; ICP, intracranial pressure.

> ### Key points: Coma
>
> - Establish a secure airway by intubation if the child is unconscious
> - Nurse child in the recovery position and aspirate any vomitus
> - Check blood sugar and give glucose if low
> - Establish the underlying cause
> - Request hourly neurological observations by an experienced nurse

## Coma at a glance

**Aetiology**
See Causes box, p. 380

**Assessment**
**Depth of coma: AVPU**
A: Alert
V: responds to Voice
P: responds to Pain
U: Unresponsive
**Pulse:** tachycardia,
    bradycardia, dysrhythmia
**Breathing:** depressed
    respiration, Kussmaul,
    tachypnoea
**Colour:** cyanosis, pallor

**Blood pressure**
**Neurological**
    **examination:**Pupils
Papilloedema, retinal
    haemorrhage
Focal signs
Fever
Focus of infection
Signs of trauma

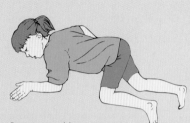
Recovery position

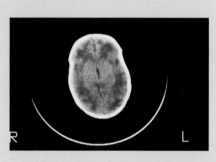

**Investigations**
Dextrostix and blood glucose
Infection screen with LP
Drug screen
Urea and electrolytes
Blood gases
Chest X-ray
CT or MRI scan (prior to LP)

**Management**
Intubate if unconscious
Recovery position
Treat hypoglycaemia
Hourly neurological
    observations

# The generalized convulsion

### Causes of convulsions in children

Febrile convulsions
Meningitis
Epilepsy
Hypoglycaemia
Hypocalcaemia
Head injury
Asphyxia

Convulsions are a very common symptom and occur in approximately 20% of children in the first 5 years of life. They are often solitary and do not indicate either that the child will have further convulsions or that he or she will develop epilepsy. The terms 'fit' and 'seizure' are often used synonymously with convulsion. In this chapter, 'convulsion' will be used consistently.

This section deals with the acute investigation and management of the generalized convulsion. The management of epilepsy is discussed in Chapter 11. Neonatal convulsions are dealt with in Chapter 22.

Convulsions are caused by synchronous discharge of electrical activity from a group of neurones that have an excitatory or inhibitory function. Cerebral activity is the result of a fine reciprocal balance between these two types of control. Factors that either stimulate a group of excitatory neurones or depress inhibitory ones may throw the system out of balance and precipitate rhythmical firing, which in turn causes a clinically observed convulsion. The immature brain is particularly liable to be subject to imbalance, as a variety of insults may disturb the equilibrium and precipitate convulsions.

A convulsion is the clinically apparent manifestation of the discharge through the central and peripheral nervous system. A generalized convulsion is associated with loss of consciousness and will often involve the face and all four limbs. A focal convulsion is not associated with loss of consciousness, and often just one side, or one limb, is involved. Epilepsy is by definition a condition of *recurrent* convulsions that are unrelated to fever or an acute cerebral insult.

The commonest trigger factor for generalized convulsions in children is fever, and these are referred to as febrile convulsions (see p. 393). Convulsions can also be triggered in sensitive children by lack of sleep, a flickering television screen or fast-moving computer games. This is sometimes referred to as reflex epilepsy.

## Clinical features of a generalized convulsion

The generalized convulsion or grand mal classically follows a stereotypic sequence:

- aura;
- cry;
- tonic phase (short period of generalized stiffening);
- clonic phase (intermittent muscle contraction and relaxation);
- sleep or drowsiness.

The aura may be visual, auditory or sensory, but is often indescribable in young children – but the parent can often recognize a typical pattern of behaviour. The aura may be absent in febrile convulsions. The cry stage is common in adolescents, but is not a common feature of younger children. The tonic phase is brief: the child loses consciousness, falls over and becomes stiff.

During the clonic phase, spasms of rhythmical muscle contraction and relaxation of the limb and facial muscles occur. The usual timing of the jerking movements is 1–2 per second. During the clonic phase, the child may be incontinent. Clonic movements usually last an average of 2–3 minutes, but in some cases the clonic stage of the convulsion is prolonged lasting more than 20 minutes. The clonic phase is followed by a period of deep sleep or drowsiness (postictal phase). The child may appear to be confused or irritable after this.

## Status epilepticus

Status epilepticus is defined as continuous seizure activity lasting for 20 minutes or more, or a series of shorter convulsions with failure to regain consciousness between them. It may occur as the result of a febrile convulsion or in a child with known epilepsy, or it may be secondary to other acute conditions. It needs to be terminated by administration of anticonvulsants.

## History – must ask!

- *Description of the convulsion.* It is very important to obtain an eye witness account of the convulsion so that a 'video' image of the episode can be visualized in the clinician's mind. Particular features to enquire about include:
  1  Duration of the convulsion.
  2  Did the convulsion start focally (confined to one side or one limb) and then spread to become generalized?
- *Triggers.* Was the child unwell or pyrexial before the convulsion? Is drug ingestion or poisoning a possibility?
- *Past history.* Is there a previous history of convulsions and any medication for these? Was the child neurologically and developmentally normal prior to the convulsion?

## Physical examination – must check!

- *Vital signs.* Assess the child's pulse, respiratory rate and general condition. If the child is cyanosed, immediately ascertain the patency of the airway.
- *Fever.* Record the child's temperature. Pyrexia may suggest that the child has had a febrile convulsion.
- *Focus of infection.* If the child is pyrexial, look for a source of infection, including examination of the tympanic membranes, throat and chest.
- *Central nervous system examination.* Neurological examination is particularly important as a convulsion may be the first sign of meningitis or other neurological disorders.

## Investigations (Table 21.7)

The possibility of meningitis must be considered in any child with a convulsion and fever, and a lumbar puncture is the rule. However, if the child is older than 18 months, has made a full recovery, is not postictal and has no focal neurological signs or neck stiffness, then it is likely that the diagnosis is a febrile convulsion and a lumbar puncture can be avoided.

Investigations are not necessary in all cases of convulsion, particularly if the child is having repeated febrile convulsions. Advisable investigations are shown in Table 21.7.

An electroencephalogram (EEG) is not indicated in every child with a first convulsion. The following are indications for EEG:

- any convulsion lasting more than 20 minutes;
- focal (atypical) convulsions;
- second afebrile generalized convulsions.

**Table 21.7** Investigations and their relevance in the child with a generalized convulsion

| Investigation | Relevance |
|---|---|
| Full blood count | Signs of bacterial infection |
| Throat, urine and blood culture, CXR | Occult bacterial infection |
| Lumbar puncture | Meningitis |
| Blood glucose | Hypoglycaemia (diabetic or metabolic disorder) |
| U&E, calcium, magnesium | Hyponatraemia, hypocalcaemia or hypomagnesaemia |
| EEG | Epilepsy |
| CT/MRI scan | Injury, or focal neurological signs suggest intracranial bleed or tumour |

**Box 21.4 Emergency treatment of the convulsing child**

- Check airway
- Lay the child on the floor in the recovery position (Figure 21.4)
- Do not insert objects into the child's mouth
- Ensure a responsible person stays with the child if a telephone call to a doctor or ambulance is made
- The child needs medication to abort the convulsion if it lasts longer than 5–10 minutes

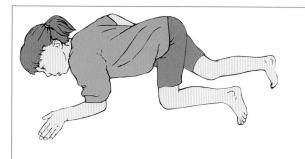

**Figure 21.4** The recovery position.

A convulsion causes considerable disturbance of the EEG, and follow-up EEG should be performed more than 6 weeks after the last convulsive episode.

Computer tomography or magnetic resonance imaging brain scans are not indicated unless the child shows focal convulsive activity.

### Management of the child with convulsions (see Box 21.4)

First place the child in the recovery position and secure the airway (Figure 21.4). The unconscious or semiconscious child should be nursed in the recovery position until he or she recovers or arrives in hospital. If the convulsion is prolonged, it should be aborted by anticonvulsants. The next step is to ascertain the cause of the convulsion.

### Status epilepticus

If the child is in status epilepticus, lorazepam or diazepam can be given intravenously by slow injection until the convulsion stops. A side effect of diazepam infusion is respiratory depression, but this should not deter adequate and effective treatment of the convulsion. If respiratory depression occurs, the child will need mechanical ventilation in an intensive care unit.

### Subsequent management

It is most important to spend time explaining the cause of the fit, first-aid procedures and prognosis to the parents. Reassure them that death is extremely unlikely during a convulsion and by following simple first-aid measures it can be avoided. Parents whose child has had a convulsion should be instructed in the first-aid management of a convulsion, including the use of rectal diazepam or buccal midazolam (see Box 21.6). The management of epilepsy is covered in Chapter 11.

### Prognosis

Children of 5 years of age and below have only a 50% chance of having further convulsions after the first episode. High risk of further convulsions is seen in children with the following adverse features:

- atypical convulsions;
- pre-existing neurological abnormality (cerebral palsy, tuberose sclerosis, structural brain anomaly);
- strong family history of childhood convulsions;
- prolonged convulsion.

A prolonged convulsion (>20 minutes) carries an increased risk of the child's developing temporal lobe epilepsy in later life. The temporal lobe has a high metabolic rate, and prolonged convulsing causes a 150% increase in oxygen consumption in that part of the brain. This very high metabolic demand may outstrip the delivery of oxygen and glucose to the area, causing autoinfarction of parts of the temporal lobe. This subsequently scars and forms the focus of temporal lobe epilepsy.

---

**🔑 Key points: Convulsions**

- Place the child in the recovery position and abort the convulsion if it lasts >10 minutes
- Obtain an eyewitness account of the convulsion
- Exclude hypoglycaemia and hypocalcaemia
- Consider investigating for infection (including an LP),
- Don't diagnose epilepsy unless convulsions are recurrent
- Teach parents how to administer buccal midazolam or rectal diazepam if convulsions are recurrent and/or prolonged
- Only request an EEG according to indications

---

# Dehydration

**Commoner causes of dehydration**

|  | Site of loss | Cause |
|---|---|---|
| Excess losses | Stool | Gastroenteritis |
|  | Urine | Diabetes mellitus |
|  | Vomiting | Pyloric stenosis Gastroenteritis |
|  | Sweat | High fever Cystic fibrosis Hot climate Extended dancing (probably in the presence of drugs) |
|  | Other body fluids | Acute surgical losses Fluid loss from burns |
| Decreased intake | Inability to drink | Stomatitis |
|  |  | Tonsillitis |

---

**👁 Generalized convulsions at a glance**

**Aetiology**
See Causes box, p. 382

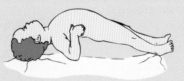

**Clinical features**
Obtain eyewitness account
History of:
- previous seizures
- diabetes
- trauma
- fever
- drug ingestion
- developmental disabilities
- perinatal problems

Signs of:
- focus of infection
- neurological abnormality

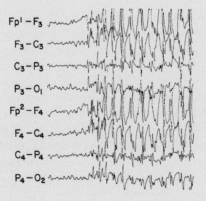

**Investigations**
Dextrostix and blood glucose
Electrolytes, calcium, magnesium
Drug levels (if on anticonvulsants or suspected ingestion)
Blood gases
Others as indicated: infection screen, FBC, MRI, liver function tests, toxic screen, skull X-ray, CT scan, EEG

**Management**
Nurse in recovery position
Suction secretions, oxygen by mask
Assess and treat hypoglycaemia
**Anticonvulsants:** Oral midazolam or rectal diazepam at home
In hospital IV lorazepam is the drug of first choice
Mechanical ventilation if respiratory depression occurs

Water is the major constituent of the human body, and a reduction in body water by more than 5% represents significant dehydration. As much as 80% of an infant's body weight is made up of water, and this proportion falls to about 65% by 3 years. Loss of body fluids is therefore poorly sustained, and dehydration occurs much more readily in infants than in older children and adults. In addition, the physiological mechanisms to prevent excessive fluid losses are less efficient in infants, so further predisposing them to dehydration.

Body water is distributed between the cells (intracellular) and the extracellular compartments. The extracellular compartments can be further divided into the intravascular and the extravascular (interstitial) spaces, separated by the capillary endothelium. Dehydration may occur as the result of depletion of fluid from any of these compartments. Acute loss of fluid from the intravascular compartment may be associated with shock (see p. 378).

The clinical signs of dehydration also depend on the concentration of electrolytes in the intracellular and extracellular compartments. Sodium and bicarbonate are the major ions within the extracellular compartment, and potassium is the major intracellular cation.

Normal body fluid is maintained by a balance between intake and output and depends on the following:

- fluid intake;
- urine volume;
- stool volume;
- sweating;
- insensible loss (water vapour in breath).

Dehydration occurs where the losses exceed the input.

Gastroenteritis is the commonest cause of excessive fluid loss. Sodium may be lost in the same proportion as water; this is called isonatraemic (isotonic) dehydration. Sometimes sodium is lost but is replaced by water, so resulting in hyponatraemic dehydration. More rarely, less sodium than water is lost, or a relative excess of sodium is replaced, causing hypernatraemic dehydration.

When you evaluate a child who presents with dehydration, you need to assess how severe the dehydration is so that you can calculate how much fluid replacement is required. You also need to identify the cause of the dehydration.

The extent of the fluid loss is principally determined by clinical history and physical examination, and by the end of your assessment you should have decided if the child is:

- mildly dehydrated, in which case you can estimate that the child has experienced <5% losses
- moderately dehydrated, in which case you can estimate that the child has experienced 5–10% losses
- severely dehydrated, in which case you can estimate that the child has experienced >10% losses.

### History – must ask!

- *Causes of dehydration.* Enquire about diarrhoea, vomiting or excessive drinking (polydipsia is a common symptom in acute-onset diabetes, see pp. 274, 281). Projectile vomiting in a young infant suggests pyloric stenosis.
- *Severity of dehydration.* Enquire into how many loose stools and how long the diarrhoea has persisted. Ask if the child is passing less urine, and how many wet nappies there have been in last 24 hours. If the child has been vomiting, enquire how often and for how long.

### Physical examination – must check!

You need to assess both the severity of the dehydration and its most likely cause.

- *Weight.* Weighing the child is extremely important. Acute water loss can be estimated from the difference between actual weight and a recent weight made before dehydration occurred (1 g of body weight is roughly equivalent to 1 mL of water). Even if a recent weight is not available, regular weighing (twice daily in the acute situation) will allow accurate management of fluid replacement.
- *Causes of dehydration.* A thorough examination should identify foci of infection or other causes of dehydration. You need to examine the ears, throat, chest and abdomen. In the young infant, pay particular attention to detecting a pyloric 'tumour' if vomiting has been a feature.
- *Severity of dehydration* (Figure 21.5 and Table 21.8). Examine the child for the following specific features to determine how severely dehydrated he or she is:
    - mental state;
    - dryness of the mucous membranes of the mouth;
    - skin turgor;
    - fontanelle;

- eye turgor;
- skin perfusion;
- pulse rate and character.

In *mild dehydration* the only physical sign may be a dry mouth. In *moderate dehydration* the child is lethargic, with inelastic skin, a sunken fontanelle and sunken eyes. The pulse may be fast, but is usually of normal volume, and when the skin is blanched by finger pressure there may be some delay in refilling. Eye turgor may be a useful sign. You can assess eye turgor by pressing on your own eyeball through closed lids. Then compare the child's eye turgor. In moderate or severe dehydration the eyeball is soft.

In *severe dehydration* the child may be very confused and only semiconscious. The skin is mottled and there is no refilling when blanched. The fontanelle and eyes are deeply sunken and the eye turgor is poor.

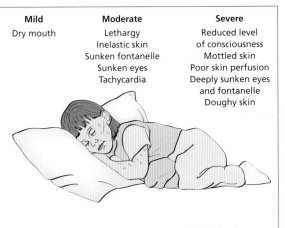

| Mild | Moderate | Severe |
|---|---|---|
| Dry mouth | Lethargy | Reduced level |
| | Inelastic skin | of consciousness |
| | Sunken fontanelle | Mottled skin |
| | Sunken eyes | Poor skin perfusion |
| | Tachycardia | Deeply sunken eyes |
| | | and fontanelle |
| | | Doughy skin |

**Figure 21.5** Estimating the severity of dehydration.

When the skin is pinched between the examiner's finger and thumb it remains in a pinched position for some time. The pulse is thready and fast.

### Investigations

In the child who is ill, investigations are required to determine the type of dehydration and the presence of acidosis, and may also be required to determine the cause.

**Plasma electrolytes and blood gas.** Measure the serum sodium, potassium, chloride, bicarbonate, urea and creatinine. A differential loss of sodium may occur, leading to hyper- or hyponatraemia, and the management will then differ. Bicarbonate may be lost as a result of diarrhoea, causing a metabolic acidosis. If excessive vomiting occurs, excessive hydrogen ions are lost, which may cause an initial metabolic alkalosis (see pyloric stenosis, p. 176). Disturbances in acid–base balance are discussed on p. 94.

**Urine assessment.** Assess the urine for specific gravity or osmolality, and consider measuring urinary electrolytes. An assessment of urinary volume over a known period of time is helpful, but difficult to collect. Treatment must not be delayed in order to measure urine output.

### Determining the type of dehydration
Isotonic dehydration, where there are equal losses of sodium and water, is the commonest type of dehydration. Hyponatraemic and hypernatraemic dehydration may also occur.

| Table 21.8 Clinical features in estimating the severity of dehydration | | | |
|---|---|---|---|
| **Clinical feature** | **Mild** | **Moderate** | **Severe** |
| Mucosa of mouth | Dry | Dry | Dry |
| Reported urine output | Normal (at least 3 × in last 24 hrs) | Reduced in last 24 h | No urine in last 12 h |
| Mental state | Normal | Lethargic or stuporous | Irritable |
| Pulse | Normal | Tachycardic | Tachycardic |
| Blood pressure | Normal | Normal | Low |
| Capillary refilling | Normal | Slow | Very slow |
| Fontanelle | Normal | Sunken | Very sunken |
| Skin and eye turgor | Normal | Reduced | Very reduced |
| Percentage dehydrated | <5% | 5–10% | >10% |

- *Isotonic dehydration.* The serum sodium is normal and children show physical signs commensurate with the degree of fluid loss.
- *Hyponatraemic dehydration.* This is defined as dehydration with serum sodium <130 mmol/L. It generally occurs when fluid losses have been replaced with hypotonic solutions such as water or fizzy drinks. The child is lethargic and the skin is dry and inelastic.
- *Hypernatraemic dehydration.* This is defined as dehydration with serum sodium >150 mmol/L. It can occur through severe and acute water loss, but more commonly is seen in breast-fed babies in the first 2 weeks of life if there is difficulty establishing feeds, or caused by a parent giving concentrated formula feeds having incorrectly measured out scoops of powdered milk. The infant initially appears to be very hungry, but has fewer clinical signs of dehydration. The skin feels doughy. Metabolic acidosis is a common feature of this condition.

### Managing the dehydrated child

#### Oral rehydration therapy

A child who is only mildly (5%) dehydrated may be treated at home using oral hydration therapy. The iller child needs to be admitted to hospital. If vomiting is not a major feature, oral rehydration is usually successful and should be tried before intravenous therapy is considered. Commercially available oral rehydration solutions, such as Dioralyte or Rehidrat, should be used as they have the correct electrolyte balance. These are dispensed as oral solutions, effervescent tablets or powders, and are reconstituted with freshly boiled and cooled water.

Breast-feeding should be maintained while using these solutions. If the baby is bottle-fed, normal milk feed can be given once the diarrhoea has settled. Regrading onto formula milk feeds is no longer recommended. Recurrence of diarrhoea on refeeding is most likely to be caused by lactase deficiency, and if >0.5% reducing substances are found in the stool, a lactose-free milk should be used.

#### Intravenous therapy

In a child with more significant dehydration, particularly if there is vomiting, you need to assess the fluid balance frequently. This involves maintaining an accurate input–output chart, weighing the child twice daily and frequent measurements of serum electrolytes.

The principles of rehydration are simple and require three calculations:

1 an estimate of the acute fluid loss;
2 an estimate of maintenance fluid requirements;
3 an estimate of on-going losses.

These three estimates are added together to determine the volume of fluid that you need to replace over the next 24 hours. An example is shown in Box 21.5.

**Estimate of acute fluid loss.** The difference between actual weight and a recent normal weight is a good approximate method of estimating acute water loss. If the normal weight is unknown, rely on your clinical assessment of the dehydration. If the child is thought to be 10% dehydrated clinically, the estimate of fluid loss is:

$$(\text{actual weight in grams} \times 110\%) - \text{actual weight}$$
$$= \text{deficit (mL)}$$

**Estimate of maintenance requirements.** Maintenance water and sodium intake depends on the age of the child. The requirements are shown in Table 21.9.

**Estimate of ongoing losses.** If possible, ongoing losses must be carefully measured on an hourly basis and added to the fluid regimen every 4 hours.

#### Rehydration protocol

The rate of rehydration depends on the type of dehydration. If the child is shocked, the circulation must be restored by boluses of colloid. If the child is not shocked, the dehydration should be corrected over 24 hours. Hypernatraemic dehydration must be corrected more slowly, over 48 hours, to avoid rapid shifts of water within the brain and resulting cerebral oedema.

**Table 21.9** Maintenance requirements of water and sodium at different ages

| Age (months) | Water (mL/kg/24 hours) | Sodium (mmol/L/kg/day) |
| --- | --- | --- |
| 0–6 | 150 | 2.5 |
| 6–12 | 120 | 2.5 |
| 12–24 | 100 | 2.5 |
| >24 | 80 | 2.0 |

## Box 21.5 Example of the calculation used for replacement fluids

A 3½ year old boy with severe gastroenteritis for 3 days is admitted. He is estimated on clinical grounds to be 10% dehydrated. On admission his weight is 15 kg.

### Step 1 Assess the fluid deficit
His estimated weight = 15 × 110% = 16.5 kg
The estimated fluid deficit is therefore 16.5 – 15 = 1500 mL

### Step 2 Assess the maintenance fluids required in next 24 hours
The requirements are 80 mL/day (see Table 21.9) = 16.5 × 80 = 1320 mL/24 hours

### Step 3 Give maintenance plus deficit
Total fluid = 1500 + 1320 = 2820 mL
Aim to give these fluids over the next 24 hours = 2820 ÷ 24 = 118 mL/hour
*In hypernatraemic dehydration it is vital to rehydrate more slowly* (for example, to give maintenance plus half the deficit over the first 24 hours), because *if the serum sodium falls too rapidly, cerebral oedema can occur.*
The most appropriate fluid initially is 0.45% saline with 5% dextrose. The electrolyte content can be adjusted once serum electrolytes are known.

### Step 4 Assess continuing fluid losses
Estimate the volume lost every 4 hours and add this volume to the next 4-hourly volume given.

Ongoing losses (estimated) = 1000 mL
Total fluids over the next 24 hour = 4315 mL
Hourly requirement for first 8 hours = 270 mL
Hourly requirement for next 16 hours = 135 mL

## Dehydration at a glance

**Epidemiology**
Infants are the most vulnerable

**Aetiology**
Gastroenteritis is the commonest cause

**Physical examination**
- Excessive losses – vomiting, diarrhoea
- Inadequate replacement of fluids
- Lethargic
- ↓ level of consciousness (**a**)
- Sunken fontanelle and eyes (**b**)
- Dry mucous membranes (**c**)
- ↓ blood pressure (**d**)
- Tachypnoea (**e**)
- Oliguria (**f**)
- Reduced skin turgor (**g**)
- Cold (shut-down) peripheries (**h**)
- Tachycardia (**i**)

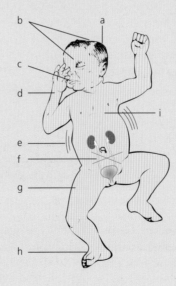

**Confirmatory investigations**
Examination findings and body weight
Estimate severity of dehydration
Serum and urinary electrolytes
Determine whether iso-, hypo- or hypernatraemic

**Management**
Replace deficit and ongoing losses and give maintenance fluids

**Prognosis**
Good
Convulsions most likely in hypernatraemic dehydration

> ### 🔑 Key points: Dehydration
>
> - Determine the percentage dehydration on the basis of clinical signs, urine output and vital signs
> - Identify the underlying reason for the dehydration
> - Replace fluid according to:
>   - the severity of fluid loss (<5%, 5–10%, >10%)
>   - whether dehydration is iso-, hypo-, or hypernatraemic
>   - the ongoing losses and maintenance needs
> - Treat the underlying cause if one is identified

## Poisoning

### Common poisons ingested by children

| Drugs | Household agents |
|---|---|
| Aspirin | Disinfectants |
| Paracetamol | Bleach |
| Iron | Weedkiller |
| Antidepressants | Paraffin or white spirit |
| | Dishwasher tablets |

Accidental drug poisoning in children has become progressively less common in recent years. This is a result of better education of parents about the risks of accidental ingestion in children and the introduction of child-proof containers for the storage of medicines. Accidental ingestion of poisonous household agents remains a problem usually caused by careless storage or putting dangerous compounds such as weedkillers into soft-drink bottles which are very attractive to small children. Poisoning is more likely to occur when a child is at the grandparents' home, where security of dangerous items may not be as strict as at home.

Accidental ingestion of poisons usually occurs in toddlers. It is common to find toddlers playing with tablets without the adult knowing whether they have ingested any or how many. Similarly, household agents such as turpentine may be smelt on the child without knowing whether he or she has swallowed any.

In older children and adolescents deliberate overdose of tablets is common, particularly among girls.

### History – must ask!

In older children who have taken a deliberate overdose, accurate information of the poisonous agent may not be forthcoming, but a friend may be able to give more reliable information. The following points must be ascertained either from the child or from a responsible adult.

- *Identify the agent.* Any tablet or medicine that may have been taken by the child must be identified. Reference manuals showing the appearance of all pharmacological agents are available, or a Poisons Reference Unit will be able to give advice by telephone.
- *Quantity of ingestion.* Establish from the adult what is the maximum number of tablets that the child may have taken.
- *Time from ingestion.*

### Physical examination – must check!

The following points must be assessed carefully on the physical examination.

- The child's conscious level must be initially assessed and reassessed regularly (Figure 21.3, p. 380).
- Look for signs of caustic burns or skin irritation around the lips and mouth, which suggest ingestion of an irritant substance.
- Does the child smell of petrol, turpentine or glue, which would give a clue to the ingested substance?
- Cardiac dysrhythmias may occur as a result of tricyclic antidepressant ingestion. Blood pressure and heart rhythm should be regularly measured. If there is any doubt, the child should be monitored by a cardiorater from the time of first admission to hospital.

### Investigations

If the nature of the poisonous agent is in doubt, urine should be taken for toxic screen to eliminate or confirm possibilities. If aspirin or paracetamol overdose is suspected, measurement of serum levels of these drugs should be performed (see p. 394).

### Management

- Refer to up-to-date guidance from the National Poisons Unit (e.g. www.toxbase.org for the UK).
- In the majority of cases, management consists of careful monitoring and observation. Historically, removal of the poison was commonly attempted by giving the child ipecacuanha syrup. However, the risks

of inducing vomiting usually outweigh any potential benefits, and induction of vomiting is absolutely contraindicated in the following circumstances:

**1** If the child is semiconscious or unconscious, as aspiration may occur if vomiting is induced.

**2** If caustic or corrosive substances have been ingested, vomiting may exacerbate the oesophageal injury.

**3** Paraffin, turpentine or petrol may be aspirated during vomiting and cause lipoid pneumonia.

• Activated charcoal, an absorbent, is occasionally recommended to reduce the absorption of some drugs such as carbamazepine and theophylline, but is often poorly tolerated by children.

• Specific antidotes or therapy for the poison should be instituted if appropriate (e.g. naloxone for opiate poisoning).

• Supportive management. Respiratory and/or cardiovascular failure are important and common complications of many forms of poisoning. If the child is comatose, hypotensive or unwell, a drip should be inserted and the child nursed in an environment where he or she can be very closely observed and respiratory support can be instituted if necessary.

• Advice to parents concerning the prevention of further accidents or ingestions in the home.

• In a child who has attempted suicide or parasuicide, appropriate psychiatric advice should be obtained.

For the specific management of salicylate and paracetomol poisoning, see p. 394.

---

### 👁 Poisoning at a glance

**Epidemiology**
Accidental ingestion – toddlers
Deliberate ingestion – adolescents

**Aetiology**
Commonest ingestions are
    salicylates, paracetamol and
    household agents

**Clinical evaluation**
Time of ingestion
Calculate quantity ingested
Inspect product container
Vital signs
Level of consciousness
Signs of perioral irritation
Smell of organic substances

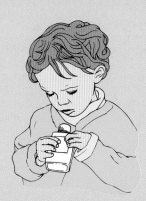

**Investigations**
Urine toxicology screen
Serum levels if identity of drug
    ingested is known

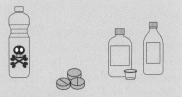

**Management**
Ring National Poisons Unit/access
    online (e.g. www.toxbase.org)
Consider charcoal
Antidotes
Supportive
Prevention of accidents in future
Psychiatry for adolescent

# Emergency paediatric conditions

## Septicaemia and severe infections

Infectious agents may cause septicaemia with a rapid deterioration in the child leading to shock. Certain bacteria are particularly likely to cause shock, including group B beta-haemolytic streptococcus in the newborn (p. 423) and *Neisseria meningitidis* in the older child (p. 128). Some bacteria (e.g. certain staphylococci) produce a toxin which causes massive vasodilatation and shock. Young babies are particularly vulnerable to severe infection as a result of their impaired immunity (p. 409).

Infection must be considered to be the underlying cause in any ill child. This is because infection is common and amenable to treatment with antibiotics if detected early enough.

**Clinical features.** Serious infection in children usually causes a prodromal illness before either focal signs develop or the child collapses. The commonest symptom is fever; the febrile child is discussed in Chapter 7. In neonates, pyrexia may not occur, but the baby's temperature may become unstable with periods of hypothermia. Worrying symptoms in babies within the first 6 months of life are discussed in Table 21.2.

Physical signs such as purpuric rash or foci of infection may be evident on examination.

**Management.** Severe infection must be treated in two ways:

**1** *Resuscitate,* i.e. support the vital signs. This means that the child must be very carefully monitored, particularly for changes in blood pressure. Severe infection often causes shock, and the key to management is to give prompt and adequate intravenous fluid resuscitation (see p. 379). The management of meningococcaemia is discussed on p. 129.
**2** *Antibiotic therapy.* The precise organism causing the child to collapse is often unknown and the choice of broad-spectrum antibiotics is most appropriate. Cefotaxime is the first-line antibiotic to be used in presumed bacterial meningitis.

## Anaphylactic reaction

Anaphylaxis is a very severe, life-threatening allergic reaction. It is fortunately rare, but signs may occur very rapidly, and it is potentially fatal as a result of laryngeal oedema. It occurs as a type I allergic reaction to a large number of allergens. The most common are drugs (e.g. penicillin), blood transfusions, food (eggs, peanuts, etc.) and insect stings. In some cases no allergen can be identified.

**Clinical features.** The allergic reaction usually starts with pruritus, urticaria and wheeze. In many cases the reaction is not severe and does not progress. In some cases bronchospasm becomes very severe and laryngeal oedema causes acute stridor. Rarely, circulatory collapse occurs.

**Management.** A severe allergic reaction should be treated rapidly. If the airway is compromised, the child should be intubated. Drug treatment includes:

- *Adrenaline* given as an emergency intramuscular injection.
- *Corticosteroids* (hydrocortisone intravenously). These may take several hours to have an effect.
- *Antihistamines.*
- *Aminophylline* if bronchospasm develops (p. 144).

In children who have had one episode of anaphylaxis, the parents should be given an adrenaline auto-injector pen to administer subcutaneously and oral antihistamine to keep with them to treat the child following a subsequent inadvertent exposure to the allergen. In addition, they must be taught basic life support techniques.

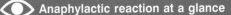
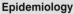

## Anaphylactic reaction at a glance

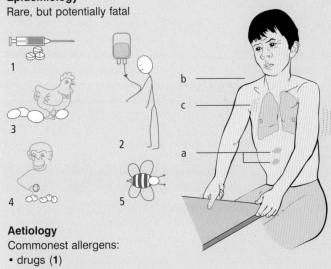

**Epidemiology**
Rare, but potentially fatal

**Aetiology**
Commonest allergens:
- drugs (**1**)
- blood transfusion (**2**)
- eggs (**3**)
- peanuts (**4**)
- bee stings (**5**)

**Clinical features**
Difficulty swallowing
Tightness in chest
Pruritus, urticaria (**a**)
Angioedema (oedema of submucosal
    and subcutaneous tissues)
Hoarseness, stridor due to laryngeal
    oedema (**b**)
Bronchospasm (**c**)
Circulatory collapse rare

**Management**
Intubation if airway compromised
Drugs:
- Adrenaline
- Hydrocortisone IV (takes hours for
    effect)
- Antihistamines
- Aminophylline for bronchospasm
Identify allergen
Adrenaline kit for family to administer
    SC at next exposure

# Febrile convulsions

Febrile convulsions are seizures which occur in children between the age of 6 months and 5 years and are caused by fever. The immature brain is more susceptible to environmental factors, and fever may precipitate a grand mal convulsion. They occur in 5% of all children in this age group, and the risk is higher if there is a family history.

**Clinical features.** Fever precedes the convulsion, but there may be a sudden rise in body temperature immediately before the convulsion which may not be recognized by the parent. Fever may occur as a result of convulsive activity, and fever with convulsion does not necessarily allow the diagnosis of febrile convulsion to be made. The convulsion is usually short-lived, lasting only a few minutes. Status epilepticus occurs in only about 1% of febrile convulsions. In all children with febrile convulsion a careful examination should be performed in order to identify the site of infection.

**Management.** Any convulsion lasting for more than 5–10 minutes should be terminated with buccal midazolam or rectal diazepam (Box 21.6). The child must be examined for any source of infection. In babies and very young children a lumbar puncture should be carried out to rule out meningitis. If the child is older than 18 months and has no neurological signs or neck stiffness, a lumbar puncture can usually be avoided. Parents should be reassured, but instructed about first-aid management of further convulsions (see Box 21.6). They should be told that the prognosis for brief febrile convulsions is very good and there is no increased risk of epilepsy, provided the child has not had a prolonged or atypical convulsion.

---

**Box 21.6 Advice to parents whose child has febrile convulsions**

- Undress the child
- Give paracetamol for its antipyretic effect
- An electric fan may be used, but warn the parents that this is dangerous if the child pokes a finger in it
- Give rectal diazepam or buccal midazolam if convulsion lasts more than 10 minutes
- Seek medical advice from the general practitioner if the child is asymptomatic, or through Accident and Emergency if the child has any symptoms

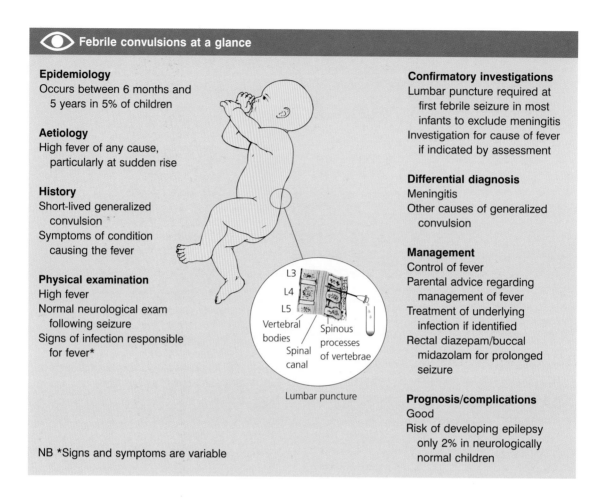

**Febrile convulsions at a glance**

**Epidemiology**
Occurs between 6 months and
5 years in 5% of children

**Aetiology**
High fever of any cause,
particularly at sudden rise

**History**
Short-lived generalized
convulsion
Symptoms of condition
causing the fever

**Physical examination**
High fever
Normal neurological exam
following seizure
Signs of infection responsible
for fever*

L3
L4
L5
Vertebral
bodies
Spinal
canal
Spinous
processes
of vertebrae

Lumbar puncture

**Confirmatory investigations**
Lumbar puncture required at
first febrile seizure in most
infants to exclude meningitis
Investigation for cause of fever
if indicated by assessment

**Differential diagnosis**
Meningitis
Other causes of generalized
convulsion

**Management**
Control of fever
Parental advice regarding
management of fever
Treatment of underlying
infection if identified
Rectal diazepam/buccal
midazolam for prolonged
seizure

**Prognosis/complications**
Good
Risk of developing epilepsy
only 2% in neurologically
normal children

NB *Signs and symptoms are variable

Continuous anticonvulsant medication for children with febrile convulsions is not recommended.

**Prognosis.** Children with uncomplicated febrile convulsions are at no greater risk of subsequent epilepsy than children without febrile convulsions. A prolonged convulsion lasting more than 20 minutes may predispose to temporal lobe seizures (see p. 211).

## Paracetamol poisoning

Owing to its easy availability in many homes, as well as the pleasant taste of childrens' liquid paracetamol preparations, paracetamol (acetaminophen) is the most common drug to be ingested accidentally by children. Paracetamol ingestion is rarely severe enough to cause serious problems, but liver failure is the major risk if >150 mg/kg is ingested.

**Clinical features.** Early symptoms are usually minimal but may include anorexia, nausea and vomiting. Signs of liver failure occur on the second day with abdominal pain, liver tenderness and hepatic failure with jaundice after 2–3 days.

Initially liver function tests are normal. The prothrombin time and liver enzymes become abnormal 12–24 hours after ingestion. The decision to treat depends on a paracetamol serum level 4 hours after ingestion.

**Management.** Successful treatment depends on early recognition and institution of adequate treatment. In patients at risk of liver damage, oral methionine or N-acetyl-cysteine reduces the severity of liver necrosis. The decision to use these agents depends on the serum level of paracetamol 4 hours after ingestion.

## Salicylate poisoning

Salicylate poisoning causes initially a respiratory alkalosis caused by stimulation of the respiratory centre, and later a metabolic acidosis as a result of the acid load of the drug. Gastric bleeding may occur as the result of its effects on the mucosa.

**Clinical features.** The earliest sign is overbreathing, often associated with vomiting and diarrhoea. Sweating may be a feature. If the overdose has been large, metabolic acidosis occurs about 6–8 hours after ingestion, with ketosis, hyperglycaemia and glycosuria. Eventually collapse may occur with loss of consciousness. The physical and laboratory findings show a considerable similarity with those found in diabetic ketoacidosis, and blood sugar levels should be measured to exclude this possibility.

A serum salicylate level helps to establish the likely severity of the overdose.

**Management.** Salicylates can be retained in the stomach for a long time, and activated charcoal is often recommended. If the patient is acidotic, sodium bicarbonate is given intravenously, which promotes renal excretion of salicylate. Haemodialysis should be used in massive overdoses to remove salicylate.

## Burns and scalds

Burns are the second commonest cause of accidental childhood death after road traffic accidents. One half of deaths are caused by smoke inhalation leading to respiratory failure (p. 374) and one half caused by thermal damage to the skin. Approximately one half of thermal injuries admitted to hospital are the result of scalds from hot water.

Thermal injuries cause death either as a result of massive fluid loss through the denuded skin or by infection. A second major problem in children who survive is scarring, which may have major psychological consequences.

**First aid.** Scalds are first treated by removing the clothes over the affected area and cooling the skin under a cold tap. Children who are scalded or burnt should be wrapped in a clean towel or cling film and brought immediately to hospital.

**Clinical assessment.** The extent of the thermal injury must be assessed. This is done by estimating the surface area involved, as illustrated in Figure 21.6. The percentage of body area affected is calculated.

If the child has suffered smoke inhalation, respiratory failure with wheeze, cyanosis and dyspnoea may occur rapidly.

**Management (see Box 21.7)** Assess the airway and respiratory function. Arterial blood gases may be necessary to decide whether mechanical ventilation is

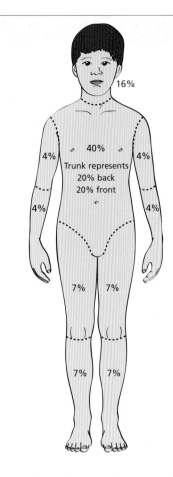

**Figure 21.6** Estimating the surface area of burns in children.

---

### Box 21.7 Management of burns

- Give intravenous fluids to compensate for severe fluid loss through burnt skin
- Analgesia to control pain
- If thermal injury to mouth or airway, assess the need for tracheostomy
- Skin grafting for full-thickness burn
- Psychological support for child and family

---

required (p. 94). Thermal injury to the airway may necessitate rapid endotracheal intubation or even tracheostomy before severe oedema causes obstruction.

If there are burns to more than 10% of the surface area, an intravenous cannula should be inserted to gain vascular access and give intravenous fluids to prevent or treat shock caused by fluid loss. Analgesia will be needed, and morphine should be administered to control pain.

Most burns victims are now treated in special burns units. Skin grafting is required for full-thickness burns. This can be assessed after a few days by testing for pain sensation: if a pinprick is not felt, the burn is full thickness. Psychological support will be needed for the child and his or her family if there is extensive scarring.

## Drowning

Most drowning incidents in Britain occur in fresh water (bath, river, swimming pool). The outcome following near-drowning in cold water (<10 °C) is significantly better than in warm water. This is probably a result of induced hypothermia from immersion.

**First aid.** The child must be resuscitated at the site of the drowning incident with mouth-to-mouth resuscitation and rapidly transferred to hospital.

**Management.**
• Clear airway and institute mechanical ventilation. Assess circulation and treat if shock is present.
• If hypothermic, slowly warm over a number of hours.

**Prognosis.** It is well known that children can recover fully despite a very prolonged period of cardiac arrest following a drowning incident, particularly if the child was rescued from cold water. Prolonged resuscitation efforts are therefore necessary until the child is rewarmed.

Hypoxic brain damage rarely occurs after near-drowning, and full recovery is the rule if the child can be resuscitated.

## Acute life-threatening events and sudden infant death syndrome

The definition of sudden infant death syndrome (SIDS) is 'the sudden death of any infant or young child, which is unexpected by history, and in which a thorough postmortem examination fails to demonstrate an adequate cause for the death.' Some children are found in a collapsed apnoeic state looking grey and mottled, but can be resuscitated. This is referred to as an 'acute life-threatening event' (ALTE).

Sudden infant death syndrome affects infants below the age of 1 year, with the peak rate at 2–4 months. It is the commonest cause of death in infancy after the first week of life. In Britain the incidence of SIDS has fallen by over 50% in the last few years, probably as a result of new advice on the sleeping position of babies (see below).

The cause of SIDS is unknown. There is no single cause; many factors are involved, including infection, cardiac dysrhythmia and accidental suffocation. It is thought by many to be caused by an environmental factor on a susceptible infant. Recently, most attention has been placed on sleeping position, the infant's temperature and exposure to tobacco smoke in the home.

It is thought that the baby's body temperature is related to sleeping position, and overheating is an important factor in the control of respiration. Babies who are nursed prone in their cots have less skin surface area exposed for heat loss. The Department of Health has issued advice to parents of young babies in the Back to Sleep health education campaign (see Box 21.8). This advice appears to be the major cause of the reduction in the number of cot deaths.

---

**Box 21.8 Back to Sleep campaign**

*Babies should be laid to sleep on their backs*
If the side position is chosen, the lower arm should be well in front of the body to prevent the child from rolling into a prone position

*Infants should not be exposed to cigarette smoke either before birth or afterwards*

*Avoid overheating the baby*
Guidance to the parents includes:
• Sleeping room temperature 16–20 °C
• Avoid excessive bedding for the temperature of the room
• Ensure bedding will not overlie the baby. Make it up so that the infant's feet come down to the end of the cot
• Avoid duvets in infants <1 year of age
• Do not increase the bedding when the child is unwell or feverish
• An infant >1 month does not require a hat for sleeping unless the room is very cold

*Infants should not sleep in the same bed as adults. Co-sleeping with an adult on a sofa carries a particularly high risk of overlay*

In babies who die of SIDS there is often a preceding history of minor illness such as a cold or a cough, but not severe enough to cause concern that the baby is seriously ill. The baby usually dies at home in his or her cot between the hours of 04:00 and 12:00. Death appears to have occurred rapidly and without warning. It is not uncommon for the child to be cold by the time he or she is found, and postmortem lividity is seen. Rarely, the baby may be found to have a major pathology at postmortem, such as pneumonia or septicaemia, but this is uncommon, and an obvious but unexpected cause for death is found in only 20% of cases.

Babies who have been found with an acute life-threatening episode are usually pale (indicating a poor circulation) and mottled in appearance. In those cases where the baby is found collapsed, but not dead in the cot, immediate first aid with mouth-to-mouth resuscitation and external cardiac massage may save the baby's life.

## Investigations

In babies who have been successfully resuscitated from acute life-threatening episodes, investigation for an underlying cause is essential. The following should be undertaken:

* infection screen, particularly blood cultures, urine culture and consider lumbar puncture;
* investigations for gastro-oesophageal reflux (p. 175);
* continuous monitoring for episodes of apnoea;
* ECG monitoring for cardiac dysrhythmias;
* metabolic investigations including blood sugar (hypoglycaemia) and inborn errors of metabolism.

## Management

The management is the same as for any baby with cardiopulmonary arrest and is described on p. 374.

### Sudden infant death syndrome at a glance

**Epidemiology**
Commonest cause of infant death (past first week)
Affects babies under 12 months, peak age 2–4 months

**Aetiology**
Related to sleep position (a), temperature (b), smoking (c) and environment
In 20%, a major unsuspected condition is found at autopsy

**Prevention**
Back to Sleep campaign has halved deaths due to sudden infant death syndrome

**History**
Normally healthy baby (preceding minor illness)
Full and careful history of last sleep required

**Physical examination**
Found dead
Examination usually unremarkable

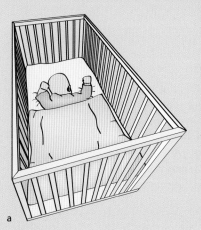
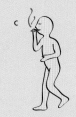

**Investigations**
As guided by history and examination

**Differential diagnosis**
Sepsis
Gastro-oesophageal reflux
Neurological abnormality
Hypoglycaemia (rare)
Cardiac arrhythmia (rare)
Inborn error of metabolism (rare)
Suffocation (rare)

**Management**
Lead paediatrician for unexpected deaths in childhood informed

### Prevention

#### The family of a previously affected child

The family of a SIDS victim will be extremely anxious about the outcome for subsequent siblings. Apnoea monitoring at home is usually offered, although there is no evidence that this will prevent further deaths. If the new baby is unwell there should be early referral to the GP with admission to hospital for close monitoring if the doctor is concerned.

#### General prevention

The advice given by the Department of Health should be given to all new parents (see Box 21.8). Additional advice includes the encouragement of breast-feeding, and warning about not overwrapping the baby if he or she develops a mild infection.

*To test your knowledge on this part of the book, see Chapter 25.*

# CHAPTER 22

# The newborn

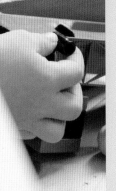

*My mother groan'd, my father wept;*
*Into the dangerous world I leapt,*
*Helpless, naked, piping loud,*
*Like a fiend hid in a cloud.*
*Struggling in my father's hands,*
*Striving against my swaddling*
*bands,*
*Bound and weary, I thought best*
*To sulk upon my mother's breast.*
*William Blake, 1793*

## COMPETENCES

### You must . . .

| Know | Be able to | Appreciate |
|------|-----------|------------|
| • The difference between prematurity and growth restriction<br>• The basics of neonatal resuscitation<br>• The key congenital and perinatal conditions that present in the newborn<br>• When a jaundiced baby requires investigation | • Examine a newborn baby<br>• Recognize a baby in need of resuscitation<br>• Recognize when a 'septic workup' is needed | • The newborn is susceptible to infection but may not show classic signs<br>• A small baby may be either premature or growth retarded or a combination of the two |

*Paediatrics and Child Health*, Third Edition. Mary Rudolf, Tim Lee, Malcolm Levene.
© 2011 Mary Rudolf, Tim Lee and Malcolm Levene. Published 2011 by Blackwell Publishing Ltd.

# The newborn

## Finding your way around . . .

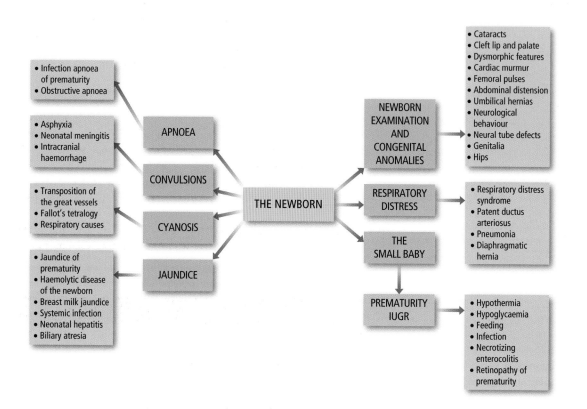

Care of the newborn infant is a very important part of paediatrics. Routine examination for occult, but treatable, abnormalities must be undertaken in all newborn infants to prevent long-term disability. Intensive care of the sick preterm and ill full-term infant has significantly improved mortality and morbidity.

Improvement in care of the newborn over recent years can be monitored by observing changes in perinatal and neonatal mortality rates (see below for definitions). The perinatal mortality rate has halved in Britain over the last 20 years and is now approximately seven per 1000 live births.

The improvement in perinatal mortality rates (which includes stillbirths) is largely a result of improvements in obstetric care. Reduction in neonatal mortality rate (now below four per 1000 liveborn infants) has been mainly a result of more effective management of congenital abnormalities by safer surgical techniques and improvements in supporting premature infants with lung disease.

This chapter is arranged in the sequence most appropriate to the way newborn babies present to paediatricians. Only a minority of babies require resuscitation, but for those who do, this must be undertaken immediately after birth and in an efficient and safe manner. All babies should be seen and examined by a doctor in the first 24 hours of life to detect occult congenital abnormalities. As a medical student you should become familiar with the newborn examination and undertake a number of such examinations on your own. You should know the common congenital abnormalities described in this section.

Only 7% of babies are born premature, but these account for the vast majority of the time that paediatricians spend caring for the newborn. The small baby and his or her problems are the final and major section of this chapter.

## Definitions and terminology

It is important to know the definitions of a number of widely used terms in perinatal statistics, as shown in Table 22.1.

# Neonatal resuscitation and asphyxia

Rapid and effective resuscitation must be available for every newborn baby, wherever birth takes place. The need for resuscitation can be anticipated in many cases. The Red Flag box shows situations where there is a high risk that resuscitation will be needed and a paediatrican needs to be present at delivery. However, despite careful fetal surveillance in labour, babies may still be born in poor condition and unexpectedly require resuscitation.

> **High-risk situations where a paediatrician needs to be present at delivery**
>
> Prematurity
> Fetal distress
> Thick meconium staining of the amniotic fluid
> Emergency caesarean section
> Vacuum, mid or high forceps delivery
> Abnormal fetus
> Multiple birth
> Prolonged rupture of the membranes

The infant's condition after birth can be described by the Apgar score (Table 22.2). This records five features, each of which can be scored with either 0, 1 or 2 points. The baby can obtain a maximum of 10 points or a minimum of 0 (no signs of life).

A normal score at 1 minute is 7–10, a score of 4–6 at 1 minute represents a moderately depressed baby and an Apgar score of 0–3 at 1 minute indicates severe depression. Babies who require active resuscitation at

**Table 22.1** Definitions used in perinatal statistics

| Term | Definition |
| --- | --- |
| Full-term | An infant born between 37 and 42 weeks of gestation |
| Preterm | An infant born before 37 completed weeks of gestation |
| Post-term (postmature) | An infant born after 42 completed weeks of gestation |
| Low birthweight | This is an old-fashioned term which has little value in modern terminology. It refers to infants whose birthweight is 2500 g or less. This term makes no distinction between prematurity and intrauterine growth retardation as the cause for the baby's being of low birthweight (see below) |
| Very low birthweight | A baby born with a birthweight of 1500 g or less |
| Extremely low birthweight | A baby born with a birthweight of 1000 g or less |
| Small for gestational age | A baby of birthweight below the 10th centile for the duration of gestation |
| Stillborn infant | A baby who shows no signs of life (including no heart beat) after delivery. 'Stillbirth' is a term used only if the infant is of 24 weeks' gestation or above |
| Perinatal mortality rate | The number of stillbirths and neonatal deaths in the first week of life per 1000 liveborn and stillborn infants |
| Neonatal mortality rate | The number of deaths of liveborn infants in the first 28 days of life per 1000 liveborn infants |
| Infant mortality rate | The number of deaths of all liveborn infants in the first year of life per 1000 liveborn infants |

**Table 22.2** The Apgar score

| Sign | 0 | 1 | 2 |
|---|---|---|---|
| Heart rate | Absent | <100/min | >100/min |
| Respiratory rate | Absent | Weak cry | Strong cry |
| Muscle tone | Limp | Some flexion | Good flexion |
| Reflex irritability (suctioning pharynx) | No response | Some motion | Cry |
| Colour | White | Blue periphery | Pink all over |

birth can be divided broadly into one of two groups on the basis of their appearance.

- *Primary apnoea.* In this group the babies are blue as a result of failure to establish spontaneous respiration, but their cardiovascular system is intact with good circulation. This corresponds to an Apgar score at 1 minute of 4–6.
- *Secondary apnoea.* These babies appear white at birth as a result of failure of the circulation as well as of respiration. Without vigorous resuscitation these babies will die. This group corresponds to a 1-minute Apgar score of 0–3.

Resuscitation in the newborn is different from resuscitation of older children and adults. The primary reason for resuscitation in children and adults is usually circulatory or cardiac, whereas in the newborn the establishment of ventilation is the major issue. The baby is born with lungs full of amniotic fluid, much of which is expelled during chest compression that occurs with vaginal delivery. Most babies breathe spontaneously at birth. After delivery, spontaneous breathing is usually rapidly established with the following procedures:

- Dry with a warm towel.
- Gently suck out the oropharynx.
- Give to the mother to put to the breast or cuddle.

A baby who is apnoeic within the first minute of life requires basic resuscitation. The colour will guide you to what resuscitation is required. A *blue* baby indicates that there is adequate circulation, and the cyanosis results from not breathing (primary apnoea or blue asphyxia). These babies will start to gasp even if nothing is done. They require lung inflation only and no cardiac support. A pale, *white* baby implies there is inadequate circulation. These babies will have slow

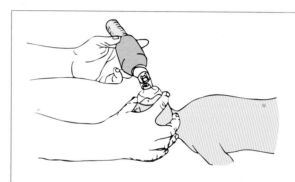

**Figure 22.1** Bag and mask resuscitation.

or absent heart rate (secondary (terminal) apnoea or white asphyxia), and if nothing is done they will die. Both lung inflation and cardiac support are required.

### Primary apnoea after 60 seconds (blue but with good heart rate)

The main aim is to replace the lung fluid with air by giving inflation breaths.

Open the baby's airway by laying the baby on his back and:

- put the head in a neutral position with the face up;
- hold the baby's jaw forward;
- ensure that the neck is not over-flexed or extended.

The inflation breaths are given by a self-inflating bag and a close-fitting mask applied around the baby's mouth and nose (Figure 22.1). Five inflation breaths each lasting 2 seconds are given and the chest movement is observed during the inflations. There should be good and symmetrical chest wall movement. If this does not occur, the technique is not working and the baby's position needs to be checked:

- Is the head in a neutral position?
- Is the jaw held forward?
- Is the neck over flexed or extended?

Readjust the baby's position and apply another five inflation breaths. If the chest wall moves, lung inflation is successful. Recheck the heart rate – if it is above 100 bpm, observe the baby for spontaneous respiratory efforts. If there are none, give short inspiratory breaths (30/minute) with the bag and mask and await spontaneous respirations. If the baby is pink but still not breathing, consider whether the baby's respiratory centre is depressed by maternal opiates. If this is a possibility (mother has received pethidine or morphine within 4 hours of delivery), give the opiate antagonist naloxone.

### Secondary apnoea (white with slow or absent heart rate)

Apply a close-fitting mask, give five inflation breaths and ensure good chest movement. This is followed by shorter breaths at 30/minute. You will require an assistant to give cardiac resuscitation. This requires cardiac compressions whilst lung inflation is being carried out, giving three compressions to one breath. Intubation may be necessary for more prolonged resuscitation.

If the heart rate remains low, intravenous sodium bicarbonate is needed to correct the metabolic acidosis and adrenaline is given intravenously or via the trachea to stimulate the heart.

### Asphyxia

Physiologically asphyxia is caused by tissue hypoxia with the production of lactic acid and carbon dioxide. This results in tissue acidosis. The healthy fetus can withstand asphyxia for some time, but eventually physiological compensatory mechanisms become exhausted and the fetus decompensates, with potential irreversible injury to a number of organ systems, most importantly the brain.

**Diagnosis.** There is no generally accepted clinical definition of asphyxia. The following are commonly used:

- cord blood acidosis with pH <7.05;
- severe depression of Apgar scores (0–5 at 10 minutes);
- delay in establishing spontaneous respiration (>10 minutes);
- hypoxic–ischaemic encephalopathy (a sequence of abnormal neurological signs including convulsions lasting for more than 2 days).

**Management.** Rapid and effective resuscitation must be available wherever babies are born. Measures are taken to avoid cerebral oedema and to treat ensuing convulsions.

**Prognosis.** Death and severe handicap occur in approximately 25% of all severely asphyxiated full-term infants. Carefully controlled therapeutic cooling can improve neurological outcome in survivors.

---

**⚙ Key points: Resuscitation and asphyxia**

- Resuscitation is needed rapidly and effectively
- Provide ventilatory support if the baby fails to establish adequate spontaneous respiration
- Provide circulatory support if the baby is hypotensive
- Give anticonvulsants for severe or persistent convulsions
- Controlled therapeutic cooling in severe asphyxia

---

## The newborn examination

Every newborn baby should be carefully examined in the first 24 hours of life. The newborn is closely inspected by his or her mother, and many congenital abnormalities will be detected by her and brought to medical attention. The purpose of the physician's examination is to detect occult abnormalities not obvious to the mother, or where the significance of an apparently minor deviation from normal is unrecognized.

The reason for the neonatal examination must be explained to the parents, and they should be present during the examination if at all possible. The baby should be fully undressed in a warm room prior to examination.

### History – must ask!

Ask the mother whether the baby is feeding well and if she has any worries about the baby.

### Physical examination – must check!

The physical examination must be systematic so that nothing is omitted. First observe the baby, then systematically start at the head and work down to the toes. Figure 22.2 summarizes the main features of the newborn examination, and particular attention must be paid to potentially treatable abnormalities which, if missed, may cause irreversible damage to the baby.

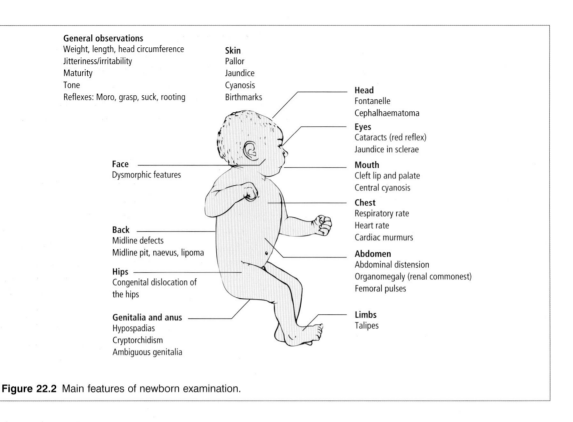

**General observations**
Weight, length, head circumference
Jitteriness/irritability
Maturity
Tone
Reflexes: Moro, grasp, suck, rooting

**Skin**
Pallor
Jaundice
Cyanosis
Birthmarks

**Head**
Fontanelle
Cephalhaematoma

**Eyes**
Cataracts (red reflex)
Jaundice in sclerae

**Face**
Dysmorphic features

**Mouth**
Cleft lip and palate
Central cyanosis

**Chest**
Respiratory rate
Heart rate
Cardiac murmurs

**Back**
Midline defects
Midline pit, naevus, lipoma

**Abdomen**
Abdominal distension
Organomegaly (renal commonest)
Femoral pulses

**Hips**
Congenital dislocation of
the hips

**Limbs**
Talipes

**Genitalia and anus**
Hypospadias
Cryptorchidism
Ambiguous genitalia

**Figure 22.2** Main features of newborn examination.

## Vital signs and general observation

- *Respiratory rate.* Count the respirations. A rate above 60 breaths per minute (tachypnoea) may be abnormal, but is normal after a feed or if the baby has been crying.
- *Colour.* Central cyanosis (involving the tongue) is always abnormal, and if it is present the baby must be rapidly investigated (see p. 411). Jaundice in the first 24 hours is always abnormal and suggests haemolytic disease (see p. 425).
- *Spontaneous movements.* Normally full-term babies have frequent smooth movements. They are often reciprocal so that when a leg extends the other flexes.
- *Jitteriness.* This refers to spontaneous movements which are stimulus-independent; jitteriness is not necessarily abnormal, but hypocalcaemia and hypoglycaemia should be excluded as a cause.
- *Irritability* Irritability is a stimulus-sensitive phenomenon and is always abnormal, suggesting a neurological problem.

## Measurement

Carefully measure the head circumference, length and birthweight, record the measurements in the notes and plot them onto centile charts to ensure that the baby has grown symmetrically. Accurate measure-ments of occipitofrontal head circumference and length in the newborn are not easy to make and require some training. These techniques are discussed in Chapter 4.

## Dysmorphic features

A *dysmorphic feature* is a variation from normal and is often subtle. Many normal people have at least one or two dysmorphic features, but the more such features coexist, the more likely it is that a recognizable dysmorphic syndrome is present. A *syndrome* is a consistent pattern of dysmorphic features which is usually recognized to be of genetic origin. The commonest syndrome recognizable in the neonatal period is Down's syndrome (p. 246).

Palpate the head and feel for the anterior and posterior fontanelles. A cephalhaematoma may be present due to subperiosteal bleeding. These resolve without treatment.

## Eyes

Newborn infants keep their eyes closed much of the time. They can see, respond to changes in light and can fix their gaze on objects. The earliest possible detection and treatment of *cataracts* is essential for normal visual development. Examination of cataracts is described in detail on p. 23.

## Mouth

Look for central cyanosis and examine the palate for a cleft. The most reliable way is to insert your *clean* little finger into the baby's mouth and palpate with the soft part of your finger. A cleft is easily felt, and this method may also detect the rare submucous cleft with a bony defect but intact mucosa.

## Chest

Cardiac murmurs are commonly heard in the neonatal period and are usually innocent. In contrast, some very severe cardiac anomalies may not be associated with a murmur at the 24-hour examination. The following features suggest that a murmur is more likely to indicate cardiac pathology:

- diastolic or gallop murmur;
- an active praecordium;
- the presence of cyanosis or breathlessness;
- absence of femoral pulses (see below).

## Femoral pulses

Palpate the femoral pulses in the groin. Absence of a femoral pulse suggests severe *coarctation of the aorta* (see Figure 10.5). Less severe coarctation, which leads to hypertension in later life, is not associated with absent pulses at the neonatal examination.

## The abdomen

A distended abdomen suggests bowel obstruction. Bile-stained vomiting must always be rapidly investigated as it is often the first sign of obstruction. The causes of bowel obstruction are discussed on p. 419.

Organomegaly is detected by careful abdominal examination. Enlargement of a single kidney as a result of pyeloureteric junction obstruction is the most common cause of a mass in the abdomen. Hepatosplenomegaly is not a common finding in the newborn infant.

*Umbilical hernias* are common, particularly in low-birthweight and black infants. They are not seen until the umbilical cord separates and the cord stump heals. The hernia appears as a soft swelling that protrudes during crying, coughing or straining and is usually easily reducible. Strangulation is very rare, and most umbilical hernias disappear spontaneously by 1 year of age.

## The back and limbs

Examine the spine carefully. Look for midline defects, naevi and lipomas. When severe, *neural tube defects* (see p. 428) are obvious. However, spina bifida occulta is harder to detect and, if missed, can lead to severe complications. Examine the limbs for deformities and extra digits.

## Genitalia and anus

The testes are present in the scrotum in 95% of full-term male infants. Most *undescended testicles* (see p. 315) enter the scrotum during the first year of life with no treatment. *Hypospadias* is a condition where the urethra is abnormally sited, with the meatal opening lying anywhere from the ventral aspect of the glans penis to the perineum (see p. 316 and Fig 16.3). With severe hypospadias, the penis is curved ventrally (chordee). Rarely, babies are born with *ambiguous genitalia* and indeterminate sex. This should be considered to be a medical emergency because of the risk of severe electrolyte imbalance and also for social reasons (see p. 316).

## Abnormal neurological behaviour

Abnormal findings on neurological examination are rarely specific for particular forms of central nervous system pathology. The main features suggestive of serious neurological abnormality are the following:

- hypotonia (floppiness) or hypertonia (stiffness);
- irritability;
- loss or asymmetry of the Moro reflex;
- feeding problems.

## The skin

Look for birth marks.

## The hips

Leave the examination of the hips to the end as it usually causes the baby to cry. It is important to detect if a hip is dislocated or dislocatable. Both these abnormalities require early treatment to prevent permanent maldevelopment of the hip joints. The Ortolani and Barlow tests are described on p. 430.

# Signs and problems presenting in the newborn period

## The small baby

The low birthweight infant may have three causes for being abnormally small:

- prematurity;
- intrauterine growth retardation (IUGR);
- a combination of both of these.

As the causes, management and prognosis of these conditions are different, it is important to determine into which of these three categories any small baby falls.

### Prematurity

A premature baby is one whose gestation falls short of 37 completed weeks. Approximately 7% of all babies are premature, and 1% of births are severely premature with birthweight below 1500 g (very low birthweight).

## Assessment of gestation

Gestational age is determined by the following techniques:

- Calculation of gestational age from the maternal last menstrual period.
- Assessment of fetal maturity from early antenatal ultrasound scans.
- Assessment of neonatal maturity by clinical assessment of gestation after birth. This is based on observation of both external physical criteria and neurological criteria. External criteria include skin development, nipple and genitalia appearance and ear form. Neurological criteria include posture, neck and limb tone and joint mobility.

## Disorders of prematurity

Table 22.3 lists the conditions most likely to occur in premature infants. It is generally the case that the more severe the prematurity, the more likely it will be that these complications will occur and the more severe they are likely to be.

**Table 22.3** A comparison of the risk of problems for premature babies and those who have intrauterine growth retardation (IUGR)

|  | Prematurity | Intrauterine growth retardation |
|---|---|---|
| Hypothermia | ++ | +++ |
| Hypoglycaemia | ++ | +++ |
| Jaundice | ++ | – |
| Infection | ++ | + |
| Respiratory distress syndrome | +++ | Reduced risk |
| Necrotizing enterocolitis | ++ | ++ |
| Retinopathy of prematurity | +++ | – |
| Intracranial haemorrhage | +++ | – |
| Feeding difficulties | +++ | – |

## Prematurity at a glance

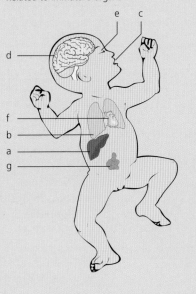

**Definition**
Birth at less than 37 weeks'
   gestation

**Epidemiology**
7% of births are premature
1% are severely premature

**Clinical features**
Thin, transparent skin
Immature nipples, genitalia and
   ear shape
Hypotonic posture with limbs in
   extension
Increased joint mobility

**Management**
Maintain environmental
   temperature
Non-oral feeding if too immature
   or sick
Management of complications
   as indicated

Related to immature organs

**Complications**
• Hypothermia
Metabolic: hypoglycaemia,
   hypocalcaemia, jaundice (**a**)
Respiratory: respiratory distress
   (**b**) syndrome, apnoea and
   bradycardia
• Feeding problems (**c**)
• Intracranial haemorrhage (**d**)
• Infection
• Retinopathy of prematurity (**e**)
• Patent ductus arteriosus (**f**)
• Necrotizing enterocolitis **g**)

**Prognosis**
Excellent if born beyond 32
   weeks' gestation
Premature babies are now
   viable from 24 weeks'
   gestation
Babies weighing less than
   1500 g are at risk for
   neurodevelopmental
   problems; 5–10% have
   serious disability

---

### *Intrauterine growth retardation*

Impaired fetal growth will cause the baby to be born smaller than expected for the duration of gestation. These babies are referred to as 'small for gestational age' (SGA). In order to make the diagnosis of an SGA baby, it is necessary to make a careful assessment of gestational age and to plot the baby's weight on a centile chart to determine whether the baby's weight is below the 10th centile for the gestational age. SGA infants can be described as symmetrically or asymmetrically small.

### Symmetrical growth retardation

A symmetrically small infant is one whose weight, head circumference and length all fall below the 10th centile in the same proportion (Figure 22.3). It is possible that a symmetrically small baby is simply a normal baby whose measurements happen to fall below the 10th centile: by definition, 10% of normal babies will have weight and other measurements below the 10th centile. The further the measurements are below the 10th centile, the more likely it is that the baby has a pathological reason for being small. The baby who is symmetrically growth retarded suggests that an insult causing impaired growth of both body and head occurred *early* in gestation. The commonest cause for this is infection in early pregnancy. Other causes for symmetrical intrauterine growth retardation (IUGR) are shown in Table 22.4.

### Prenatal infection

Prenatal infection occurs as the result of a number of organisms. These are usually described by the acronym TORCH infection:

**T**oxoplasma
**O**ther (syphilis)
**R**ubella
**C**ytomegalovirus
**H**erpes.

Toxoplasma, syphilis and rubella are now very rare in Britain as causes of significant illness in the newborn. Cytomegalovirus is much more common, but rarely causes severe disabling sequelae. Babies present in the neonatal period with hepatosplenomegaly, purpura (caused by thrombocytopenia) and conjugated hyperbilirubinaemia.

The long-term sequelae of TORCH infection include microcephaly, cerebral palsy, mental retardation, blindness and deafness.

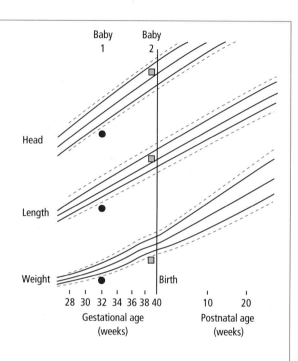

**Figure 22.3** Growth chart showing baby 1 born at 32 weeks of gestation with symmetrical growth retardation and baby 2 born at 39 weeks of gestation with asymmetrical growth retardation.

## Asymmetrical growth retardation

In asymmetrical growth retardation the baby's weight is affected most, followed by length, with head growth being least impaired (Figure 22.3, baby 2). In this case the cause of the growth retardation has occurred relatively *late* in fetal development, most usually as a result of placental insufficiency. Weight gain is affected first, and fat is not laid down. Brain growth is affected least, as in the presence of relative starvation the brain is spared and continues to obtain the major share of available nutrition.

The asymmetrically growth-retarded infant looks long and thin. There is little subcutaneous fat and the baby is scrawny. His or her skin is dry and often cracks and peels in the days after birth. If adequate nutrition can be introduced immediately after birth, postnatal catch-up weight gain is often rapid.

## Management of intrauterine growth retardation

After delivery the main problem to anticipate in the SGA infant is the development of hypoglycaemia. Early and effective feeding is also important. An estimate must be made of the expected weight of the infant had IUGR not occurred, by reading the expected weight for the gestational age from a growth chart. Feeds should then be given according to the expected weight rather than the actual weight. Feeding to the actual weight will only extend the period of inadequate nutrition.

The growth-retarded baby has a reduced risk of developing respiratory distress syndrome. The reason for this is that prenatal stress resulting from the underlying cause of the growth retardation causes endogenous corticosteroid release, with the effect of

**Table 22.4** Causes of symmetrical and asymmetrical growth retardation

| Symmetrical intrauterine growth retardation | Asymmetrical intrauterine growth retardation |
| --- | --- |
| Chromosomal abnormalities | Toxaemia of pregnancy |
| Prenatal infection | Multiple pregnancy |
| Maternal disease | Placental insufficiency |
| Maternal alcoholism | Maternal smoking |

maturing the fetal lung and enhancing surfactant production (see p. 421).

## Outcome of intrauterine growth retardation

Very severely growth-retarded babies may never catch up in terms of growth despite attempts at optimal postnatal feeding. Severe IUGR is a cause of short stature in children (p. 253).

There is evidence that severe growth retardation, particularly where there has been restriction in brain growth, is associated with long-term intellectual impairment.

### Problems of the small baby

The small baby is particularly prone to a number of problems, depending on the degree of prematurity and the severity of the growth retardation (see Table 22.3).

## Hypothermia

A small baby has a larger surface area from which heat can be lost. Heat loss must be minimized by drying the baby at birth and nursing in an incubator. Very immature babies have little or no waterproofing keratin layer and water is easily lost through the skin. Nursing in high ambient humidity and under a Perspex heat shield minimizes this effect.

## Hypoglycaemia

The definition of hypoglycaemia is a blood sugar <2.6 mmol/L. It is a particular problem for small babies because of their lack of glycogen and fat stores. They have fewer reserves of mobilizable glucose on which to draw. Hypoglycaemia is particularly a problem in babies who have suffered IUGR as they have fewer fat stores than babies who are premature alone. Hypoglycaemia must be anticipated in small infants and regular assessment of blood sugar made. This is most conveniently carried out on capillary blood by glucose-sensitive stick tests. Low levels of blood sugar must be treated rapidly with additional milk feeds or intravenous glucose (dextrose) solution.

The prognosis of hypoglycaemia depends on whether the baby was symptomatic. Infants with asymptomatic hypoglycaemia have an excellent prognosis, but those with severe neurological symptoms and convulsions have a poor prognosis. One half of infants who have sustained neonatal convulsions as a result of hypoglycaemia will develop severe neurological disability (cerebral palsy, p. 236, and/or learning disability, p. 242).

## Feeding

Actual or functional immaturity of the gastrointestinal tract is a common problem that prevents early gastric feeding in small babies. The suck reflex does not develop until 35 weeks of gestation. Therefore, premature babies cannot breast- or bottle-feed and the milk must be given through a nasogastric tube. Ill premature infants are at increased risk of necrotizing enterocolitis and gastric feeding may be contraindicated. Growth-retarded and asphyxiated premature infants may be at additional risk because of impaired blood flow to the bowel prior to delivery. These babies may benefit from delayed onset of milk-feeding.

## Infection

Both premature and growth-retarded newborn infants have impairment of their immune function and are more prone to infection than full-term and appropriately grown infants. Great attention must be paid to avoidance of cross infection, and broad-spectrum antibiotics must be used if infection is suspected (see p. 423).

## Apnoea of prematurity

Premature babies may experience apnoea, which results from immaturity of the respiratory system. They usually show a periodic pattern of respiration, with periods of hyperventilation alternating with periods of hypoventilation eventually leading to brief apnoeic episodes. Apnoea of prematurity is diagnosed by excluding other causes of apnoea in otherwise well premature infants. The management is with a xanthine-based drug (caffeine, aminophylline or theophylline) and the prognosis is excellent.

## Small for gestational age (intrauterine growth retardation) at a glance

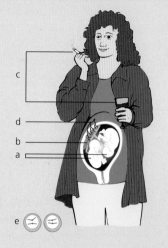

### Definition
Weight less than 10% for gestational age (but problems are more common if less than 3rd centile). Growth retardation may be symmetrical or asymmetrical

### Aetiology
Multiple pregnancy (a)
Placental insufficiency (b)
Maternal smoking/alcohol intake (c)
Congenital infection (TORCH infections) (d)
Genetic syndromes (e)
Normal small babies

### Clinical features
Low birthweight
Mature ears, genitalia, breast tissue
Good muscle tone
*Symmetrical IUGR:* length and head circumference proportional to weight
*Asymmetrical:* long and thin, little subcutaneous fat, dry peeling skin, sparing of head growth

### Investigations
TORCH screen

### Complications
Hypoglycaemia
Birth asphyxia
Hypothermia

### Management
Monitor blood glucose
Early and increased feeds

### Prognosis
At risk for poor growth in childhood
At risk for intellectual impairment if poor head growth has occurred

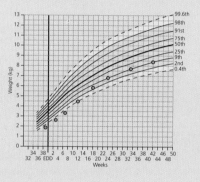

# Respiratory distress

## Causes of acute respiratory distress in premature infants

Respiratory distress syndrome
Pneumonia (congenital or acquired)
Pneumothorax
Surgical conditions (diaphragmatic hernia)
Cardiac causes

Respiratory disease is a very common symptom in premature infants and requires careful assessment in all cases in order to determine the diagnosis and whether specific treatment is required. Respiratory distress occurs in approximately 5% of full-term infants and in over 50% of very low birthweight infants.

In prematurely born infants, respiratory distress syndrome is the most common diagnosis, although infection must be considered in all infants because if treatment is delayed the baby may die very rapidly of overwhelming infection. The commonest surgical cause is diaphragmatic hernia (p. 426).

## Clinical evaluation – must check!

The clinical features of respiratory distress include the following:

- tachypnoea;
- recession (subcostal, intercostal, sternal);
- cyanosis;
- expiratory grunting.

Chest X-ray is the best method to distinguish between the various causes and to make a definitive diagnosis. Respiratory distress syndrome has a characteristic radiological appearance (see Figure 22.6), and an X-ray will distinguish it from a number of other common causes.

### Management

Management depends on the diagnosis, but there are general principles of management of the baby with respiratory distress. These include:

* *Monitoring vital signs.* Babies with respiratory distress are potentially if not actually very ill. Early deterioration may be detected by monitoring respiratory rate, heart rate and blood pressure. Maintenance of normal blood pressure is particularly important in avoiding cerebral complications.
* *Monitoring blood gases.* This is essential in all infants with respiratory distress. Pulse oximeters may guide oxygen therapy requirements, but must not be relied on completely to assess what inspired oxygen concentration is needed. It is only possible to determine what the appropriate oxygen concentration is for an individual baby by measuring the partial pressure of oxygen in arterial blood ($Pa\mathrm{o}_2$) and titrating the inspired oxygen to maintain the arterial oxygen concentration in the normal range. The decision as to whether a baby requires respiratory support is deter-

mined by the blood pH and by the partial pressure of carbon dioxide in arterial blood ($Pa\mathrm{co}_2$).
* *Respiratory support.* Babies with deteriorating lung disease, particularly those who are very small and weak, require respiratory support. This takes the form of either continuous positive airway pressure (CPAP) or intermittent positive pressure ventilation (IPPV).
* *Treat infection.* The possibility of infection must always be considered. Blood cultures and antibiotics are given until the cultures are known to be negative.

## Cyanosis in the neonatal period

### Causes of neonatal cyanosis

*Cardiac*
Transposition of the great arteries
Other right to left shunt defects

*Respiratory*
Respiratory distress syndrome
Pneumonia
Pneumothorax
Diaphragmatic hernia

---

### 👁 Neonatal respiratory distress at a glance

**Epidemiology**
50% premature infants
5% full-term infants

**Aetiology**
* Respiratory distress syndrome (surfactant deficiency) in premature infants (**a**)
* Pneumonia (**b**)
* Pneumothorax (**c**)
* Diaphragmatic hernia (**d**)
* Cardiac causes (**e**)
* Meconium aspiration

**Clinical features**
* Tachypnoea
* Recession (intercostal, subcostal, sternal)
* Cyanosis
* Expiratory grunting

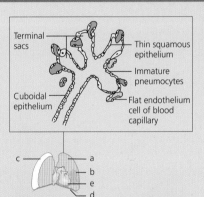

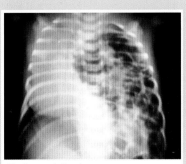

Diaphragmatic hernia

**Confirmatory investigations**
Chest X-ray
Infection screen
Blood gases

**Management**
Monitor vital signs
Titrate inspired oxygen concentration against baby's oxygen saturation
Surfactant in respiratory distress syndrome
CPAP and/or IPPV for respiratory failure
Antibiotics for infection
Monitor function of other organ systems

**Prognosis**
Depends on underlying causes and infant's maturity

Peripheral cyanosis involving hands and feet is very common in the neonatal period, and is referred to as acrocyanosis. This is of no clinical significance providing the baby has no central cyanosis (tongue involvement). Central cyanosis is always significant and indicates respiratory or cardiac disease. It must be rapidly investigated. If there is doubt about clinical cyanosis, a short period of oxygen saturation monitoring is required.

The commonest cardiac cause of cyanosis presenting in the neonatal period is transposition of the great vessels. This is a surgically remediable condition with a good prognosis. Cardiac failure rarely presents in the neonatal period other than in premature infants with patent ductus arteriosus (p. 426). They are not cyanosed. Fallot's tetralogy (p. 200), the commonest cause of cyanotic heart disease in childhood, rarely presents with cyanosis in the neonatal period.

### Clinical evaluation – must check!

Cyanosis caused by respiratory disease can be differentiated in most cases from that caused by cardiac disease by the presence of respiratory distress, which suggests the presence of lung disease. Occasionally, babies (particularly those born prematurely) may have both respiratory and cardiac disease.

The helpful clinical distinguishing features between cardiac and lung disease are shown in the Clues box.

A nitrogen wash-out test is sometimes used to determine whether the baby has cyanotic heart disease or lung disease where diagnosis is difficult (Figure 22.4). This involves monitoring oxygen saturation while the baby is breathing oxygen as close to 100% as possible. If the oxygen saturation exceeds 95% there cannot be a significant right to left shunt.

Investigations of a child with suspected cyanotic heart disease include chest X-ray, electrocardiogram (ECG) and echocardiography, which should define the structural anatomy.

### Management

The management of cyanotic lesions depends on the underlying diagnosis. Oxygen, CPAP and mechanical ventilation (p. 411) may be of considerable benefit for respiratory disease, but are usually of little benefit in cardiac disease. Prostaglandin infusion to maintain the ductus arteriosus open may be life-saving in infants with a duct-dependent cyanotic cardiac lesion.

---

**Clues to the differential diagnosis of cyanosis**

| Causes of cyanosis | Features on clinical evaluation |
| --- | --- |
| *Cardiac* | |
| Transposition of the great vessels | Murmur<br>Characteristic chest X-ray<br>Echocardiogram |
| Other congenital cardiac lesions with right to left shunt | Murmur<br>Echocardiography<br>Chest X-ray may be diagnostic |
| *Respiratory* | |
| Respiratory distress syndrome | Signs of respiratory distress<br>Characteristic chest X-ray |
| Other causes of respiratory distress | Chest X-ray<br>Blood cultures |

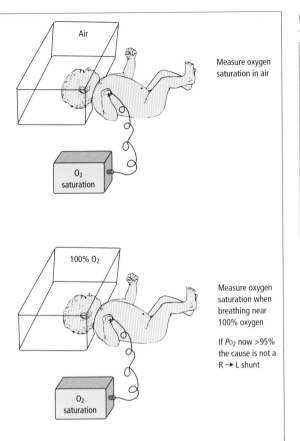

Air

Measure oxygen saturation in air

O₂ saturation

100% O₂

Measure oxygen saturation when breathing near 100% oxygen

If $P_{O_2}$ now >95% the cause is not a R → L shunt

O₂ saturation

**Figure 22.4** The nitrogen wash-out test.

# Convulsions

## Causes of neonatal convulsions

Asphyxia
Hypoglycaemia
Hypocalcaemia
Meningitis
Congenital brain anomalies
Intracranial haemorrhage
Maternal drug withdrawal (neonatal abstinence syndrome)
Inborn errors of metabolism (rare)
Unknown (idiopathic)

Neonatal convulsions are very common and occur in 0.5–1.0% of all babies. It is sometimes very difficult to interpret whether unusual movements in premature infants are convulsive in nature. Jitteriness is not a sign of cerebral dysfunction and is described on p. 404. Neonatal convulsions are usually clonic and fragmentary, often involving different limbs for a short time. Less commonly, neonatal convulsions may be tonic or myoclonic. Idiopathic epilepsy does not occur in the neonatal period.

## 👁 Cyanosis in the newborn period at a glance

**Epidemiology**
Cyanosis due to respiratory disease is common; due to cardiac disease is rare. See Causes box, p. 411

**Clinical features**
Cyanosis of the lips and tongue (distinguish from acrocyanosis)
Respiratory distress if cyanosis is respiratory
Heart murmur if cyanosis is cardiac*

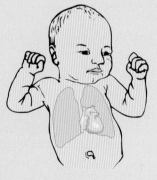

**Confirmatory investigations**
Blood gases – low arterial O₂
Nitrogen wash-out to distinguish cardiac from respiratory disease
Chest X-rays
ECG and echocardiography if cardiac cyanosis is suspected

**Management**
Oxygen, CPAP and ventilation for respiratory cyanosis
Investigate cardiac disease
Cardiac surgery usually required for cyanotic heart disease

**Prognosis**
Good for most respiratory causes and operable cardiac lesion

NB *Signs and symptoms are variable.

### History – must ask!

A careful maternal and perinatal history is required in all cases. Pay particular attention to maternal illness (diabetes predisposes the baby to hypoglycaemia), evidence of fetal distress, symptoms of neurological abnormality prior to the convulsion (feeding problems, irritability, stiffness) and whether there is a family history of neonatal convulsions. Ask the mother if she took any illicit drugs in pregnancy.

### Physical examination – must check!

• *Extensive bruising.* This may be suggestive of birth trauma.
• *Dysmorphic features.* These are suggestive of an underlying brain anomaly.
• *Intrauterine growth retardation.* If the baby is SGA this increases the risk of hypoglycaemia and hypocalcaemia.
• *Hepatosplenomegaly and purpura.* These suggest prenatal infection (TORCH).

### Investigations

The investigations listed in Table 22.5 should be undertaken in all neonates with convulsions. These include:

• metabolic tests;
• tests for infection;
• brain imaging.

### Management

Management should be directed towards treating the underlying cause of the convulsions (meningitis, hypoglycaemia, etc.) as well as therapy to prevent further convulsions if a specific cause cannot be found.

Phenobarbitone is the first-line anticonvulsant used in the neonatal period.

### Prognosis

The prognosis depends on the underlying cause for the convulsions. A very poor prognosis is likely if a major congenital brain anomaly is detected, and there is a 50% chance of poor outcome if the fits are caused by meningitis, asphyxia or major intracranial haemorrhage.

**Table 22.5** Investigations and their significance in neonates with convulsions

| Investigations | Significance |
| --- | --- |
| Full blood count | Abnormal white cell count suggestive of infection |
| Blood cultures | Infection |
| Lumbar puncture | Meningitis |
| Blood glucose | Hypoglycaemia |
| Serum calcium | Hypocalcaemia |
| Ultrasound brain imaging | Intracranial haemorrhage Periventricular leucomalacia Congenital anomaly |
| Metabolic screen | Inborn error of metabolism |

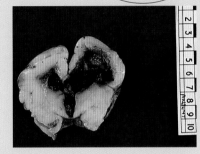

### Neonatal convulsions at a glance

**Epidemiology**
0.5–1% of all neonates

**Aetiology**
Causes are intracranial (asphyxia, meningitis, malformation or haemorrhage), metabolic (hypoglycaemia, hypocalcaemia) or idiopathic

**Clinical features**
Usually clonic and fragmentary movements
Less commonly tonic or myoclonic
May be difficult to differentiate from jitteriness*
Apnoea and bradycardia*
History of intrapartum asphyxia*
Bilateral intraventricular haemorrhage. There is a clot distending the ventricular system with extensive involvement into the right hemisphere (grade IV haemorrhage)

NB *Signs and symptoms are variable.

**Confirmatory investigations**
• Blood glucose, electrolytes, calcium
• Infection screen, including lumbar puncture to exclude meningitis
• Ultrasound for haemorrhage or cerebral malformations
• Metabolic screen

**Management**
Treat underlying cause
Prevent further convulsions with phenobarbitone

**Prognosis**
Depends on underlying cause
If none identified, the prognosis is usually good

## Apnoea

### Causes of apnoea in the neonate

*Central apnoea*
Apnoea of prematurity
Hypoglycaemia
Infection
Intracranial haemorrhage
Necrotizing enterocolitis
Convulsions
*Obstructive apnoea*
Small jaw
Thick oropharyngeal secretions
Congenital blockage of the posterior nares (very rare)

Apnoea is a very common symptom in the neonatal period and is particularly seen in premature infants. The definition of apnoea is a pause in respiration lasting for 20 seconds or more. It is a non-specific symptom and the baby requires careful assessment to discover the underlying cause.

Apnoea may be central or obstructive in origin. Central causes may involve the brainstem or higher cortical structures. Obstructive causes occur as a result of airway obstruction and can sometimes be recognized by observing the episode.

Apnoea of prematurity is a diagnosis of exclusion.

### Clinical evaluation – must check!

In *obstructive apnoea* the baby continues to make respiratory efforts despite increasing cyanosis or bradycardia, suggesting that the airway is becoming blocked and the baby is fighting to overcome this effect. Obstructive apnoea can be excluded by passing a tube through the nares and evaluating whether the baby has a small jaw.

In *central apnoea* the baby usually shows periodic respiration with slowing in the respiratory rate until apnoea occurs. It is always important to consider infection as the cause of apnoeic episodes and to investigate this rapidly and institute treatment as early as possible. Other investigations should be performed to exclude or confirm the causes of the apnoea.

## Management

The acute apnoeic episode should be treated rapidly. Infants presenting with a significant apnoea should normally be admitted for careful observation for at least 24 hours. The management depends on the severity and frequency of the attacks. Initially, tactile stimulation is effective, and nasopharyngeal suction may be necessary in obstructive causes. Severe apnoeic episodes may require bag and mask resuscitation.

Treatment should also be directed towards the cause of the condition if this is known. Where the cause is thought to be apnoea of prematurity, non-specific therapy involves administration of a xanthine-based drug to stimulate the respiratory system. Aminophylline, theophylline and caffeine are most widely used. Continuous positive airway pressure may be useful in more refractory cases, and the most severe cases require mechanical ventilation.

Rarely, no known cause for the acute life-threatening events will be found. In these cases induced illness should be considered. Some families find an apnoea monitor reassuring, though recurrent 'false alarms' are often problematic.

---

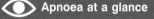 **Apnoea at a glance**

**Epidemiology**
Common symptom, particularly in premature infants

**Aetiology**
Apnoea may be due to partial obstruction of the airway or central causes (see Causes box, p. 415)

**Clinical features**
Pause in breathing lasting longer than 20 seconds
Often associated with periodic breathing
Bradycardia
Cyanosis*

Central: factors affecting respiratory centre

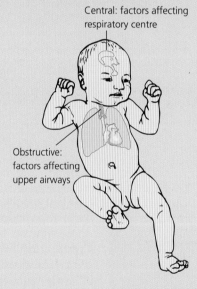

Obstructive: factors affecting upper airways

**Confirmatory investigations**
Infection screen in all cases
Assess for anatomic problems of upper airway
Assess for brain pathology

**Management**
Treat all apnoeic episodes with stimulation
Treat underlying cause, where possible
Xanthine derivatives if apnoea is persistent
CPAP or IPPV if apnoea is very severe
Home apnoea monitors are rarely indicated except for severe life-threatening apnoeic episodes (see p. 396)

**Prognosis**
Good except where there is major central pathology

NB *Signs and symptoms are variable.

# Neonatal jaundice

| Causes of neonatal jaundice |
|---|
| *Unconjugated hyperbilirubinaemia* |
| Rhesus and ABO incompatibility |
| Bacterial infection |
| Excessive bruising |
| Internal haemorrhage |
| Prematurity |
| Hypothyroidism |
| Breast-milk jaundice |
| Physiological |
| |
| *Conjugated hyperbilirubinaemia* |
| Neonatal hepatitis |
| Cystic fibrosis |
| Biliary atresia |

Jaundice in the neonatal period is a very common feature; it is usually caused by the physiological immaturity of the liver, and is self-limiting over the first week of life as liver function matures. Neonatal jaundice (hyperbilirubinaemia) can be classified depending on whether it is conjugated or unconjugated.

Jaundice occurs as a result of the build-up of bilirubin – which may be caused by prehepatic, hepatic or posthepatic causes.

- *Prehepatic.* This is a result of excessive breakdown of red blood cells, as occurs in haemolysis. The bilirubin is all unconjugated.
- *Hepatic.* An abnormality in liver function, such as occurs in neonatal hepatitis, will cause a build-up of conjugated bilirubin.
- *Posthepatic.* This is a result of absent or atretic bile ductules extending to main branches of the bile ducts, and causes conjugated hyperbilirubinaemia. This condition is referred to as biliary atresia (see below).

Jaundice may be clinically significant for two reasons:

**1** High levels of unconjugated bilirubin may cause irreversible brain damage, referred to as kernicterus. Bilirubin toxicity (kernicterus) causes nerve deafness, choreoathetoid cerebral palsy and mental retardation.
**2** Prolonged jaundice may indicate severe underlying disease.

## History – must ask!

Neonatal jaundice occurs in almost all newborn infants to some degree. Jaundice may cause the baby to become lethargic and feed less well. Conversely, those babies who become somewhat dehydrated appear more jaundiced as a result of haemoconcentration and so may feed less well, thus causing more severe dehydration.

In conjugated hyperbilirubinaemia, specific enquiries include family history of cystic fibrosis, metabolic disorders and liver disease.

## Physical examination – must check!

On examination the distribution of the jaundice may help in estimating the total bilirubin level:

- Limited to head and neck: mild.
- Over lower trunk and thighs: moderate.
- Extending to hands and feet: may require treatment.

Examination should also identify petechial or purpuric lesions, anaemia and hepatosplenomegaly.

## Investigations

Total and unconjugated levels of bilirubin should be measured. The Coombs' test determines whether there is antibody on the red blood cell membrane. It is positive in rhesus incompatibility.

There are four circumstances which indicate that a baby should be investigated rapidly for serious causes of the jaundice:

- Early evidence of jaundice appearing in the first 24 hours of life. This suggests that there is underlying haemolysis.
- Clinical evidence of deep jaundice.
- Prolonged conjugated jaundice lasting more than 2 weeks, which suggests a serious underlying cause.
- Increasing levels of conjugated bilirubin. This suggests a severe hepatic cause of the jaundice.

Further investigations are indicated for prolonged jaundice and increasing conjugated bilirubinaemia to diagnose the causes listed in Table 22.6.

## Management

The aim of treatment for unconjugated hyperbilirubinaemia is to avoid kernicterus. The level of unconjugated bilirubin which causes brain damage is not known for certain and depends on the gestational age of the baby and how sick the baby is. Charts are

**Table 22.6** Investigations and their relevance in a jaundiced neonate

| Investigations | Relevance |
| --- | --- |
| Full blood count | Neutrophilia or neutropenia suggests infection<br>Thrombocytopenia suggests TORCH infection |
| Maternal and neonatal blood groups and Coombs' test | ABO and rhesus incompatibility |
| Urine cultures | Infection |
| Lumbar puncture | Meningitis |
| Ultrasound scans | Internal haemorrhage<br>Biliary atresia |
| Thyroid function tests | Hypothyroidism |
| Hepatitis B antigen | Hepatitis B infection |
| Metabolic screen | Inborn errors of metabolism |
| Sweat test | Cystic fibrosis |

available which indicate the level of unconjugated bilirubin at which babies of different gestational age should be treated.

Treatment is initially by phototherapy, which degrades the unconjugated bilirubin to non-toxic soluble compounds and these are excreted in the urine. If levels continue to rise to a potentially toxic level, a series of exchange transfusions are necessary. The management of conjugated hyperbilirubinaemia depends on the underlying cause.

## 👁 Neonatal jaundice at a glance

**Epidemiology**
All premature infants, also common in full-term infants
1–2% of babies require treatment

**Aetiology**
Jaundice may be caused by conjugated or unconjugated hyperbilirubinaemia
See Causes box, p. 417

**Clinical features**
Yellow pigmentation of skin
Yellow sclerae
Lethargy*
Bruising*
Poor feeding*
Hepatomegaly*

**Confirmatory investigations**
Conjugated and unconjugated bilirubin
FBC and smear
Blood group
Coombs' test

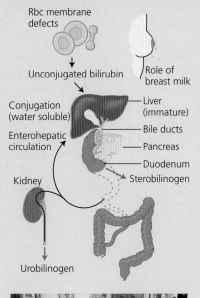

Rbc membrane defects
Unconjugated bilirubin
Role of breast milk
Conjugation (water soluble)
Enterohepatic circulation
Liver (immature)
Bile ducts
Pancreas
Duodenum
Kidney
Sterobilinogen
Urobilinogen

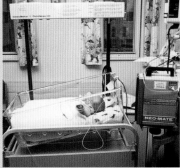

**Features of concern**
Presentation less than 24 hours
Severe jaundice
Prolonged (greater than 2 weeks) jaundice
Increased conjugated bilirubin

**Management**
Identify cause
*Unconjugated hyperbilirubinaemia:*
Phototherapy
Exchange transfusion to avert kernicterus if very high bilirubin
Hearing assessment if levels indicate risk of kernicterus
*Conjugated hyperbilirubinaemia:*
Treatment depends on cause

**Prognosis/complications**
Danger of kernicterus (athetoid cerebral palsy) and neurosensory deafness if unconjugated bilirubinaemia rises to high levels
Prognosis for severe conjugated bilirubinaemia is poor

NB *Signs and symptoms are variable.

## 🔑 Key points: Neonatal jaundice

• Identify the cause
• If it is a self-limiting condition, strongly reassure the parents
• Avoid kernicterus in unconjugated hyperbilirubinaemia with phototherapy and exchange transfusions
• The management of conjugated jaundice depends on the cause
• If high levels of unconjugated bilirubin occur, follow-up is necessary for neurological complications
• Babies jaundiced beyond 2 weeks of age require urgent investigation in hospital

# Bowel obstruction

**Causes of bowel obstruction in the neonate**

*Anatomical abnormalities*
Oesophageal atresia
Duodenal atresia
Jejunal atresia
Anal atresia

*Functional abnormalities*
Hirschsprung's disease
Meconium ileus
Volvulus secondary to malrotation

Congenital intestinal obstruction occurs in one in 1000 babies. Causes can be divided into anatomical obstruction (e.g. duodenal atresia) and functional obstruction, where the bowel is patent but the peristaltic function is abnormal (e.g. Hirschsprung's disease, see below).

### Clinical features – must check!

There are four major features of intestinal obstruction:

- bile-stained vomiting;
- failure to pass meconium;
- abdominal distension;
- visible peristalsis.

If the obstruction is high in the gastrointestinal tract, abdominal distension may not be obvious and the infant may pass copious amounts of meconium from below the obstruction. The stool, however, does not show a change from meconium to products of milk digestion (the changing stool).

Bile-stained vomiting is always abnormal and strongly suggests obstruction. An emergency surgical opinion is required.

### Investigations and management

Assessment for dehydration with serum electrolytes is important in the vomiting neonate. A plain abdominal X-ray shows fluid levels and dilated bowel in complete obstruction. In duodenal atresia the classical 'double bubble' is seen (Figure 22.5), with air in the stomach and first part of duodenum.

Surgery is required to relieve the site of obstruction.

**Clues to the differential diagnosis of neonatal bowel obstruction**

*Anatomical abnormalities*

| | |
|---|---|
| Oesophageal atresia | Mucusy, chokes on first feed. Associated with tracheo-oesophageal fistula in 95% of cases |
| Duodenal atresia | Bile-stained vomiting, 'double bubble' seen on abdominal X-ray |
| Jejunal atresia | Commonest cause of congenital bowel obstruction. Abdominal distension and bile-stained vomiting |
| Anal atresia | Detected on routine examination |

*Functional abnormalities*

| | |
|---|---|
| Hirschsprung's disease | Delayed passage of meconium and marked abdominal obstruction |
| Meconium ileus | Delayed passage of meconium. Very thick tenacious meconium |
| Volvulus secondary to malrotation | Intermittent episodes of partial obstruction. Bile-stained vomiting |

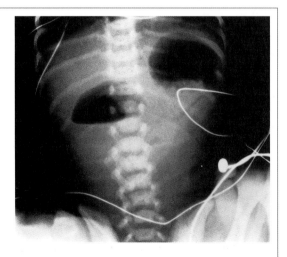

**Figure 22.5** Abdominal X-ray showing the 'double bubble' in duodenal atresia.

## Neonatal conditions

## Respiratory distress syndrome

Respiratory distress syndrome (RDS) has in the past been referred to as hyaline membrane disease (HMD), a condition recognized on histological examination. The condition is caused by surfactant deficiency in the immature lung. Although babies now rarely die in the acute phase of RDS, complications such as brain damage and chronic lung disease mean that it remains generally the commonest cause of death in premature infants and the commonest cause of disability in infants who survive the condition.

The incidence of RDS is inversely related to the degree of prematurity. Approximately 70% of infants born at 26 weeks' gestation will develop RDS, 25% at 32 weeks and 0.5% at term.

## Aetiology

Respiratory distress syndrome is caused by surfactant deficiency. Surfactant is a phospholipid which causes reduction in surface tension of the alveolus. It is produced by type II alveolar cells, which, although they are present from an early stage in fetal development, do not start to produce surfactant until close to term. Consequently, premature birth is associated with deficiency of surfactant and the development of RDS. The stress of premature birth and developing RDS causes release of corticosteroids from the infant's own adrenal glands, and this will in turn cause surfactant to be produced. RDS is therefore a self-limiting condition as endogenous surfactant will eventually resolve the clinical condition, but it may take 7 days or more for sufficient endogenous surfactant to be produced to resolve the lung disorder. The challenge of neonatology is to manage the baby in optimal condition and prevent any complications of treatment until the RDS resolves.

The fetal lung is a stiff structure as a result of lack of surfactant. At birth the baby takes a deep breath which expands the lungs with air, but if surfactant is not present the stiff alveoli collapse down to their fetal size and the next breath is another massive inspiratory effort. This increased work of breathing continues until the baby becomes exhausted. Surfactant molecules produce a molecular monolayer within the alveolus and prevent the alveolus from collapsing down to its unexpanded state.

The antenatal administration of a corticosteroid for 48 hours to the mother who is at risk of delivering a premature infant is the most effective treatment in preventing RDS in her baby by stimulating surfactant release. Endogenous corticosteroid release, as occurs in the growth-retarded fetus, also reduces the risk of the SGA baby developing RDS. Infants of diabetic mothers are at considerably increased risk of RDS because hyperinsulinaemia inhibits surfactant development.

## Clinical features

The baby presents with signs of respiratory distress as described above. There is no specific clinical feature of RDS, but it is rare in mature infants and common in the severely premature baby. A major feature of RDS is recession, which may be very severe in small infants with a soft rib cage. Sternal recession is marked, with the appearance of the sternum meeting the spine. Grunting is uncommon in premature infants and is mainly a feature of full-term babies.

## Investigations

Diagnosis of RDS is confirmed by chest X-ray which is usually diagnostic (Figure 22.6). It shows two characteristic features:

**1** An air bronchogram (radiolucent air in the bronchi seen against the airless lung)
**2** Ground glass appearance of the lung fields as a result of alveoli collapse

## Management

Specific treatment for this condition includes the following:

- *Titration of the inspired oxygen level against oxygen saturations measured by pulse oximetry.* If the baby is breathing spontaneously, the oxygen can be administered via a headbox.
- *Continuous positive airway pressure.* Respiratory support can be given in a spontaneously breathing baby by applying CPAP via either a facemask or nasal prongs. This technique maintains constant positive

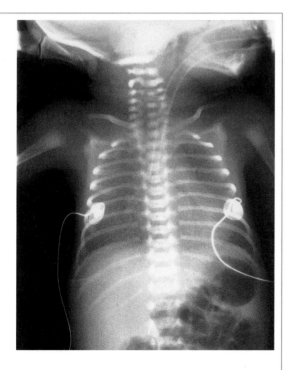

**Figure 22.6** X-ray showing the features of respiratory distress syndrome (RDS).

distending pressure on expiration, which prevents alveolar collapse.

• *Mechanical ventilation.* Very small babies will require immediate mechanical ventilation because they are too weak to breathe spontaneously. Larger babies who do not improve on CPAP or those having severe apnoeic episodes will also require mechanical ventilation (IPPV). Mechanical ventilation is applied by intubating the baby and connecting the endotracheal tube to a ventilator.

• *Administration of exogenous surfactant.* Natural or synthetic surfactant is given directly into the baby's lungs by instillation through the endotracheal tube. This therapy has reduced the mortality of RDS by 40%.

## Complications

The major complications of RDS and its treatment are listed in Table 22.7.

| Table 22.7 Complications of respiratory distress syndr.ome |
| --- |
| Pneumothorax |
| Pneumonia |
| Intracranial haemorrhage |
| Hydrocephalus |
| Patent ductus arteriosus |
| Necrotizing enterocolitis |
| Retinopathy of prematurity |
| Chronic lung disease |
| Cerebral palsy |

## Prognosis

Approximately 80% of small babies with RDS survive, but a proportion have major sequelae. The two most important are cerebral palsy and chronic lung disease. Approximately 5% of infants surviving RDS will develop severe cerebral palsy (see p. 236). Chronic lung disease is defined by the requirement of additional oxygen beyond 28 days of age. With increasing numbers of babies surviving RDS, chronic lung disease is becoming more common. Approximately 40% of babies weighing 1 kg at birth develop chronic lung disease. It is usually a self-limiting condition, since the oxygen requirement falls as the baby's lung grows, but a small proportion may be sent home on additional oxygen. Babies with chronic lung disease are much more likely to wheeze in the first 2 years of life and a few may develop long-term respiratory problems.

## Respiratory distress syndrome at a glance

**Epidemiology**
Increasing risk with degree of prematurity
70% of 28-week infants,
0.5% of full-terms

**Aetiology**
Due to surfactant deficiency

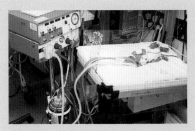

**Prevention**
Corticosteroids for mother 48 hours prior to delivery if at risk for premature birth

**Clinical features**
Tachypnoea
Intercostal, subcostal, sternal recession
Cyanosis
Expiratory grunting

**Confirmatory investigations**
Chest X-ray shows air bronchogram, ground glass appearance of lung fields

**Differential diagnosis**
Infection
Pneumothorax
Diaphragmatic hernia
Cardiac causes

**Management**
Titration of inspired $O_2$ against baby's $O_2$ saturation
CPAP or IPPV for respiratory failure
Surfactant for intubated infants
Monitor vital signs and blood pressure

**Complications**
See Table 22.7

**Prognosis**
Babies who are ventilated are at risk for bronchopulmonary dysplasia (chronic lung disease)
Very premature babies receiving high $PO_2$ are at risk of retinopathy
80% of babies survive severe respiratory distress syndrome, but 5% develop severe cerebral palsy

## Infection

The newborn, and particularly the premature infant, is particularly susceptible to infection because of immaturity of the immune system. An important factor in the integrity of the immune response is maternal IgG, which crosses the placenta to the fetus in the last 3 months of pregnancy. Babies who are born severely preterm miss the maternal IgG contribution.

Infection in the newborn is usually bacterial and may be acquired either at birth from the maternal genital tract during delivery (perinatally) or by cross-infection (nosocomial) from medical and nursing staff. Perinatally acquired early infection is most commonly caused by group B beta-haemolytic streptococcus and *E. coli*. Nosocomial infection is most commonly caused by *Staphylococcus epidermidis* and *Pseudomonas*.

### Clinical features

There are no specific signs of infection in the newborn, and infection must always be considered to be a pos-

sible cause of any compromise in all newborn infants. Signs of infection are shown in the Red Flag box.

### Clinical signs suggestive of acquired neonatal infection

Unstable temperature
Lethargy
Apnoeic or bradycardic episodes
Hypotonia
Irritability
Convulsions
Poor feeding
Respiratory distress
Jaundice
Vomiting
Abdominal distension

### Investigations

Infection must be considered to be a cause of almost any acute symptom or sign in the neonate and requires rapid investigation. Infection screen includes the following:

- full blood count;
- C-reactive protein
- blood and urine cultures;
- swabs from skin, throat, trachea and rectum;
- lumbar puncture
- Chest X-ray.

## Management

Antibiotic treatment is most effective if started early. Bacteriological confirmation of infection will take 24–48 hours from taking the specimens and consequently, if infection is suspected, broad-spectrum antibiotics should be started immediately. They can be stopped if microbiological surveillance is negative. If it is positive, a full course should be given for 5–7 days.

## Meningitis

Meningitis occurring in the neonatal period is sufficiently different from meningitis in older children to be considered separately. The incidence of neonatal meningitis is one in 4000 babies. The neonate is relatively immunocompromised by immaturity, which predisposes to meningitis. Any organism may cause neonatal meningitis, but the most common are group B beta-haemolytic streptococci and *Escherichia coli*.

The neonate does not develop specific symptoms of meningitis such as a stiff neck, and the signs of infection are often very non-specific. This is why meningitis must be considered in any baby with unexpected deterioration. Signs include cyanotic and apnoeic spells, unstable temperature, irritability and convulsions. Lumbar puncture is essential in any neonate with unexplained deterioration to confirm or exclude the diagnosis.

Treatment is directed towards the causal organisms. Broad-spectrum antibiotics should be given prior to isolation of the infecting bacterium. The prognosis depends on how quickly the diagnosis is made and appropriate antibiotic treatment started. In general, it is not good. Approximately 25% of babies die and a further 25% become severely handicapped. Hydrocephalus is a common complication after neonatal meningitis.

## Pneumonia

Pneumonia develops shortly after birth if infection is acquired from the mother during passage down the genital tract (perinatal infection). Group B beta-haemolytic streptococcus is usually the causative organism. Pneumonia may also occur in mechanically ventilated babies who acquire nosocomial infection from their carers. Pseudomonas or *Staphylococcus aureus* is the most likely infectious agent for late pneumonia.

**Clinical features.** The baby presents early with respiratory distress and shock. The chest X-ray may show an identical appearance to that of RDS, so pneumonia must always be considered as a differential diagnosis in RDS. Group B beta-haemolytic streptococcus is identified in blood cultures. Pneumonia must always be considered in any infant who deteriorates on mechanical ventilation.

**Management and prognosis.** An appropriate antibiotic is curative if given early enough. Group B beta-haemolytic streptococcus is always sensitive to penicillin. Supportive care is necessary to manage the circulation until the baby recovers. Prognosis is good with early diagnosis. Death occurs in rapidly progressive cases.

## Intracranial haemorrhage

Intracranial haemorrhage is very common in premature newborn infants. In particular, intraventricular haemorrhage (IVH) occurs in up to 40% of very low birthweight infants. Intracranial haemorrhage develops in the floor of the lateral ventricle and usually ruptures into the lateral ventricle. In only 25% of cases does further rupture occur into the periventricular white matter. This form of parenchymal haemorrhage is the most severe, and if the child survives there is a high risk of cerebral palsy (p. 236).

Periventricular leucomalacia (PVL) is caused by cerebral ischaemia and frequently occurs in babies with IVH. It is less common than IVH, but PVL is the commonest cause of severe cerebral palsy in surviving premature infants. Poor outcome is particularly likely if the baby develops cystic PVL.

**Clinical features.** Many babies who develop IVH show no symptoms, but convulsions are not uncommon in babies with parenchymal haemorrhage. The diagnosis is made by ultrasound examination.

**Management and prognosis.** There is no specific treatment, but post-haemorrhagic hydrocephalus occurs in 10% of babies following IVH. Cerebral palsy (see p. 236) occurs in 80% of babies with cystic PVL, and is usually severe. Cerebral palsy may also occur in infants with parenchymal haemorrhage, but this is usually less severe than that seen with PVL.

## Necrotizing enterocolitis

This is a rare complication of newborn infants. It is caused by impaired blood flow through the bowel, which predisposes the mucosa to invasion by enteric organisms. The babies present with acute deterioration, apnoea, abdominal distension and bloody diarrhoea. In 20% of cases bowel perforation occurs, followed by signs of peritonitis.

The diagnosis is confirmed on abdominal X-ray, when gas produced by the invading organisms can be seen in the bowel. Management is initially expectant. Enteral feeds are stopped for at least 10 days and broad-spectrum antibiotics started. If bowel perforation has occurred, laparotomy is indicated. Most babies make a full recovery, but 10% later develop bowel stricture in the area of necrotizing enterocolitis involvement.

## Jaundice of prematurity

All premature infants become visibly jaundiced in the few days after birth. This is caused by immaturity of the liver and failure of the hepatocytes to conjugate the bilirubin adequately. Jaundice of prematurity never reaches levels high enough to consider an exchange transfusion and the babies are well.

The diagnosis is made by excluding other conditions. The jaundice is self-limiting. Moderately high levels of bilirubin may require phototherapy, but no other treatment is necessary.

## Haemolytic disease of the newborn

Haemolysis occurs in the fetus as a result of maternal antibodies reacting with antigen on the fetal red blood cell. The two commonest reasons for this are rhesus incompatibility and ABO blood group incompatibility.

In rhesus disease the mother is rhesus negative and the fetus rhesus positive. The mother has been sensitized to rhesus-positive cells in earlier pregnancies, when fetal cells cross into the maternal circulation. This causes the mother to develop anti-rhesus antibodies, which cross the placenta and cause haemolysis of fetal red blood cells. This tends to be worse in successive pregnancies.

In ABO blood group incompatibility, the mother is most commonly blood group O and the baby is blood group A. The mother's natural anti-A antibodies react with the fetal cells causing, haemolysis and jaundice. This condition cannot be detected antenatally.

**Clinical features.** Fetal haemolysis causes the fetus to be anaemic initially, and if untreated, severe oedema (hydrops) occurs. At birth the severely affected baby is very oedematous and anaemic with rapid development of jaundice. Less severely affected infants show anaemia at birth with development of jaundice in the first 24 hours after birth. Babies with rhesus disease are more likely to develop RDS.

**Management.** The aim of management is to deliver the baby before severe haemolysis has occurred and then undertake a series of exchange transfusions to wash out the antibodies as well as the toxic bilirubin. Rhesus-negative women are now immunized with anti-D antibody and consequently rhesus haemolytic disease is now very rare.

The treatment of infants with ABO incompatibility is similar and is aimed at preventing dangerously high levels of unconjugated hyperbilirubinaemia. Late anaemia (6–8 weeks after birth) is common in haemolytic conditions, and the baby may require a top-up blood transfusion.

**Prognosis.** If kernicterus is avoided, the prognosis is excellent. Sensorineural hearing impairment may be the only sign of bilirubin toxicity.

## Breast-milk jaundice

This is a benign condition and requires no treatment. It is generally diagnosed by excluding other more serious conditions. In this condition the baby is being breast-fed, develops mild to moderate hyperbilirubinaemia in the second week of life and remains well. Breast-feeding should continue with appropriate reassurance for the parents.

## Neonatal hepatitis

This is a rare condition. It is usually caused by either a virus (hepatitis B, cytomegalovirus), cystic fibrosis or a metabolic cause. There is no specific treatment.

An avoidable cause of morbidity from hepatitis B is when the baby contracts the infection from the mother. The baby is most at risk if the mother contracts hepatitis B in the last trimester of pregnancy. The baby should be immunized immediately after birth with hepatitis B vaccine and again at 6 months, as well as receiving hepatitis immunoglobulin at birth and again at 3 and 6 months of age.

## Biliary atresia

Biliary atresia is an important but rare condition and is caused by atresia of intrahepatic or extrahepatic bile ducts. The babies present with increasing conjugated hyperbilirubinaemia from 4 weeks of life. If undiagnosed, there is rapid progression to liver failure and death, but if the diagnosis is made within 3 months of birth, surgery may restore liver function to near normal. This condition should be considered in any baby presenting with conjugated jaundice beyond 2 weeks of age.

## Patent ductus arteriosus

Patent ductus arteriosus (Figure 22.7) is a common complication of infants who require mechanical ventilation. During fetal life, the ductus arteriosus shunts blood from right to left away from the unexpanded lungs. In premature infants with lung disease, particularly RDS, the increased pulmonary resistance and hypoxia makes it more likely that the ductus will reopen. In neonatal life the direction of the blood shunt is reversed and is more likely to be left to right, therefore increasing the work of breathing. This may make it difficult to wean the baby from the ventilator.

The baby has a systolic murmur and collapsing pulses (p. 194). If the left to right shunt is large, the

chest X-ray shows plethoric lung fields. Diagnosis is confirmed by echocardiography.

Fluid restriction and diuretics may encourage the ductus to close. Indomethacin is a prostaglandin synthetase inhibitor and is used to close the ductus if standard treatment fails. Rarely, surgical ligation may be required. With appropriate treatment the prognosis is excellent.

## Obstructive apnoea

This condition occurs in babies with either anatomical or functional problems.

*Anatomical obstruction* of upper airway structures occurs, for example, in posterior nasal obstruction (choanal atresia). Babies born with a small jaw (micrognathia) are subject to obstructive apnoea when the tongue falls back and causes the upper airway to be occluded.

*Functional obstruction* occurs in premature infants who may have hypotonia of the oropharyngeal musculature, which predisposes to collapse of the upper airway structures during breathing.

Obstructive apnoea may be recognized by the effort of breathing that the baby makes to overcome upper airway obstruction. Anatomical obstruction caused by choanal atresia is diagnosed by an inability to pass a cannula through both nostrils. You can see if the baby has micrognathia by looking at the face in profile.

Anatomical obstruction requires surgical correction, and the prognosis is generally good. Obstruction in premature infants is best treated by nasal CPAP. This improves the patency of the upper airway until the baby grows and the tone improves spontaneously. Premature babies usually grow out of the problem.

## Diaphragmatic hernia

This is a congenital defect in the left hemidiaphragm that allows bowel to herniate into the left chest, with compression of the lungs and deviation of the heart to the right. If herniation occurs early in pregnancy, severe lung hypoplasia develops as a result of the compression and the baby dies rapidly in the neonatal period. Management is directed towards respiratory support, and surgical repair of the hernia is performed once the lung is stabilized.

## Hirschsprung's disease

Hirschsprung's disease is caused by the absence of ganglion cells in the bowel wall nerve plexus. The

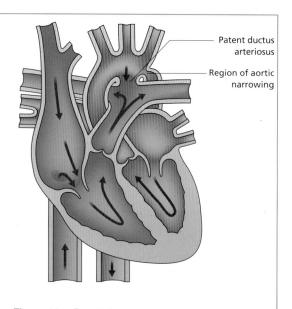

Patent ductus arteriosus

Region of aortic narrowing

**Figure 22.7** Patent ductus arteriosus.

colon is most commonly affected, and although presentation in the neonatal period is most common, mild cases may present later in infancy with severe constipation (p. 171).

The baby presents with delay in passage of meconium and abdominal distension. Rectal examination reveals an empty rectum. The diagnosis is suspected by abdominal X-ray, which shows dilated loops of bowel with an airless rectum, but can only be confirmed at biopsy when the abnormal nerve plexus is identified.

Management is surgical and in two stages. A defunctioning colostomy in a normal section of the bowel is first performed and the abnormal bowel resected later with closure of the colostomy.

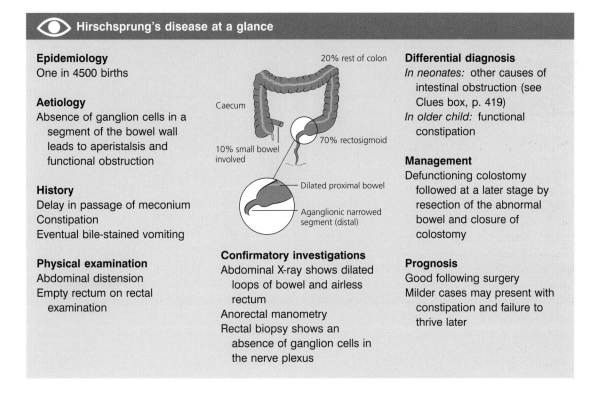

### Hirschsprung's disease at a glance

**Epidemiology**
One in 4500 births

**Aetiology**
Absence of ganglion cells in a segment of the bowel wall leads to aperistalsis and functional obstruction

**History**
Delay in passage of meconium
Constipation
Eventual bile-stained vomiting

**Physical examination**
Abdominal distension
Empty rectum on rectal examination

Caecum
10% small bowel involved
20% rest of colon
70% rectosigmoid
Dilated proximal bowel
Aganglionic narrowed segment (distal)

**Confirmatory investigations**
Abdominal X-ray shows dilated loops of bowel and airless rectum
Anorectal manometry
Rectal biopsy shows an absence of ganglion cells in the nerve plexus

**Differential diagnosis**
*In neonates:* other causes of intestinal obstruction (see Clues box, p. 419)
*In older child:* functional constipation

**Management**
Defunctioning colostomy followed at a later stage by resection of the abnormal bowel and closure of colostomy

**Prognosis**
Good following surgery
Milder cases may present with constipation and failure to thrive later

## Hydronephrosis

'Hydronephrosis' refers to a grossly enlarged kidney caused by urinary tract obstruction. It is the commonest cause of abdominal organomegaly. Commonest sites of obstruction are:

- pelviureteric junction (usually unilateral);
- junction of ureter and bladder (ureterocoele);
- posterior urethra.

Unilateral hydronephrosis is common, as a result of obstruction at the pelviureteric junction (PUJ obstruction). Bilateral hydronephrosis and distended bladder in a boy is caused by bladder neck obstruction that results from obstruction at the posterior urethra (posterior urethral valves). Severe reflux may cause hydronephrosis.

Nephromegaly is usually the only sign of hydronephrosis. If there has been long-standing urinary outflow obstruction, there is usually a history of maternal oligohydramnios and the baby may be born with severe respiratory distress caused by lung hypoplasia (Potter's syndrome). This is usually a fatal condition.

Ultrasound examination is particularly good at defining the diagnosis and site of obstruction. Surgical excision of the obstruction is curative in most cases. Severe renal impairment may occur if the obstruction has been long-standing.

## Cleft palate and lip

Cleft lip (Figure 22.8), a distressing congenital abnormality in view of the cosmetic implications, occurs in one in 1000 children and tends to recur in families, although there is no single gene inheritance. Cleft palate is seen in association with a cleft lip in 70% of cases.

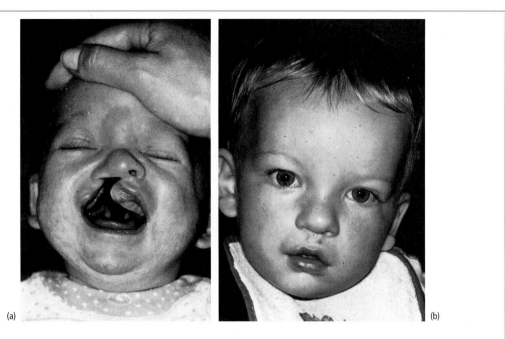

(a)                                                                    (b)

**Figure 22.8** (a) Baby with cleft lip and (b) the same baby after plastic surgical repair.

**Table 22.8** Problems to be anticipated in babies with cleft palate

Difficulties in establishing milk feeding

Milk aspiration

Speech difficulties caused by nasal escape

Conductive hearing loss as a result of eustachian tube dysfunction

Dental problems as a result of gingival margin maldevelopment

The parents of children with cleft palate must be seen as soon after birth as possible and the nature of the condition discussed with them. Cleft palate is associated with the problems listed in Table 22.8.

The cosmetic appearance is excellent following plastic surgery and photographs of treated cases are particularly helpful in allaying parents' anxieties (see Figure 22.8). Surgical correction is usually undertaken at about 9 months of age. The parents may need specialized advice to ensure effective feeding. It is important to involve speech therapists, an orthodontic and plastic surgeon and to arrange regular audiology assessment to prevent sequelae of the disorder.

## Neural tube defects (spina bifida)

Spina bifida is a very important cause of severe disability and is a result of the failure of the neural tube to close normally in early pregnancy. The introduction of periconceptual folic acid supplementation has reduced the incidence of spina bifida lesions by 75%. Routine screening of almost all women in early pregnancy by either ultrasound or alpha-fetoprotein with selective termination of pregnancy has made open spina bifida a rare condition.

Various degrees of severity of neural tube disorder exist and are illustrated in Figure 22.9.

- *Anencephaly.* This is the most severe form of neural tube disorder, where there is complete failure of the development of the cranial part of the neural tube and the brain does not develop.
- *Myelomeningocoele.* This refers to an open lesion with the malformed and exposed spinal cord (myelocoele) being covered by a thin membrane of meninges (meningocoele). This is associated with severe neurological abnormality of the lower limbs, bladder and anal innervation together with hydrocephalus in 90%. Surviving children have major disabilities requiring lifelong supervision.
- *Meningocoele.* In this condition the spinal cord is intact and functions normally, but the defect involves

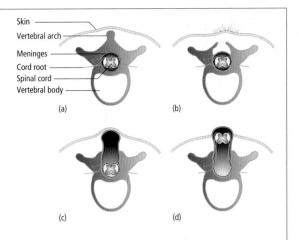

Skin
Vertebral arch
Meninges
Cord root
Spinal cord
Vertebral body

(a)          (b)

(c)          (d)

**Figure 22.9** Varieties of neural tube disorders: (a) normal, (b) spina bifida occulta, (c) meningocoele with intact cord, (d) meningomyelocoele.

an exposed bag of meningeal membranes which ruptures easily. Meningitis and hydrocephalus are a major risk in these cases. Rapid surgical closure is necessary to avoid infection.
• *Spina bifida occulta.* This refers to a 'hidden' abnormality of the developing neural tube which, if unrecognized and untreated, may later cause serious neurological disability.

The first three conditions are very obvious at birth and the mother will draw them immediately to medical attention. Spina bifida occulta may be missed on cursory examination and has very severe implications.

### Spina bifida occulta

Spina bifida occulta (SBO) may be the only visible feature of tethering of the spinal cord within the spinal canal, with eventual stretching of the cord. This is associated with the development of bladder dysfunction and pyramidal tract signs in the lower limbs as the child grows. Spina bifida occulta is suggested by a subtle abnormality of the midline over the spine. In particular these include:

• a deep pit over the lower back;
• a tuft of hair;
• a naevus;
• a fatty tumour (lipoma) at or near the midline.

Ultrasound is the best investigative technique to exclude tethering of the spinal cord, and all babies with the possibility of SBO should be referred for scanning.

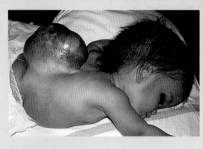

## Neural tube defects (spina bifida) at a glance

### Epidemiology
Now rare as a result of antenatal screening and folic acid supplementation preconceptually

### Aetiology/pathophysiology
Failure of neural tube closure early in pregnancy. The defects range from anencephaly to spina bifida occulta (Figure 22.9), with complications related to the severity of the lesion

### Clinical features
Open midline lesion with malformed and exposed spinal cord and meninges
Variable paralysis and sensory loss of legs
In spina bifida occulta a pit, hair tuft, naevus or lipoma may be found in the midline of the back (a)

### Confirmatory investigations
Ultrasound can detect significant spina bifida occulta

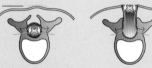

Spina bifida occulta    Spina bifida with meningomyelocele

### Complications
(Vary according to severity of lesion)
Neurogenic bladder
Neurogenic bowel
Hydrocephalus (in 90% with meningomyelocoele)
Scoliosis

### Management
Immediate surgical closure
*Mobility:*
Physiotherapy to prevent joint contractures
Walking aids
*Bladder and bowel:*
Intermittent urinary catheterization to allow regular, complete emptying of the bladder
Prophylactic antibiotics for UTI
Regular toileting, laxatives, suppositories
*Hydrocephalus:*
Ventriculoperitoneal shunt
*Skin care:*
Avoidance of ulceration due to sensory loss

### Prognosis
If the defect is severe there is likely to be significant physical and some intellectual impairment

## Congenital dislocation of the hip

Congenital dislocation of the hip (CDH) is diagnosed at birth and occurs in 0.2% of neonates. Factors associated with increased risk of CDH are shown in Table 22.9. Routine examination of the hips at birth will detect babies in whom the hips are either dislocated or dislocatable, and both these abnormalities require early treatment to prevent permanent maldevelopment of the hip joints with severe impairment in walking. The hips are also routinely checked at 6 weeks and 6–9 months (p. 24). Increasingly, assessment of hip stability is performed by ultrasound screening. If any abnormality is detected on clinical examination, the baby should be referred for ultrasound assessment.

There are three components of the clinical examination:

**1** *Observation.* Is there any asymmetry of gluteal folds around the buttocks? Is there any difference in leg length or posture?

**2** *The Ortolani test* (Figure 22.10). This is a test to see whether the hip is already dislocated. Examine the baby on his or her back with the knees flexed. Grasp the infant's thigh with your middle finger on the greater trochanter and the thumb on the lesser trochanter and gently abduct the hip. If the hip is dislocated, you will be unable to do this. The Ortolani test attempts to relocate the already dislocated hip by lifting the thigh upwards and gently abducting it to bring the hip from its dislocated position back into the acetabulum. This is associated with a 'clunk' as the head of the femur is relocated in the acetabulum.

**3** *The Barlow test* (Figure 22.11). This test detects the hip that is in joint but is dislocatable because of underdevelopment of the acetabulum. Place the baby in the same position as for the Ortolani test and grasp the thigh in the same way. Place the hip an abducted position. The aim of the test is to use downward and lateral force via your thumb to attempt to dislocate the hip posteriorly. You will feel the femoral head slip over the posterior lip of the acetabulum.

**Table 22.9** Factors associated with increased risk of congenital dislocation of the hip

Family history

Breech delivery increases risk 10-fold

Female sex

Neurological defects associated with impaired lower limb movement, e.g. spina bifida

If an abnormality is detected, or if the hip feels stable but there is a ligamentous 'click' on abduction, an ultrasound scan of the hip is performed to look for an abnormally shallow acetabulum. There is no value in X-raying the neonatal hip as the hip joint is not ossified until 3–4 months of age.

Treatment involves immobilizing the hip joint in abduction by a special splint for 3 months, in order to allow normal development of the acetabular rim.

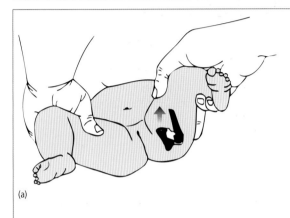
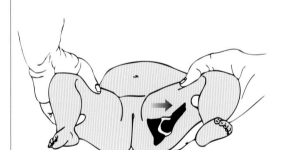

(a)　　　　(b)

**Figure 22.10** The Ortolani test.

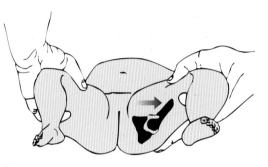
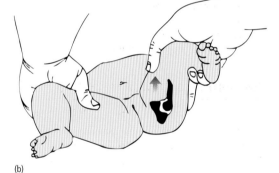
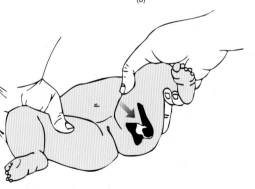

(a)　　　　(b)

(c)

**Figure 22.11** The Barlow test.

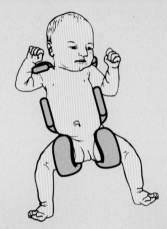

## 👁 Congenital dislocation of the hips at a glance

**Epidemiology**
One and a half per 1000 births
Commoner in girls and breech
    births

**Aetiology/pathophysiology**
Dysplasia of the acetabulum
    leading to laxity, subluxation
    or dislocation

**Clinical features**
Positive Ortolani/Barlow
    screening test
Restricted hip abduction if the
    hip is dislocated
Asymmetric leg skin folds*
Shortening of the affected leg*

**Confirmatory investigations**
Ultrasound of the hip

**Management**
Immobilization of the hip in
    abduction by splinting for
    several months
Monitor progress by ultrasound
    or
X-ray
Surgery if conservative
    measures fail

**Prognosis**
Good with treatment
If undetected, leads to
    permanent limp or waddling
    gait

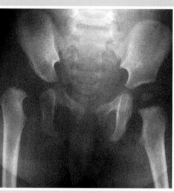

NB *Signs and symptoms are variable.

## Retinopathy of prematurity

Retinopathy of prematurity is a common condition of very premature infants. It occurs in 50% of babies with birthweight <1500 g, but resolves spontaneously in the vast majority of cases. In Britain retinopathy of prematurity (ROP) causes blindness in 1% of severely immature infants.

The cause of ROP is incompletely understood, but iatrogenic oxygen toxicity is a factor, although in premature infants probably not a major factor. The retina becomes ischaemic and, if this is severe, fibrosis and eventually retinal detachment occur with resulting blindness.

The condition can only be recognized by regular ophthalmoscopy. If the condition appears to be rapidly progressive, retinal detachment can be avoided by laser therapy to the back of the eye. However, most babies require no treatment and the prognosis is good.

*To test your knowledge on this part of the book, see Chapter 25.*

# CHAPTER 23
# Adolescence and puberty

*Adolescence is the interruption of peaceful growth.*
*Anna Freud*

## Changes occurring in adolescence

## Conditions

## COMPETENCES

### You must . . .

| Know | Be able to | Appreciate |
|---|---|---|
| • The tasks that characterize adolescence<br>• The physical changes that occur and how they are 'staged'<br>• About the common and important conditions affecting adolescents | • Relate to adolescent patients | • That adolescents can agree to treatment without parental consent if the doctor deems they are mature enough to understand the implications<br>• Adolescence is a time when individuals rarely present to doctors |

*Paediatrics and Child Health*, Third Edition. Mary Rudolf, Tim Lee, Malcolm Levene.
© 2011 Mary Rudolf, Tim Lee and Malcolm Levene. Published 2011 by Blackwell Publishing Ltd.

## Finding your way around . . .

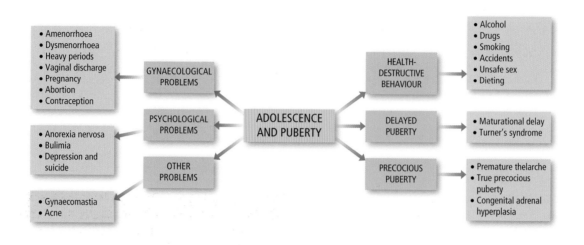

Until recently, the health care of the adolescent has been somewhat neglected in Britain, with the responsibility for this age group falling somewhere between the paediatrician and the physician. Even in general practice, adolescents gain little attention between the needs and demands of young children and the elderly. The problem is compounded by the fact that, as a group, adolescents tend not to seek out health care, although it is well reported that they have considerable needs which are not being met.

In paediatrics, there is increasing awareness that these needs should be met, and it is important that you develop an awareness of the health issues facing adolescents, and acquire the special skills needed in relating to them.

As adolescents infrequently present with a 'problem' which requires a differential diagnostic approach, the issues covered in this chapter for the most part are not problem orientated.

### Changes occurring in adolescence

Adolescence can be defined as the period between childhood and maturity during which the process of growing up occurs. During this period the individual undergoes physical, psychological and social changes.

### Physical changes

The adolescent's body undergoes rapid change, and over the course of a few years secondary sexual characteristics are acquired, fertility is achieved and there is an accompanying growth spurt.

### Psychological changes

Psychological changes occur of both an emotional and intellectual nature. Cognitively, adolescents develop a widening scope of intellectual activity and a capacity for insight. As compared with younger children, they begin to use abstract reasoning and logic, and develop an increased sophistication in moral reasoning. These skills are used in questioning the fundamental values of parents and other adults, and developing a critical awareness of social injustices and the world around.

Emotional changes also occur, often with conflict and turmoil. There is a search for independence, and relationships change with both parents and peers. Experimentation and exploration occur and may result in risk-taking behaviour and a need to test limits.

### Social changes

Significant changes occur for the individual socially, although most adolescents today remain financially and physically dependent on their parents. At school the adolescent is given greater freedom and flexibility, and more emphasis is placed on self-motivation and self-discipline. Peer relationships gain increasing importance, heterosexual interests and activities increase, and the majority of adolescents experience some form of sexual activity. By the end of adolescence, the individual has to face leaving school and moving towards further education, earning and financial independence or unemployment.

### The tasks of adolescence

By the end of adolescence, it is expected that the individual will have succeeded in completing the tasks required to become a competent adult. In order to do so, all of the physical, cognitive, emotional and social

| **Table 23.1** Tasks of adolescence |
| --- |
| Establishing a sense of identity |
| Achieving a degree of independence |
| Achieving sexual maturity |
| Taking on adult responsibility |
| Development of an adult thinking pattern |

| **Table 23.2** Vulnerable adolescents |
| --- |
| Chronic illness |
| Physical and mental handicap |
| Victims of physical, emotional and sexual abuse |
| Homeless and unemployed |
| Pregnant |
| Disrupted homes |
| Minority groups |

changes must have been integrated into some sort of meaningful whole. The individual should have achieved sexual maturity, established a stable sense of identity, achieved a degree of independence, developed an adult pattern of thinking and taken on adult responsibilities (Table 23.1).

## Health care for the adolescent

Adolescence is in general a healthy period of life, and the incidence of illness in this age group is lower than at any other time. As a result, there is a very low rate of contact with doctors.

### Health issues during adolescence

The health issues of this age group can be divided into medical problems, health concerns (which may well not be related to those perceived by health professionals) and health promotion. The medical problems broadly relate to health-destructive behaviour, psychological problems, concerns around pubertal changes and gynaecological issues. The extent of adolescents' worries are often underestimated and seem to focus particularly on weight gain, nutrition, exercise and sexual matters. Health promotion is an important issue, in part because destructive behaviour is particularly prevalent at this age, and also because adolescents are more amenable to changes in lifestyle than they are likely to be later in life.

There are certain adolescents who are especially vulnerable, either for medical or psychosocial reasons (Table 23.2). These are the very individuals who are likely to have difficulty in accessing health care and it is important that efforts are made to reach them.

### Health care facilities

Adolescents' health care may be delivered via their GP's surgery, at school, in hospital outpatients, family planning clinics, or in special adolescent centres. Whatever the facility, the service needs to be

| **Box 23.1 Goals of teenage health clinics** |
| --- |
| • Immediate help and advice on all health issues<br>• Counselling for emotional and personal problems<br>• Advice about sexually transmitted diseases and safer sex<br>• Contraceptive advice and availability<br>• Pregnancy testing and counselling |

relevant and specific to adolescents' particular needs (see Box 23.1).

The ideal service needs to be friendly, discreet, multidisciplinary, attractive and easily accessible. Outpatients clinics in hospital often fail, in that adolescents are faced with toys and toddlers in the waiting room, and inadequate attention is paid to their need for privacy. The GP may also fail in that adolescents may not believe that the doctor they have known since infancy is going to supply them with confidential care. Schools too may fail through lack of facilities and personnel. In recognition of the particular needs for this age group, a new concept of the 'drop-in' clinic is developing, whereby adolescents can attend a conveniently located, easy-to-find centre, at times that fit in with school and where anonymity is more likely to be attained. These centres aim to provide immediate help and advice on all health matters, counselling for emotional and personal problems, and contraceptive advice and supplies.

### Approach to the adolescent

More important than the physical facility is the approach to be taken by health personnel in seeing an adolescent in any health context (see Box 23.2). Principles include a respect for the adolescent's emerging maturity and his or her need for privacy.

**Box 23.2 Guidelines for relating to adolescents**

- Take time to listen
- Show respect for the adolescent's emerging maturity
- Allow the adolescent to express his or her concerns
- Avoid judgemental statements
- Assure confidentiality (provided the well-being of the patient or another is not jeopardized)
- Respect the need for privacy

Time must be allowed for concerns to be expressed and the effort made to listen well. A sympathetic non-judgemental approach is usually appreciated. Confidentiality should be provided and made explicit, although the adolescent should know that this would have to be broken if his or her own well-being or that of another is jeopardized.

Adolescents often do not initially state the problems that are most troubling them, even though they may be very depressed, troubled by delayed puberty or bad acne. They may be grateful if the doctor broadens the context of any visit to address these concerns.

If the adolescent is accompanied by a parent, as commonly occurs in the hospital setting, it is important that the patient is always given the opportunity to see the doctor alone, both to address private concerns and to encourage them to take responsibility for their own health needs. The doctor may need to strike a balance between the adolescent's need for autonomy, privacy and confidentiality and his or her parent's concern and wish to be informed.

### Consent to treatment

In most circumstances consent is not a problematic issue, although the doctor should be aware that legally a young person under the age of 16, in the absence of mental incapacity, or a younger child who in the doctor's view is of sufficient understanding to make an informed decision, is entitled to refuse to submit to any examination, assessment or treatment.

The problem for doctors tends to centre on the prescription of contraceptives, treatment for sexually transmitted diseases and abortion, in cases where the adolescent does not wish the parent to be involved. Although the doctor may be uncomfortable, the law indicates that an individual under the age of 16 years is capable of giving his or her own consent, provided the doctor deems the individual to be mature enough to make an informed decision regarding risks and benefits.

## Physical changes in adolescence

Puberty can be defined as the process of gonadal maturation which results in the acquisition of secondary sexual characteristics, a growth spurt and fertility. These occur under the influence of the sex hormones (Figure 23.1). Gonodotrophin-releasing hormone (GnRH) is released from the hypothalamus and stimulates the synthesis of follicle-stimulating hormone (FSH) and luteinizing hormone (LH), which in turn stimulate the gonads to produce testosterone or oestrogen. These hormones are responsible for development of breasts and the uterus in girls and all the secondary sexual characteristics in boys. Androgens secreted by the adrenal glands are responsible for sexual hair in girls and contribute to sexual hair development in boys. The key ages at which pubertal events are usually seen are shown in Table 23.3.

For the purpose of clinical description, puberty has been divided into five stages, known as Tanner stages. These range from Tanner stage 1 (prepuberty) to Tanner stage 5 (full maturity). They are useful for monitoring the progress of puberty in children where there are concerns about growth or puberty. The five

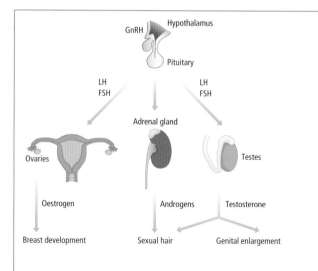

**Figure 23.1** Hormonal events leading to the development of secondary sexual characteristics.

| Table 23.3 Key ages in puberty | Boys | Girls |
| --- | --- | --- |
| Normal pubertal range from start to completion | 11–16 years | 10–14 years |
| First signs of puberty | Testicular enlargement | Breast budding |
| Precocious puberty | Onset <9.5 years* | Onset <8.5 years |
| Delayed puberty | Onset >14 years | Onset >13 years |
| Delayed menarche | – | Onset >16 years |

* High likelihood of pathological rather than physiological cause for precocious puberty in boys.

stages for breast, gonadal and pubic hair development are illustrated in Figure 23.2.

## Pubertal development in boys

Puberty in boys usually starts between the ages of 11 and 14 years. The first sign is testicular enlargement, which is followed by pigmentation and thinning of the scrotum and growth of the penis. As puberty progresses, pubic, axillary and facial hair develop, the voice deepens and the ability to ejaculate develops. The growth spurt, which is accompanied by an increase in body size and muscle bulk, occurs when puberty is well under way and is maximal from 14 to 16 years, reaching its peak 2 years after that of girls.

## Pubertal development in girls

Puberty tends to start earlier in girls than boys. The first sign is usually breast budding, which develops at around 10–11 years, and is followed by pubic and axillary hair development. The growth spurt occurs early, and is virtually completed by menarche (the onset of periods) which usually occurs at 11–13 years. The interval between onset of puberty and menarche is on average 2.0–2.5 years.

# Health-destructive behaviour

Many of the medical problems incurred by this age group relate to health-destructive behaviour, which includes alcohol, smoking, substance abuse, injuries and unsafe sex. This behaviour results from the desire to explore and experiment, which is characteristic of adolescents in their challenge to achieve independence and assert their individuality.

## Alcohol

Surveys show that children become familiar with alcohol at an early age, and by their teens drinking is

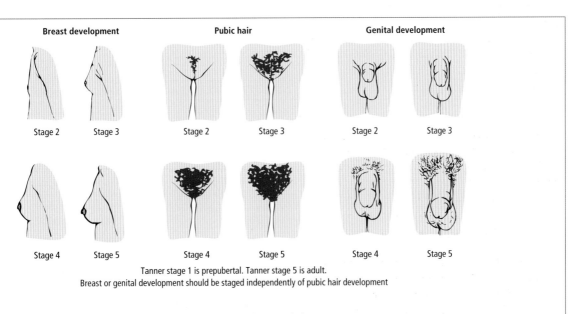

Tanner stage 1 is prepubertal. Tanner stage 5 is adult.
Breast or genital development should be staged independently of pubic hair development

**Figure 23.2** Tanner staging of secondary sexual characteristics.

a regular part of their lives. By the age of 15, 77% boys and 66% girls are drinking up to 10 and 6 units per week, respectively. Alcohol has a greater effect on judgement and control in young, inexperienced drinkers. Interestingly, the principal place where alcohol is obtained is the home.

## Drugs

Studies of drug and solvent misuse among secondary school children suggest misuse levels of about 16% of which 5% represent hard drugs. Peer group influence is important in terms of experimentation. Misusers are more likely to come from single-parent families and be involved in truancy, vandalism, smoking and drinking. Most involvement is temporary, but a minority progress to multiple drug use, chronic use and addiction. Table 23.4 summarizes the signs of drug taking, and Table 23.5 describes the commoner drugs of abuse, their effects and clinical features.

Educational initiatives are provided in schools and focus on providing information on the abuse and misuse of drugs, promoting self-esteem, decision-making skills and coping with adverse situations.

## Smoking

The earlier a person begins to smoke, the greater the risk of chronic bronchitis, emphysema, cardiovascular

disease and lung cancer. As compared with adults, where the prevalence of smoking is decreasing, it is increasing in this age group, and 10% of 11- to 15-year-olds smoke regularly. Girls are more likely to be smokers than boys, and those who smoke are more likely to try other drugs, sniff solvents, drink alcohol and go out partying. Smokers are often underachievers and truants.

## Accidents

Car and motorcycle accidents are the leading causes of adolescent morbidity and mortality. The majority of these incidents involve vehicles driven by adolescents. Alcohol and failure to wear seat belts and motor

**Table 23.4** Signs of drug taking

| |
|---|
| Sudden changes of mood |
| Loss of appetite |
| Loss of interest in appearance, school work, leisure interests |
| Drowsiness or sleeplessness |
| Furtive behaviour |
| Unusual stains/smells on clothing |

**Table 23.5** Common forms of substance abuse

| Substance | Epidemiology | Effects | Physical signs |
|---|---|---|---|
| *Solvent* (sniffing) – toluene based glues, aerosols, fuel gases and solvents | Mainly boys 100 deaths per year from heart failure, suffocation and injuries | Intoxication, excitement, hallucination | Disorientation, slurred speech, blurred vision Skin irritation around the nose and mouth Solvent smells on breath or clothing |
| *Cannabis* (generally smoked as a hand-rolled cigarette) | Most widely used illicit drug | Pleasurable feelings of relaxation, altered sensory perception | Red eyes and tachycardia |
| *Cocaine* (sniffed through a tube or injected). 'Crack' refers to a less refined form of cocaine | | Exhilaration, indifference to pain and hunger, residual depression and fatigue | Tachycardia, hypertension, hyperthermia Teratogenic effect on the fetus |
| *Opiates* (swallowing, injecting, sniffing and smoking) | Leading cause of drug-related death Consequences of injecting include thrombophlebitis, AIDS and hepatitis B | Euphoria and contentment | Sedation, depression of respiration, heart rate and bowel activity Skin scars |

cycle helmets are factors underlying most fatalities. Sports injuries and drowning are additional prominent causes of serious injury.

## Unsafe sex

Sexual activity is occurring at younger ages. Thirty-five per cent of girls and 46% of boys have experienced sexual intercourse before the age of 16. The majority do not seek contraceptive advice for some time, and casual sexual relationships are particularly likely to be unprotected. Unsafe sex can lead to pregnancy and sexually transmitted diseases including AIDS, and have a deleterious effect on future fertility.

The highest rate of sexually transmitted disease is found amongst adolescents. This is in part a result of the sexual behaviour characteristic of this age group, which includes multiple partners, failure to use barrier contraception, reluctance to consider that a partner may have venereal disease, and lack of communication skills to discuss the issue. There are also physiological differences that render the adolescent vaginal epithelium more susceptible to infection.

Gonorrhoea, chlamydia and human papilloma virus are the commonest sexually transmitted diseases in adolescence. HIV infection is on the increase, although because of the long latency period it may not manifest itself in the teenage years. Risk factors for contraction of HIV include unprotected intercourse and intravenous drug use.

## Dieting

A preoccupation with appearance and body shape is characteristic of adolescence. Dieting is an almost universal activity among teenage girls, and often takes the form of extreme starvation diets. Eating disorders are an increasing problem. A further concern is that girls as young as 8 or 9 years commonly have a distorted sense of body image, and are increasingly involved in dieting behaviour.

## Problems of puberty

### Delayed puberty

Puberty is defined as being delayed if there are no signs of puberty by the age of 14 in a boy, 13 in a girl or if menarche has not occurred by the age of 16 (Table 23.3). Adolescents may present either because of concerns about the absence of sexual development or because of short stature (see p. 253). The causes of delayed puberty are shown in Table 23.6. The com-

**Table 23.6** Causes of delayed puberty

| |
|---|
| *Boys and girls* |
| Maturational delay (commonly familial) |
| Pituitary lesions |
| Gonadal failure |
| Chronic and severe disease |
| *Girls* |
| Turner's syndrome |
| Intense athletic training |
| Anorexia nervosa |

monest cause of pubertal delay is maturational delay, which is commonly familial. Other causes to be considered are Turner's syndrome in girls, and anorexia nervosa or intense athletic training, both of which can suppress the hypothalamus. Any chronic and severe disease can delay puberty, and rare causes include pituitary or gonadal failure.

### Maturational delay (constitutional delay)

Maturational delay of puberty (see p. 266) is commonly familial. Although a normal variant, it can cause considerable distress, particularly in boys. The diagnosis is based on the pattern of growth (short but steady, see p. 256), a family history of delayed menarche in the women or delayed growth in the men of the family, a delayed bone age and the absence of any evidence of central nervous system pathology. Reassurance is usually all that is required, but if the adolescent (nearly always a boy) is suffering socially, puberty can be triggered by a low dose of testosterone given for a few months.

### Turner's syndrome (see p. 272)

In Turner's syndrome, which is caused by an abnormality or absence of one of the X-chromosomes, puberty does not occur, as the gonads, which are just streaks of fibrous tissue, fail to secrete oestrogen. Girls with Turner's syndrome should have been identified earlier in childhood because of short stature, but still occasionally present with delayed puberty. It is important to remember that many girls with Turner's syndrome are normal phenotypically and do not have the classic features of the syndrome, so a karyotype is indicated in any girl with either delayed puberty or short stature.

**Table 23.7** Causes of precocious puberty

*Hypothalamic–pituitary*

Maturational advance (true precocious puberty)

Central nervous system lesions

*Ovarian*

Premature thelarche

*Adrenal*

Congenital adrenal hyperplasia

Adrenal tumours

## Precocious puberty

Puberty is defined as being precocious if secondary sexual characteristics occur before the age of 8.5 years in a girl or 9.5 years in a boy (Table 23.3). The causes of precocious puberty are shown in Table 23.7. Precocious puberty in girls is usually idiopathic; boys are far more likely to have an underlying pathological lesion, and so require especially thorough evaluation.

The child with precocious puberty suffers on two accounts. First, he or she has to contend with physical, emotional and social changes at an inappropriately young age and, secondly, adult height is jeopardized as a result of premature fusion of the bones.

Pubertal signs may occur precociously as a result of premature activation of the hypothalamic–pituitary axis ('true' precocious puberty) or inappropriate secretion of oestrogen or androgens. These can be distinguished clinically. In the former, the full picture of puberty occurs. In the latter, oestrogen secretion causes breast development (thelarche) but no pubic hair; androgen secretion causes pubic hair but no testicular or breast enlargement.

Accompanying features of precocious puberty (with the exception of premature thelarche) include acceleration of growth, advance of skeletal maturation and emotional changes.

Investigations should be directed by the findings on physical examination and should include hormone levels, a karyotype in girls, X-ray for bone age, pelvic ultrasound, and computed tomography (CT) or magnetic resonance imaging (MRI) of the head.

### Premature thelarche

Premature thelarche (isolated premature breast development) is not uncommon and occurs in the first 2 years of life. It is a benign condition thought to be caused by a maturational aberration of the hypothalamic–pituitary axis. It does not cause acceleration of growth, and investigations are normal, although ovarian ultrasound may show a few small cysts. The breasts regress spontaneously over some months. Accidental ingestion of maternal contraceptive pills can also cause thelarche.

### True precocious puberty

True precocious puberty refers to puberty that is triggered early by premature activation of the hypothalamic–pituitary axis. In girls, the underlying cause is usually idiopathic, but in boys there is commonly an underlying central nervous system lesion such as a tumour or trauma. Treatment includes therapy for the underlying lesion if there is one, and administration of a hormonal analogue which suppresses the secretion of the gonadotrophins.

### Congenital adrenal hyperplasia

Congenital adrenal hyperplasia is an autosomal recessive disorder which results in a block in the adrenal production of corticosteroids. As a consequence, a build-up of androgenic precursors occurs, which can result in either ambiguous genitalia (detected at birth, see p. 316) or precocious development of pubic hair. Diagnosis is confirmed by the finding of elevated corticosteroid precursors, and treatment consists of life-long steroid replacement therapy.

### Gynaecomastia

Gynaecomastia (breast development in boys) is very common, occurring in 65% of adolescent boys, and is thought to be caused by an oestrogen–androgen imbalance which occurs at puberty. It may be unilateral or bilateral, and spontaneous regression occurs over time. Reassurance is usually all that is required, but if there is significant social embarrassment, hormonal or surgical treatment can be given.

### Acne

Acne is virtually universal in adolescence. Its development is linked to the onset of sebaceous gland activity and the production of free fatty acids. Inflammation occurs as a result of colonization by micro-organisms.

**Clinical features.** The skin lesions consist of a mixture of comedones (white heads and black heads), pustules and nodulocystic lesions, which may be interspersed with scarring. Lesions may be confined to the face or involve the chest and upper back. As adolescents become preoccupied with their appearance, acne assumes great importance. It can cause much distress, may dominate life and may even give rise to self-imposed isolation.

**Management.** Offering treatment for even mild acne can enhance self-image and is therefore important. Diet plays no significant part in the development of acne, although a healthy diet should be encouraged for reasons of general health. Greasy cosmetic and hair preparations should be discontinued. Mild cleansing agents can help by drying the skin and suppressing skin flora. In more severe cases topical antibiotics and retinoic acid, which acts by eliminating the keratinous

plug, may be required. The adolescent should be warned that all topical treatment requires several weeks to have an effect. In severe pustular or nodulo-cystic acne, oral antibiotics (usually tetracycline) are indicated.

# Psychological problems of adolescence

## Eating disorders

Eating disorders commonly begin as innocent dieting behaviour, which progresses to become a serious condition which may be life-threatening. Girls are far more commonly affected than boys, and the age of onset is decreasing so that as many as one fifth are

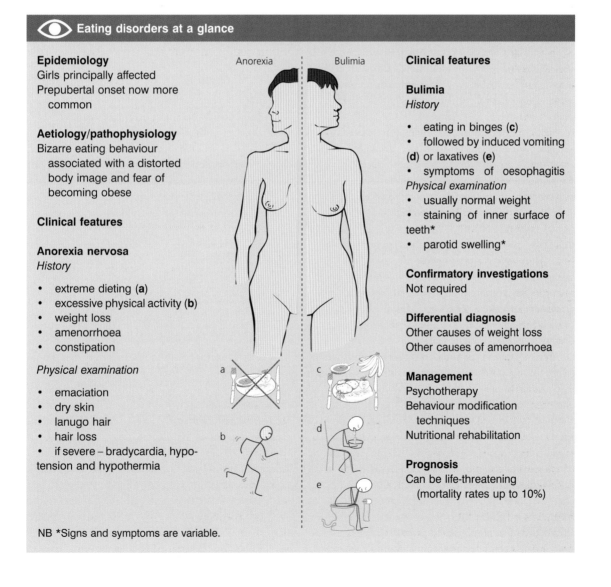

**Eating disorders at a glance**

**Epidemiology**
Girls principally affected
Prepubertal onset now more
  common

**Aetiology/pathophysiology**
Bizarre eating behaviour
  associated with a distorted
  body image and fear of
  becoming obese

**Clinical features**

**Anorexia nervosa**
*History*

- extreme dieting (**a**)
- excessive physical activity (**b**)
- weight loss
- amenorrhoea
- constipation

*Physical examination*

- emaciation
- dry skin
- lanugo hair
- hair loss
- if severe – bradycardia, hypotension and hypothermia

Anorexia          Bulimia

**Clinical features**

**Bulimia**
*History*

- eating in binges (**c**)
- followed by induced vomiting
(**d**) or laxatives (**e**)
- symptoms of oesophagitis
*Physical examination*
- usually normal weight
- staining of inner surface of
teeth*
- parotid swelling*

**Confirmatory investigations**
Not required

**Differential diagnosis**
Other causes of weight loss
Other causes of amenorrhoea

**Management**
Psychotherapy
Behaviour modification
  techniques
Nutritional rehabilitation

**Prognosis**
Can be life-threatening
  (mortality rates up to 10%)

NB *Signs and symptoms are variable.

under the age of 13 years. The eating disorders are characterized by an intense fear of becoming obese, and a distorted body image, so that even emaciated affected individuals perceive themselves as being fat. In an attempt to achieve the desired weight there is a denial of hunger, preoccupation with food and bizarre eating behaviours.

## Anorexia nervosa

Girls with anorexia nervosa restrict their intake of carbohydrate- and fat-containing foods by extreme dieting in order to control their weight. This is usually accompanied by excessive physical activity.

An arbitrary definition of anorexia nervosa has been taken to be a loss of more than 20% body weight in relation to height. The clinical features found are those of malnutrition, with emaciation, amenorrhoea, constipation, dry skin, lanugo hair and hair loss. As body weight decreases, bradycardia, hypotension and hypothermia are found.

## Bulimia

The girl with bulimia has bouts of eating in binges and then purges herself by inducing vomiting or using laxatives.

These girls, in contrast to anorexics, often are of normal weight or slightly obese. Oesophagitis, parotid swelling and staining of the internal surface of the teeth can occur as a result of frequent vomiting.

Eating disorders, particularly anorexia, can be life-threatening and mortality rates are as high as 10%, so the condition must be taken seriously. The approach involves a combination of psychotherapy, behaviour modification techniques and nutritional rehabilitation. Antidepressants are sometimes prescribed.

## Depression and suicide

Adolescence is naturally a time of moods which swing from the depths of depression to the heights of elation. It is often difficult therefore to decide which adolescent is at risk for true depression. Factors associated with an increased risk include a disturbed or disrupted home life, poor functioning at school, low self-esteem, antisocial and aggressive behaviour, substance misuse, stressful life events and a family history of affective disorder.

Suicide is increasing in incidence and is a leading cause of death in this age group. The method most

---

### 👁 Depression and suicide at a glance

**Epidemiology**
Suicide: a leading cause of death in teenagers
Commonest method is drug ingestion
Risk factors
• disturbed home life
• poor functioning at school
• low self-esteem
• antisocial behaviour
• substance misuse
• family history of affective disorder

**Clinical features**
Insomnia and difficulty falling asleep*
Altered appetite*
School failure and absenteeism*
Alcohol and drug use*

**Management**
Identify sources of stress
Counselling/psychotherapy for adolescent and family
Antidepressants with caution
Attempted suicide: hospitalize for medical treatment and psychosocial assessment

**Prognosis**
Seriousness of attempted suicide is related to the degree of premeditation and likelihood of rescue, rather than drug dose
Most successful suicides follow an earlier attempt

NB *Signs and symptoms are variable.

commonly used in adolescence is ingestion of medication, either their own or a parent's. The seriousness of an attempt cannot be related to the lethality of the dose, but is related to the degree of premeditation and the likelihood of rescue.

**Clinical features.** Depression has been defined as a persistently lowered mood and misery that is severe enough to interfere with everyday life. It is accompanied by feelings of worthlessness, a sense of hopelessness, anxiety, pessimistic thoughts and often suicidal ideas or acts. The depressed adolescent may experience insomnia and difficulty falling asleep, sometimes to the extent of being awake all night and sleeping through the day, and appetite may be altered. Falling school grades, increase in school absenteeism, and the use of alcohol and drugs are common.

**Management.** Sources of stress should be identified and dealt with as far as possible. Counselling, psychotherapy and, where appropriate, family therapy may be helpful. The parents, too, need help, especially in dealing with uncooperative behaviour, and providing additional care and affection. At this age, treatment with antidepressants should only be prescribed by specialists.

Any attempt at suicide must be taken seriously, as most successful suicides occur among those who have made earlier attempts. Short-term hospitalization is usually indicated to attend to pharmacological sequelae, to assess the psychosocial situation and to impress on the family the need to attend to underlying problems.

# Gynaecological problems

## Menstrual complaints

### Amenorrhoea

Amenorrhoea, or the absence of periods, may be primary or secondary. The term 'primary amenorrhoea' indicates that menarche has never occurred, and is discussed on p. 439 ('Delayed puberty'). Secondary amenorrhoea refers to the cessation of periods for more than 3 months after regular cycles have been established. Its causes are listed in Table 23.8.

Most amenorrhoea in adolescence is physiological. After menarche it is usual for periods to be scanty or irregular for several months, and several months may elapse between periods. Stress, such as starting a new school, can disrupt periods, and girls undergoing intense athletic training can experience amenorrhoea as a result of hypothalamic–pituitary axis suppression.

| Table 23.8 Causes of secondary amenorrhoea |
| --- |
| *Physiological* |
| Hormonal cycle immaturity |
| Stress |
| Intense athletic training |
| Pregnancy |
| *Pathological* |
| Anorexia nervosa |
| Chronic illness |
| Brain tumour |
| Hyperthyroidism |

Pregnancy should always be considered as a cause of amenorrhoea in the teenage girl.

The commonest pathological cause of amenorrhoea is anorexia nervosa or dieting. Interestingly, amenorrhoea can precede the weight loss. Any chronic illness can cause amenorrhoea, but particularly those associated with malnutrition or tissue hypoxia, such as diabetes mellitus, inflammatory bowel disease, cystic fibrosis or cyanotic congenital heart disease.

When you evaluate a girl with amenorrhoea, you should take a complete history, focusing on diet, potentially stressful events, exercise, sexual activity, medical history and neurological symptoms. You need to look for signs of anorexia nervosa, pregnancy and neurological abnormality on physical examination. Baseline investigations include a full blood count, plasma viscosity and pregnancy test, and if these are negative, consider gonadotrophin levels, thyroid function tests, pelvic ultrasound and imaging of the head.

### Dysmenorrhoea

Adolescent girls commonly experience painful menstrual cramps, and dysmenorrhoea is the commonest cause of short-term school absenteeism. The mechanism is thought to be caused by high levels of endometrial prostaglandins. Effective treatment can be given prophylactically using prostaglandin synthetase inhibitors. An alternative is the oral contraceptive pill, if contraception is desired.

### Heavy periods

Excessive menstrual bleeding is most often secondary to the anovulatory cycles that normally occur in the first year postmenarche. Without ovulation, oestrogen

**Table 23.9** Causes of vaginal discharge

Physiological

Poor perineal hygiene

Foreign body

Candida

Sexually transmitted diseases*

* Indicative of sexual abuse if found in a prepubertal child.

unopposed by progesterone causes endometrial pro-liferation with eventual massive shedding. Hormonal treatment is required if there is anaemia or hypovol-aemia. Other causes of heavy periods include bleeding disorders and aspirin ingestion.

### Vaginal discharge

A normal physiological increase in vaginal discharge (Table 23.9) occurs in the year prior to menarche. In childhood, discharge secondary to poor perineal hygiene is common and may be accompanied by dysuria, frequency and pruritus. The treatment is as described for dysuria (p. 296). If the discharge is persistent and foul smelling, a foreign body (usually toilet paper) should be suspected. In the prepubertal girl candida is not common, although it may follow antibiotic therapy. Sexually transmitted diseases must be suspected in the sexually active girl, and a high index of suspicion maintained even in the prepubertal child as, if found, it is indicative of sexual abuse.

### Sexually transmitted diseases

Coverage of sexually transmitted diseases is beyond the scope of this book. However, they are a significant and prevalent cause of morbidity in the adolescent years, and should not be overlooked when working with teenagers.

### Pregnancy

It has been reported that almost 15% of sexually active teenagers become pregnant within 2 years of initiating intercourse, and over half the pregnancies result in live births. The rise in live births is particularly increasing among younger adolescents, many of whom become pregnant deliberately. Girls most at risk are those who lack self-esteem, become sexually active early, come from unhappy or unstable backgrounds, and those in care.

Adolescent pregnancy carries increased risks for both the mother and the baby. Contributing factors obstetrically include late booking for antenatal care, poor attendance at clinic and antenatal classes, and poor nutrition. The babies tend to suffer from higher infant and perinatal mortality rates, an increased incidence of sudden infant death syndrome (SIDS), low birthweight (both pre- and post-term), gastrointestinal problems, accidental and non-accidental injury, behaviour problems and delayed psychomotor development.

An adolescent mother is more likely to suffer from postnatal depression, and is less likely to marry ultimately, finish her secondary school education or gain employment.

Reducing the teenage pregnancy rate is a key aim of the UK government, who have published a Teenage Pregnancy Strategy.

### Abortion

Abortion remains a major form of contraception in this age group, and one third of teenage pregnancies end in legal abortion. Apart from the medical risks of abortion, there are considerable emotional effects for the teenage girl. Follow-up, careful counselling and support are particularly important as many become pregnant again within a year.

### Contraception

More adolescents are engaging in sexual intercourse at younger ages, often without any form of contraception. Studies show that fewer than 50% of teenagers use any form of contraception at the time of first intercourse, and the lag between becoming sexually active and seeking effective contraception usually exceeds 1 year. Unfortunately, the first visit to a family planning clinic is frequently because of a pregnancy scare.

Reasons why adolescents commonly fail to seek contraceptive advice include their conviction that sexual intercourse is an unpremeditated and infrequent act, fear that their parents will find out and doubt that any advice they seek will be confidential.

Information, access to contraception and motivation are all necessary for successful pregnancy prevention. Interestingly, in contrast to common expectations, sex education, far from increasing sexual activity, has been shown to delay the onset of first intercourse, increase contraceptive use and reduce numbers of pregnancies. Advice to the teenager should be based on frequency and circumstances of sexual activity, past experience and compliance with both contraceptive and non-contraceptive chronic medications. Emphasis needs to be placed on the need for protection against sexually transmitted disease as well as pregnancy. The risk of any contraceptive method should be weighed against the risk of pregnancy, which for young adolescents is a significant one. If contraception is to be successful, every effort must be made to individualize the method to the needs of the patient. The advantages and disadvantages of the various types of contraception for adolescents are shown in Table 23.10.

Parental consent is not required for the prescription of contraception, provided the doctor has grounds to believe that the adolescent is mature enough to appreciate the risks (and benefits) of contraception.

**Table 23.10** The advantages and disadvantages of various contraceptive methods during adolescence

| Contraceptive method | Advantages | Disadvantages |
|---|---|---|
| Condom | Effective in preventing transmission of STD including HIV Low price Available without prescription Little need for advanced planning No side effects | Inadequate protection in preventing pregnancy if used alone Acceptance low in younger adolescents |
| Oral contraceptive pill | Reliable method if taken effectively Method unrelated to episode of intercourse Relief of dysmenorrhoea Decreased risks of benign breast disease, anaemia and ovarian cysts | Not good for chaotic adolescents Less suitable if intercourse is infrequent Post-pill amenorrhoea more common in adolescence Raises levels of high-density lipoproteins (major side effects are exceedingly rare in adolescents) |
| Depot (parenteral) contraceptive | Reliable with the advantage that compliance is not an issue. Some preparations give protection for as much as 3 years | Maybe unsuitable if intercourse is infrequent Some concern regarding osteoporosis in the long term |
| Intrauterine contraceptive systems (IUS) | Effective in preventing pregnancy Requires no motivation | Increased menstrual bleeding and dysmenorrhoea Increased risk of pelvic infection and future infertility |
| Postcoital contraception | Taken after unprotected sex has taken place | Adolescent needs to know how to access |

STD, sexually transmitted disease.

*To test your knowledge on this part of the book, see Chapter 25.*

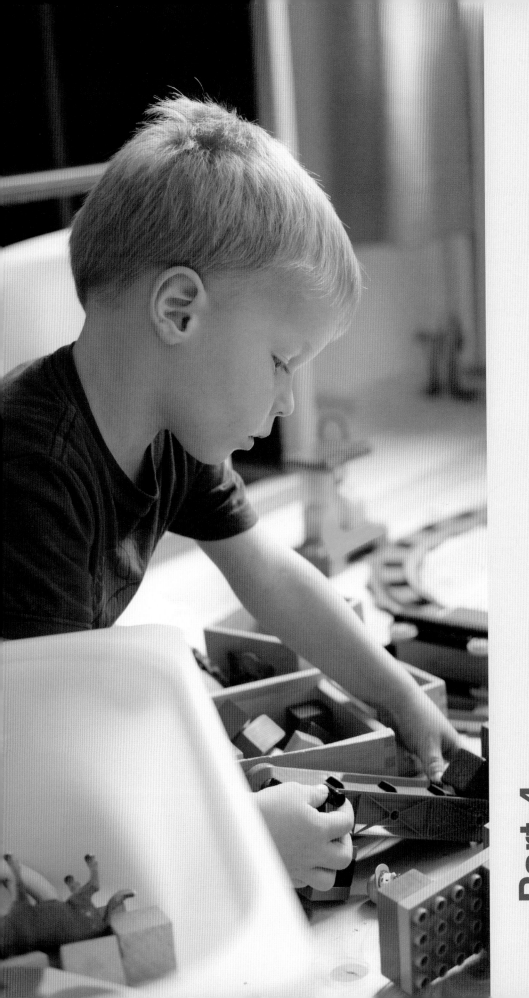

Part 4
Your paediatric rotation and exams

# CHAPTER 24

# Getting the most out of your paediatric rotation and achieving good marks

*Paediatrics and Child Health*, Third Edition. Mary Rudolf, Tim Lee, Malcolm Levene.
© 2011 Mary Rudolf, Tim Lee and Malcolm Levene. Published 2011 by Blackwell Publishing Ltd.

# How to get the most out of your paediatric rotation

The aim of undergraduate medical training in paediatrics is to give students a broad understanding of the common and important illnesses and disorders of childhood. The purpose is to make sure that medical graduates, whatever speciality they choose to work in, are able to identify when children need investigation or intervention and to manage them appropriately. Your paediatric course is likely to focus on how children present with disorders and illnesses, and the initial management, rather than covering specialist management in great detail. The ability to take a good paediatric history and conduct an effective examination of infants and children is absolutely fundamental to making an accurate diagnosis, and so undergraduate courses examine these skills in detail.

In order to make the most of your paediatric attachment, you should study the course material carefully at the start of the placement. This usually lists the core curriculum and key skills that you need to acquire during the attachment. The types of assessment used to judge progress should also be provided. They vary from course to course, but may include the following:

• *Student logbooks.* Logbooks encourage you to record your various educational experiences; for example, conditions or investigations that you have witnessed and clinics you have attended. They may need to be countersigned by supervising clinicians and submitted at the end of the course to demonstrate that you have achieved appropriate clinical experience.

• *Workplace-based assessments (WPBA).* Students are often required to conduct a number of clinical examinations – for example, a respiratory examination, developmental examination, etc. – under direct observation of a supervising clinician, who then fills out a formal WPBA feedback form. You will be required to submit these forms at the end of the course to demonstrate that you have acquired good clinical examination skills.

• *Multi-source feedback (MSF).* Occasionally you will be asked to arrange a multi-source feedback, where members of a multi-disciplinary team provide feedback which focuses on your clinical skills, communication skills and professional attitude.

• *Written case reports.* Case reports require a detailed history and examination, followed by the differential diagnosis and initial management plan. They are generally written in a similar way to entries made in a child's medical record. Case reports allow for assessment of many of the key skills that you are expected to acquire during the attachment.

• *Written feedback from supervising clinicians/course teachers.* These reports are often helpful in identifying if you have excellent skills and attitude, as well as if you may be struggling with the course.

• *Written examination.* Most courses have some form of written examination, usually extended matching questions (EMQ), or multiple choice questions (MCQ). Some of the questions may be based on slide images, or on written stems. Stem questions usually focus on testing diagnostic reasoning, and you are required to choose the most likely diagnosis or next intervention, based on a short clinical description or 'stem'.

• *Objective Structured Clinical Examination (OSCE).* OSCEs consist of a circuit of short 5- to 10-minute stations, mostly with an examiner at the station and a real or simulated parent and/or child. They focus on key clinical skills such as history taking, counselling or clinical examination. Some may include video clips, photographs or investigations that you need to interpret. Students rotate through all of the stations in turn.

# Preparing for examinations

In order to make sure that you perform well in written examinations, you need to work at acquiring a broad knowledge of the whole syllabus (Box 24.1). The best way to prepare is to attend the whole course and its seminars and workshops. It is especially worthwhile to spend a good amount of time seeing children in any setting – community and hospital, acutely via the accident and emergency department, and in outpatient clinics.

Many multiple choice questions (MCQs) and extended matching questions (EMQs) test your ability to link symptoms and signs to particular diagnoses. Reading through the chapters in this book will be good preparation. Each chapter starts with a 'symptoms and signs' section, guiding you systematically to link particular presentations to relevant diagnoses. A box lists the most significant symptoms and signs providing you with clues as to how to come to a differential diagnosis.

An important aspect of preparation is to practise some exam questions, such as those provided in this book. Many courses provide mock questions or past papers. This enables you to familiarize yourself with the question structure and technique, as well as check-

## Box 24.1 Tips to performing well in paediatric assessments and examinations

- Read the course material carefully at the start of the attachment
- Check through all the ways you will be assessed and how these assessments contribute to your final mark
- Take every opportunity to meet children and parents, and take a history and perform an examination as often as you can
- Attend all of the available course seminars and workshops, as these will often cover much of the course syllabus
- When you have seen a child with a particular condition, read the appropriate section of this textbook and consider the differential diagnoses
- Watch the video on the companion website showing how to examine children section by section and practise the technique on children on the ward
- Try and complete your in-course assessments as soon as you can, rather than doing them all in a rush at the end of the attachment
- Practise written exam questions (MCQ, EMQ) and read through the topics for questions you get wrong
- Practise OSCE scenarios with colleagues and give feedback to each other

ing your knowledge. In order to learn from questions that you get wrong, you should try to understand why you chose the wrong answer. Reading through the section of this book appropriate to the question stem will help. Chapter 25 provides you with sample questions to try. If you get any wrong, you are guided to the section of the book that will provide you with the correct answer.

## Preparing for Objective Structured Clinical Examinations

OSCEs assess basic clinical skills. At each of the stations you are asked to interact with a patient or a simulated patient. Your performance is scored by an examiner with a check list or rating scale. Sometimes the patients themselves score you too.

Most students get exceptionally nervous prior to OSCEs. The rigid time limits for each station, and the

need to move on rapidly to a completely new station tend to fill students with apprehension, especially if there has been a mishap on a previous station.

The key to OSCEs is to ensure that during the paediatric course you practise all the skills you may have to perform in the OSCE in real life, with real children and parents. It helps if you aim to perform at least one detailed history and examination every day during your paediatric attachment, so that the skill becomes second nature by the time of the examination. The website associated with this book provides videos to demonstrate the correct technique for examining children, and you will find it most helpful if you watch it section by section rather than in one go. In addition, the specific aspects of the history and physical examination relevant to each presenting symptom and sign are provided for you at each chapter's opening. Remember, too, it is always helpful to spend time observing how experienced clinicians counsel parents and children.

Try to practise the scenarios with student colleagues prior to the exam. Common counselling scenarios should be listed in your course documentation; they often include immunization, enuresis, soiling, febrile convulsion, asthma and constipation. Remember that marks are given not only for appropriate content, but also for good counselling skills such as active listening, eye contact and emotional empathy. Practise by counselling a student colleague and then asking them to give you feedback.

On the day of the OSCE, try to channel your nerves into performing well. Often there is a 'change-over' minute between each station, so make the most of this by trying to forget your performance on the previous station, and focusing on the next station. There may be some written information outside the station for you to read. If so, use this to plan how you will approach the next station. For example, if the written information suggests the station concerns the examination of the lower limbs in a child with an abnormal gait, then think what the differential diagnosis might be. Plan to ask if the child is able to walk for you to demonstrate the gait, as well as planning to observe the child's legs and assess tone, power and reflexes. Remember, as you enter the station, to take time to introduce yourself well to both parents and children, as a good friendly start really helps the rest of the station go well and will help you make the most of the time available.

# CHAPTER 25

# Testing your knowledge

This chapter provides you with the opportunity to test your knowledge by working through multiple choice questions. The aim is to help you identify what you have yet to learn as well as serving as an aid to help you pass examinations. The first set of questions covers each section of the book. Two practice papers follow, covering the full range of topics that you are likely to receive in a paediatric examination.

## Multiple choice questions

*Please note that there may be more than one correct answer for each statement. Give yourself one mark for each correct answer, and do not subtract marks for incorrect answers. Answers are provided at the end of the end of the chapter, along with a reference that will lead you back to the topic for more information.*

### Part 1: About children

Answers begin on p. 470.

1 The following is helpful advice for a mother who wants to breast-feed:
   a) Place the baby on the breast immediately after delivery
   b) Allow demand feeding
   c) Have an undisturbed night's rest the first night
   d) If mastitis seems to be developing, give that breast a rest from sucking
   e) Drink plenty of fluids

2 Which of the following statements are true?
   a) Children should be encouraged to eat a low-fat, high-fibre diet
   b) Iron deficiency is a problem, as young children often fail to eat iron-rich foods
   c) Children should have at least 30 oz (900 mL) milk per day
   d) Pregnancy during the teenage years has nutritional consequences for both mother and baby
   e) Drinks machines are no longer permitted on school premises

3 The following statements concerning weaning are correct:
   a) Weaning should be delayed until the infant is 12 months old
   b) Breast milk is the only food a baby requires for the first 6 months
   c) Avoid introducing new tastes to the baby in its first year

d) Multivitamins should be started at birth
e) The baby should not eat with the family until he or she can feed him- or herself with a spoon

4 The following statements about a child's development are true:
   a) Bonding is more difficult if the baby is separated from the mother at birth
   b) A baby begins to sustain eye contact by 6 months
   c) It usually takes several months before sleep–wake cycles emerge
   d) Babies begin to smile by 6 weeks
   e) Children only begin to learn rules of games once they are school age

5 The following practices are against the law:
   a) Giving morphine with the intention of the baby dying
   b) Not treating a life-threatening condition
   c) Prescribing contraception to a 12-year-old
   d) Giving diamorphine to a premature neonate for pain relief
   e) Withholding nutrition from a baby with bowel obstruction

6 Poverty is known to be associated with:
   a) Prematurity
   b) Learning difficulties
   c) Iron deficiency anaemia
   d) Lower educational achievement
   e) More hospitalizations as a child

7 The following represent a definite contra-indication to breast-feeding:
   a) Maternal administration of penicillin
   b) Maternal depression
   c) Severe maternal hypertension
   d) Anti-retroviral medication given to the mother
   e) Mastitis

8 The following are advantages of including disabled children in mainstream school:
   a) Social support for parents
   b) Cheaper in terms of therapeutic services
   c) Better socialization
   d) Improved academic results
   e) Benefits for children of normal ability

9 At the 6- to 8-week child health assessment the following should be checked:
   a) Hips for congenital dislocation
   b) Distraction test of hearing

c) Tooth decay

d) Immunization record

e) Developmental assessment

10 The following immunization times are part of the national immunization schedule:

a) Oral polio during infancy

b) Meningitis C at high school

c) One injection for diphtheria, tetanus, pertussis, polio and HiB at 2, 3, 4 months

d) BCG for all at birth

e) MMR at high school

11 Immunizations should not be given in the following circumstances:

a) Live attenuated vaccines to severely immuno-compromised children

b) If the child is older than the age indicated on the schedule

c) If the child has a fever

d) If there has been a serious reaction to a previous dose of the same vaccine

e) A history of developmental delay

12 The following are true about child protection:

a) All professionals are required to report suspected cases of child abuse

b) Health visitors are in a good position to follow at-risk children

c) Children in care need regular review

d) The child health service has a role in prevention of abuse and neglect

e) Health professionals should liaise with social care

## Part 2: A paediatric tool kit

Answers begin on p. 470.

1 The following are important causes of error in measuring children:

a) Not correcting the weight of a 9-month-old for prematurity when the baby was born 3 months premature

b) Weighing babies wearing a nappy

c) Using cloth tape to measure head size

d) Extending the child's neck when measuring height

e) Measuring length with a tape measure

2 The following comments about growth charts are correct:

a) Two children in 100 would be expected to have their height below the second centile

b) Correction should be made for prematurity until the child starts school

c) A small cross should mark the child's measurement

d) The UK 1990 charts are not appropriate for babies of immigrants from Asia

e) Plateauing of height or weight requires evaluation

3 Clubbing is associated with the following conditions:

a) Severe asthma

b) Ulcerative colitis

c) Cystic fibrosis

d) Bronchiectasis

e) Atrial septal defect

4 The following statements are true concerning the examination of a child with respiratory symptoms:

a) Alar flaring, tachypnoea and recessions are all indications of respiratory distress in children

b) Babies have slower respiratory rates than older children

c) Auscultation is reliable in locating the site of consolidation in young children

d) Upper airway sounds in young children can be mistaken for crepitations and rhonchi when auscultating

e) Wheezing is always present in a child with severe asthma

5 The following are helpful signs when examining a boy's genitalia:

a) Transillumination is a good way to differentiate hydrocoeles from hernias

b) It helps to have the boy sit crossed-legged if you cannot feel the testes

c) Hydrocoeles extend into the groin

d) A swelling in the groin could be a testis

e) Both undescended testes and hernias are commoner in premature babies

6 The following findings are abnormal in children:

a) Sinus arrhythmia

b) Delay of the femoral pulses when compared with the radial

c) A systolic ejection murmur

d) A thrill

e) Pulse rate of 150 bpm at 8 weeks of age

7 The following are true of lymphadenopathy:
   a) Shotty mobile nodes are common and not concerning
   b) If you find nodes, you should look for an enlarged liver and spleen
   c) A focus of infection may be found proximal to the node
   d) A way of differentiating infectious mononucleosis from tonsillitis is by the size of the cervical nodes
   e) A blood count may be helpful in diagnosis

8 Peripheral muscle disease is suggested by the following abnormal signs:
   a) Limb hypotonia
   b) Absent deep tendon jerks
   c) Positive Babinski reflex
   d) Gower's sign
   e) Tachycardia

9 In a child suspected of having a squint, the following tests should be performed:
   a) Corneal light reflex
   b) Range of eye movements
   c) Corneal reflex
   d) Test of colour vision
   e) Cover test

10 A normal child of 9 months should have achieved the following milestones:
   a) Stranger anxiety
   b) Walks with one hand held
   c) Finger feeds
   d) Builds a tower of two blocks
   e) Has three words with meaning

11 A normal child of 15 months should have achieved the following milestones:
   a) Copies a circle
   b) Builds a tower of two blocks
   c) Can recognize three different colours
   d) Runs
   e) Plays interactively with other children of the same age

12 Warning signs that development is not progressing normally include:
   a) Regression of skills that have been acquired
   b) First smiling at 6 weeks
   c) Unintelligible speech at 3 years
   d) Not walking by 18 months
   e) A pincer grip at 12 months

13 Common causes of microcytic anaemia in children include:
   a) Thalassaemia trait
   b) Sickle cell disease
   c) Lead poisoning
   d) Folate deficiency
   e) Iron deficiency

14 The following features on a blood film suggest viral infection:
   a) Leucopenia
   b) Lymphocytosis
   c) Increased reticulocytes
   d) Spherocytes
   e) Atypical lymphocytes

15 The following are important causes of hypernatraemia:
   a) Severe diarrhoea
   b) Dehydration
   c) Inappropriate formula milk preparation
   d) Diabetes mellitus
   e) Overhydration

16 Causes of metabolic acidosis include:
   a) Pyloric stenosis
   b) Severe gastroenteritis
   c) Diabetic ketoacidosis
   d) Severe neonatal respiratory distress syndrome
   e) Shock

17 The following laboratory results are consistent with the diagnosis of diabetic ketoacidosis:
   a) pH 7.13
   b) $P_{CO_2}$ 3.5 kPa
   c) Bicarbonate 12 mmol/L
   d) Blood sugar 3.5 mmol/L
   e) Potassium 6.9 mmol/L

18 The following laboratory results are consistent with the diagnosis of pyloric stenosis:
   a) pH 7.49
   b) Bicarbonate 11.5 mmol/L
   c) Potassium 2.9 mmol/L
   d) Chloride 87 mmol/L
   e) Sodium 139 mmol/L

19 You expect to find the following in viral meningitis:
   a) Cloudy CSF fluid
   b) Four lymphocytes/mm$^3$
   c) No growth

**d)** Low glucose
**e)** High protein

**20** The following are supportive findings for a urinary tract infection:
**a)** Cola-coloured urine
**b)** The presence of nitrites
**c)** White cells >50/mm³
**d)** Positive ketones
**e)** $10^4$ cfu/mL *E. coli*

**21** The following statements about children's chest X-rays are true:
**a)** The heart diameter is normally 50% of the diameter of the chest
**b)** The right diaphragm is normally higher than the left
**c)** Consolidation of the right middle lobe causes loss of definition of the right heart border
**d)** There is excess penetration if you can just see the vertebrae through the heart shadow
**e)** Blunting of the costophrenic angles indicates a small pleural effusion

**22** The following results from a sweat test fulfil the criteria for cystic fibrosis:
**a)** Sweat 120 mg
**b)** Sodium 50 mmol/L
**c)** Chloride 30 mmol/L
**d)** Potassium 6 mmol/L
**e)** Bicarbonate 20 mmol/L

**Part 3: An approach to problem-based paediatrics**

Answers begin on p. 470.

**1** A 4-week-old baby with a fever of 38.5 °C should have the following:
**a)** Chest X-ray
**b)** Lumbar puncture
**c)** Blood culture
**d)** Urine culture
**e)** Admission to hospital

**2** The following abnormalities on a full blood count usually suggest acute infection:
**a)** Immature neutrophils
**b)** High white cell count
**c)** Thrombocytopenia
**d)** Low mean cell volume
**e)** High plasma viscosity

**3** Common complications of otitis media include:
**a)** Sensorineural deafness
**b)** Vertigo
**c)** Glue ear
**d)** Perforation of the tympanic membrane
**e)** Quinsy

**4** Factors which predispose to pneumonia include:
**a)** Inhaled foreign body
**b)** Immunocompromise
**c)** Gastro-oesophageal reflux with aspiration
**d)** Cystic fibrosis
**e)** Inhaled steroids for moderately severe asthma

**5** A lumbar puncture should usually be carried out in the following circumstances:
**a)** Febrile convulsion in a 3-year-old child
**b)** Febrile convulsion in a 9-month-old child
**c)** Positive Kernig's sign
**d)** Temperature >40 °C
**e)** Presence of papilloedema

**6** The following are signs of respiratory distress:
**a)** Alar flaring
**b)** Subcostal recession
**c)** Tachypnoea
**d)** Pallor
**e)** Dry cough

**7** Cough is a common symptom in the following conditions:
**a)** Asthma
**b)** Inhaled foreign body
**c)** Bronchiolitis
**d)** Cystic fibrosis
**e)** Acute laryngotracheobronchitis (croup)

**8** The following are common causes of wheezing in childhood:
**a)** Acute laryngotracheobronchitis (croup)
**b)** Gastro-oesophageal reflux
**c)** Aspiration of a foreign body
**d)** Acute cardiac failure due to a ventricular septal defect
**e)** Coeliac disease

**9** Link the following condition with its characteristic cough:
**a)** Croup
**b)** Asthma

c) Habit
d) Bronchiectasis
e) Pertussis
  1 Disappears on sleep
  2 Productive
  3 Paroxysm ended by vomiting
  4 Nocturnal
  5 Barking

**10** The following are features of pyloric stenosis:
a) Anaemia due to blood in the vomitus
b) Bile in the vomitus
c) Presents in the first day of life
d) Projectile vomiting
e) Needs a barium swallow to confirm the diagnosis

**11** In a 2-year-old child with chronic diarrhoea, the following are common causes:
a) Threadworms
b) Severe constipation
c) Lactose intolerance
d) Irritable bowel syndrome
e) Appendicitis

**12** Lactose intolerance:
a) Is most commonly a result of an autosomal recessive genetic defect
b) Often follows an episode of acute gastroenteritis
c) Is treated by giving lactase to a baby
d) Can be detected by testing the stool for reducing substances
e) Is routinely diagnosed by hydrogen breath test

**13** The following are causes of blood in the stool:
a) Salmonella infection
b) Giardia infection
c) Crohn's disease
d) Henoch–Schönlein purpura
e) Anal fissure

**14** The following are true about constipation:
a) Likely to be the diagnosis if a breast-fed baby does not open his or her bowels for 5 days
b) It may cause an anal fissure
c) Prescribing laxatives may cause long-term dependency
d) It can be seen in association with recurrent urine infections

e) Hirschsprung's should be considered if the patient is an infant

**15** Which of the following features are consistent with a diagnosis of migraine?
a) Band-like pain
b) Vomiting
c) History of travel sickness
d) Photophobia
e) Onset before age 5

**16** Management of children experiencing idiopathic recurrent abdominal pain should include:
a) Reassurance
b) Explaining to the parent that the child is malingering
c) A letter to school suggesting that the child is allowed home when the pain starts
d) Checking a blood count periodically
e) Scheduling a return appointment

**17** In a 6-year-old child with nocturnal enuresis, the following should be performed:
a) Renal ultrasound scan
b) Serum creatinine
c) Urine for microscopy and culture
d) Referral to a psychologist
e) Referral to a urologist

**18** In a bag specimen of urine, the following features are indicative of a urinary tract infection:
a) $10^4$ organisms
b) >50 white blood cells
c) Protein +
d) Nitrites negative
e) Ketones +

**19** The following are causes of diurnal enuresis in a 7-year-old child:
a) Constipation
b) Neurogenic bladder
c) Urinary tract infection
d) Spina bifida
e) Cystic fibrosis

**20** Link the following skin lesion with its characteristic feature:
a) Strawberry naevus
b) Café-au-lait spots
c) Mongolian blue spot
d) Molluscum contagiosum

**e)** Henoch–Schönlein purpura
1 Associated with neurofibromatosis
2 Resolves without treatment
3 Rash, mainly on the buttocks and thighs
4 Occurs on base of spine and buttocks
5 Self-limiting papule

**21** The following conditions are associated with a macular or maculopapular rash:
**a)** Measles
**b)** Scabies
**c)** Henoch–Schönlein purpura
**d)** Rubella
**e)** Fifth disease

**22** Link the statements that follow with the appropriate purpuric condition:
**a)** Idiopathic thrombocytopenic purpura
**b)** Henoch–Schönlein purpura
**c)** Meningococcaemia
(Note: Each condition may have more than one answer)
1 Platelet count <10 000
2 Rapid development of shock
3 Bleeding gums
4 Danger of intracerebral bleed
5 Abdominal pain
6 Need to check urine for protein
7 Treated with IV broad-spectrum antibiotic

**23** The following are recommended for facial eczema:
**a)** A fluorinated steroid cream
**b)** Use of a medicated soap
**c)** A low-protein diet
**d)** An emollient cream
**e)** Emulsifying ointment in the bath

**24** The differential diagnosis of joint swelling in a child includes:
**a)** Leukaemia
**b)** Sickle cell disease
**c)** Trauma
**d)** The effects of a streptococcal sore throat
**e)** Ulcerative colitis

**25** Swellings in the neck can be caused by:
**a)** Parotitis
**b)** Infectious mononucleosis
**c)** Thyroiditis
**d)** Crohn's disease
**e)** Otitis media

**26** The following are features of nephrotic syndrome:
**a)** Frank haematuria
**b)** High serum albumin
**c)** Low serum cholesterol
**d)** Facial oedema
**e)** Ascites

**27** The following features are characteristic of a hernial swelling:
**a)** Transilluminates
**b)** Extends from the groin to the scrotum
**c)** Exacerbated by crying
**d)** Commonly strangulates
**e)** Resolves by 1 year of age

**28** The following statements are true of short stature in children:
**a)** In most cases it is a variant of normal
**b)** There is often early puberty
**c)** The short stature is present from birth in cases of growth hormone deficiency
**d)** It may be caused by chronic renal failure
**e)** Rarely it may be due to Cushing's syndrome

**29** The following are important investigations to perform in a child who presents with signs of failure to thrive:
**a)** Lower bowel endoscopy
**b)** Detailed nutritional assessment
**c)** Sweat test
**d)** Chromosome analysis
**e)** Brain scan

**30** The following are common causes of obesity in children:
**a)** Endocrine disease
**b)** Chromosome disorders
**c)** Lifestyle factors
**d)** Autosomal recessive condition
**e)** Type II diabetes

**31** The following features indicate that a large head demands urgent investigation:
**a)** One parent with a large head
**b)** Irritability
**c)** Bulging fontanelle
**d)** A family history of epilepsy
**e)** Previous head trauma

**32** The following are features of concern:
**a)** Not walking by 18 months
**b)** Not crawling by 9 months

**c)** Right-handed dominance at 18 months
**d)** Not smiling by 6 weeks
**e)** Not appearing to see by 2 weeks

**33** In a child of 18 months, the following may be an important sign of organic disease:
**a)** Not walking
**b)** Only eight words with meaning
**c)** Not talking in sentences
**d)** Persistent mouthing
**e)** Unable to hop

**34** The following are important causes of language delay:
**a)** Down's syndrome
**b)** Turner's syndrome
**c)** Visual impairment
**d)** Deafness
**e)** Autism

**35** The following statements are true:
**a)** Masturbation is a sign of sexual abuse
**b)** Temper tantrums become a feature at 12 months
**c)** Most babies sleep through the night by 4 months
**d)** Encopresis is a sign of disturbed behaviour
**e)** Dyslexia and attention deficit disorder are causes of school failure

**36** In a child who will not sleep, the following represent standard management:
**a)** Prescription of chloral
**b)** Keep the child up until they fall asleep
**c)** Encourage them to sleep in the parental bed
**d)** Ignore the child's cries for at least 15 minutes
**e)** Allow the child a milky drink when he or she wakes

**37** The following are true of bullying:
**a)** An average child is bullied at school once per week
**b)** <10% of school children are bullies
**c)** The school often colludes with bullying
**d)** The bullying child usually has low self-esteem
**e)** Bullying is a common cause of school avoidance

**38** The following statements are true of attention deficit disorder:
**a)** Is more common in girls than boys
**b)** The child finds it difficult to stay sitting still

**c)** Is usually associated with impaired intelligence
**d)** Symptoms deteriorate during adolescence
**e)** Methylphenidate is of proven benefit in selected cases

**39** Link the following statements:
**a)** Breath-holding spells
**b)** Syncope
**c)** Hyperventilation
**d)** Myoclonic epilepsy
**e)** Absence spells
1 Precipitated by anger
2 Mainly teenagers
3 Jerking
4 EEG shows 3 per second spike and wave
5 Treated by breathing into a brown paper bag

**40** An abnormal EEG is commonly seen in:
**a)** Reflex anoxic seizures
**b)** Simple absence seizures
**c)** Breath-holding spells
**d)** Facial tics
**e)** Infantile spasms

**41** Important complications of a ventricular septal defect include:
**a)** Cyanosis at birth
**b)** Cardiac failure at birth
**c)** Bacterial endocarditis
**d)** Pulmonary hypertension
**e)** Intellectual impairment

**42** Anaemia commonly presents with the following features:
**a)** As an incidental finding on a blood count
**b)** Hypertension
**c)** Cyanosis
**d)** Purpura
**e)** Pallor

**43** The following are features that should arouse suspicion of non-accidental injury:
**a)** Extensive bruising on a 5-year-old child's shins
**b)** Failure to thrive
**c)** Spiral fracture of the femur in an 18-month-old
**d)** Torn frenulum of the tongue in a 6-month-old
**e)** Two different explanations from the parents as to how the injury happened

**44** The following are causes of amblyopia:
**a)** Genetic
**b)** Retinoblastoma

**c)** Colour blindness
**d)** Squint (strabismus)
**e)** Unilateral cataract

**45** In a child with a squint, the following conditions should be excluded:
**a)** Malalignment of the ocular muscles
**b)** Muscular dystrophy
**c)** Blindness in one eye
**d)** Facial nerve palsy
**e)** Cataract

**46** Important factors predisposing to severe illness in children include:
**a)** Early nursery entry within the first year of life
**b)** HIV/AIDS infection
**c)** Preterm infant
**d)** Diabetes mellitus
**e)** Splenectomy

**47** The following are reasons to admit a child with a fever to hospital:
**a)** High fever
**b)** Suspicion of non-accidental injury
**c)** Age <6 weeks
**d)** Maculopapular rash
**e)** Petechial rash

**48** A 2-year-old is admitted with a convulsion. The following investigations are indicated:
**a)** Blood sugar
**b)** Calcium
**c)** Blood culture
**d)** Liver function tests
**e)** EEG

**49** In an 8-year-old child with severe acute respiratory failure, the following are possible causes:
**a)** Cerebral palsy
**b)** Drug ingestion
**c)** Non-accidental injury
**d)** Diabetic ketoacidosis
**e)** Meningitis

**50** The following blood gas abnormalities indicate the need to intubate and ventilate the child:
**a)** $P_{CO_2}$ of 2.35 kPa
**b)** pH 7.08 and $P_{CO_2}$ of 8.76 kPa
**c)** pH 7.37 and $P_{CO_2}$ 8.76 kPa
**d)** $Pa_{O_2}$ 3.76 kPa and $P_{CO_2}$ 5.12 kPa
**e)** pH 7.21 and $P_{CO_2}$ 9.26 kPa

**51** In a shocked child, the following should be rapidly undertaken:
**a)** Admit to intensive care after initial assessment if no response to fluid boluses
**b)** Immediately obtain venous access and give fluid replacement before obtaining laboratory results
**c)** A blood transfusion
**d)** If the child is conscious, management is less urgent
**e)** Give inotropes if cardiac function is impaired

**52** Common causes of coma in a child aged 12 months include:
**a)** Drug overdose
**b)** Near-miss cot death
**c)** Prolonged febrile convulsion (status epilepticus)
**d)** After simple partial seizures
**e)** Hypoglycaemia

**53** The following are common causes for a convulsion in a 5-year-old child:
**a)** Hypocalcaemia
**b)** Hyperglycaemia
**c)** Fever
**d)** Head injury
**e)** Meningitis

**54** The following statements are true about febrile convulsions:
**a)** They are rare after the age of 6 years
**b)** Epilepsy is a common sequela
**c)** The fit tends to occur when there is a sudden rise in temperature at the start of an illness
**d)** Anticonvulsants should be prescribed
**e)** Antibiotics are indicated, as the cause is usually a bacterial infection

**55** The following clinical features are important in determining the severity of dehydration:
**a)** Reduced eye turgor
**b)** Depressed anterior fontanelle
**c)** Doughy feel to the skin
**d)** Capillary refill time >3 seconds
**e)** Weight on admission

**56** The following conditions are common causes of severe dehydration in a 2-year-old child:
**a)** Prolonged febrile convulsion
**b)** Anorexia nervosa
**c)** Rotavirus gastroenteritis

**d)** Bronchiolitis
**e)** Severe tonsillitis

**57** The following are important clinical signs suggestive of an acute surgical abdomen in a 2-year-old child:
**a)** Pain referred to the periumbilical area
**b)** Intermittent screaming episodes
**c)** Guarding
**d)** Cough
**e)** 'Redcurrant jelly' stool

**58** The following statements are true of acute intussusception:
**a)** Most frequently occurs in 5-year-old children
**b)** Is often associated with joint pain
**c)** Requires urgent laparotomy and surgical reduction
**d)** Is often relieved by contrast enema
**e)** Recurrence is common

**59** The following statements are correct when referring to chronic asthma:
**a)** It should not be diagnosed before 6 months of age
**b)** Skin testing is a reliable method for detecting allergy
**c)** It has an incidence of 10% in childhood
**d)** A chest X-ray should be performed at every admission to hospital
**e)** It is rare to note a family history

**60** Important principles in the management of chronic asthma include:
**a)** A diary of symptoms
**b)** Avoidance of cigarette smoking at home
**c)** Taking up carpets in the child's room
**d)** A cow's-milk-free diet reduces symptoms
**e)** Advice to the child to avoid all sport at school

**61** The commonest presenting features of diabetes mellitus in childhood include:
**a)** Itching
**b)** Thirst and weight loss
**c)** Loss of consciousness due to hypoglycaemia
**d)** Smell of acetone on breath
**e)** Abdominal pain

**62** Absence seizures:
**a)** There are usually accompanying involuntary movements

**b)** The EEG characteristically shows 3 per second spike and wave abnormality
**c)** They are most common in intellectually impaired children
**d)** The children grow out of the condition
**e)** Sodium valproate is effective medication

**63** The following statements about infantile spasms are correct:
**a)** They commonly present in the first 4 weeks of life
**b)** They may be the first feature of muscular dystrophy
**c)** They usually have a poor prognosis
**d)** They are also referred to as 'salaam' spasms
**e)** Treatment involves giving steroids

**64** The following statements about infective endocarditis are correct:
**a)** It is unlikely to occur with ventricular septal defect
**b)** It is usually due to infection with staphylococcus
**c)** Antibiotics should be given immediately prior to any investigations
**d)** Being tattooed is a risk factor for developing subacute bacterial endocarditis
**e)** It presents with prolonged fever

**65** The following statements about acute lymphoblastic leukaemia in childhood are correct:
**a)** It is the commonest malignancy in children
**b)** <50% of children survive for 5 years
**c)** Short stature is a recognized complication of treatment
**d)** Radiotherapy is rarely required
**e)** It occurs most commonly in children <2 years old

**66** In cystic fibrosis (CF), the following statements are true:
**a)** The prevalence of the recessive gene is 1:25 of the Caucasian population
**b)** A sweat test sodium of 25 mmol/L is diagnostic
**c)** Meconium ileus is the presenting feature in the majority of cases
**d)** Pancreatic enzyme replacement should be used to treat all children with CF
**e)** Prognosis of children with CF is 50–60 years

**67** The following statements about thalassaemia are true:
a) It is a form of haemoglobinopathy
b) It is due to an autosomal dominant condition
c) Hypochromic microcytic anaemia occurs in thalassaemia trait
d) HbF is greatly increased in children with thalassaemia disease
e) Blood transfusion must be avoided to prevent iron overload

**68** The definition of cerebral palsy includes the following features:
a) It is a disorder of movement
b) Spasticity is the commonest form
c) It is due to an insult in the developing brain
d) The physical signs remain constant throughout childhood
e) It is a form of neurodegenerative disorder

**69** The following are features of spastic cerebral palsy:
a) Increased limb tone
b) Athetoid movements
c) Persistence of a grasp reflex in an 8-month-old infant
d) Development of a parachute reflex at 9 months
e) Brisk deep tendon reflexes

**70** The following complications are common in children with severe cerebral palsy:
a) Limb shortening in spastic hemiplegia
b) Dislocation of the hip joints
c) Carpal tunnel syndrome
d) Migraine
e) Epilepsy

**71** In regard to severe learning disability, the following statements are correct:
a) The child never develops speech or language
b) The diagnosis for the condition is usually obvious
c) Down's syndrome is a cause
d) Diagnosis is usually made in the first month of life
e) Many of these children are able to lead independent adult lives

**72** Causes of severe sensorineural hearing impairment include:
a) Very high levels of unconjugated bilirubin
b) Secretory otitis media
c) Meningitis
d) Head injury
e) Exposure to high noise levels

**73** Recognized risk factors for deafness in childhood include:
a) Premature delivery
b) Cleft palate
c) Family history of deafness
d) Epilepsy
e) Learning disability

**74** The need for neonatal resuscitation should be anticipated in the following:
a) Elective caesarean section
b) Thick meconium staining of the liquor
c) Suspected intrauterine growth retardation
d) Multiple delivery
e) Delivery at 31 weeks' gestation

**75** In a neonate, the following statements about bile-stained vomiting are correct:
a) It is a common and benign finding
b) Hirschsprung's disease is a common cause
c) A barium enema should be performed urgently
d) Small bowel malrotation is an important cause
e) It is a feature of pyloric stenosis

**76** Common causes of intrauterine growth retardation (IUGR) include:
a) Maternal diabetes mellitus
b) Maternal hypertension
c) Fetal chromosome abnormality
d) Multiple pregnancy
e) Maternal smoking

**77** Important complications to anticipate in IUGR infants are:
a) Respiratory distress syndrome
b) Neonatal jaundice
c) Hypothermia
d) Hypoglycaemia
e) Cerebral palsy

**78** The following statements about neonatal hypoglycaemia are correct:
a) May cause cerebral palsy
b) May be asymptomatic
c) Can be anticipated in small-for-gestational-age infants
d) Is common in babies born to diabetic mothers
e) Is associated with diabetes in later life

**79** The following statements about respiratory distress syndrome in premature babies are correct:
   a) Is usually associated with brain damage in surviving babies
   b) Occurs in >50% of infants born at <30 weeks' gestation
   c) Can be avoided by giving antenatal corticosteroids
   d) Is treated by postnatal corticosteroids
   e) Is diagnosed by a ground-glass appearance on chest X-ray

**80** Important causes of neonatal jaundice include:
   a) Sickle cell disease
   b) Prematurity
   c) Intrauterine growth retardation
   d) ABO incompatibility
   e) Alpha thalassaemia

**81** In neonatal jaundice, the following investigations suggest haemolysis as its cause:
   a) Mother group O, baby group A
   b) Mother group A, baby group O
   c) Baby rhesus-negative
   d) Coomb' test positive
   e) Low neonatal T4

**82** Causes of neonatal convulsions include:
   a) Hypoglycaemia
   b) Hypocalcaemia
   c) Severe hyponatraemia
   d) Meningitis
   e) Hyperkalaemia

**83** Causes of neonatal apnoeic spells include:
   a) Prematurity
   b) Intrauterine growth retardation
   c) Convulsions
   d) Side effect of caffeine treatment
   e) Infection

**84** The following are important signs of neonatal infection:
   a) Convulsions
   b) Apnoea
   c) Vomiting
   d) Poor feeding
   e) Lethargy

**85** The following statements are true of puberty:
   a) The first sign in girls is menstruation
   b) The growth spurt occurs prior to the onset of puberty
   c) The interval between the onset and menarche is on average 2 years
   d) First sign in boys is testicular enlargement
   e) Is significantly delayed if not started by 12 years in boys

**86** Risk-taking behaviour in adolescents may lead to:
   a) Unwanted pregnancy
   b) Venereal disease
   c) Infertility in girls
   d) Blindness
   e) Drug abuse

**87** Common causes of pubertal delay include:
   a) Anorexia nervosa
   b) Intense athletic training
   c) Down's syndrome
   d) Cerebral palsy
   e) Maturational delay

## Practice examination papers

In this section, you have the opportunity to take an exam under exam conditions. Allow yourself 45 minutes to complete each paper. *Note that there may be more than one correct answer for each statement.* Mark the paper by giving yourself one mark for each correct answer, and do not subtract marks for incorrect answers. There are 35 questions in each paper with the potential of 175 correct answers per paper. Answers are provided at the end of the end of the chapter, along with a reference that will lead you back to the topic for more information.

### Examination paper 1

Answers begin on p. 472.

**1** The following are important influences on a child's eventual height:
   a) Weight of the mother during pregnancy
   b) Height of the father
   c) Whether the child is breast-fed
   d) A family history of cystic fibrosis
   e) The child required frequent foster care placements

**2** Principles of good nutrition in children include:
a) Toddlers should not be given snacks between meals
b) Added salt should be avoided
c) The child should be encouraged to finish all meals
d) Add a level teaspoon of sugar to a bottle of cow's milk each day
e) Avoid giving fatty foods such as cheese before the child is 18 months old

**3** The following are known to be associated with poverty:
a) Prematurity
b) Frequent respiratory infections
c) Learning difficulties
d) Hearing impairment
e) Iron deficiency anaemia

**4** The following statements are correct concerning measurement of blood pressure:
a) Choose a cuff size one-third of the length of the child's upper arm
b) It is not possible to accurately measure blood pressure in infants <1 year of age
c) Systolic blood pressure in a neonate should be above 100 mmHg
d) A systolic pressure of 100–120 mmHg is abnormal in a child of 13 years
e) A wide pressure difference between systole and diastole is a feature of patent ductus arteriosus

**5** The following are true when examining the abdomen of young children:
a) A protuberant abdomen in a toddler is a worrying sign
b) You can usually feel the liver edge in toddlers
c) A rectal examination should always form part of the examination
d) An enlarged spleen extends towards the left iliac fossa
e) It is never acceptable to examine the abdomen of a child who is standing

**6** The following neurological signs are suggestive of an upper motor neurone lesion:
a) Limb hypotonia
b) Clasp-knife rigidity of the arm

c) Clonus
d) Absent tendon reflexes
e) Positive Babinski reflex

**7** The following are normal developmental milestones:
a) Smile at 8 weeks
b) Sitting unsupported at 7 months
c) Pincer grip by 12 months
d) First words by 12 months
e) Two- to three-word sentences at 2 years

**8** Common causes of microcytic anaemia in children include:
a) Thalassaemia trait
b) Sickle cell disease
c) Iron deficiency
d) Lead poisoning
e) Folate deficiency

**9** Causes of metabolic acidosis include:
a) Pyloric stenosis
b) Severe gastroenteritis
c) Diabetic ketoacidosis
d) Severe neonatal respiratory distress syndrome
e) Shock

**10** You expect to find the following in bacterial meningitis:
a) Cloudy CSF fluid
b) Four lymphocytes/mm$^3$
c) No growth
d) Low glucose
e) High protein

**11** The following are true about chest X-rays of children:
a) The heart diameter is normally 80% of the diameter of the chest
b) The right diaphragm is normally higher than the left
c) Consolidation of the right middle lobe causes loss of definition of the right heart border
d) The penetration is appropriate if you can just see the vertebrae through the heart shadow
e) Blunting of the costophrenic angles indicates a small pleural effusion

**12** The following are true of fever:
a) The height of the temperature correlates with the severity of the illness
b) Sponging with cold water is an effective antipyretic

c) Blood cultures are best taken at a dip in the fever

d) Swinging pyrexia suggests septicaemia

e) Pyrexia of unknown origin is defined as a raised temperature for >1 week in an infant

**13** The following are signs of respiratory distress:

a) Alar flaring

b) Tachypnoea

c) Subcostal and intercostal recessions

d) Wheezing on inspiration

e) Barking cough

**14** The following suggest that there is significant pathology underlying persistent diarrhoea for 3 months:

a) Poor weight gain

b) Abdominal pain

c) Blood in the diarrhoea

d) Undigested food

e) Iron deficiency

**15** Clinical features of colic include the following:

a) Crying that characteristically occurs in the morning

b) Usually persists for the first year of life

c) Distended abdomen

d) Excessive flatus

e) Is worse during weaning

**16** The diagnosis of idiopathic recurrent abdominal pain is suggested if:

a) A child also has headaches and leg pain

b) Pain is suprapubic

c) It causes the child to miss school frequently

d) It is accompanied by diarrhoea

e) There is good weight gain

**17** The following conditions are associated with a purpuric rash:

a) Measles

b) Scabies

c) Meningococcal septicaemia

d) Fifth disease

e) Severe thrombocytopenia

**18** The following statements are true regarding swellings in the neck:

a) It is best to palpate cervical lymph nodes standing behind the child

b) If cervical lymph nodes are swollen, the liver and spleen should be palpated

c) Mumps obscures the bony angle of the jaw

d) Mastoiditis pushes the ear upwards

e) Thyroiditis can cause a goitre and either hypo- or hyperthyroidism

**19** The following are relevant investigations to perform in a child who presents with signs of failure to thrive:

a) Full blood count

b) Detailed nutritional assessment

c) Jejunal biopsy

d) Chromosome analysis

e) Brain scan

**20** The following symptoms and signs are suggestive of autism:

a) Delay in language development

b) Poor eye contact

c) History of not being a 'cuddly' baby

d) Failure to thrive

e) Father who enjoys train spotting

**21** In a child with temper tantrums, the following are all standard features of management:

a) Ignore the tantrum

b) Take the child out of the room for a short period of time during the tantrum

c) Avoid tantrums by giving the child what he or she wants

d) Take away all the child's toys during the tantrum

e) Blame the mother for 'spoiling' the child

**22** The following are features of significant heart disease:

a) Pansystolic murmur

b) A murmur that changes with the child's position

c) There is no radiation

d) Associated with a thrill

e) Diastolic murmur

**23** Radiological features that are particularly suggestive of child abuse include:

a) A skull fracture in a 12-year-old child

b) Spiral fracture of the femur

c) Two rib fractures

d) Two fractures of different ages

e) Colles fracture of the wrist in a 3-year-old

24 The following signs require immediate treatment and transfer to hospital:
   a) A petechial rash
   b) Shock
   c) Dehydration
   d) Coma
   e) Chest pain

25 In a child who is shocked, the following investigations should be performed after initial stabilization:
   a) Lumbar puncture
   b) Electrolytes and urea
   c) Saturation monitoring
   d) Blood cultures
   e) Blood sugar

26 The following suggest that a baby is significantly dehydrated (10%):
   a) Dry mouth
   b) Urinating four times a day
   c) Lethargy
   d) Sunken eyes
   e) Sunken fontanelle

27 'Back to sleep' advice includes:
   a) Babies should be laid to sleep in the prone position
   b) Ensure that the child's bedroom is well heated
   c) Avoid duvet covers <1 year of age
   d) Ensure infant's feet come to the end of the cot
   e) Avoid cigarette smoke in the house

28 Important principles of management of hypoglycaemia in diabetic children include:
   a) Increase dose of short-acting insulin
   b) Change insulin dosage to a sliding scale
   c) Give glucose gel per rectum
   d) If unconscious, give glucagon intramuscularly
   e) Intravenous glucose (dextrose) must be given urgently as the first-line management

29 Common complications of cystic fibrosis include:
   a) Biliary cirrhosis
   b) Male infertility
   c) Bronchiectasis
   d) Failure to thrive
   e) Diabetes

30 The following are common associated disabilities in children with cerebral palsy:
   a) Epilepsy
   b) Hearing impairment
   c) Cortical visual impairment
   d) Feeding difficulties
   e) Speech and language problems

31 The following statements are true of severe sensorineural hearing impairment:
   a) The prognosis for hearing is best if the diagnosis is made before the child is 3 months old
   b) Deaf children should be discouraged from learning sign language
   c) Severely deaf children do best if educated with normal hearing peers
   d) The incidence is 1%
   e) Glue ear is a common cause

32 Important complications to anticipate in premature infants include:
   a) Respiratory distress syndrome
   b) Neonatal jaundice
   c) Hypothermia
   d) Hypoglycaemia
   e) Apnoea

33 The following are important signs of neonatal infection:
   a) Convulsions
   b) Apnoea
   c) Constipation
   d) Poor feeding
   e) Lethargy

34 Causes of secondary amenorrhoea include:
   a) Pregnancy
   b) Anorexia nervosa
   c) Epilepsy
   d) Urinary tract infection
   e) Brain tumour

35 The following form part of the child health promotion programme:
   a) Annual height and weight
   b) Screening for neurosensory deafness
   c) Immunizations
   d) Health education
   e) Accident prevention

## Examination paper 2

Answers begin on p. 472.

1 Breast-feeding has the following advantages:
   a) It prevents HIV transmission from mother to baby
   b) It reduces the risk of enteric infections in the baby
   c) Mothers who breast-feed more than three babies are more likely to develop breast cancer
   d) Promotes maternal 'bonding' with her baby
   e) Enhances the infant's IQ

2 The following practices are against the law:
   a) Not to treat life-threatening infections
   b) Not to ventilate a very premature infant
   c) To give diamorphine to a premature neonate for pain relief
   d) To give morphine with the intention of the baby dying
   e) To withhold nutrition from a baby with bowel obstruction

3 The following comments about growth charts are correct:
   a) Two children in 100 would be expected to have their height above the 98th centile
   b) Correction should be made for prematurity until the age of 24 months
   c) A small cross should mark the child's measurement
   d) The UK 1990 charts are not appropriate for babies of immigrants from Asia
   e) Plateauing of height or weight requires evaluation

4 The following statements are true when examining a child with respiratory symptoms:
   a) You may not hear wheezing in a child with severe asthma
   b) Babies have slower respiratory rates than older children
   c) Auscultation is reliable in locating the site of consolidation in young children
   d) It is easy to differentiate upper airway sounds from crepitations and rhonchi by auscultation
   e) Alar flaring, tachypnoea and recessions are reliable signs of respiratory compromise in children

5 The following are helpful signs when examining a boy's genitalia:
   a) Hydrocoeles transilluminate, whereas hernias do not
   b) It helps to have the boy sit crossed-legged if you cannot feel the testes
   c) A hernia extends into the groin
   d) A swelling in the groin could be a testis
   e) Both undescended testes and hernias are commoner in premature babies

6 In a child suspected of having a squint the following tests should be performed:
   a) Corneal light reflex
   b) Range of eye movements
   c) Corneal reflex
   d) Test of colour vision
   e) Cover test

7 Warning signs that development is not progressing normally include:
   a) Regression of skills that have been acquired
   b) First smiling at 6 weeks
   c) Unintelligible speech at 3 years
   d) Not walking by 18 months
   e) Persistent primitive reflexes

8 The following features on a blood film suggest bacterial infection:
   a) Leucocytosis of $>15 \times 10^9$ white cells/L
   b) Lymphocytosis
   c) Increased reticulocytes
   d) A preponderance of immature white cells ('shift to the left')
   e) Atypical lymphocytes

9 The following blood gas results are consistent with respiratory acidosis:
   a) pH 7.42
   b) $P\text{CO}_2$ 9.4 kPa
   c) Bicarbonate 23 mmol/L
   d) Arterial saturation 85%
   e) $P\text{aO}_2$ 3.5 kPa

10 The following are supportive findings for a urinary tract infection:
   a) The absence of nitrites
   b) White cells $>50/\text{mm}^3$
   c) Positive ketones
   d) *E. coli* $>10^5$ cfu/mL
   e) Haematuria

**11** The following are recognized complications of meningitis in children:
a) Sensorineural deafness
b) Conductive deafness
c) Hydrocephalus
d) Cataracts
e) Acute adrenal failure

**12** The following features suggest asthma as a cause:
a) Night cough
b) Wheezing after vigorous exercise
c) Wheezing after choking on a peanut
d) Bronchiolitis
e) A productive cough

**13** A breast-fed baby aged 7 months develops gastroenteritis. You should tell the mother to:
a) Stop breast milk
b) Give Dioralyte
c) Try rice cereal when the vomiting stops
d) Give an antidiarrhoeal medication if it continues more than 3 days
e) Change to soy formula

**14** The following are features of concern in a child with headaches:
a) Vomiting
b) Increased headache on sitting up
c) Fall-off in school performance
d) Waking at night with headache
e) Hypotension

**15** The following are true of nocturnal enuresis:
a) Occurs in 10% of 6-year-olds
b) The most effective treatment is an enuresis alarm
c) Treatment with DDAVP for 3 months causes long-term remission
d) It is usually precipitated by a urinary tract infection
e) There is often a family history

**16** The following advice is appropriate for eczema:
a) Encourage the mother to breast-feed subsequent infants for 6 months
b) Steroid cream should be used sparingly
c) Bath oil
d) Dress the child in nonsynthetic clothing
e) Ensure a dust-free environment

**17** The following statements are true if growth is found to be 'falling off':
a) The parents are often short
b) It always merits investigation
c) Crohn's disease may be a cause
d) The bone age is delayed in endocrinological causes
e) It is of no concern in adolescence

**18** The following are relevant in a child with developmental delay:
a) A family history of consanguinity
b) Microcephaly
c) Loss of developmental milestones
d) A hearing evaluation
e) A history of prematurity

**19** The following are common causes of global developmental delay:
a) Fragile X syndrome
b) Turner's syndrome
c) Congenital HIV infection
d) Alcohol during pregnancy
e) Muscular dystrophy

**20** The following are features of breath-holding spells:
a) Usually associated with an aura
b) May occur when asleep
c) Often precipitated by pain or anger
d) Persist into school age
e) Loss of consciousness may occur

**21** The differential diagnosis of anaemia in a 5-year-old includes:
a) Leukaemia
b) Idiopathic thrombocytopenic purpura
c) Chronic lead poisoning
d) Thalassaemia minor (trait)
e) Threadworm infection

**22** The following are features of severe illness in a 3-month-old baby:
a) High-pitched cry
b) Reduced skin perfusion
c) Purpura
d) Wheeze
e) Bile-stained vomiting

**23** Shock is a well-recognized feature of:
a) Anaphylactic reaction following exposure to peanuts
b) A burn involving 5% surface area
c) Meningococcal septicaemia
d) Rotavirus infection
e) Prolonged febrile convulsion

**24** The following are common causes of a convulsion in a 5-year-old child:
a) Hypocalcaemia
b) Hyperglycaemia
c) Fever
d) Head injury
e) Phenylketonuria

**25** Common causes of acute abdominal pain in a 2-year-old child include:
a) Lower lobe pneumonia
b) Upper lobe pneumonia
c) Mesenteric adenitis
d) Urinary tract infection
e) Constipation

**26** In the management of asthma, the following statements are correct:
a) Administration of most treatments is best by inhaler
b) Sodium cromoglycate is the first-line drug
c) There is no place for the use of oral steroids
d) All children with chronic asthma should be referred to a respiratory paediatrician
e) Leukotriene medication should be used as first-line management

**27** Correct advice to epileptic children and their families includes:
a) Anticonvulsant levels need to be monitored on a regular basis
b) They will never be able to apply for a driver's licence
c) They must not swim
d) They will continue to have convulsions all their life
e) Some careers may not be possible

**28** Long-term effects of childhood cancer include:
a) >50% chance of death within 5 years of diagnosis
b) Significant risk of second malignancy
c) Short stature resulting from radiotherapy

d) Survivors need annual follow-up
e) About 25% of survivors have major depression in later life

**29** The following statements are correct concerning sickle cell disease:
a) The diagnosis is made by bone marrow aspiration
b) It is inherited as an autosomal recessive condition
c) It can present with painful swollen hands
d) Massive splenomegaly is a common finding
e) Diagnosis is by haemoglobin electrophoresis

**30** The following are common causes of cerebral palsy:
a) Muscular dystrophy
b) Epilepsy
c) Birth asphyxia (hypoxic–ischaemic insult)
d) Congenital toxoplasmosis infection
e) Neonatal meningitis

**31** The following are true regarding children with disabilities:
a) Where possible, they should attend special schools
b) There is usually an underlying genetic cause
c) Respite care should be arranged for all children
d) Stages in parental adjustment to the disability are similar to bereavement
e) Once the child starts school, therapeutic input is generally provided there

**32** Important causes of neonatal respiratory distress include:
a) Diaphragmatic hernia
b) Pneumothorax
c) Pneumonia
d) Fallot's tetralogy
e) Rhesus incompatibility

**33** The following statements about puberty are true:
a) The first sign in girls is menstruation
b) The growth spurt occurs prior to the onset of puberty
c) Menarche is delayed if it has not occurred by age 16
d) First sign in girls is usually breast budding
e) It is significantly delayed if not started by 12 years in boys

**34** At the 6- to 8-week child health assessment, the following should be checked:
   **a)** Hips for congenital dislocation
   **b)** Distraction test of hearing
   **c)** Testicular descent
   **d)** Immunization record
   **e)** Developmental assessment

**35** Contraindications to immunization include:
   **a)** The child has a cold
   **b)** The child has missed the previous immunization
   **c)** The child has a fever
   **d)** A serious reaction to a previous immunization with the same vaccine
   **e)** A history of developmental delay

## Answers to multiple choice questions

References to boxes, tables and/or relevant pages are provided to lead you back to the topic for more information, and an explanation for the answers. T = true, F = false.

### Part 1

| | | | | | |
|---|---|---|---|---|---|
| **1** | a) T | b) T | c) F | d) F | e) T | Box 1.2 |
| **2** | a) F | b) T | c) F | d) T | e) F | pp. 14–16 |
| **3** | a) F | b) T | c) F | d) F | e) F | Box 1.3; pp. 12–14 |
| **4** | a) T | b) F | c) T | d) T | e) F | pp. 6–7 |
| **5** | a) T | b) F | c) F | d) F | e) T | Box 2.1; pp. 32–4 |
| **6** | a) F | b) T | c) T | d) T | e) T | Table 1.5; p. 16 |
| **7** | a) F | b) F | c) F | d) T | e) F | p. 11 |
| **8** | a) F | b) T | c) T | d) F | e) T | pp. 46–7 |
| **9** | a) T | b) F | c) F | d) T | e) T | Table 2.1 |
| **10** | a) F | b) F | c) T | d) F | e) F | Table 2.4 |
| **11** | a) T | b) F | c) T | d) T | e) F | p. 26 |
| **12** | a) T | b) T | c) T | d) T | e) T | pp. 30–2 |

### Part 2

| | | | | | |
|---|---|---|---|---|---|
| **1** | a) T | b) T | c) T | d) F | e) T | p. 56 |
| **2** | a) T | b) F | c) F | d) F | e) T | Box 4.3; p. 58 |
| **3** | a) F | b) T | c) T | d) T | e) F | Table 4.1 |
| **4** | a) T | b) F | c) F | d) T | e) F | pp. 63–6 |
| **5** | a) T | b) T | c) F | d) T | e) T | p. 70 |
| **6** | a) F | b) T | c) F | d) T | e) F | pp. 60–3 |
| **7** | a) T | b) T | c) F | d) F | e) T | pp. 69–70 |
| **8** | a) T | b) T | c) F | d) T | e) F | Box 4.9 |
| **9** | a) T | b) T | c) F | d) F | e) T | Box 4.12 |
| **10** | a) T | b) F | c) T | d) F | e) F | pp. 85–8 |
| **11** | a) F | b) T | c) F | d) F | e) F | pp. 85–8 |
| **12** | a) T | b) F | c) F | d) T | e) F | Table 5.2 |
| **13** | a) T | b) F | c) T | d) F | e) T | pp. 91–2 |
| **14** | a) F | b) T | c) F | d) F | e) T | p. 92 |
| **15** | a) T | b) T | c) T | d) F | e) F | Table 6.4 |
| **16** | a) F | b) T | c) T | d) F | e) T | Table 6.6 |
| **17** | a) T | b) T | c) T | d) F | e) T | Table 6.7; p. 95 |
| **18** | a) T | b) F | c) T | d) T | e) T | Table 6.7; p. 96 |
| **19** | a) F | b) T | c) T | d) F | e) F | Table 6.8 |
| **20** | a) F | b) T | c) T | d) F | e) F | pp. 96–8 |
| **21** | a) T | b) T | c) T | d) F | e) T | pp. 98–100 |
| **22** | a) T | b) F | c) F | d) F | e) F | p. 103 |

### Part 3

| | | | | | |
|---|---|---|---|---|---|
| **1** | a) T | b) T | c) T | d) T | e) T | Table 7.1 |
| **2** | a) T | b) T | c) F | d) F | e) T | Table 7.1 |
| **3** | a) F | b) F | c) T | d) T | e) F | p. 120 |
| **4** | a) T | b) T | c) T | d) T | e) F | p. 151 |
| **5** | a) F | b) T | c) T | d) F | e) F | p. 208 |
| **6** | a) T | b) T | c) T | d) F | e) F | p. 134 |
| **7** | a) T | b) T | c) T | d) T | e) T | Table 8.1 |
| **8** | a) F | b) F | c) T | d) F | e) F | p. 136 |
| **9** | a) 5 | b) 4 | c) 1 | d) 2 | e) 3 | Table 8.1 |

| | | | | | |
|---|---|---|---|---|---|
| **10** | a) F  b) F  c) F  d) T  e) F | pp. 176–7 |
| **11** | a) F  b) T  c) T  d) F  e) F | pp. 162–3 |
| **12** | a) F  b) T  c) F  d) T  e) F | p. 180 |
| **13** | a) T  b) F  c) T  d) T  e) T | p. 172 |
| **14** | a) F  b) T  c) F  d) T  e) T | p. 171 |
| **15** | a) F  b) T  c) T  d) T  e) F | p. 217 |
| **16** | a) T  b) F  c) F  d) F  e) T | p. 182 |
| **17** | a) F  b) F  c) T  d) F  e) F | p. 299 |
| **18** | a) F  b) T  c) F  d) F  e) F | pp. 96, 303 |
| **19** | a) T  b) T  c) T  d) T  e) F | p. 297 |
| **20** | a) 2  b) 1  c) 4  d) 5  e) 3 | Clues Box p. 323; Clues Box p. 327; pp. 320–7 |
| **21** | a) T  b) F  c) F  d) T  e) T | Table 17.1 |
| **22** | a) 1, 3, 4,  b) 5, 6  c) 2, 7 | pp. 320–1; Clues Box p. 323 |
| **23** | a) F  b) F  c) F  d) T  e) T | p. 330 |
| **24** | a) T  b) T  c) T  d) T  e) F | p. 286 |
| **25** | a) T  b) T  c) T  d) F  e) F | pp. 113–4 |
| **26** | a) F  b) F  c) F  d) T  e) T | Table 15.3, p. 310 |
| **27** | a) F  b) T  c) T  d) F  e) F | Clues box and all of p. 313 |
| **28** | a) T  b) F  c) F  d) T  e) T | p. 253 |
| **29** | a) F  b) T  c) T  d) T  e) F | Table 13.2 |
| **30** | a) F  b) F  c) T  d) F  e) F | p. 259 |
| **31** | a) F  b) T  c) T  d) F  e) T | pp. 263–4 |
| **32** | a) T  b) F  c) T  d) T  e) T | p. 226 |
| **33** | a) T  b) F  c) F  d) T  e) F | p. 226 |
| **34** | a) T  b) F  c) F  d) T  e) T | p. 229 |
| **35** | a) F  b) F  c) F  d) T  e) T | Chapter 19 |
| **36** | a) F  b) F  c) F  d) T  e) F | Box 19.2 |

| | | | | | |
|---|---|---|---|---|---|
| **37** | a) F  b) T  c) F  d) T  e) T | p. 359 |
| **38** | a) F  b) T  c) F  d) F  e) T | pp. 236, 361 |
| **39** | a) 1  b) 2  c) 5  d) 3  e) 4 | Clues boxes pp. 204, 205 |
| **40** | a) F  b) T  c) F  d) F  e) T | Clues boxes pp. 204, 205 |
| **41** | a) F  b) F  c) T  d) T  e) F | p. 193 |
| **42** | a) T  b) F  c) T  d) F  e) T | p. 343 |
| **43** | a) F  b) T  c) T  d) T  e) T | Box 20.1 & pp. 363–367 |
| **44** | a) F  b) F  c) F  d) T  e) T | p. 223 |
| **45** | a) T  b) F  c) T  d) F  e) T | p. 207 |
| **46** | a) F  b) T  c) T  d) F  e) T | Table 21.1, p. 371 |
| **47** | a) F  b) F  c) T  d) T  e) T | p. 371 |
| **48** | a) T  b) T  c) T  d) F  e) F | Table 21.7, p. 384 |
| **49** | a) F  b) T  c) F  d) F  e) T | p. 347 |
| **50** | a) F  b) T  c) F  d) F  e) T | pp. 94–5, 375 |
| **51** | a) T  b) T  c) T  d) F  e) T | Box 21.3; pp. 378–9 |
| **52** | a) F  b) F  c) T  d) T  e) F | p. 380 |
| **53** | a) F  b) F  c) T  d) T  e) T | p. 382 |
| **54** | a) T  b) F  c) T  d) T  e) F | pp. 393–4 |
| **55** | a) T  b) T  c) T  d) T  e) T | Table 21.8 |
| **56** | a) F  b) T  c) F  d) F  e) T | p. 385 |
| **57** | a) F  b) T  c) T  d) T  e) T | p. 170 |
| **58** | a) F  b) F  c) F  d) T  e) F | pp. 184–6 |
| **59** | a) T  b) F  c) F  d) F  e) F | p. 141 |
| **60** | a) T  b) T  c) T  d) F  e) F | pp. 141–6 |
| **61** | a) F  b) T  c) F  d) T  e) T | p. 274 |
| **62** | a) F  b) T  c) F  d) T  e) T | pp. 210–13 |
| **63** | a) F  b) F  c) T  d) T  e) T | p. 211 |

64  a) F  b) F  c) F  d) T  e) T      p. 201

65  a) T  b) F  c) T  d) F  e) F      p. 351

66  a) T  b) F  c) F  d) F  e) F      pp. 149–51

67  a) T  b) F  c) T  d) T  e) F      pp. 346–7

68  a) T  b) T  c) T  d) F  e) F      pp. 236–8

69  a) T  b) F  c) T  d) F  e) T      pp. 237–8

70  a) T  b) T  c) F  d) F  e) T      pp. 238–41

71  a) F  b) F  c) T  d) F  e) F      pp. 242–4

72  a) T  b) F  c) T  d) T  e) F      Table 12.6

73  a) T  b) T  c) T  d) F  e) F      Table 12.5

74  a) F  b) T  c) F  d) T  e) T      p. 401

75  a) F  b) F  c) F  d) T  e) F      p. 420

76  a) F  b) T  c) T  d) T  e) T      Table 22.4

77  a) F  b) F  c) T  d) T  e) F      Table 22.3

78  a) T  b) T  c) T  d) T  e) F      p. 409

79  a) F  b) T  c) T  d) F  e) T      pp. 410–11

80  a) F  b) T  c) F  d) T  e) F      p. 417

81  a) T  b) F  c) F  d) T  e) F      Table 22.6, p. 418

82  a) T  b) T  c) T  d) T  e) F      p. 431

83  a) T  b) F  c) T  d) F  e) T      p. 415

84  a) T  b) T  c) T  d) T  e) T      p. 423

85  a) F  b) F  c) T  d) T  e) F      Table 23.3, p. 437

86  a) T  b) T  c) T  d) F  e) T      pp. 437–9

87  a) T  b) T  c) F  d) F  e) T      Table 23.6

# Answers to practice examination papers

T = true, F = false.

## Paper 1

1  a) F  b) T  c) F  d) F  e) T      Box 1.1. p. 4–5

2  a) F  b) T  c) F  d) F  e) F      Box 1.5, p. 14

3  a) F  b) T  c) T  d) T  e) T      Table 1.5, p. 16

4  a) F  b) F  c) F  d) F  e) T      p. 63, Table 4.4

5  a) F  b) T  c) F  d) F  e) F      pp. 66–8

6  a) F  b) T  c) T  d) F  e) T      Box 4.9

7  a) F  b) T  c) T  d) T  e) T      Table 5.1

8  a) T  b) T  c) T  d) T  e) F      pp. 91–2

9  a) F  b) T  c) F  d) F  e) T      Table 6.6

10  a) T  b) F  c) F  d) T  e) T      Table 6.8

11  a) F  b) T  c) T  d) T  e) T      pp. 98–100

12  a) F  b) F  c) F  d) T  e) T      pp. 108–10, 115–16

13  a) T  b) T  c) T  d) F  e) F      p. 134

14  a) T  b) T  c) T  d) F  e) T      Clues Box p. 165

15  a) F  b) F  c) F  d) T  e) F      p. 178

16  a) T  b) F  c) F  d) F  e) T      p. 166, Table 9.4, p. 168

17  a) F  b) F  c) T  d) F  e) T      Table 17.1

18  a) F  b) T  c) T  d) F  e) T      pp. 113–14

19  a) T  b) T  c) T  d) T  e) F      Table 13.2

20  a) T  b) T  c) T  d) F  e) F      p. 236

21  a) T  b) T  c) F  d) F  e) F      Box 19.4

22  a) T  b) F  c) F  d) T  e) T      Table 10.1

**23** a) F  b) T  c) T  d) T  e) F    Fig 20.3, pp. 365–6

**24** a) T  b) T  c) T  d) T  e) F    p. 372

**25** a) F  b) T  c) T  d) T  e) T    Table 21.5

**26** a) F  b) F  c) T  d) T  e) T    Table 21.8

**27** a) F  b) F  c) T  d) T  e) T    Box 21.8

**28** a) F  b) F  c) F  d) T  e) F    p. 278; Box 13.2

**29** a) T  b) T  c) T  d) T  e) T    p. 149

**30** a) T  b) T  c) T  d) T  e) T    p. 238

**31** a) T  b) F  c) F  d) F  e) F    pp. 247–9

**32** a) T  b) T  c) T  d) T  e) T    Table 22.3

**33** a) T  b) T  c) F  d) T  e) T    p. 423

**34** a) T  b) T  c) F  d) F  e) T    Table 23.8

**35** a) F  b) T  c) T  d) T  e) T    p. 19, Table 2.1

**Paper 2**

**1** a) F  b) T  c) F  d) T  e) T    Table 1.2, pp. 10–11

**2** a) F  b) F  c) F  d) T  e) T    pp. 32–3

**3** a) T  b) T  c) F  d) F  e) T    pp. 58–9, Box 4.3

**4** a) T  b) F  c) F  d) F  e) T    pp. 64–6

**5** a) T  b) T  c) T  d) T  e) T    p. 70, Clues Box p. 313

**6** a) T  b) T  c) F  d) F  e) T    Box 4.12

**7** a) T  b) F  c) F  d) T  e) T    Table 5.2

**8** a) T  b) F  c) F  d) T  e) F    p. 92

**9** a) F  b) T  c) T  d) T  e) T    Table 6.7

**10** a) F  b) T  c) F  d) T  e) T    p. 98, Table 6.9

**11** a) T  b) F  c) T  d) F  e) T    p. 210

**12** a) T  b) T  c) F  d) F  e) F    p. 138

**13** a) F  b) T  c) T  d) F  e) F    p. 161

**14** a) T  b) F  c) T  d) T  e) F    p. 206 Clues Box, p. 207

**15** a) T  b) T  c) T  d) F  e) T    pp. 306–7

**16** a) T  b) T  c) T  d) F  e) F    Box 17.1

**17** a) F  b) T  c) T  d) T  e) F    p. 256

**18** a) T  b) T  c) T  d) T  e) T    pp. 226–8

**19** a) T  b) F  c) F  d) T  e) F    p. 233

**20** a) F  b) F  c) T  d) F  e) T    Clues Box p. 204

**21** a) T  b) F  c) T  d) T  e) F    p. 343

**22** a) T  b) T  c) T  d) T  e) T    Table 21.2

**23** a) T  b) F  c) T  d) F  e) F    p. 378

**24** a) F  b) F  c) T  d) T  e) F    p. 382

**25** a) T  b) F  c) T  d) T  e) T    p. 169

**26** a) T  b) F  c) F  d) F  e) F    Box 8.2; p. 142

**27** a) F  b) F  c) F  d) F  e) T    p. 214–15

**28** a) F  b) T  c) T  d) T  e) F    p. 42–3

**29** a) F  b) T  c) T  d) F  e) T    p. 347–8

**30** a) F  b) F  c) T  d) T  e) T    Table 12.3

**31** a) F  b) F  c) F  d) T  e) T    pp. 45–8

**32** a) T  b) T  c) T  d) F  e) F    p. 410

**33** a) F  b) F  c) T  d) T  e) F    Table 23.3

**34** a) T  b) F  c) T  d) T  e) T    Table 2.1

**35** a) F  b) F  c) T  d) T  e) F    p. 27

# Index

In this index tables, figures and photographs are indicated in bold type